Human Malformations

and Related Anomalies

OXFORD MONOGRAPHS ON MEDICAL GENETICS

General Editors
ARNO G. MOTULSKY   MARTIN BOBROW
PETER S. HARPER   CHARLES SCRIVER

Former Editors
J. A. FRASER ROBERTS   C. O. CARTER

OXFORD MONOGRAPHS ON MEDICAL GENETICS NO. 27

Human Malformations
and Related Anomalies

VOLUME I

Edited by

ROGER E. STEVENSON
Greenwood Genetic Center
Greenwood, South Carolina

JUDITH G. HALL
The University of British Columbia
Vancouver, British Columbia
Canada

RICHARD M. GOODMAN
The Chaim Sheba Medical Center
Tel-Hashomer, Israel

New York   Oxford
Oxford University Press
1993

Oxford University Press

Oxford   New York   Toronto
Delhi   Bombay   Calcutta   Madras   Karachi
Kuala Lumpur   Singapore   Hong Kong   Tokyo
Nairobi   Dar es Salaam   Cape Town
Melbourne   Auckland   Madrid

and associated companies in
Berlin   Ibadan

Library of Congress Cataloging-in-Publication Data
Human malformations and related anomalies / edited by Roger Stevenson.
Judith Hall, Richard Goodman.
p. cm.   Includes bibliographical references and index.
ISBN 0-19-506232-9
1. Abnormalities, Human.   I. Stevenson, Roger E., 1940–   .
II. Hall, Judith G.   III. Goodman, Richard M. (Richard Merle), 1932–1989
[DNLM: 1. Abnormalities.   2. Genetics.   QS 675 H918]
QM691.H88   1993
616'.043—dc20   DNLM/DLC
for Library of Congress   92-48933

1 3 5 7 9 8 6 4 2

Printed in the United States of America
on acid-free paper

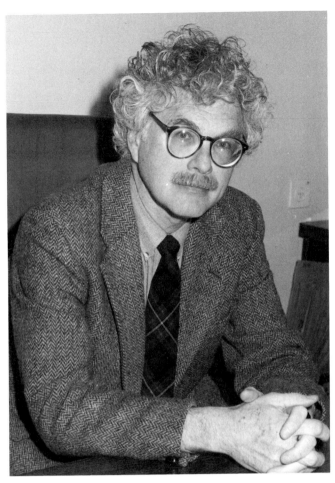

Richard M. Goodman (1932–1989)

To Richard M. Goodman, scholar, humanitarian, teacher, husband, father, friend. Rich gave of his energy and enthusiasm to many endeavors. He engaged in lively discussion of all issues facing the world and found solitude in archaeology, history and art, poetry, and observing children at play. He had keen insight into the world of children—those with mental and physical impairments and those not burdened with these handicaps.

Rich found great joy in writing and through writing shared his wit, his reverence for mankind, and the discoveries of an inquiring mind. He spent many months in planning for these volumes. Their completion reminds us how much we miss him.

Preface

Justice requires that . . . all infants have the . . . right to be born with sound mind and body.

Supreme Court of New Jersey, 1960

The statement with which this preface begins expresses the ideal that society holds for the health of its offspring. It equates malformations and mental retardation with injustices that warrant redress by society. The benevolence of the concept notwithstanding, actual means of assuring that all infants are born free of physical and mental defects are not available. Even with the greatest diligence, parents cannot entirely avoid the risk that their offspring will have a congenital anomaly or mental impairment. Using present technology, the cause of abnormal embryonic development can be determined postnatally in only 50 percent of infants with malformations, and the likelihood that an infant was affected could have been predicted prenatally in only a minority of cases. While acknowledging the desire to avoid birth defects, society must recognize that birth defects are a risk inherent in childbearing, a risk that may be reduced but that cannot be eliminated for many generations to come.

Abnormally formed infants have always captured people's attention. Human malformations are depicted among the oldest drawings and carvings; the meanings of malformations are discussed in the earliest writings (see Volume I, Chapter 1). In virtually all cultures, they have evoked some medical, educational, or societal efforts toward prevention. Nevertheless, malformations continue to occur and continue to arouse curiosity and consternation.

In 1900, congenital anomalies ranked fourth among causes of death in the first year of life. These defects now have become the leading cause of infant mortality.[1] Their growing influence on infant mortality does not reflect a greater incidence of structural abnormalities at birth, but rather a reduction in the impact of premature birth, infectious diseases, respiratory distress syndrome, trauma, and other common maladies of infancy. Efforts to understand, treat, and prevent human malformations have been less successful.

Congenital anomalies are experiments of nature and may, if investigated, provide insight into normal development. They constitute the major reason for referral of infants and children under three years of age for genetic evaluations (Table 1).[2] Throughout the childhood years structural defects continue as a major cause of morbidity and mortality. Between years 3 and 5, developmental impairment becomes the most common reason for genetic evaluation. In some cases, developmental impairment leads to the recognition of occult anomalies in the brain. In other cases, the brain appears to be normally formed but it fails to function normally.

The goal in *Human Malformations and Related Anomalies* is to consider each significant human anomaly from the perspective of the clinician and to examine it within the context of what is known about embryonic and fetal development. What is the nature of the anatomical defect? What related anomalies and syndromes must be considered? What are possible treatment and prevention strategies?

This book is intended to provide a body of information on specific anomalies and to connect individual anomalies to the malformation syndromes in which they are known to occur, primarily through the use of tables. Volumes on syndrome identification and computerized data banks have become valuable resources to clinicians seeking a diagnosis, range of expression, natural history of the growing number of recorded malformation syndromes. *Recognizable Patterns of Human Malformations;*[3] *Syndromes of the Head and Neck;*[4] *Radiology of Syndromes, Metabolic Disorders, and Skeletal Dysplasias;*[5] *The London Dysmorphology Database;*[6] *Birth Defects Information Series;*[7] and *Pictures of Standard Syndromes and Undiagnosed Malformations (POSSUM)*[8] are among the most commonly used references and resources.

Contemporary understanding of human anomalies has been advanced by several efforts. During the 1960s and 1970s, Victor McKusick organized series of conferences sponsored by the National Foundation–March of Dimes on the clinical delineation of birth defects. These popular conferences benefited from the heightened awareness of birth defects engendered by the identification of the cytogenetic basis for Down syndrome and other malformation syndromes (1959–1960), recognition of thalidomide as the cause of an epidemic of limb anomalies (1958–1962), observation of the large number of infants born with birth defects following the rubella pandemic (1964), and elucidation of the metabolic basis for storage diseases and other disorders with distinctive morphologic features. Participants in the March of Dimes conferences were drawn from a wide range of disciplines. The first of those conferences focused on anomalies in a single anatomical system, helping to define the state of knowledge about that system. Since the initial series, the meetings have continued with varying emphases.

During the same period, David W. Smith brought a new perspective to the study of human anomalies—which he termed *dysmorphology.* His focus was on the mechanisms by which anomalies occurred, and the spirit of his inquiry has been perpetuated by an annual Workshop on Malformations and Morphogenesis named after him. This workshop has demonstrated the benefits of collaboration among clinicians, pathologists, embryologists, and other basic scientists. With the application of the emerging technologies of molecular biology and developmental genetics, we can anticipate signifi-

Table 1. Reasons for referral for genetic evaluation[a]

	n	Age (yr) 0–1	1–3	3–5	5–12	12–20	>20
	n	485	274	134	237	194	176
Structural anomalies							
Malformations	445(30%)	47%	22%	20%	25%	24%	14%
Dysmorphic features	178(12%)	18	13	8	7	12	4
Cutaneous feature(s)	106(7%)	6	5	7	8	8	11
Growth							
Defect	117(8%)	6	8	6	13	9	5
Excess	21(1%)	1	2	0	2	3	<1
Developmental impairment	281(19%)	8	31	37	23	14	16
Special sense impairment	21(1%)	1	2	<1	2	0	2
Neurologic signs	105(7%)	4	8	11	9	4	11
Precocious/delayed puberty	20(1%)	—	<1	<1	<1	7	2
Metabolic disturbance	58(4%)	4	4	5	4	4	3
Other[b]	66(4%)	2	3	2	26	10	6
Family history of							
Physical defect	24(2%)	1	1	2	<1	2	5
Functional defect	25(2%)	1	<1	2	1	3	4
Parents of child with							
Physical defect	9(<1%)	—	—	—	—	—	5
Functional defect	3(<1%)	—	—	—	—	—	2
Repeated pregnancy loss	14(<1%)	—	—	—	—	—	7
At risk[c]	7(<1%)	<1	—	—	—	—	3

[a]1500 cases: excludes agency referrals, prenatal diagnosis, and postmortem examinations. From Stevenson and Dean.[2]

[b]Includes single minor anomalies, behavioral problems, hematologic disorders, etc.

[c]At risk because of environmental exposure, consanguinity, race, ethnicity, etc.

cant advances in understanding of normal and abnormal embryonic fetal human development before the end of this century.

Human Malformations and Related Anomalies continues the tradition of ordering birth defects according to anatomical systems. This format first appeared in the philosophical and medical literature of the seventeenth century. Regional anatomy was also used in part as the outline for the catalogues of anomalies published by Taruffi,[9] Lowne,[10] and Ballantyne[11] at the beginning of the twentieth century. More recently, anatomical systems formed the framework for the International Classification of Diseases and various modifications of this classification[12] and for Josef Warkany's classic book, *Congenital Malformations, Notes and Comments* (1971).[13]

The historically important texts of Taruffi, Ballantyne, and Warkany represent monumental efforts by individuals who had vast experience with human anomalies. *Human Malformations and Related Anomalies* draws from still wider experience of a group of contributors with diverse scientific backgrounds. They bring to these volumes the knowledge and perspectives of contemporary physicians and scientists who are actively expanding the understanding, treatment, and prevention of human anomalies.

Volume I is devoted to general issues related to the evaluation and understanding of birth defects. Contributions from embryology, experimental teratology, anthropology, genetics, and the medical specialties combine to give a broad analysis of the history and influence of malformations on human society. Appropriate attention is given to the history of con-

cepts as well as to contemporary principles and practices related to birth defects.

Volume II gives detailed accounts of human anomalies arranged by the anatomical systems. An orderly format in each section permits the reader to find information on the incidence, diagnosis, pathogenesis, and causes of human anomalies. Most significant anomalies have separate entries in the appropriate system. Some anomalies are grouped together to reduce repetition. The occurrence of each anomaly in various associations and syndromes is documented, often in table form. The natural history, approaches to treatment, and prevention strategies are given in the final subsection of each entry. A Syndrome Index for the various syndromes that have anomalies in multiple systems precedes the Subject Index.

It seems unlikely that the prevention of all congenital anomalies is close at hand. Families will continue to face the difficulty of having children with birth defects. Physicians will continue to face the tasks of evaluating the extent of the defect, identifying the cause, planning treatment and long-term management, and assisting the family members as they adapt to raising a malformed child. Scientists will continue to be challenged by the need to understand the defects that occur and to develop strategies for their management and prevention. We trust that these volumes will be a useful resource to all who provide assistance to infants born with congenital anomalies and to their families.

Greenwood, South Carolina   R. E. S.
Vancouver, British Columbia   J. G. H.

References

1. Lynberg ML, Khoury MJ: Contribution of birth defects to infant mortality among racial/ethnic minority groups, United States, 1983. MMWR 39(SS-3):1, 1990.
2. Stevenson RE, Dean J: Malformations as a reason for referral for genetic evaluations. Proc Greenwood Genet Center 11:3, 1992.
3. Jones KL: Smith's Recognizable Patterns of Human Malformations, ed 4. WB Saunders, Philadelphia, 1988.
4. Gorlin RJ, Cohen MM Jr, Levin LS: Syndromes of the Head and Neck, ed 3. Oxford University Press, New York, 1990.
5. Taybi H, Lachman RS: Radiology of Syndromes, Metabolic Disorders, and Skeletal Dysplasias, ed 3. Year Book Medical Publishers, Chicago, 1990.
6. Winter RM, Baraitser M, Douglas JM: A computerized data base for the diagnosis of rare dysmorphic syndromes. J Med Genet 21:121, 1984.
7. Buyse M: Center for Birth Defects Information Services. BDOAS XVI(5):83, 1980.
8. Murdoch Institute: POSSUM Newsletter. September, 1987.
9. Taruffi C: Storia della teratologia, vol I–VIII. Regia Tipographia, Bologna, 1881–1894.
10. Lowne BT: Descriptive Catalogue of the Teratological Series in the Museum of the Royal College of Surgeons of England. Taylor and Francis, London, 1893.
11. Ballantyne JW: Manual of Antenatal Pathology and Hygiene, The Embryo. William Green and Sons, Edinburgh, 1904; Reprinted by Jacobs Press, Clinton, SC, 1991.
12. International Classification of Diseases, Revision 9, Clinical Modification (ICD-9-CM). U.S. Department of Health and Human Services Publication Number 91-1260, 1991.
13. Warkany J: Congenital Malformations: Notes and Comments. Year Book Medical Publishers, Chicago, 1971.

Acknowledgments

The concept of *Human Malformations and Related Anomalies* emerged from discussions between Richard Goodman and Roger Stevenson at the 1984 Short Course in Medical and Experimental Mammalian Genetics at the Jackson Laboratory in Bar Harbor, Maine. After several seasons of planning, a large number of colleagues were invited to contribute chapters for the two volumes. To them we are most indebted. The chapter narratives are based on the experience of the authors and the vast literature on human anomalies. After the premature death of Rich Goodman in May 1989, Judith Hall assumed the responsibilities of co-editor.

Illustrations from the files of the authors and editors were supplemented with illustrations from the archives of Charles Scott (clinical photography), Will Blackburn (pathology), Mike Thomason, and Rodney Macpherson (radiology). Numerous other authors and publishers permitted the use of previously published illustrations. Individual credits are given in the figure legends. Most of the figures on embryological development were adapted from the O'Rahilly and Müller, Patten, Moore, and Sadler textbooks. Original illustrations were prepared by John Wesley Lewis, Caroline Stevenson, and Milton Burroughs.

Numerous libraries provided searches, reprints, and citation verifications. We specifically acknowledge assistance from the libraries of the Upper Savannah Area Health Education Consortium (SC), the British Museum, the New York Academy of Medicine, Lander University, the Medical University of South Carolina, and the Medical College of Georgia. In addition, the *London Dysmorphology Database, Mendelian Inheritance in Man,* and *POSSUM* were valuable sources of references. Thomas Hill, Ellen Dewkett, Angela Stevenson, Daniel Lee, and Julia Gilmer responded to thousands of library inquiries during the course of manuscript preparation. Leslie Stevenson, Bess Stevenson, and Ericka Stevenson prepared the index.

The editors' work was aided immensely by the efficiency and good humor of the secretaries and staffs of all contributors in meeting the various deadlines and in preparation of manuscript copy and computer disks. We are especially indebted to Rhonda Erneston and Mary Lynn Lyle for the organization and preparation of the final manuscript copy.

Throughout the project we have benefited from the counsel and encouragement of Jeffrey House and Susan Hannan of Oxford University Press. Their experience and cooperation have contributed to making a formidable task into an enjoyable undertaking.

Finally, we wish to thank our colleagues at the Greenwood Genetic Center and the University of British Columbia. They have made suggestions regarding format and content, reviewed manuscripts, and taken on additional responsibilities to give us time to devote to this project.

R. E. S.
J. G. H.

Contents

Volume I

Contributors

Gary M. Albers, M.D.
Pediatric Pulmonary Medicine
University of North Carolina
Chapel Hill, North Carolina

Judith E. Allanson, M.B., Ch.B.
Children's Hospital of Eastern Ontario
Ottawa, Ontario
Canada

Arthur S. Aylsworth, M.D.
Department of Pediatrics and The Brain and
    Development Research Center
University of North Carolina
Chapel Hill, North Carolina

Dagmar Bauer-Hansmann, M.D.
Universitats-Frauenklinik Bonn
Abteilung fur Prenatale Diagnostik und Therapie
Bonn, Germany

Will R. Blackburn, M.D.
University of South Alabama College of Medicine
Mobile, Alabama

Ellen Boyd, M.D.
Greenwood Genetic Center
Greenwood, South Carolina

John C. Carey, M.D., M.P.H.
University of Utah
Salt Lake City, Utah

M. Michael Cohen, Jr., D.M.D., Ph.D.
Dalhousie University
Halifax, Nova Scotia
Canada

Nelson Reede Cooley, Jr.
Department of Pathology
University of South Alabama College of Medicine
Mobile, Alabama

Cynthia J. R. Curry, M.D.
Medical Genetics/Prenatal Detection
Valley Children's Hospital
Fresno, California

Vazken M. Der Kaloustian, M.D.
Montreal Children's Hospital
McGill University
Montreal, Quebec
Canada

Katherine C. Donahue, Ph.D.
Department of Social Science
Plymouth State College
Plymouth, New Hampshire

Luis F. Escobar, M.S., M.D.
Indiana University
Indianapolis, Indiana

Richard H. Finnell, Ph.D.
Department of Veterinary Anatomy and Public
Health
College of Veterinary Medicine
Texas A & M University
College Station, Texas

David B. Flannery, M.D.
Department of Pediatrics
Medical College of Georgia
Augusta, Georgia

Mitchell S. Golbus, M.D.
Reproductive Genetics Unit
University of California Medical Center
San Francisco, California

Richard M. Goodman* (Editor)
Department of Human Genetics
University of Tel Aviv
Tel Aviv, Israel

Robert J. Gorlin, D.D.S., M.S., D.Sc.
University of Minnesota
Minneapolis, Minnesota

John M. Graham, Jr., M.D., Sc.D.
Medical Genetics Birth Defects Center
Cedars-Sinai Medical Center
Los Angeles, California

Judith G. Hall, M.D. (Editor)
Department of Pediatrics
B.C. Children's Hospital
Vancouver, British Columbia,
Canada

James W. Hanson, M.D.
Department of Pediatrics
University of Iowa
Iowa City, Iowa

*Deceased.

Louis H. Honoré, B.Sc., M.B., Ch.B.
Department of Pathology
University of Alberta Hospital
Edmonton, Alberta
Canada

H. Eugene Hoyme, M.D.
Department of Pediatrics
Section of Genetics and Dysmorphology
University of Arizona
Tucson, Arizona

Alasdair G. W. Hunter, M.Sc., M.D., C.M.
Children's Hospital of Eastern Ontario
Ottawa, Ontario
Canada

Malcolm C. Johnston, D.D.S.
Dental Research Center
University of North Carolina
Chapel Hill, North Carolina

Kenneth L. Jones, M.D.
School of Medicine
University of California, San Diego
San Diego, California

Ronald L. Jorgenson, D.D.S., Ph.D.
South Texas Genetics Center
Austin, Texas

Ian Leck, M.B., Ph.D., D.Sc.
University of Manchester, U.K.
Pembury
Woodstock
Oxon
England

John T. Lettieri, M.D.
Western Carolina Cleft Lip/Palate and
    Craniofacial Center
Spartanburg, South Carolina

Barbara C. McGillivray, M.D.
Department of Medical Genetics
University of British Columbia Hospital
Vancouver, British Columbia
Canada

Patrick M. MacLeod, M.D.
Department of Pediatrics
Queen's University
Kingston, Ontario
Canada

Leslie C. Meyer, M.D.
Shriners Hospitals for Crippled Children
Greenville, South Carolina

Eberhard Passarge, M.D.
Institut für Humangenetik
Universitätsklinikum
Essen, Germany

Mary C. Phelan, Ph.D.
Greenwood Genetic Center
Greenwood, South Carolina

Leo Plouffe, Jr., M.D., C.M.
Department of Obstetrics and Gynecology
Medical College of Georgia
Augusta, Georgia

Donald A. Riopel, M.D.
The Sanger Clinic
Charlotte, North Carolina

Robert A. Saul, M.D.
Greenwood Genetic Center
Greenwood, South Carolina

R. Neil Schimke, M.D.
Department of Medicine
Kansas University Medical School
Kansas City, Kansas

Richard J. Schroer, M.D.
Greenwood Genetic Center
Greenwood, South Carolina

Charles I. Scott, Jr., M.D.
A.I. DuPont Institute
Wilmington, Delaware

Heddie O. Sedano, D.D.S., Dr. Odont.
School of Dentistry
University of Minnesota
Minneapolis, Minnesota

Joe Leigh Simpson, M.D.
University of Tennessee
Memphis, Tennessee

Kathleen Sulik, Ph.D.
Department of Cell Biology and Anatomy
University of North Carolina
Chapel Hill, North Carolina

Roger E. Stevenson, M.D. (Editor)
Greenwood Genetic Center
Greenwood, South Carolina

Helga V. Toriello, Ph.D.
Butterworth Hospital
Grand Rapids, Michigan

Elias I. Traboulsi, M.D.
The Wilmer Ophthalmological Institute
The Johns Hopkins Center for Hereditary Eye Diseases
Baltimore, Maryland

Margot I. Van Allen, M.D., M.Sc.
Department of Medical Genetics
University Hospital
Vancouver, British Columbia
Canada

Michael van Waes, M.Sci.
Division of Biological Sciences
University of Montana
Missoula, Montana

Marion S. Verp, M.D.
Department of Obstetrics and Gynecology
The University of Chicago
Chicago, Illinois

Wladimir Wertelecki, M.D.
Department of Medical Genetics
University of South Alabama College of Medicine
Mobile, Alabama

Golder N. Wilson, M.D., Ph.D.
Division of Pediatric Genetics
University of Texas
Southwestern Medical Center
Dallas, Texas

Robin M. Winter, B.Sc.
Institute of Child Health
London
United Kingdom

Robert E. Wood, Ph.D., M.D.
Pediatric Pulmonary Medicine
University of North Carolina
Chapel Hill, North Carolina

Hans Zellweger, M.D.*
Department of Pediatrics
University of Iowa
Iowa City, Iowa

*Deceased.

Human Malformations
and Related Anomalies

1

Causes of Human Anomalies: An Overview and Historical Perspective

ROGER E. STEVENSON

The preimplantation, embryonic, and fetal periods are the most complex and vulnerable 9 months of the life cycle. During this time, the unique combination of genes distributed to each human conception will be accorded a single opportunity to form a structurally and functionally adequate organism. Early embryonic cells possess developmental potency that will be lost in the generations of cells to follow. Activity of genes that will be needed at no other time in life is required at specific intervals during the prenatal months. Environmental influences that are innocuous for the mature organism can be remarkably destructive prenatally. Protection against such noxious influences from without and within depends to a great extent on the health and lifestyle of the maternal custodian. Malformations, if they are to occur, will arise during the first few months of pregnancy. Constitutional impairments to growth and function will be established during this period also even though they may not be overtly discernible. It should not be surprising that human conceptions are lost at an astounding rate. Of the world's 1 million conceptions each day, less than one-half reach a stage of development compatible with extrauterine survival. No small part of this natural decimation of life can be attributed to malformations.

Loss of human conceptions steadily decreases from the time of implantation (day 7 postfertilization) to the stage of postnatal viability, 24 weeks postfertilization at the present time.[1-3] It should be recognized that postnatal viability is an arbitrary assignment and one that changes with changes in postnatal care. Advances in obstetric and neonatal care during the past two decades have consistently lowered the gestational age at which extrauterine survival of the preterm infant can be expected.

It is known that certain genetic and environmental influences can prevent the orderly division of the fertilized egg and preparation for implantation. With certainty, some conceptions fail to implant, but the exact incidence of this phenomenon cannot be given. No reliable means of determining conception (fertilization prior to implantation) has been developed. Roberts and Lowe,[4] calculated that perhaps as many as one-half of fertilized ova fail to implant.

Fully one-third of conceptions are lost after implantation (day 7 postfertilization) but before the pregnancy is recognized by the mother. Hertig et al.[5] were able to examine 26 early postimplantation conceptuses obtained at the time of hysterectomy and found 6 to show abnormalities of organization and implantation. A similar incidence of defective embryos has been documented in material from induced abortion.[6] It is likely that these defective embryos would be spontaneously aborted very early. Implantation can now be determined by measuring maternal secretion of urinary human chorionic gonadotropin (hCG), which is produced

only by the trophoblast of the conceptus. Spontaneous abortion before clinical evidence of pregnancy occurs in 8%–33% of pregnancies with hCG evidence of implantation.[3,7,8] These very early abortions commonly show disorganization, with discordance of size between embryo and placenta, degeneration of tissues, and a high incidence of chromosome abnormalities.[1,5,6,9]

Once pregnancy becomes clinically recognized, pregnancy loss becomes less frequent, occurring in 10%–25% of pregnancies (Fig. 1–1).[10,11] The earlier the pregnancy loss, the greater the likelihood of chromosome abnormality and of specific malformations being identified as the cause of the abortion.[12-15] The later the abortion, the higher the probability that environmental forces were responsible.

Stillbirths account for 1 of every 100 deliveries after 24 weeks postfertilization. Stillborn infants have a high incidence of anomalies. About 15%–20% of stillborn babies will have major anomalies, one-third of which will be due to chromosome abnormalities.[16-18]

Prenatal mortality eliminates most human conceptions affected with major anomalies. Yet liveborn infants are not free of congenital anomalies, 2%–3% of them having defects detectable at birth and a greater number having anatomic variants or minor malformations that pose no significant threat to health or psychosocial well-being.[18-24]

It has become increasingly evident that prenatal mortality in the form of abortion and stillbirth is the major force that keeps the malformation rate among liveborn infants at its low level. This discriminating force applies to conceptions malformed for all reasons. The high fetal mortality rate among malformed conceptions prevents the increase in frequency of genetic defects that would occur over time if these conceptions were to survive.

Human destiny depends on precise performance of the genetic endowment in reproducing the human likeness reliably, predictably, efficiently, and fault-free. It depends no less on an environment secure from forces that would throw normal genetic instructions off course. Human life is fragile, and nowhere is this fragility more dramatically exposed than in the occurrence of malformations. The same mutational process that over time has brought humans to their present state of evolution through subtle, small increments of change can also make great changes in the organism as well. Single mutant changes involving but a minor biochemical alteration in the genetic code or chromosome modification barely visible under the microscope can produce major structural changes incompatible with life and longevity. Likewise can human fragility be seen in a susceptibility to environmental forces. No genomic strengths are known to protect against the malforming propensity of thalidomide, German measles infection, and many other noxious insults from the environment.

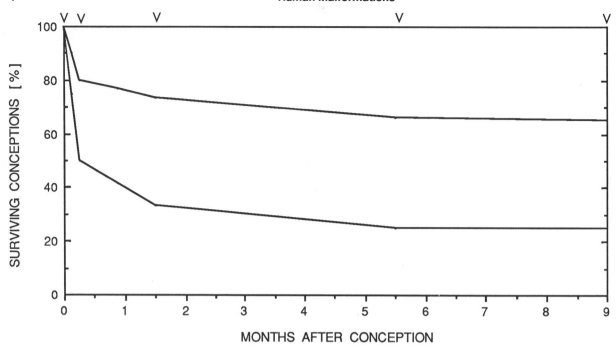

Fig. 1–1. Estimates of maximal (upper curve) and minimal (lower curve) survival rates of human conceptions. Loss rates are highest before implantation (20%–50%), less between implantation and recognition of pregnancy (8%–33%), and still less after pregnancy rec- ognition (10%–25%) and after 24 weeks (1%). Arrowheads indicate, respectively, conception, implantation, pregnancy recognition, 24 weeks gestation, and term.

Humans hold the reproductive process in some awe, correctly amazed that the complex transition from a single fertilized cell to the normally formed and functioning human can be repeatedly successful. Each conception, a unique combination of genes in an ever-changing environment, has but a single chance in this olympic event. There are no trials. A single misstep, timing error, or failure to execute can render the organism either incapable of completing its transformation or impaired by malformation or dysfunction. Human reproductive failures number perhaps twice the successes. Most of the failures take the form of abortion or stillbirth, but a minority occur in the individuals with morphologic and functional impairments.

Numerous difficulties are encountered in gaining insights into human development. Because of reverence for prenatal life and commitment to do no harm, experiments to test hypotheses regarding normal and abnormal developmental processes cannot be carried out. Advantage can be taken of animal experiments in which embryos are subjected to various noxious influences or in which genetic material is manipulated, but extrapolation from these models to humans must be offered with some reservation. Humans usually have but a single offspring at a time, have a long generation time, and in total have a small number of offspring. Psychological and cultural taboos can also hinder access to and study of malformations. These difficulties aside, a large body of information about malformations in humans is available, and there are means to obtain even more data. In developed countries all human births are registered, malformations are identified, and, as a general course, treatment permits most infants with malformations to survive. Without planning it, there are adequate numbers of pregnant women who drink,

or smoke, or acquire syphilis, or are otherwise exposed to harmful substances to provide reasonable evidence if these environmental insults produce malformations. There are enough babies born with any one of the most frequent 25 malformations to provide collectively a formidable body of information on their phenotypes, natural histories, epidemiologies, and causation. For a condition that occurs once in every 50,000 births, 2100 cases occur annually in the worldwide newborn population. For a condition with an incidence much rarer, e.g., 1/500,000, over 200 new cases are added to the world's population each year. Granted, these conditions may not be easy to find given the worldwide political, social, and medical inequities. Yet the malformations occur and are there to be studied, even those that are extremely rare. Understanding rare human anomalies becomes possible only when clinicians make careful observations on every infant born with an anomaly and share these observations in the medical literature.

History

Few events evoke the emotions of humans as greatly as the birth of a baby with malformations. At once, sympathy, disbelief, fear, guilt, imagination, and curiosity are expressed. Humans have come to expect orderly and predictable events in all of nature. Malformations dramatically deviate from the expected and demand an explanation. And humans, because of their capacity to reason, imagine, and fabricate, will not be found wanting for explanations. They will utilize the best of their lore, history, observations, and experience to identify a basis or cause for every occurrence. To fill the void in scientific understanding, humans often have called upon the supernatural as an explanation. With increasing scientific understanding, concepts involving faulty embryogenesis, genetic aberrations, and specific influences from the environment have become recognized as causes of malformations.

For generations before the middle of this century, large families were the rule, in part as necessity for survival, protection, and work force, in part as the response to exhortation by religious and governmental leaders, and in part as happenstance in the absence of efficient birth control. Before this century, one of every five infants born would succumb to childhood illness or other maladies before reaching maturity.[25] Malformation was but one phenomenon that claimed the lives of infants, but one that came with great drama and suddenness. It would not seem unexpected in this situation to find malformations interpreted as carrying great importance, a message beyond the immediate.

Early peoples, of course, did not understand the biologic basis of reproduction. To be sure, they observed that offspring followed sexual union between man and woman. But the concepts of gametes, fertilization, embryogenesis, and the like are relatively recent. Aristotle thought that embryos arose from material in menstrual blood, being activated, controlled, and molded by semen.[26] Others before and after him envisioned the embryo was formed from elements collected from all parts of the body and transmitted through the reproductive fluids.[27,28] Still others regarded the embryo as fully formed in sperm or egg.[29,30]

Accounts of humankind's occupation with the nature and meaning of malformations exist among the earliest written records. The oldest writings that deal with malformations are the cuneiform tablets from the Library of Nineveh, which probably date from 2000 BC.[31] The written records covering four millennia since these tablets were produced contain a rich heritage of observations on malformations.

Interest in malformations, however, did not begin with civilizations having written language. Pre-graphic humans gave expression to their knowledge of malformations by weaving them into folklore, by depicting them in drawings and other art work, and by transforming individuals with structural anomalies into gods and mythical creatures.[32–36] Folklore was passed verbally from one generation to the next for unknown periods of time before being permanently recorded in written form. No doubt the folklore changed a bit with each generation, depending on the imagination and the purpose of the storyteller and perhaps compensating for a lack of details of the original event.

There is no reason to think that malformations have not existed for as long as humans have existed, perhaps 3–5 million years. Archaeological findings that predate modern humans do not include examples of specific structural malformations, although the morphology and size of their forerunners may now be viewed as "malformed." Certainly the height and skull circumference of early hominids would constitute short stature and microcephaly according to contemporary anthropology.[37]

Depictions of conjoined twins represent the oldest evidence of malformations among humans. The conjoined goddess of Anatolia has been dated at 6500 BC (Fig. 1–2).[32] A chalk drawing and a sculpture of dicephalics by primitive artists in the South Pacific have yet to be specifically dated but are thought to have been produced between 4000 and

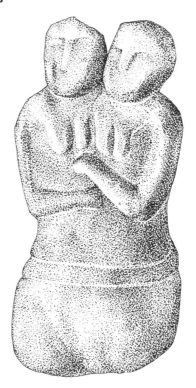

Fig. 1–2. White marble figure of conjoined goddesses dated about 6500 BC from a shrine at the Catal Hüyük site in Anatolia (Turkey).

5000 BC (Fig. 1–3).[34] Statues of individuals with achondroplasia and other dwarfing dysplasias are among Egyptian treasures from 2000 BC.[36]

Concepts regarding the causes of congenital anomalies can be traced through the folklore, art, writings, and scientific advances of the past four millennia. These concepts have been held for varying periods of time by varying cultures. Some eventually blended into a new generation of thought or vanished entirely. Some concepts would be readily discarded by the contemporary scientific community whereas others have been proved to some degree by scientific means. These concepts of causation include

1. Supernatural forces
2. Celestial bodies
3. Abnormal reproductive components
4. Hybridization with animals
5. Maternal impressions
6. Arrest of embryonic processes
7. Mechanical influences
8. Fetal diseases
9. Heredity
10. Environmental insults

Supernatural forces

Malformations numbered among the many natural phenomena attributed to the will of god(s). Early humans saw special meaning in malformations, as they did in earthquakes, floods, droughts, and celestial events.

Early philosophers expressed the concept that god(s) created malformations with sportive intent.[33,38,39] One aspect of this interpretation was that malformations represented

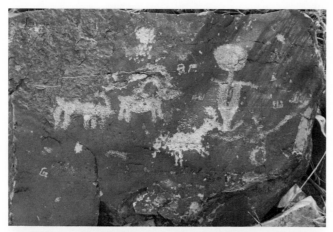

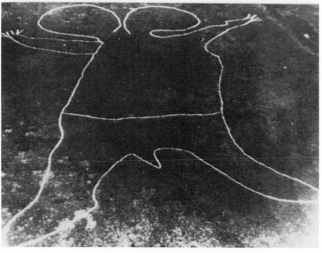

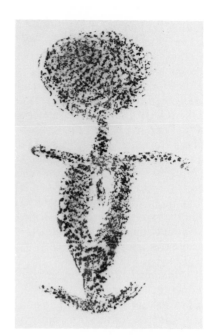

Fig. 1–3. Rock drawing (top) from Utah (USA) showing sireno-melia and possibly ectopia cordis. The drawing has not been dated but presumably is pre-Columbian. Courtesy of Dr. Charles E. Schwartz, Greenwood Genetic Center, Greenwood, SC. Engraving of dicephalic conjoined twins (bottom) on a rock platform near Berowra Waters on the outskirts of Sydney, Australia. Although this figure has not been dated accurately, it is assumed to be 4000–5000 yr old. Note presence of six digits on right hand and four digits on left hand. Courtesy of the *Medical Journal of Australia,* © 1943.

merely a demonstration of god(s)' creative repertoire. Malformations were made because they could be made. Similarly, some interpreted malformations to be the result of god(s) at play, amusing themselves by manipulating human morphology. At the same time malformations served to confound humans. As Pliny[39] wrote, "Nature creates monsters for the purpose of astonishing us and amusing herself".

A more serious intent underpinned the concept that god(s) used malformations to convey messages. Messages so conveyed were generally those of grave nature, constituting warnings or admonitions rather than expressions of pleasure.[40] Implicit in this concept was the possibility that humans could avoid a personal or societal calamity by timely atonement or action. Only subtle distinctions perhaps separate this concept from the belief that malformations represented the demonstration of displeasure or punishment from god(s). Variations of these concepts were held among all early civilizations and indeed are not uncommonly heard today. Linguistic connections can be found for both aspects of this interpretation: *monsters,* the term historically used for malformed infants, may derive from *monstrare,* to show, or *monere,* to warn.

In the foregoing discussion, the creation of monsters was considered as one action by the same god who controlled good happenings as well. Supernatural beings can be separated on the basis of having a good or evil nature, and it is not surprising to see malformations attributed to the influence of evil spirits. This influence gave authority for the destruction of infants with congenital anomalies, a common practice in many civilizations. Not uncommonly, the mother's life was in peril as well.

That a reciprocal relationship of sorts may exist between malformed beings and the supernatural has been suggested by several authors.[33,41] Rather than being the creators of malformed humans, the gods have themselves been created with the likeness of malformed humans. Certain gods have clearcut likenesses to human malformations. Among these are the conjoined twin goddess of the shrine of neolithic Anatolia (6500 BC) and Bes and Pthah, the achondroplastic gods of the Egyptians.[32,36]

Euhemerus, a Sicilian historian of the fourth century BC, held that god(s), mythological creatures, and extraordinary subjects of folklore may have been patterned after individuals who had malformations.[33] One can see in the Greek gods and other mythological beings features reminiscent of malformed humans. Atlas may represent an individual with an encephalocele (Fig. 1–4). Polyphemus may have been derived from a cyclopic infant, Prometheus from one with omphalocele or gastroschisis, the Siren from one with sympodia, and the Centaur from a syncephalus dilecanus conjoined twin.[41] The transformation of individuals with other anomalies into gods may require more imagination. But a plausible account holds that malformed infants were seen, and as descriptions of their appearance were transmitted through the generations they were embellished, exaggerated, or altered and eventually transformed into gods.

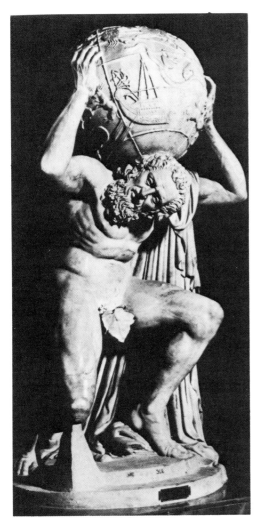

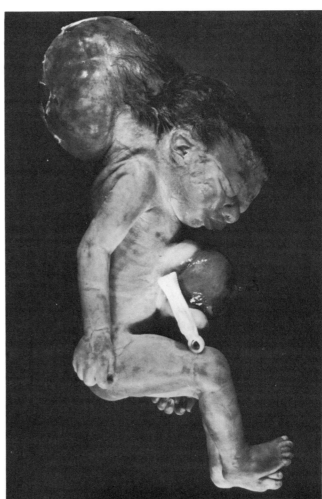

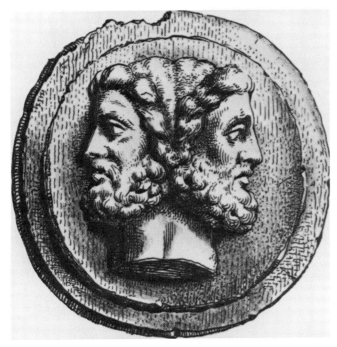

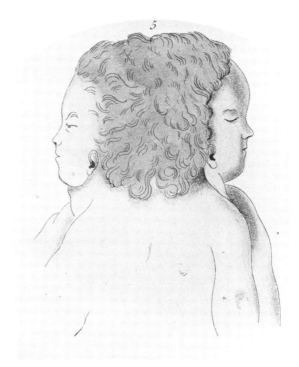

Fig. 1–4. Gods that may have derived their images from malformed humans. Top figures show Atlas supporting the sky on his shoulders (left; courtesy of National Archaeological Museum, Naples) compared with an infant with a large encephalocele (right). Bottom figures show the two faces of the Roman god Janus (left) compared with drawing of a conjoined twin from Guering's *Anatomical Monstrosities* (1837). Courtesy of Dr. Will Blackburn and N. Reede Cooley, Jr., University of South Alabama College of Medicine, Mobile.

Celestial bodies

Closely related to the concept that supernatural forces could cause human malformations was the belief that the heavenly bodies wielded similar powers. These two concepts were given equally prominent places in the early written records. Although astrological observations and predictions may have been made over hundreds of centuries, the creation of astrology has been attributed to the Sumerians, occupants of that region in the Middle East known in biblical times as Babylonia and today as Iraq.[42] The Sumerians refined the concept of astrological influences, kept written records of their observations, and disseminated their philosophy over the known world.

According to astrology, the destinies of humans and nations are controlled by the position of the celestial bodies. Malformations were but one of the human infirmities produced by the "inevitable and irremedial" consequences of unfavorable positions of the stars.[33,42] Because other earthly events were likewise determined by star positioning, the birth of a baby with a malformation came to be used as an earthly sign of events to follow.

A remarkable library of clay tablets that, among other things, catalog human and animal malformations and their meanings was excavated near the Tigris River in the nineteenth century.[31,42,43] The tablets, part of the Royal Library of Nineveh, probably date to ~2000 BC and represent beliefs held long before that time. On the two sides of one tablet (K2007) is a listing of 62 human malformations and the meanings attached to them by the Chaldeans (Fig. 1–5). Thirteen malformations affected the ear, 13 affected the mouth and nose, 5 the upper limbs, 10 the lower limbs, 4 the genitalia, and 17 involved other structures.

Examples of the portents as given by Ballantyne[31] include

When a woman gives birth to an infant—
(2) that wants a right ear, the days of the master (king) will be prolonged (reach old age);
(4) whose right ear is small, the house of the man (in whose house the birth took place) will be destroyed;
(13) that has no mouth, the mistress of the house will die;
(16) whose jaws are absent, the days of the master (king) will be prolonged, but the house (where the infant is born) will be ruined;
(22) whose upper lip overrides the lower, the peoples of the world will rejoice (or good augury for the troops);
(25) that has no right hand, the country will be convulsed by an earthquake;
(31) that has the heart open and that has no skin, the country will suffer from calamities;
(32) that has no penis, the master of the house will be enriched by harvest of his field;
(35) whose anus is closed, the country will suffer from want of nourishment;
(56) that has some teeth already through (cut), the days of the king will arrive at old age; the country will show itself powerful over (against) strange (feeble) lands; but the house where the infant is born will be ruined.

Potency as a cause for malformations was shared by all of the visible heavenly bodies, including comets, planets, stars, and the moon. Certain powers were partitioned to various of the heavenly bodies. The term *moon calf* has dual meaning, that of a monster or malformed being and that of a molar pregnancy. Both attest to belief in the influence of the moon on reproductive matters. Pliny[44] interpreted molar pregnancy as being generated without impregnation. This is remarkable in light of current knowledge that complete hydatidiform moles lack any maternal chromosomes, their diploid nuclei being constituted from two sperm or from duplication of a single sperm.[45]

Adherence to the astrological concepts persisted throughout the Middle Ages. Among those who subscribed to these views are Ptolemy, Albertus Magnus, Thomas Aquinas, and Bartholin.[33] In the seventeenth century other theories began to crowd astrological concepts out of favor, but even today many depend on horoscopic predictions in the conduct of their lives and reproductive practices.

Abnormal reproductive components

Even before the rudiments of reproductive physiology were understood, aberrations of the reproductive components were suspected of giving rise to malformations. Abnormalities of the sperm and egg are now known to consist predominantly of mutations and chromosomal imbalances. Earlier concepts, however, attributed abnormalities less to the genetic capacity and more to the source, quantity, vigor, or age of the reproductive components.[40,46] Early philosophers recognized male semen and female menses to be the two main reproductive components.[26,39,40,46–52] Some held that the capacity to produce a baby and hence to produce abnormalities resided entirely or predominantly in the semen, others thought this only to be a property of the menses, and still others believed in some collaboration between the two sexual fluids.

Semen, it was commonly held by early physicists, provided all the substance necessary for producing a new being.[47,49] The maternal role in reproduction was to provide incubation, nourishment, and a safe haven until birth. Being wholly dependent for its form on the semen, the infant was subject to the vagaries of semen production. Too much semen, too little semen, or aged semen were all accepted as reasons for a baby to be malformed. Not unexpectedly, too little semen was thought to result in deficiencies of various parts of the body; too much semen to duplication, overgrowth, multiple pregnancies, and the like (Fig. 1–6). According to Empedocles, malformations could result from a deficiency in or excess of the semen or to its faulty movement.[47] This popular concept with some modification was held through the Greek and Roman civilizations and through the Middle Ages. Paré,[40] in 1573, cites too great a quantity of seed (semen), too little a quantity of seed, and rotten or corrupt seed among the 13 causes of malformations.

A less popular interpretation held that menses was preeminent in formative powers and that excessive or deficient menstrual flow could produce malformations.[50] This concept may have influenced or been influenced by the religious prohibition against coitus during the time of menstruation.

Consistent with these concepts, males were thought to be produced by semen produced in the right testis and females from semen produced in the left testis and hermaphrodites from fluid from both testes.[51] An alternative interpretation was that males developed when the conceptus implanted in the right side of the uterus, females when implanted in the left, and hermaphrodites when implanted in the middle of the uterus.[51,52]

Aristotle did not accept the unisexual interpretation of formation of a baby, favoring instead the joint contribution of

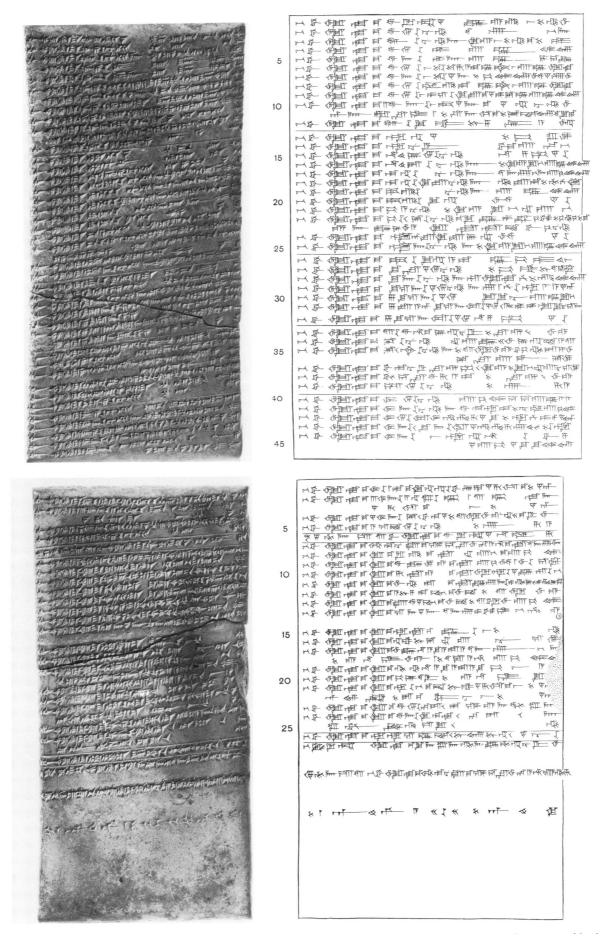

Fig. 1–5. Clay tablet (K2007) from Royal Library of Nineveh lists 62 human malformations and their interpretations. Top figures show obverse of the 6 inch tall tablet and a transcript of the cuneiform text. Bottom figures show the reverse side. Note the scribe's erasure following line 14. Courtesy of The Trustees of the British Museum.

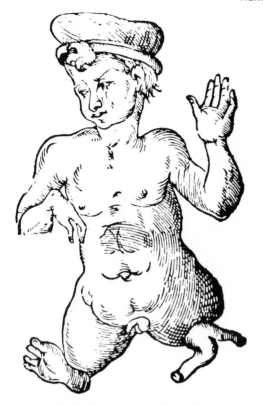

Fig. 1–6. In the sixteenth century, Paré[40] depicted this child with limb reduction defects, which he attributed to insufficient quantity of semen.

male and female to the baby and to malformations as well. "The blood of the menses is the marble, the semen is the sculptor, and the fetus is the statue" seems to imply that Aristotle may have considered the menses to be the more important of the two, however.[26] Following the same concept, Pliny[39] thought that the menses was "the material substance of generation: and the man's seed serveth instead of a runnet to gather it round into a curd; which afterwards in process of time quickeneth and groweth to the form of a body."

Hybridization with animals

Cross-fertilization between humans and animals offered a convenient explanation when babies were born with features resembling animals or when animals were born with features resembling humans. Some authorities held that cross-fertilization could only occur between different species or between humans and animals of similar size and gestational period.[26,33] The concept, more ancient than the written record, remained viable into the eighteenth century. Looked upon as a sordid happenstance, such unions constituted a sufficient breech of acceptable behavior that the presumed parents and the child were often put to death.[40,53−55]

Lucky the accused who could find another plausible explanation. Albertus Magnus is said to have intervened in one such circumstance in the year AD 1200.[54] The event followed the birth of a malformed calf, one with human features, thought to be the product of the cow and her shepherd. The shepherd, under sentence of burning, was freed upon explanation by Magnus that the malformed calf was caused by the

position of the stars, an equally potent explanation for the times.

Less lucky were others, including one George Spencer of pre-revolutionary America. In the year 1641, a cyclopic pig with a proboscis ("butt one eye in the middle"), above which "a thing of flesh grew forth and hung downe, it was hollow, and like a mans instrum' of gen'ation" was born in the New Haven colony. George Spencer, a servant, who was unfortunately affected with cataract ("butt one eye for vse, the other hath a pearle in itt") was accused, tried, and convicted as the father of the malformed pig. George Spencer was executed for this crime after the malformed pig was "slaine in his sight, being run through wth a sworde."

Cross-hybridization seems to have been a matter of disgust for mortals only, since there are numerous instances of god–animal hybrids.[33]

Maternal impressions

"Special watch should be kept over our pregnant women during the year of their pregnancy to guard the expectant mother against the experiences of frequent and violent pleasures—or pains either—and insure her cultivation of a gracious, bright, and serene spirit."[56] In this admonition to his countrymen, Plato gave credence to the thought that emotional experiences could influence the outcome of pregnancies. It is a thought that has attracted disciples from the cultures of all ages and all geographic regions.

During the height of the Greek and Roman empires, pregnant women were advised to view public artworks, those graceful and strong statues in the public squares, in order to claim for their offspring similar characteristics.[57] When a baby was born with a malformation it was to be assumed that the mother was not diligent in this duty or that she came upon unfavorable images that were incorporated into defective development. It is the production of visible abnormalities through maternal experiences during pregnancy that conveys the idea of marking.

Although malformations related to maternal impressions were usually generated by visual experiences, they were not the exclusive domain of this sense. Pliny, among others, indicated that auditory and tactile experiences as well as the experiences of the imagination could provoke malformations in the unborn infant.[39,58−65] With this explanation, observers could interpret many unusual birthing events. In the Greek novel *Aethiopic* the birth of the white baby, Charliceae, to the black king and queen of Ethiopia, was attributed to the viewing of a marble of Andromeda at the time of conception.[59] Conversely, the birth of a black infant to Roman parents was credited to the presence of a picture of a Moor over their bed, according to the account given by Quintilian.[60] The birth of a hirsute baby with the likeness of John the Baptist was thought to have resulted from the mother's preoccupation with a picture of John the Baptist pictured as a hirsute individual clothed in animal skins.[61] For the same reason, Eng and Chang, the famous conjoined twins of the 1800s were banned from exhibition in France for fear that pregnant women would deliver babies of similar nature or worse (Fig. 1–7).[62] None other than Etienne Geoffroy Saint-Hilaire, the father of experimental teratology, had requested the entry visa for the twins.

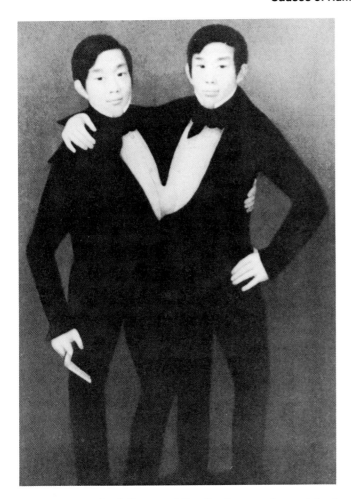

Fig. 1-7. Portrait of Chang and Eng Bunker, popular conjoined twins in the nineteenth century. The artist painted Chang on the right, the reverse of his position in life.

Witnessing acts of violence was believed to carry sufficient emotional impact to be responsible for the birth of malformed babies. The birth of a baby with multiple fractures (presumably osteogenesis imperfecta) in France was attributed to the mother's witnessing the fracturing of a criminal's limbs at the wheel.[63] Congenital amputation of an infant's hand was thought to be related to observing the spectacle of amputation of a thief's hand.[64] By one account the disfigurement present in Joseph Merrick, the "elephant man," could be attributed to the mother's encounter with an escaped carnival elephant rampaging the streets of London.[65]

Malformations that bore any resemblance to an animal were likely to be attributed to the viewing of that animal during the course of pregnancy. By this means anencephaly and microcephaly were believed related to the viewing of monkeys, claw hands to bears, cleft lip to rabbits, and hirsutism to any furry animals.[33]

Physical contact was also considered in interpretations of the influence that experiences during pregnancy could have on the fetus. An anecdote from the Middle Ages tells of a pregnant woman who bumped heads with another woman, resulting in the birth of conjoined twins attached at the vertex.[66] A similar causal connection was made between the occurrence of a skull fracture in a pregnant woman and the later birth of an infant with an occipital skull defect.[67] More subtle fetal changes could be wrought through tactile sense as well.

Marking of a fetus could also result from imagination or dreams. A most extraordinary tale relates the birth of a baby with a shell-like head to the longing of the mother for mussels during the pregnancy.[68] The offspring, so the story goes, took nourishment in liquid form and survived about 11 yr, dying following a fracture of the bivalve cranium. Even conception itself could be achieved through maternal imagination. A relevant story relates the conception of Magdalena in seventeenth century France during the absence of her husband, Hieronymus Augustus.[69] Her claims that she imagined her husband's presence and thereby became pregnant were sufficient to convince medical and legal authorities that the child was fathered in absentia by the husband.

In some cases, the phenomenon of marking depended on maternal imagery at the time of conception, but in other cases marking resulted from experiences later in pregnancy. Paré[40] noted that maternal impressions could transform the unborn only during the first 42 days after conception, during that period of time when the baby was not yet formed. Such restrictions were not posed by many other authorities. Emotional experiences of the father could mark infants as well, but this possibility was limited to the period surrounding conception.[70]

The mechanism by which maternal or paternal impressions could produce developmental abnormalities was of little concern in most cultures, but became necessary to support the concept against criticism in the eighteenth century. Most advocates of the concept argued that emotional experiences were conveyed through nerve connections between the mother and babies; others, through alterations in the blood or body humors, and still others through spiritual connections.[63,71-73] For some, leaving the explanation to the occult was sufficient.

However colorful these interpretations may be, they lack scientific validity. It cannot be argued that the fetus is exempt from influence by maternal emotion. If such influence exists, however, it must find expression in some as yet undefined measure of fetal health rather than in a specific malformation or malfunction related to the maternal impression.

Arrest of embryonic development

The invention of the microscope in the late seventeenth century forced fundamental changes in the concepts of human reproduction and malformations. While not immediately eliminating the ideas held for centuries, it made possible a scientific perspective based on anatomic observations. Gametes could be examined, fertilization visualized, and the changes of embryologic development followed in experimental animals. Observations could be repeated and convincingly communicated to other workers. Dependence on anecdotal experience and on conjecture could now be decreased.

One of the earliest principles to come from the microscopic age was that embryogenesis proceeds from a simple amorphous form to the complex. This principle replaced the widely held belief that embryos were fully formed miniature humans, residents of the invisible world of the sperm or egg. Aristotle had recognized that embryonic development progressed from simple form based on observations in chick embryos, but his thoughts had been lost in the intervening centuries prior to development of the microscope.[26]

William Harvey[74] noted the likeness of cleft lip and the absence of midline facial fusion in early human embryos and suggested that they were in some way related:

> In the fetuses of all animals, indeed that of man inclusive, the oral aperture without lips or cheeks is seen stretching from ear to ear; and this is the reason, unless I am much mistaken, why so many are born with the upper lip divided as it is in the hare and camel, whence the common name of harelip for the deformity. In the development of the human fetus the upper lip only coalesces in the midline at a very late period.

Later, microscopic observations were to document that embryos pass through stages of development during which the anatomy of other structures might simulate the anatomy of a recognized malformation.[33,75–77] To this point, syndactylous digits were found to resemble those of the embryonic hand or foot before postfertilization day 50, phocomelias to limb configuration at a similar embryonic time, ectopic cordis to the heart position before day 22, cranial and spinal schises to incompletely fused neural folds before day 26, omphalocele to the midgut location in the umbilical cord prior to day 75, and so forth.

The basic tenet of the concept of arrest of embryonic development is that progress toward a finished anatomic structure is halted at an intermediate and incomplete stage. Structures that arise separately but are destined to fuse fail to do so. Structures that arise singularly and are destined to divide into separate structures fail to complete the division. Structures that are destined to disappear are retained. Structures that undergo refinement of the morphology retain their primitive appearance.

As part of the overall concept of arrest of development, some investigators of the nineteenth century considered that the human embryo ascends a phylogenetic scale, passing through various lower animal forms in the process of embryonic maturation.[77] To them, arrest of development during an early stage of this ascent could result in a malformation resembling the features of an animal.

The phenomenon of arrest of embryonic development is misplaced as a cause of human malformation. Knowledge of the phenomenon helps in understanding why certain malformations take a particular form, but tells nothing about the cause except that it was operational at a given time in embryonic development.

Mechanical forces

Certain congenital defects invite the notion that mechanical forces may alter the anatomy of the developing fetus. Perhaps most obvious among these are amputations, dislocations, fractures, deformations of body parts, and constriction rings or bands. Early writers accepted this belief and passed it along for centuries to those observers who followed.[26,33,40,70,78–80] Although periodically criticized, the idea has resurged in some form in every generation to claim a place among the causes of human malformations.

Mechanical forces account for 3 of the 13 major causes of human malformations accepted by Paré in *Monsters and Marvels* (Fig. 1–8).[40] As the sixth cause he lists "the narrowness or smallness of the womb"; as the seventh "the indecent posture of the mother, as when, being pregnant, she has sat

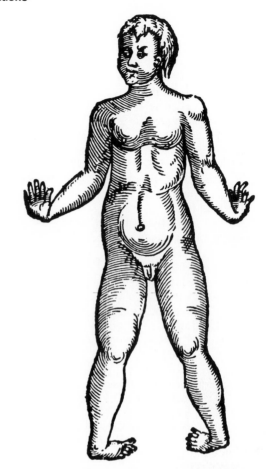

Fig. 1–8. In the sixteenth century Paré[40] depicted this child with deformations of the hands and feet, which he attributed to excessive intrauterine pressure.

too long with her legs crossed, or pressed against her womb"; and as the eighth "through a fall, or blow struck against the womb of the mother, being with child." Paré likened the uterus to a mold which if "rough or in some other way badly disposed—the medal or effigy that issued from it is defective, hideous, and deformed."

Hippocrates[78] covered a similar gamut of possibilities by which mechanical forces could influence the form of the unborn:

> As to the infant crippled in the womb, I say that it is crippled in consequence of a contusion, the mother having been struck on the place corresponding to the fetus, or having had a fall or having sustained some other form of violence. If the infant experienced a contusion, it becomes crippled in the part contused; if the contusion be greater, the membrane that surrounds it ruptures and the woman aborts. Or yet again, infants become crippled in the following way: when in the womb there is a narrowness at the part where in fact the crippling is produced, it is inevitable that the body moving in a narrow place shall be crippled in that part. It is thus that trees which in the earth have not enough space, and are hindered by a stone or other thing, become bent during growth, or rather become large in one part and small in another. The infant experiences the same thing when, in the womb, a portion is relatively too narrow for the corresponding part of the infant.

It is obvious from the foregoing that stresses on the fetus could be placed by external or internal mechanical forces. The most obvious and violent of the external forces was trauma to the pregnant abdomen. While falls and blows were widely accepted as a cause for malformation, one of the more interesting controversies regarding mechanical forces relates to the wearing of corsets.[53,80-82] Tightly laced corsets were popular in the nineteenth century, and some observers attributed malformations of the fetus to this practice. It seems that this cause was particularly incriminated when the corset was worn to conceal the pregnancy.

Internal forces were thought to have equal potency in producing malformations. Ballantyne[33] summarized the various internal structures and conditions in which malforming forces might be exercised against the fetus. He included abdominal and pelvic tumors, pelvic contraction, small or malformed uterus, uterine fibroids, bands of amnion, and the umbilical cord. He also recognized that twins could exert deforming pressure on a co-twin and that one part of a fetus could exert pressure on another part.

Certain defects attributed to mechanical forces in previous times would be viewed today as imaginative and without scientific foundation. That conjoined twins resulted from intrauterine pressure that caused fusion of two separate fetuses was widely held during the seventeenth and eighteenth centuries.[53,82,83] Aristotle[26] probably was expressing this concept as well when he described the fusion of chick embryos into conjoined forms.

In similar manner, certain physical forces that were accepted in prior centuries as the cause of malformations would not be found tenable today. Linkage of anencephaly to injury to a pregnant woman's head, or fetal scarring to an animal bite during pregnancy, or hand malformations to injury to the mother's hand, or spina bifida to a maternal back injury all represent such unlikely associations. In fact, these anecdotes of trauma distant from the mother's abdomen bring to mind the concept of maternal impressions rather than mechanical influences.

Diseases of the embryo

Processes of growth, maturation, and functional refinement consume the energies and resources of the fetus and infant. These are the same processes that can be impeded by a variety of pathologic insults (inflammation, infection, ischemia, metabolic disturbance, and so forth) during this epoch of the life cycle. In contrast, formation of structures is the primary activity of the embryo. Pathologic insults during the period of embryogenesis can impair this primary activity, causing malformations. Timing is the essence of the consideration that diseases affecting embryonic tissues may be causally related to malformations.

That a causal relationship existed between embryonic disease and malformations required an understanding that complex anatomic structures are formed from simple precursors.[84] Thus the concept received widespread attention only during the nineteenth century. Like other considerations, the roots of the concept can be found centuries earlier, but only after 1800 did it sprout into the mainstream of thought. A number of pathologic processes came to be suspected as the cause of malformations during this period.

Inflammatory processes of whatever cause were accepted as a basis for certain malformations.[85-87] Accordingly, it was held that peritonitis could result in umbilical, diaphragmatic, or inguinal hernias; pericarditis could cause cardiac malformations; and pleuritis could cause defects of the respiratory system. In the view of J. Y. Simpson,[87] a nineteenth century Scottish obstetrician, inflammatory diseases acted by arresting development at some incomplete state or by destroying structures more or less fully formed. An inflammatory process was also suspected as the basis for the formation of amniotic adhesions. In this regard, amniotic adhesions were likened to intraabdominal adhesions associated with peritonitis. Amniotic adhesions could attend inflammation of the amnion, cutaneous diseases, or both.[33]

Pathologic processes involving the central nervous system were often incriminated as a cause of malformation. Both major and minor malformations were attributed to convulsive states. Beclard[88] thought that virtually any type of malformation could be caused by diseases of the nervous system. He gave as possibilities the formation of cyclopia from destruction of the olfactory nerve, loss of facial structures from disease of the medulla oblongata, and diaphragmatic hernia from destruction of the vagus nerve.

Perhaps the most argued concept was the relationship between hydrocephaly and anencephaly.[89,90] Well before the nineteenth century, when embryonic disease became a widely accepted cause of malformations, Morgagni[90] had contended that rapidly increasing hydrocephaly in the embryo could rupture the cranium, resulting in anencephaly.

It is possible to see in this theory a maturation toward contemporary thought. While specific relationships between pathologic processes and malformations envisioned by nineteenth century observers might not be accepted, the general principle that the consequence of pathologic processes during embryonic life is malformation would be acknowledged.

Heredity

Although the physicochemical basis for heredity has been determined only during the past century, there can be little doubt that earlier physicians and philosophers accepted a view that normal morphology and malformations could be inherited from parents. That they lacked an understanding of how hereditary characteristics were transmitted is equally certain.

Two contrasting views prevailed. The oldest and most popular, *pangenesis,* held that anatomic characteristics of the parents flowed from all parts of the body to constitute the semen or menses.[27-29] Some form of this basic idea dates to before Hippocrates. It was strongly advocated in the mid-nineteenth century by Charles Darwin, who named the units of inheritance that derived from various parts of the body *gemmules.*[27] According to pangenesis, acquired characteristics could be transmitted to offspring and in so doing were converted into heritable traits. Related to this concept was the idea that offspring existed as fully formed miniatures within the sperm or egg.[29]

The alternative view of hereditary transmission, that of Aristotle, held that the material necessary for formation of a new being existed in the menstrual blood, but required activation by semen. After such activation, embryos differentiated from formless masses into the distinctive form of the parents.[25] Unusual features or malformations arose from failure of the semen to control formation of the embryo.

Paré[40] includes heredity among his 13 causes of malformations. He accepted as common knowledge the direct transmission of intellectual abilities, physical characteristics and mannerisms, and diseases like gout and leprosy but ac-

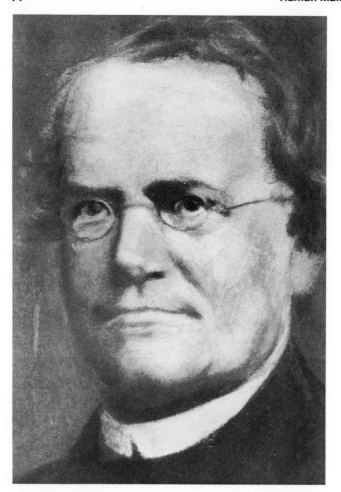

Fig. 1–9. Johann Gregor Mendel[91] (1822–1884), an Augustinian monk from Moravia, who set forth the principles of single gene inheritance in 1865.

knowledged that some traits of parents could be corrected by the "formative power" of reproduction.[40]

By the beginning of the twentieth century, heredity was widely accepted as a cause of some malformations, although the traits that could be inherited as well as the manner of transmission were not agreed upon. Ballantyne[33] accepted that "all hereditary tendencies are already in the ovum and spermatozoon before fertilization," but had a faulty view of how genetic characteristics became represented in the sex cells. He thought that some hereditary characteristics, those conveying the qualities of the parent, were naturally incorporated into the germ cells while other characteristics became impressed on the germ cells by the parent in whom they were found. He accepted the production of malformations as one of the seven influences of heredity on offspring.

Laws of unit inheritance were set forth by Johann Gregor Mendel,[91] an Augustinian monk from Moravia, in a little recognized publication in 1865 (Fig. 1–9). Mendel's studies on the hybridization of *Pisum* led him to conclude that various characteristics were inherited independently and that the integrity of an individual characteristic was maintained even though its expression might be masked by the presence of an alternative characteristic in the hybrid. Mendel's principles were rediscovered some 30 years later and were rapidly ap-plied to the inheritance of traits of all living beings, including humans.[92–94]

The linkages between *nuclein,* discovered in 1869 by Friedrich Miescher, chromosomes observed by Walther Flemming and others in the 1870s, and the transmission of heritable traits was made in the following century.[95,96] W. S. Sutton[97] noted the correlation between the presence of a certain chromosome and the presence of a specific characteristic in the grasshopper *Brachystola magna.* He further speculated that "it is conceivable that the chromosomes may be divisible into smaller entities . . . and may be dominant or recessive independently." That such smaller entities or factors were located in linear arrangement on the chromosomes and that they were indeed responsible for determining heritable characteristics was demonstrated between 1910 and 1920 by T. H. Morgan using *Drosophila melanogaster.* O. T. Avery et al.[100] provided the final linkage in 1944, identifying the molecule responsible for transmission of heritable traits as deoxyribonucleic acid. The biochemical mechanism by which genes are expressed, discovered by Beadle and Tatum,[101] a model for the structure of DNA, constructed by Watson and Crick[102] and elaboration of the genetic code by Nirenberg and Matthaei[103] were to follow in the ensuing two decades.

Brachydactyly (type AI) has the distinction of being the first malformation (1905) to be attributed to single gene inheritance, it being transmitted as an autosomal dominant trait (Fig. 1–10).[104] Down syndrome became the first malformation syndrome (1959) shown to be caused by a chromosome defect, trisomy 21.[105]

Environmental influences

Centuries of observations have substantially eroded the concept that the uterus provides total security for the embryo against adverse influences from the environment. Certain influences gain access to the embryo through indulgence by the mother. Other influences reach the fetus through no fault of the mother. Injury, radiation, infection, metabolic disturbances, and certain other chemical exposures are among these insults.

Few experiments using environmental insults during embryonic development had been conducted prior to the nineteenth century. It had been noted in the 1700s that chicken eggs, artificially incubated, frequently resulted in malformed chicks, this being attributed to alterations in the incubation temperature.[106] During the first half of the nineteenth century, Etienne Geoffroy Saint-Hilaire[107] and his son Isidore[81] carried out many experiments subjecting incubating eggs to coating with occlusive liquids, shaking, pricking, and positioning. They found that growth impairment and a variety of malformations could be produced with these insults. They further noted that embryos subjected to very early insults would fail to form entirely or would be dwarfed in size. Dareste[108] and numerous contemporaries[109,110] of the mid-1800s used electrical current, heat, magnetism, and a variety of chemicals to induce malformations in the embryos of chickens and other animals. A correlation was noted between the timing of the insult and the severity of the malformation, but a variety of insults could produce the same defect. Dareste[108] accepted arrest of embryonic development as the mechanism by which the malformations arose and thought that the find-

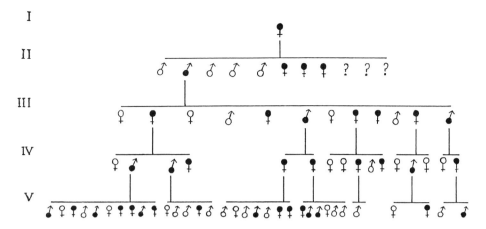

Fig. 1–10. Pedigree of family with brachydactyly inherited as an autosomal dominant trait published by Farabee[104] in 1905. This report represents the malformation attributed to single gene mutation.

ings noted in the experimental situation might apply to human development as well. Féré[110] could produce similar malformations following exposure of eggs to a variety of gases or following injection of a variety of noxious chemicals. Experiments of this nature were continued and expanded during the twentieth century by Warkany and a number of other investigators.[111–114]

Three observations in the twentieth century strengthened the view that environmental insults could penetrate whatever protective barriers exist during human pregnancy and cause, among other maladies, malformation of the developing embryo. Following the discovery of x-rays in 1895, radiation became widely used in medicine for diagnostic and treatment purposes. It became obvious during the 1920s that babies born after intrauterine radiation doses of 50–250 rads had an increased risk of birth defects, particularly growth impairments, microphthalmia, microcephaly, and other abnormalities of the central nervous system.[115] Gregg,[116] in 1941, provided the first evidence for production of congenital defects by an infectious organism. He noted the appearance of congenital cataract among infants born of mothers who had experienced rubella virus infection during the early months of pregnancy (Fig. 1–11). Independent observation of limb defects among infants born of mothers taking the sedative thalidomide during the early months of pregnancy were made in 1961 by Lenz[117] in Germany and McBride[118] in Australia (Fig. 1–12). The number of environmental influences identified that can adversely affect the developing infant has greatly expanded in the years since these observations and forms the logic for continuous scrutiny of all environmental agents for their potential to cause malformations and exists as a major focus in contemporary preventive obstetrics.[119,120]

Malformations and evolution

Entire races of malformed humans exist in the folklore and literature of many early civilizations. Hippocrates[121] described a nation of macrocephalics in which nobility was equated with the degree of elongation of the head. India was home to a race of Sciapods, who possessed a single lower limb terminating in a foot sufficiently large to provide shade against the heat of the day (Fig. 1–13).[29] Mer people, men and

women whose lower anatomy was that of a fish or other creature of the deep, occupied the central role in many a seafarer's tale (Fig. 1–14).[122,123] Among many names, they were called *sirens, tritons, nymphs, kelpies, nereids,* and *silkies.* In ancient Scythia, a tribe of cyclopic families was said to live along the Arimaspias River.[124]

To the contrary, archaeological findings lend no support to the view that groups of early humans or prehumans were affected with structural defects. The basic human form has remained the same over the several millions of years since humans took an evolutionary direction distinct from that of the great apes. Morphologic changes that have occurred over the millennia represent changes of scale. Lucy, the celebrated hominid who lived in eastern Africa 3.5 million years ago, stood 3.5 feet tall, weighed 60 pounds, and had a brain volume of 380–450 ml (Fig. 1–15).[37] Brain volume has since quadrupled, forcing alteration in the overall craniofacial appearance, and stature has increased nearly twofold. Jaw and

Fig. 1–11. Five-month-old infant with prenatal rubella infection. Infant has severe growth retardation and opisthotonus typical of severe central nervous system infection. At autopsy (7 months), infant had disseminated nervous system infection with necrosis and calcification. Courtesy of Dr. Murdina M. Desmond, Baylor College of Medicine, Houston.

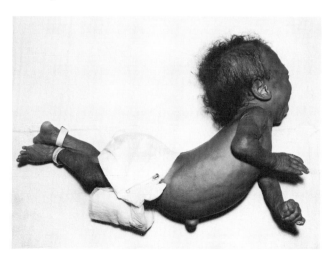

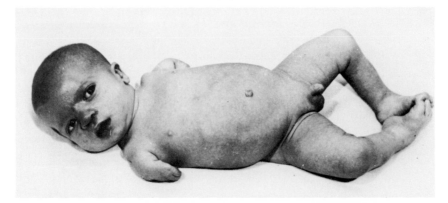

Fig. 1–12. Male infant with meromelia of upper limbs caused by prenatal exposure to thalidomide during the first trimester. About 4000 infants are known to have been affected during the 4 years thalidomide was marketed.

tooth structures have changed with diet, and the female pelvis has enlarged to permit birthing of offspring with larger heads. But the footprints cast in the volcanic ash of Olduvai gorge 4 million years ago show the same heel, arch, five toes, and forward directed hallux of modern humans. Maxillae of the earliest human show midline fusion. The skeleton of the limbs shows the same bony segmentation as that found today.[125,126]

Evolution occurs in subtle, generally imperceptible steps that add slight advantages to the species or eliminate slight disadvantage. Anatomy could be altered through the evolutionary process, resulting in a structure that by contemporary criteria would qualify as a malformation, but it would take thousands of generations, perhaps millions of years, to do so. Too narrow a band of time on the evolutionary scale can be viewed in any detail to discern major changes in the human anatomy. Malformations, as generally encountered, repre-

sent sudden and dramatic changes in anatomy. On the whole they must be considered deleterious and are selected against by natural and societal means. Heritable malformations of any magnitude are rarely transmitted for more than a few generations, and environmentally caused malformations are generally confined in a single generation. Hence malformations cannot be considered useful as evolutionary events.

Humans share with all creatures the same susceptibility to the selective forces of nature. In the human genome, evolution has produced what many view as the zenith of earthly biology. Humans do not number among the largest, the fastest, or the strongest of the earth's organisms. Numerous other creatures surpass humans on any of these scales. Nor do humans possess the most highly refined special senses. Nor have they become the most colorfully decorated of the creatures. Humans are set apart from the world's creatures by possessing the ability to reason.

It is inviting to question whether humans have optimally evolved for the existing climate, landscape, and atmosphere. Could an additional finger provide some advantage over the five-fingered hand? Could further changes in scale enhance human superiority? Would development of an additional sense or refinement of the present senses be an asset?

Humans will undoubtedly need to retain the capacity to change fundamentally to face exigencies that lie ahead. In the future, nature may exert selective forces different from those

Fig. 1–13. Drawing of a Sciapod representative of a race in India mentioned in the Hippocratic writings. Sciapods were characterized by a single lower limb terminating in a foot large enough to provide shade when held overhead.

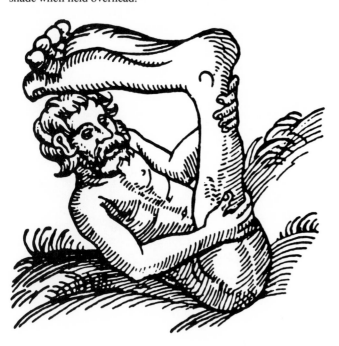

Fig. 1–14. A fifteenth century woodcut from the Nuremberg Bible showing Noah's Ark attended by a mermaid (left), a merman (right), and a merdog (lower).

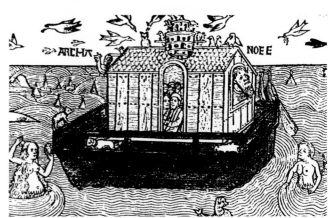

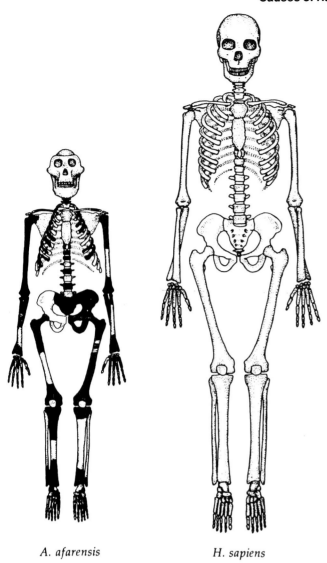

A. afarensis   *H. sapiens*

Fig. 1–15. Size comparison of Lucy, the early hominid found by Donald Johanson in the Afar region of Ethiopia, and modern human. Only portions of Lucy's skeleton (solid areas) were found, but allow estimates of size (3.5 feet in height and 60 pounds in weight).

operating at present. A crowded earth with limited foodstuffs may favor organisms of smaller size. An earth overheated by the greenhouse effect may favor those who can adapt with color change or altered thermoregulation. An environment flooded with messages to the special senses may give advantage to those protected by a dulling of the senses.

One might also wonder if eons of evolution would sufficiently refine the human genome so as to preclude the occurrence of malformations or whether such a prospect could be reasonably anticipated for future generations. Such expectations must be met with discouragement, for the same property of the human genome—mutability—that provides the grist on which evolution works is a biologic process that produces undesirable results as well, malformations being among these. Evolutionary change depends on a constant flow of mutations some of which may offer subtle advantage over existing human stock. At the same time, mutability of the human genome also allows for genetically caused mal-

formations. Hence, as long as the evolutionary process remains intact, malformations will be part of the human experience. The malformed may be eliminated in one manner or another, prenatally or postnatally, or even prevented by gamete selection or other preconceptional measures, but the system that produces genetically based malformations will be ever present.

Embryology and malformations

The human organism forms during the embryonic period. The task of putting together the human anatomy necessitates widespread collaboration among the primordial and derivative cells and a carefully orchestrated pace. This brief time, for the most part confined to the second through the eighth weeks after fertilization, has limited tolerance for errors of coordination or execution. Embryologic events follow a rigid schedule with repeated sequences of events, each dependent on the preceding and collateral events. There is little ability to backtrack, to correct, to regenerate, to compensate.

Over 500,000 conceptions are brought to the threshold of embryogenesis daily, having survived the vicissitudes of the week-long preimplantation period. In virtually all circumstances the astounding creation of the human form goes unnoticed, being largely completed by the time the mother recognizes that she has conceived. In few epochs of human life will accomplishments of such magnitude be confined to so brief a period. Perhaps only the transition from fetal to neonatal life offers equal intensity of biologic drama.

As fabrication of anatomic structures is the major activity of the embryo, malformation is the major pathology to occur during this period. Matters of growth and function, subordinate during embryogenesis, assume the major roles during fetal life.

Two principles form the basis for human, and indeed all mammalian, embryology. First, the instructions for embryologic construction derive from egg and sperm. Through these gametes, the conception gains at once representative heritable traits from each parent and instructions for producing the human form. Second, all structures regardless of their complexity must be constructed of simple cells. At the time of implantation, approximately 1 week postfertilization, the embryonic disc contains less than 100 cells.[127] From these, billions of cells must be produced, differentiated, and aggregated into tissue forms, organs of specific function, and the final human configuration.

Both principles have gained acceptance in the relatively recent past and more than anything else owe this acceptance to the discovery of the microscope. The two reproductive components, sperm and egg, were initially visualized, respectively, by van Leeuwenhoek[128] in 1670 and von Baer[129] in 1827. Spallazani[130] recognized in the early 1700s that male and female sex components were required for conception, but actual observation of fertilization of an egg by sperm awaited the investigations of Hertwig[131] in 1875. How the sex cells were formed and exactly what each brought to the conception process were not understood. Documentation that hereditary traits were determined by genes located on the chromosomes contained in sperm and egg was made by Morgan[98,99] and associates early in this century. The necessity for a reduction in the number of chromosomes distributed to the sex cells (meiosis) was first suggested by Weissman[132] in 1887.

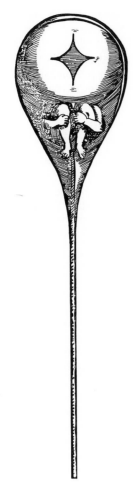

Fig. 1-16. Preformed individual (homunculus) depicted in the head of a sperm. Redrawn from Hartsoeker P: *Essay de Dioptrique,* Paris, 1964.

The doctrine of preformation of embryos dominated thought prior to the microscope and even for some years after that.[29] The doctrine essentially held that miniature humans, fully formed, were encased in the sperm or egg (Fig. 1-16). Pregnancy served to allow these preformed humans to grow in a safe place to the size necessary for extrauterine existence. Aristotle,[26] basing his views on observations of chick embryos, noted that complex structures formed from simpler beginnings and rejected the possibility of preformation. Harvey's observations[74] led him to the same conclusion in 1651 and allowed him to suspect that defects, specifically cleft lip, could be caused by failure of the simple structures to complete their development into final form. Wolff's microscopic observations[84] that complex structures arose from simple globules (the cell theory was yet a century away) provided the convincing evidence for epigenesis, i.e., the formation of large and complex fetal structures from smaller and simpler components.

References

1. Poland BJ, Miller JR, Harris M, et al.: Spontaneous abortion: A study of 1,961 women and their conceptuses. Acta Obstet Gynecol Scand Suppl 102:1981.

2. Boue J, Boue A, Lazar P: The epidemiology of human spontaneous abortions with chromosomal anomalies. In: Aging Gametes. RJ Blandau, ed. Karger, Basel, 1975, p 330.

3. Wilcox AJ, Weinberg CR, O'Connor JR, et al.: Incidence of early loss of pregnancy. N Engl J Med 319:189, 1988.

4. Roberts CJ, Lowe CR: Where have all the conceptions gone? Lancet 1:498, 1975.

5. Hertig AT, Rock J, Adams EC, et al.: Thirty four fertilized human ova, good, bad and indifferent, recovered from 210 women of known fertility. Pediatrics 23:202, 1959.

6. Shiota K, Uwabe C, Nishimura H: High prevalence of defective human embryos at the early postimplantation period. Teratology 35:309, 1987.

7. Miller JF, Williamson E, Glue J, et al.: Fetal loss after implantation. Lancet 2:554, 1980.

8. Whitaker PG, Taylor A, Lind T: Unsuspected pregnancy loss in healthy women. Lancet 1:1126, 1983.

9. Rushton DI: Examination of products of conception from previable human pregnancies. J Clin Pathol 34:819, 1981.

10. Simpson JL, Mills JL, Holmes LB, et al.: Low fetal loss rates after ultrasound-proved viability in early pregnancy. JAMA 258:2555, 1987.

11. Harlap S, Shiono PH, Ramcharan S: A life table of spontaneous abortions and the effects of age, parity, and other variables. In: Human Embryonic and Fetal Death. IH Porter, EB Hook, eds. Academic, New York, 1980, p 145.

12. Warburton D, Stein Z, Kline J, et al.: Chromosome abnormalities in spontaneous abortion: Data from the New York City study. In: Human Embryonic Fetal Death. IH Porter, EB Hook, eds. Academic, New York, 1980, p 261.

13. Shepard TH, Fantel AG, Fitzsimmons J: Congenital defect rates among spontaneous abortuses: Twenty years of monitoring. Teratology 39:325, 1989.

14. Hassold T, Chen N, Funkhouser J, et al.: A cytogenetic study of 1000 spontaneous abortions. Ann Hum Genet 44:151, 1980.

15. Kajii T, Ferrier A, Niikawa N, et al.: Anatomic and chromosomal anomalies in 639 spontaneous abortuses. Hum Genet 55:87, 1980.

16. Pitkin RM: Fetal death: Diagnosis and management. Am J Obstet Gynecol 157:583, 1987.

17. Angell RR, Sandison A, Brain AD: Chromosome variation in perinatal mortality: A survey of 500 cases. J Med Genet 21:39, 1984.

18. Marden PM, Smith DW, McDonald MJ: Congenital anomalies in the newborn infant, including minor variations. J Pediatr 64:357, 1964.

19. Chávez GF, Cordero JF, Becerra JE: Leading major congenital malformations among minority groups in the United States, 1981-1986. CDC Surveil Sum 37:17, 1988.

20. Van Regemorter N, Dodion J, Druart C: Congenital malformations in 10,000 consecutive births in a university hospital: Need for genetic counseling and prenatal diagnosis. J Pediatr 104:386, 1984.

21. Källén B: Population surveillance of multimalformed infants—Experience with the Swedish registry of congenital malformations. J Hum Genet 35:205, 1987.

22. Chung CS, Myrianthopoulos NC: Congenital anomalies: Mortality and morbidity, burden and classification. Am J Med Genet 27:505, 1987.

23. Leppig KA, Werler MM, Cann CI, et al.: Predictive value of minor anomalies. I. Association with major malformations. J Pediatr 110:531, 1987.

24. Méhes K, Stalder G: Minor Malformations in the Neonate, Akadémiae Kiadó, Budapest, 1983.

25. Spiegelman M, Erhardt CL: Mortality and longevity in the United States. In: Mortality and Morbidity in the United States. CL Erhardt, JE Berlin, eds. Harvard University Press, Cambridge, 1974, p 1.

26. Aristotle: On the Generation of Animals, book II, sect III. In: The Works of Aristotle, vol II. WD Ross, ed. Encyclopaedia Britannica, Chicago, 1952, p 179.

27. Needham J. Chemical Embryology, Cambridge University Press, Cambridge, 1931.

28. Darwin C: The Variation of Plants and Animals under Domestication, vol 2, ed 2. Appleton, New York, 1892, p 370.

29. Hartsoeker P: Essay de Dioptrique, sect 88. CJ Anisson, Paris, 1694.

30. Gautier d'Agoty: Zoogénésie ou generation de l'homme et des animaux. Paris, 1750.

31. Ballantyne JW: The teratological records of Chaldea. Teratologia 1:127, 1894.

32. Mellaart J: Deities and shrines of neolithic Anatolia. Archaeology 16:29, 1963.

33. Ballantyne JW: Manual of Antenatal Pathology and Hygiene. The Embryo, vol 2. William Green and Sons, Edinburgh, 1904.

34. Brodsky I: Congenital abnormalities, teratology and embryology: Some evidence of primitive man's knowledge as expressed in art and lore in Oceania. Med J Austr 1:417, 1943.

35. Barnett RD: Six fingers in art and archaeology. Bull Anglo-Isr Archeol Soc 6:5, 1986–7.

36. Kunze J, Nippert I: Genetics and Malformations in Art. Grosse Verlag, Berlin, 1986.

37. Johanson DC, Edey MA: Lucy, the Beginnings of Humankind. Simon and Schuster, New York, 1981.

38. Montaigne ME: Essays. Translated by C Cotton. Encyclopaedia Britannica, Chicago, 1952, p 343.

39. Pliny C: Natural History, vol II, book VII. Translated by H Rackham. Harvard University Press, Cambridge, 1963, p 527.

40. Paré A: On Monsters and Marvels. Translated by JL Pallister. University Chicago Press, Chicago, 1982.

41. Schatz F: Die Griechischen Gotter und die Menschlichen Missgeburten. Bergmann, Wiesbaden, 1901.

42. Lenormant F: La Divination et la science des présages chêz les Chaldéens. Maisonneuve, Paris, 1875, p 103.

43. Leichty E: The Omen Series, Summa Izbu. JJ Augustin Publishers, Locust Valley, NY, 1970.

44. Pliny C: Natural History, vol 2. Translated by P Holland. A Islip, London, 1601, p 397.

45. Surti U, Szulman AE, O'Brien S: Dispermic origin and clinical outcome of three complete hydatidiform moles with 46,XY karyotype. Am J Obstet Gynecol 144:84, 1982.

46. Lucretius: On the Nature of Things, book IV. Translated by HAJ Munro. Encyclopaedia Britannica, Chicago, 1952.

47. Empedocles: The Fragments of Empedocles. Translated by WE Leonard. Open Court, Chicago, 1908.

48. Marcus Aurelius: Meditations, book X. Translated by G Long. Encyclopaedia Britannica, Chicago, 1952, p 299.

49. Diels H: Die Fragmente der Vorsokrakiter, ed 3. Weidmann, Berlin, 1912, p 140.

50. Esdras II: Chapt 5, verse 8. In: The Oxford Annotated Apocrypha. BM Metzger, ed. Oxford University Press, New York, 1965.

51. Galen: On the Usefulness of the Parts of the Body, book 14, chapt 7. Translated by MT May. Cornell University Press, Ithaca, 1968.

52. Avicenna: A Treatise on the Canon of Medicine. Translated by DC Gruner. AM Kelley Publishers, New York, 1970.

53. Licetus: De Monstris, book II, C 68–72. P Frambotti, Patavii, 1668.

54. Albertus Magnus: De animalibus, book XVIII, C6. J and G de Gregoriis, Venetiis, 1495.

55. Hoadley CJ: Records of the Colony and Plantation of New Haven from 1638 to 1649. Case, Tiffany, Hartford, 1857.

56. Plato: Laws, book VII, p 792e. Translated by AE Taylor. In: The Collected Dialogues of Plato. E Hamilton, H Cairns, eds. Princeton University Press, Princeton, 1961.

57. Plutarch: Lives of the Noble Grecians and Romans: Lycurgus. Translated by J Dryden. Encyclopaedia Britannica, Chicago, 1952.

58. Ploss HH, Bartels M, Bartels P: In: Woman: An Historical, Gynaecological and Anthropological Compendium. EJ Dingwall, ed. W Heinemann, London, 1935, p 461.

59. Heliodorus: An Ethiopian Romance. Translated by M Hadas. Greenwood Press, Westport, CT, 1976, p 94.

60. Quintilian MF: Institutiones Oratoricae. Translated by HE Butler. Harvard University Press, Cambridge, 1958.

61. Montaigne ME: Essays, book I, chapt 20. Translated by C Cotton. Encyclopaedia Britannica, Chicago, 1952.

62. Wallace I, Wallace A: The Two. Simon and Schuster, New York, 1978, p 97.

63. Malebranche N: Treatise Concerning the Search after Truth, book 2, chapt 7. Translated by T Taylor. Oxford, 1694.

64. Taruffi C: Storia della Teratologia, vol 1. Regia, Bologna, 1881, p 242.

65. Howell M, Ford P: The True History of the Elephant Man, chapt 4. Penguin, New York, 1980.

66. Munster S: Cosmographie universelle, book iii. CP L'Huillier, Paris, 1575.

67. Kerkring T: Spicilegium Anatomicum, obs xxiii, SA Frisii, Amsterdam, 1670, p 56.

68. Fienus T: De viribus imaginationis tractatus, questions xiii to xxiii. G Rivii, Louvain, 1608.

69. Bartholin T: Anatomicarum et Medicarum Rariorum, cent V, hist 61. P Havboldi, Hafniae, 1661, p 296.

70. Licetus F: De la nature, des Causes, des Differences des Monstres. Translated by H Houssay. Paris, 1937, p 61.

71. Turner D: A Treatise on Diseases Incident to the Skin, ed 5, part I, chapt XII. London, 1712.

72. Cardanus J: Opera Omnia, book i, chapt 9. Huguetan and Ravaud, Lugduni, 1663.

73. Krause KC: Quaenam sit causa proxima mutans corpus fetus, non matris gravidae, hujus mente a causa quadam violentiore commota. St. Petersburg, 1756.

74. Harvey W: On Animal Generation, exercise 69. Translated by R Willis. Encyclopaedia Britannica, Chicago, 1952, p 482.

75. von Autenrieth JHT: Observationum ad historiam embryonis facientium, Schrammianis, Tubingae, 1797, p 38.

76. Stockard CR: Developmental rate and structural expression: An experimental study of twins, "double monsters" and single deformities, and the interaction among embryonic organs during their origin and development. Am J Anat 28:115, 1921.

77. Meckel JF: Handbuch der pathologischen Anatomie. CH Reclam, Leipzig, 1812, p 48.

78. Hippocrates: De la Generation. In Oeuvres Completes D'Hippocrate, vol 7. Translated by E Littre. AM Hakkert, Amsterdam, 1979, p 485.

79. Ormrod F: Influence of maternal impressions on the foetus. Lancet 1:393, 1875.

80. Geoffroy Saint-Hilaire E: Mem Soc Med d'emulation de Paris, IX, 1826, p 65.

81. Geoffroy Saint-Hilaire I: Histoire de Anomalies vol 3. J-B Bailliere, Paris, 1836, p 534.

82. Scharfius B: Miscellanea curiosa sive ephemeridum medicophysicarum germanicarum Academie naturae curiosorum, Dec ii, Ann ii, obs cii. Norimb, E Streck, 1684, p 254.

83. Lemery: Histoire de l'Academie Royale des Sciences. Paris, 1724, 1726, p 44; 1740, pp 260, 305; 1742, pp 109, 210, 324, 433, 517, 607.

84. Wolff CF: Über die Bildung des Darm Kanals im befruchteten Hühnchen. Translated by JF Meckel. R Buchhandlung, Halle, 1812.

85. Simpson JY: Obstetric Memoirs and Contributions, vol 2. JP Lippincott, Philadelphia, 1856, p 176.

86. Ahlfeld F: Die missbildungen des Menschen. FW Grunow, Leipzig, 1882, p 284.

87. Simpson JY: Contributions to intra-uterine pathology. Edinb Med Surg J 52:17, 1839.

88. Beclard PA: Elements of General Anatomy. Translated by J Togno. Carey & Lea, Philadelphia, 1830, p 105.

89. Cleland J: Contribution to the study of spina bifida, encephalocele, and anencephalus. J Anat Physiol 17:257, 1883.

90. Morgagni GB: de sedibus et causis morborum, vol 1. Translated by B Alexander. Remondiniana, Venetiis, 1761, p 251.

91. Mendel G: Experiments in Plant Hybridisation. Translated by The Royal Horticultural Society of London. Harvard University Press, Cambridge, 1965.

92. Corcos AF, Monaghan FV: Role of DeVries in the recovery of Mendel's work. J Hered 76:187, 1985; 78:275, 1987.

93. Corcos AF, Monaghan FV: Tschermak, a non-discoverer of Mendelism. J Hered 77:468, 1986; 78:208, 1987.

94. Corcos AF, Monaghan FV: Correns, an independent discoverer of Mendelism? J Hered 78:330, 1987; 78:404, 1987.

95. Miescher F: Ueber die chemische Zusammensetzung der Eiterzellen. Hoppe-Seylers Med-Chem Untersuch 4:441, 1871.

96. Flemming W: Beitrage zur Kenntniss der Zelle und ihrer Lebenserscheinungen. Arch Mikrosk Anat Entwickl 20:1, 1882.

97. Sutton WS: On the morphology of the chromosome group in *Brachystola magna*. Biol Bull 4:24, 1902.

98. Morgan TH: Random segregation versus coupling in Mendelian inheritance. Science 34:384, 1911.

99. Morgan TH: On the mechanism of heredity. Proc R Soc Biol 94:162, 1922.

100. Avery OT, MacLeod CM, McCarty M: Studies on the chemical nature of the substance inducing transformation of pneumococcal types. I. Induction of transformation by a desoxyribonucleic acid

fraction isolated from pneumococcus type III. J Exp Med 79:137, 1944.

101. Beadle GW, Tatum EL: Genetic control of biochemical reactions in *Neurospora*. Proc Natl Acad Sci USA 27:499, 1941.
102. Watson JD, Crick FHC: A structure of deoxyribose nucleic acid. Nature 171:737, 1953.
103. Nirenberg MW, Matthaei HJ: The dependence of cell-free protein synthesis in *E coli* upon naturally occurring or synthetic polyribonucleotides. Proc Natl Acad Sci USA 47:1589, 1961.
104. Farabee WC: Inheritance of digital malformations in man. In: Papers of the Peabody Museum of American Archaeology and Ethnology, vol 3. Harvard University Press, Cambridge, 1905, p 69.
105. Lejeune J: Le mongolisme. Premier example d'aberration autosomique humaine. Ann Gen Semaine Hop 1:41, 1959.
106. Birch T: History of the Royal Society of London, vol 3. A Millar, London, 1757, p 455.
107. Geoffroy Saint-Hilaire E: Sur les déviations organiques provoquées et observées dans un établissement d'incubation artificielle. Mem Mus Hist Nat 13:289, 1825.
108. Dareste C: Recherches sur La Production Artificielle de Monstruosites, ed 2. C Reinwald, Paris, 1891.
109. Windle BCA: On the effects of electricity and magnetism on development. J Anat Physiol 29:346, 1895.
110. Féré C: Tératogénie experimentale et Pathologie générale. In Cinquantenaire de la Société de Biologie, Vol Jubilaire. Masson, Paris, 1899, p 360.
111. Warkany J, Nelson RC: Appearance of skeletal abnormalities in offspring of rats reared on deficient diet. Science 92:383, 1940.
112. Warkany J: Congenital malformation induced by maternal nutritional deficiency. J Pediatr 25:476, 1944.
113. Gillman J, Gilbert C, Gillman T: Preliminary report on hydrocephaly, spina bifida and other congenital anomalies in rat produced by trypan blue. S Afr J Med Sci 13:47, 1948.
114. Fraser FC, Fainstat TD: The production of congenital defects in the offspring of pregnant mice treated with cortisone. Progress report. Pediatrics 8:527, 1951.
115. Goldstein L, Murphy DP: Etiology of ill-health in children born after maternal pelvic irradiation. II. Defective children born after postconception pelvic irradiation. Am J Roentgenol 22:322, 1929.
116. Gregg NM: Congenital cataract following German measles in the mother. Trans Ophthalmol Soc Aust 3:35, 1941.
117. Lenz W: Thalidomide and congenital abnormalities. Lancet 1:45, 1962.
118. McBride WG: Thalidomide and congenital abnormalities. Lancet 2:1358, 1961.
119. Stevenson RE: The Fetus and the Newly Born Infant, ed 2. CV Mosby Co, St. Louis, 1977.
120. Shepard TH: Catalog of Teratogenic Agents, ed 6. Johns Hopkins University Press, Baltimore, 1989.
121. Hippocrates: On air, waters, and places. In Hippocratic Writings. Translated by F Adams. Encyclopaedia Britannica, Chicago, reprint, 1952, p 15.
122. Kampmeier OF: On sireniform monsters, with a consideration of the causation and the predominance of the male sex among them. Anat Rec 34:365, 1927.
123. Fleming CB: Maidens of the sea can be alluring, but sailor, beware. Smithsonian 14:86, 1983.
124. Born W: Monsters in art. Ciba Symp 9:684, 1947.
125. Clark WELG: The Fossil Evidence for Human Evolution, University of Chicago Press, Chicago, 1972.
126. Isaac GL, McCown ER: Human Origins: Louis Leakey and the East African Evidence. WA Benjamin, Menlo Park, CA, 1976.
127. Hardy K, Handyside AH, Winston RML: The human blastocyst: Cell number, death and allocation during late preimplantation development in vitro. Development 107:597, 1989.
128. van Leeuwenhoek A, Hammen S: Observationes de natis e semine genetal: Animalculis. Philos Trans R Soc (No. 142) 12:1040, 1677.
129. von Baer KE: De ovi mammalium et hominis genesi. L Voss, Leipzig, 1827.
130. Spallanzani L: Prodomo di un'opera da imprimersi sopra le riproduzioni animali. G Montanari, Modena, 1768.
131. Hertwig O: Beitrage zur Kenntnis der Bildung, Befruchtung und Theilung der thierischen Eis. Morphol Jahrb 1:347, 1876.
132. Weissman A: On the significance of the polar globules. Nature 36:607, 1887.

2

Terminology

ROGER E. STEVENSON and JUDITH G. HALL

Meaningful terminology is fundamental to communication and to most educational processes. The plethora of terms used to describe human morphologic alterations sometimes promotes but often frustrates these processes. Understandably, students may be confounded by the admixture of terms commonly used. Some provide true descriptions of the alteration *(macrocephaly)*; some bear ethnic, rank, or national connotations *(Roman nose)*; some are colored with mythological imagery *(sirenomelia, cyclopia)*; some imply a specific pathogenesis *(oligohydramnios sequence)*; some imply a specific etiology *(warfarin embryopathy)*; and some give tribute to a discoverer *(Meckel diverticulum)*. The same term can be used in a very restricted sense by one group while having a more generic meaning for the total scientific community. Terms most removed from description of the anatomic alteration are most variable and carry the greatest prospect for continued change in the future.

A universally acceptable and permanent terminology for anomalies would appear utopian. No previous system has met with full acceptance. One problem is that the needs of different groups dealing with congenital anomalies are not the same. Anthropologists, anatomists, radiologists, and pathologists focus on the description of the change; therapists, on the functional implications; embryologists and teratologists, on the mechanisms; and clinicians, on the diagnosis, cause, treatment, and prevention. In each of these areas, a jargon has arisen to serve the perceived requirements of the group. Sometimes the terms used by one group coincide with those used by colleagues with other emphases. In other situations, the terms used by one group meet indifference or rejection by others. The language of human congenital anomalies is the property of all. Exclusive claim cannot be placed on any terms, and no group can prohibit use beyond a specified definition.

Nomenclature

Anatomically based nomenclature for structural anomalies emphasizes topography and morphology. The purposes are to identify the anatomic part involved and to describe the alteration of that part. In this system, the development of new terms to describe human malformations would appear unnecessary. Human anatomy does not change, and time-honored terms for each structure are available.[1] Morphologic alterations of individual structures can also be defined with simple, biologically correct terms. Should new descriptive terms become desirable, they can be introduced without necessitating revision of the entire system. Because anatomic terms are the least likely to change, they are used in the present volumes.

Anatomic alterations include size, shape, consistency, density, continuity, patency, color, and position changes. Some are readily determined by gross inspection. Others fall into a continuum nearer the normal than the extreme. Indeed, some can be separated from the normal only by arbitrary convention. For those structural changes that fall along a continuum, one expects 5% to fall beyond 2 SD of the mean for the population: 2.5% below 2 SD of the population norm, and 2.5% above 2 SD of the norm. It is of interest that this definition of normality results in an incidence of abnormal members among the continuous traits similar to the incidence of major congenital anomalies in the population (Table 2–1). Some continuous traits, e.g., color, density, and consistency, have no standardized measurements from which their norms and standard deviations can be determined. In the clinical setting, determination of these features as abnormal is almost invariably subjective.

In an anatomically based nomenclature, no consideration is given to causation and pathogenesis, although in certain instances they may be coincidentally accommodated. *Macrocephaly* is used generically to describe large head of unknown cause and also to describe large head with large brain. *Hydrocephaly* is used to describe a large head due to ventricular enlargement. *Hydrocephaly,* however, does not necessarily imply head enlargement, since hydrocephaly can coexist with normal or even small head sizes. This type of duplicity and nuance is to be expected in any system of naming and can be tolerated by most users. *Macrohydrocephaly* or *hydromacrocephaly* to identify large head due to enlarged ventricles becomes too cumbersome.

The terminology for anomalies based on morphologic alterations is derived from the Greek language, as introduced by Malacarne in 1798,[2] but an increasing drift toward the use of Anglicized terms is evident. With English now being considered the universal scientific language, this trend will likely continue. A mix of English, Latin, and Greek terms will be found in the present volumes, with the choice of the term being based on familiarity and ease of flow.

Etiology and pathogenesis

Etiology simply means cause. For all human anomalies, the etiologic possibilities are limited to genetic (single gene, multiple genes, chromosomal) or to environmental (mechanical, infectious, chemical) causes, or to some combination of the two. Little regard for etiology is given when naming individual structural anomalies, but etiology can be found, however, in the names of many syndromes (trisomy 13 syndrome, prenatal alcohol syndrome, X-linked hydrocephaly syndrome).

Pathogenesis indicates the mechanism or process by

Table 2–1. Incidence of major and minor anomalies at birth

	Leppig et al.[11]	Marden et al.[10]	Mehes[8]	Myrianthopoulos and Chung[9]
Major malformations (%)	3.8	2.1	2.2	7.1
Minor malformations (%)	40.7	14.7	17.2	7.26
Sample size	4305	4412	4589	53,257

which a feature is produced. Again, little indication of pathogenesis is incorporated into the names of individual structural anomalies, but considerable emphasis is given in the naming of entities with multiple features (early amnion rupture, oligohydramnios sequence).

Histologic modifiers

Histologic analyses permit the description of the cellular and tissue processes underlying certain morphologic alterations. When known, these processes can be used as descriptive modifiers or to imply pathogenesis.[3]

Aplasia, hypoplasia, hyperplasia, dysplasia

Aplasia indicates absence of cellular proliferation, hence the absence of tissue mass and, consequently, of an organ or morphologic feature. *Hypoplasia* indicates insufficient cell proliferation, resulting in a deficiency of tissue mass and ultimately undergrowth of an organ or morphologic feature. Similarly, *hyperplasia* means excessive proliferation of cells, accumulation of excessive tissue mass due to the increased cell number, and overgrowth of an organ or morphologic feature. *Dysplasia* as used in clinical genetics implies disorganization of cell structure, disordered cell arrangement in tissues, and faulty tissue organization in an organ or morphologic feature.

At the tertiary (organ) level, these terms are best used only when the underlying histology is known. "Hyperplasia of [an anatomic part]" has greatest meaning when it implies that the excessive mass is due to an excessive number of otherwise normal cells. Regrettably, *hyperplasia* is often used as a mere description of overgrowth without regard to or knowledge of the histology. Worse yet, it is sometimes used to identify the larger of two parts of apparent unequal size without knowledge of the histology of either.

At some point in their natural history, many cells become aplastic; i.e., they cease to proliferate. Such cells (and tissues) can respond to injury, numerical depletion, hormone stimulation, and increased workload only by increasing their size. Muscle hypertrophy is a well-known example. Other cells retain the ability to divide actively. Endothelium, epithelium, mucosa, cartilage, bone, and connective tissues contain cells that are being constantly replenished by mitosis.

The ability to repair damage can be an important cellular response during embryogenesis.[4] Neither the point in development at which paralysis of the various human cell types occurs nor the signals that deprive cells of their ability to divide are known. Presumably most cells retain the ability to divide throughout embryogenesis and for variable periods of time thereafter. Hence embryos have the ability to repair and

recover from certain insults as long as the entire anlage is not damaged and as long as there are adequate time and resources to complete the repair before further differentiation is required.

Dysplastic cells have altered sizes, shapes, and cytostructures. To the pathologist, these abnormal cells are regressive, often induced by chronic inflammation or irritation, and may progress in a neoplastic direction. No such connotations accompany the term *dysplastic* when used to describe the cellular, tissue, and organ disorganization found in congenital structural anomalies. These forms of dysplastic change arise during development, are usually genetically determined, and do not progress to neoplasia. The inborn errors of the chondroosseous skeleton constitute a large group of disorders called *dysplasias*.[5] Multiple bones are involved, showing microscopic and radiographic evidence of disturbed growth and structure. Chondrocytes, osteocytes, connective tissue, or noncellular matrix can be abnormal, and the transition from cartilage to bone is often disorganized.[6] Clinically these skeletal dysplasias are manifested by short stature; abnormal alignment, growth, or symmetry of body segments; or, less commonly, specific malformations (cleft palate, polydactyly, and so forth).

Agenesis has been used to indicate the failure of an organ to form, and in general it implies aplasia rather than loss through atrophy or disruption. *Dysgenesis* can be used in a similar fashion to indicate anomalous structure due to disorganization of the component cells and tissues.

Atrophy, hypotrophy, hypertrophy, dystrophy

Atrophy means the degeneration of cells, usually resulting in shrinkage of tissue mass and diminished size of the affected organ or morphologic feature. Like the -*plasia* terms, atrophy and other -*trophy* terms are applied at the cellular (primary), tissue (secondary), and organ (tertiary) levels. Atrophy can be characterized by smaller than normal cell size, accumulation of intracellular pigment granules, and replacement of parenchymal cells by fat or connective tissue.

Hypotrophy indicates that cells fail to achieve a normal size, and hence tissues, organs, and morphologic features are undergrown. *Hypertrophy* is the enlargement of cells and consequent enlargement of tissue mass, organ, or morphologic feature. *Dystrophy* means a disturbance in cell or tissue growth caused by faulty nutrition. The term has been used most widely, however, for certain heritable conditions of muscle, eye, or nails (e.g., myotonic dystrophy, lattice dystrophy of the cornea, nail dystrophy). In these conditions *dystrophy* is used without implying that defective nutrition is the underlying pathogenesis.

Again, at the tertiary (organ or gross morphology) level, it may not be possible to distinguish enlargement due to hypertrophy from enlargement due to hyperplasia or to distinguish small size due to hypotrophy from small size due to atrophy, hypoplasia, or dystrophy. These distinctions require a knowledge of the histologic structure. Accumulation of intracellular or extracellular fluid may alter size without affecting any of the cellular processes. In the absence of histologic information, general terms can be used to describe alterations in tissue bulk, e.g., *enlarged muscle* to incorporate both muscle hyperplasia and hypertrophy or *small muscle* to encompass the possibilities of atrophy, hypotrophy, hypoplasia, dystrophy, and dysplasia.

For practical reasons, the structural anomalies included in this discussion are those that can be detected by clinical observation and gross measurement. It is acknowledged that there exist domains of microscopic and submicroscopic structural anomalies that are no less important than those mentioned. Histologic appearance is discussed only when those findings appear fundamental to understanding the gross structural alteration.

Types of anomalies

Malformation, disruption, deformation

Distinction between pathogenetically different types of structural anomalies is indicated by the terms *malformation, disruption,* and *deformation.*[7] Anomalies can be placed into one of these categories on the basis of the developmental stage during which the alteration took place, the process that caused the change, or the end result. Malformations arise during the initial formation of a structure. The structure can have a faulty configuration, can be incompletely formed, or can fail to form altogether. Malformations are caused by genetic or environmental influences or by a combination of the two. They result from abnormal processes during the formation of the structures (i.e., during organogenesis). For most structures, organogenesis is complete by 8 weeks postfertilization. However, teeth, brain, and genitalia are notable among the many structures whose formation extends beyond 8 weeks.

Disruptions result from destructive processes that alter structures after formation. A wide range of morphologic changes can occur secondary to disruptions, including alterations of shape and configuration, division of parts not usually divided, fusion of parts not usually fused, and loss of parts previously present. The causes of disruptions are usually environmental, but genetic causes (e.g., genetically programmed loss of blood supply) are also possible. Mechanical forces can cause compression, hemorrhage, thrombosis, emboli, and other vascular impairments that damage formed structures.

The term *deformation* indicates molding of a part through mechanical forces, usually acting over a prolonged period of time. Deformations result from loss of symmetry, altered alignment, abnormal positioning, and distorted configuration; they occur after organogenesis, often involve musculoskeletal tissues, and require no obligatory underlying tissue defect. Abnormal tissues may, however, be more susceptible to deformation. Deformations are usually reversible postnatally, depending on how long-standing they are and on how much growth has occurred subsequent to the initial compressive effects. They are usually due to external forces but can result from edema, which can exert intrinsic compressive forces.

The criteria for designating a malformation or disruption given above have been modified from those set forth by Spranger et al., who represent the International Working Group on Nomenclature of Errors of Morphogenesis.[7] According to their definitions, malformations are all genetic in etiology, disruptions occur during or after organogenesis, and deformations are caused only by extrinsic forces. The restriction of *malformation* to structural defects of genetic origin would appear unwarranted and contrary to historical usage. For instance, it seems entirely appropriate to consider the limb anomalies caused by thalidomide to be malformations since they occur during the period of morphogenesis.

While this tripartite schema was thoughtfully devised and allows for meaningful communication among many who work with human congenital anomalies, universal usage should not be anticipated. The term *malformation* will be used in a generic sense by many to indicate any structural alteration that occurs during the prenatal period. In defense of this general usage, it should be remembered that scientists and the general public alike understand the general nature of the problem when the term is used. Likewise, the term *deformity* is used by orthopedists to indicate any anomaly of the skeleton. The value to geneticists of using *malformation, disruption,* and *deformation* according to the foregoing definitions is that it allows certain generalizations to be made about the causation, pathogenesis, prognosis, and recurrence of different types of anomalies.

Major and minor anomalies

Major structural anomalies have medical and social consequences. The incidences of major defects appear highest among abortions, intermediate in stillborn infants, and lowest among liveborn infants. The incidence of major anomalies recognized at birth among liveborn infants is 2%–3% in most series (Table 2–1).[8-15] An equal number of additional major anomalies will be recognized by age 5 yr (e.g., cardiac defects, absent kidney).

No individual major anomaly has a high enough incidence in the population for it to be considered a structural polymorphism; i.e., none has an incidence of >1%. The monopodic, cyclopic, and other malformed races that exist in some noncritical accounts of ancient writers must be viewed with skepticism (see Chapter 1).

Minor anomalies are relatively frequent structural alterations that pose no significant health or social burdens (Tables 2–1 to 2–3).[8-11] They are nonetheless important because their presence prompts a search for coexistent, more important structural anomalies. The presence of two or more minor anomalies is an indication that a major defect may be present as well.[8,10-11] Minor anomalies often provide critical clues that permit the diagnosis of a specific syndrome or a specific disorder having multiple anomalies. They can also provide a clue to the timing of an insult during prenatal development.

Approximately 15% of newborn infants have one or more minor structural anomalies. A higher incidence may be found among premature infants, and babies with intrauterine growth retardation have an even higher rate. The risk of having a major birth defect increases with the number of minor defects present (Table 2–3). Infants free of minor defects have a low incidence (approximately 1%) of major malformations. Infants with one minor defect have a 3% risk of major defects. Those with two minor defects have a 10% risk of a major malformation, and those with three or more minor defects have a 20% risk of a major defect.[8,10-11]

No clear distinction exists between normal variation and minor anomalies or between minor anomalies and major anomalies. The determinations are often arbitrary. Holmes[16] separates minor anomalies from normal variants by considering as normal those features that occur in 4% or more of the population. This is a fourfold greater incidence than the

Table 2–2. Minor anomalies

Cranium and scalp	Sinuses	Skin
Triple hair whorl	Branchial	Shoulder dimples
Absence of hair whorl	Preauricular	Sacrum dimples
Patent metopic suture	Ear lobe	Dimples over other bones
Metopic fontanel	Helical	Sole crease
Sagittal fontanel	Pilonidal	Horizontal palmar crease (single)
Parietal foramen	*Face and neck*	Bridged palmar crease
Flat occiput	Synophrys	Single crease, finger V
Prominent occiput	Flat bridge of nose	Skin tags (preauricular, ear lobe, others)
Frontal bossing	Prominent bridge of nose	Hemangioma
Flat brow	Hypotelorism	Nevi
Ears	Hypertelorism	Pigmented spots
Microtia	Nostrils anteverted	Hypopigmented spots
Darwinian point	Long nasal septum	*Trunk*
Darwinian tubercle	Epicanthal fold	Extra nipples
Lack of helical folding	Iris freckles	Single umbilical artery
Bridged concha	Upward palpebral slant	Umbilical hernia
Ear lobe crease	Downward palpebral slant	Diastasis rectus
Ear lobe notched	Short palpebral fissures	Glandular hypospadias
Ear lobe bifid	Cleft uvula	Shawl scrotum
Lop ear	Cleft lip microform	Vaginal tag
Cup-shaped ear	Cleft gum	*Limbs*
Retroverted ear	Long philtrum	Cubitus valgus
Thickened helix	Short philtrum	Tapered fingers
Helix excessively folded	Smooth philtrum	Overlapping fingers
Helix attached to scalp	Microstomia	Broad thumb, great toe
	Macrostomia	Clinodactyly
	Macroglossia	Nails hypoplastic
	Microglossia	Nails hyperconvex
	Broad alveolar ridge	Increased space, toes
	Micrognathia	Syndactyly, toes 2–3
	Webbed neck	Overlapping digits
	Redundant neck skin	Heel prominent
	Ptosis	

1% usually required for a human polymorphism. The level of sensitivity to minor anomalies is set differently by different observers. This may in part be the explanation for the low incidence of minor defects (7.26%) reported by Myrianthopoulos and Chung[9] for the Collaborative Study in the United States and the high incidence (39%) reported by Leppig et al.[11]

Table 2–3. Concurrence of minor and major anomalies at birth in three series

No. of minor malformations	Percent with major malformations		
	Leppig et al.[11]	Marden et al.[10]	Mehes[8]
0	2.3	1.4	1.2
1	3.7	2.9	3.8
2	6.7	10.8	12.5
≥3	19.6	90	26

Minor morphologic features give the most consistent clues to the diagnosis of many multi-anomaly syndromes. Prenatal alcohol syndrome and prenatal hydantoin syndrome, for example, are more commonly diagnosed by a pattern of minor morphologic features than on the basis of major malformations.

Mehes[8] has found the number of minor anomalies detected to be greatest at the time of birth, with a decrease in the detection of many features by age 1 yr. This suggests that certain minor anomalies resolve or become obscured with growth and function. Downslanting palpebrae, horizontal palmar creases, asymmetric ears, preauricular skin tags, and clinodactyly are among those features with similar incidences at birth and at 1 year. A 50% or greater reduction in the prevalences of high-arched palate, low-set ears, and upslanting palpebral fissures occurs by 1 yr. This contrasts with the increased detection of major defects during the first year of life.[9]

Connectional terms

Since multiple structural anomalies often occur together, a terminology that relates the components has developed.[7,17-21] In connectional terminology, anatomic description of the anomalies has been largely abandoned because listing each anatomical feature of the composite becomes cumbersome. Greater emphasis is given to pathogenesis and causation. The terminology relating multiple anomalies has the least consensus and the greatest liability for change and perhaps for confusion. This occurs in part because new combinations of anomalies continue to be identified, in part because different observers independently describe the same entity, and in part because of the development of new insights into pathogenesis and causation. These problems have prompted attempts to develop a uniform nomenclature. Over several years, beginning in 1974, a series of workshops were held to construct a classification and nomenclature of congenital anomalies and other human morphologic changes.[7,17,22] As new rules regarding nomenclature were published, there was disagreement, and the scientific community became embroiled in a debate.[22-25] It would be premature to suggest that this debate has culminated in widely accepted terminology.

An equivalent meeting dealing with terminology is reported to have been held among persons themselves affected with congenital anomalies, in London, in 1898.[26] The term *prodigies,* which the participants are said to have found acceptable, has never been adopted in the medical field.

Syndrome, association, complex, spectrum, sequence, field defect, and *phenotype* have all been used to describe some composite of anatomic features. Johannsen[27] coined the term *phenotype* to encompass the outward manifestations produced by an individual gene. The nature of the gene itself was termed *genotype. Genotype* and *phenotype* can refer to a single gene and its manifestations (anatomic, biochemical, physiologic), to a related group of genes and their manifestations, or to the entire genetic constitution and all resulting hereditary features. In current usage, *phenotype* has become a general term for describing a composite of features without regard to the underlying cause. Consistent with this usage, environmental as well as genetic factors can contribute to the phenotype. This more general use of *phenotype* in many cases suggests that the cause of the features is uncertain or that multiple causes might produce this composite of manifestations. In some cases a modifier is added to indicate pathogenesis, e.g., *akinesia phenotype* to indicate those features that are produced by absence of prenatal movement from any cause. *Complex* is a general term that is also used to indicate a composite of manifestations. *Spectrum* is sometimes used to describe entities with multiple features, particularly those in which prominent features can be expressed with considerable variation.

Greater specificity is suggested by the term *syndrome,* which means a group of features seen together, but it also implies that the composite of features has a common, specific etiology. Use of the term indicates that a specific diagnosis has been made and that the natural history and recurrence risk are known. A well-recognized exception is to use the term to include the multiple features found in several well-delineated disorders, such as those described by de Lange and by Rubinstein and Taybi.[28-29] While the etiologies of these two disorders have not been identified, a single specific etiology is suspected for each. The reader will recognize that

syndrome is also used widely in medicine and without the specificity suggested above when used to describe structural anomalies.

Association has been used in clinical genetics to identify the nonrandom concurrence of two or more features that occur more frequently than expected by chance alone but for which no etiology has been demonstrated. VACTERL (*v*ertebral, *a*nal, *c*ardiac, *t*racheo-*e*sophageal, *r*enal, and *l*imb anomalies) and CHARGE (*c*olobomas, *h*eart defects, *a*tresia choanae, *r*etarded growth, *g*enital anomalies, and *e*ar anomalies) associations are two well-known examples. Use of *association* does not imply a specific diagnosis. Recognition of such statistically related anomalies prompts the search for other defects when one component of an association is noted. Empiric risks for recurrence may also be given even though no cause for the association can be determined.

Sequence has been used by some to indicate a pattern of anomalies that results from a single primary anomaly or from a single mechanical factor.[7,30] The anomaly or mechanical factor that initiates the sequence may produce multiple secondary anomalies or may produce a secondary anomaly that leads to a tertiary anomaly and so forth in cascade fashion. Although proposed to identify a pattern of anomalies having uniform pathogenesis (oligohydramnios sequence), in use *sequence* sometimes implies causation (athyreotic hypothyroidism sequence). Redundancy in using the term *sequence* when applied to specific disease states such as athyreotic hypothyrodism is obvious. Further confusion can arise because of the long-standing use of *sequence* for the arrangement of nucleotides and codons in the genome.

Finite areas of embryonic tissue develop into multiple and hence related morphologic structures. Damage to these finite areas or developmental fields can result in multiple structural anomalies. Use of the developmental field concept helps to explain why certain malformations occur together. Designation and understanding of developmental fields require considerable knowledge of embryonic topography and the fate of the component cells. An arbitrary time during embryogenesis must be selected at which time the dimensions of the developmental field are established and from which the developmental potential of the field is predicted. A polytopic field defect is a pattern of multiple anomalies often in different body areas resulting from disturbance of a single developmental field. The term *monotopic field* is used when the repertoire of a developmental field is limited to a single body area; *monotopic field defect* is used to describe the malformation (usually of a single anatomic structure) that results from a disturbance to that field.[18]

Many difficulties arise with the actual use of *developmental field* to define structural anomalies. Many who deal with human anomalies are not facile in linking various anomalies to their precursor embryonic cells. Considerable overlap of developmental fields occurs, depending on the dimensions selected and on the embryonic age at which the field is thought to be established. If the concept were pushed to the ultimate, the zygote would have to be considered the primary field from which the entire embryo develops.

Addition of the terms *developmental field defect* and *sequence* to the identification of entities with multiple anomalies has not appeared to clarify the pathogenesis or etiologies of these conditions. Implicit in the occurrence of such an entity are the notions that the component anomalies have a common etiology, that certain of the component anomalies may have arisen from a disturbance of common precursor cells (developmental field defect), and that certain component anomalies may be secondary to preceding anomalies or mechanical forces (sequence). *Syndrome, phenotype, spectrum,* and *association,* with appropriate modifiers, provide adequate identification of the composite entities to serve most needs.

Multiple anomalies can also be related through the time period during which they develop. A single insult during embryogenesis may affect multiple unrelated structures that are becoming formed at the time. In the absence of evidence that links the pathogenesis of widely diverse and seemingly unrelated components of conditions with multiple features, these components may be considered "pleiotropic effects" of the underlying cause.

Pinsky[19] has advocated the grouping of discrete syndromes that share a large portion of major features into communities and classes. It was suggested that grouping on the basis of multiple features could assist recall of the member syndromes, bibliographic retrieval, and computer analysis. At the same time the grouping could stimulate ideas about pathogenesis that might apply to a group of disorders sharing similar morphologic features. This system could further permit collective statements that would then apply to the group as a whole and more clearly define the similarities and differences of member syndromes. Merits aside, this polythetic system has been slow to gain popularity in part because it has been presented more as a theoretical system than as a practical system to be readily understood and utilized.

Naming

The naming of composite entities (syndromes, associations, phenotypes) follows no fixed rules nor has any committee assumed authority for naming. Authors and editors often designate a name in the initial description of an entity, or one arises in a subsequent review. For conditions of known etiology, names that acknowledge the cause would seem to be most appropriate (trisomy 13 syndrome, prenatal alcohol syndrome). This is not possible for many syndromes caused by single genes or for conditions of unknown etiology. Several different approaches have been used in these cases.

If the major components are few, their enumeration in the name is possible (hypertelorism-hypospadias syndrome). This can be misleading, however, when the identifying features are not present (e.g., absence of cryptophthalmos in the cryptophthalmos syndrome). When the major components are numerous, the name can become tiresome. Use of the first letters of the major features to form a unique acronym has been successful in several instances (LEOPARD syndrome, VACTERL association). These approaches offer the user some assistance in recalling the primary features of the entities.

Perhaps the most widely accepted practice in naming composite entities has been to use eponyms. Eponymic designation attempts to credit the individual(s) who first described an entity or who first recognized it to be a specific entity. Not uncommonly, earlier reports of an entity are overlooked or not recognized to be that entity, leading to competing names or to compound eponyms (de Lange syndrome versus Brachmann-de Lange syndrome). Problems are also encountered when a prolific investigator describes more than one entity

(Fanconi anemia syndrome and Fanconi renotubular syndrome). When heterogeneity is found to exist in an established name, renaming becomes necessary (Lawrence-Moon-Bardet-Biedl syndrome now divided into Lawrence-Moon syndrome and Bardet-Biedl syndrome). These difficulties aside, the use of eponyms appears well-established and will likely be replaced only by naming according to etiology (based on the gene or environmental insult responsible). The possessive form of eponyms has been dropped in this book in keeping with McKusick's suggestion.

One international committee has published reasonable guidelines regarding the naming of human anomalies.[17] Their suggestions include the use of etiologic agents when known (trisomy 18 syndrome), eponyms (Down syndrome), and other well-established designations. Use of the initials of patients (BBB syndrome, FG syndrome) and acronyms (EMG syndrome) was discouraged by this committee.

Timing of structural alteration

The timing at which an anomaly arises has some importance in descriptive terminology. Postnatal alteration of an anatomic part should be distinguished from prenatal alteration, and prenatal alteration during organogenesis should be distinguished from alteration after organogenesis.

Congenital means present at birth. It gives no idea of pathogenesis and causation, nor does it imply development at any particular time during prenatal life. Hence use of *congenital* with *malformation, disruption,* or *deformation* in the sense described here would be redundant. Congenital anomaly, congenital defect, or congenital abnormality would be more appropriate term combinations since their use would restrict the general terms *anomaly, defect,* and *abnormality* to those present at birth.

Embryonic staging as set forth by Mall,[32] Streeter,[33] and O'Rahilly[34] use arbitrary subdivisions of the period from fertilization to the start of fetal life to provide a description of the topographic, morphologic, and cytologic changes that take place during human development. The stages are defined by the composite of morphologic features and hence show some variability in size and chronologic age and in the progress of any single anatomic feature.

The age of an embryo is given in days following ovulation. Embryonic (postovulation) age is thus 2 weeks less than menstrual age (days or weeks following onset of last menstrual period), which is commonly used to date pregnancies in obstetrics and neonatology.

Fertilization generally occurs within 24 hours after ovulation, usually in the outer reaches of the Fallopian tubes. The initial four stages of human development take place over the first 5–6 days and span the early series of divisions of the free-floating conceptus up to and including the early implantation process. In the latter half of this period the conceptus is called a *blastocyst,* a mass of cells with an internal cavity. The period is called the *preimplantation* period.

Implantation occurs during stages 4–5, which span the period 5.5–12 days. The embryonic disc becomes bilaminar (ectoderm and endoderm), and the amniotic cavity develops on the epidermal surface and the yolk sac on the endodermal surface during these stages.

Stage 23 (56–60 days, or 8 weeks, postfertilization) was considered arbitrarily to end the embryonic period[34]. The beginning of marrow formation in the humerus was a developmental landmark used to assist in identifying this stage. The first 8 weeks after fertilization, or weeks 2–8, are generally considered the period of embryogenesis. The embryo has taken the human form, and most organs are fully formed and located in their final position by the end of this time. Exceptions exist, however, and include external genitalia, abdominal wall, heart, and dental structures.

The fetal period begins with week 9 and extends to delivery, usually 40 weeks from the last menstrual period and 38 weeks from fertilization. Growth and maturation of function are the major processes that occur during this period. However, as noted above, formation of some structures continues into this time. External genitalia do not complete differentiation until week 12, hair follicles do not form until week 12, the midgut does not return to the abdominal cavity from the body stalk until week 10, and teeth do not gain their definitive morphology until much later in fetal life.

Malformations as previously defined occur during the period of organ formation. Most will occur during the first 8 weeks, but exceptions to this are not uncommon in those structures that are still forming after 8 weeks. Disruptions and deformations occur following morphologic development and hence for the most part occur after 8 weeks postovulation.

Terms indicating prenatal environmental influences: teratogen, hadegen, trophogen

Some terms are particularly useful in defining environmental influences that act during gestation and that alter morphology, function, or growth. *Teratogen* has been used with widely variable meanings.[4,36,37] In this text a teratogen will have three features. First, as its derivation (*teratos* = monster, *gen* = produce) suggests, the end result of a teratogenic influence will be a morphologic abnormality rather than a functional one. Second, teratogens are environmental rather than genetic influences. Third, teratogens exert their influence following fertilization and before delivery. Teratogens have an effect primarily during the first 8 weeks of embryogenesis, causing malformations, but may act at a later point in pregnancy, causing disruptions or deformations as well. These late effects of teratogens can also include malformation of structures that gain their morphology after the usual 8 weeks of embryogenesis.

Those environmental influences that alter function but leave the anatomy undisturbed have been termed *hadegens.* Hades was the Greek god of the underworld. One of Hades' possessions was a helmet that permitted him to become invisible. The term *hadegen* is used to identify environmental factors that do not lead to visible structural anomalies but rather produce function abnormalities of equal importance.

Environmental agents can also alter growth. Since growth can be considered either morphologic or functional, the term *trophogen* can be used to distinguish those influences that alter growth from those that produce structural anomalies or functional disturbances.

This triad of terms can describe the results of environmental agents acting during pregnancy that cause morphologic abnormalities, growth changes, or functional impairments, these agents being teratogenic, trophogenic, or hadegenic, respectively. A given environmental agent can cause all three types of changes, or may cause one type of change during one prenatal period and a different type of change at another

time. Rubella, for example, is hadegenic, teratogenic, and trophogenic in the first trimester, and after the fourth month it is hadegenic alone. In this schema, it is inappropriate to designate a factor that impairs growth or alters mental function but causes no structural anomaly as teratogenic.

Terms with negative impact

By and large, structural anomalies are negatively viewed by medical practitioners, affected individuals, and society. Insensitive terminology can further stigmatize those affected and can separate caretakers from affected individuals, affected from family, and family from society. Terminology should be as neutral as possible while correctly identifying or defining the structural anomaly. The care needed in choosing words when dealing with families or affected members may be obvious (Chapters 8 and 9). However, use of terms employed internally in science should also be circumspect since these terms find their way to families via medical records, news articles, and courtrooms.

It should be acknowledged that some morphologic abnormalities are not viewed negatively by affected individuals. A case in point might be alteration in size caused by achondroplasia. In this circumstance it is not unusual to find affected persons wishing to have a recurrence of achondroplasia in their biologic offspring, because normal size is less desirable in these particular families.[38]

Terminology does not remain constant; the nuances and implications of terms change with the generations. Until the early 1900s *monster* and *monstrosity* were widely used terms in medical circles to describe malformations or other morphologic changes. *Monster* has now gained a different nuance, primarily because of its use in movies to depict scary creatures. The new usage does not adhere to either of the word's origins (*to show* or *to warn*), but suggests that those who look abnormal may also act in destructive, frightening, and otherwise offensive ways.

Although *monster* and *monstrosity* have been used from the first written records of human malformations and into the twentieth century, they have in this century disappeared entirely from medical terminology. Other terms have had only brief life spans. Examples from the four editions of Smith's *Recognizable Patterns of Human Malformations* will suffice to illustrate.[30,39] In a period of less than 20 years (edition 1 [1970] to edition 4 [1988]), repeated changes can be found in the preferred terminology for morphologic entities. *Potter's syndrome* (edition 1) changed to *oligohydramnios tetrad* (edition 2) and then to *oligohydramnios sequence* (edition 3). The preferred term for *amniotic bands* changed with each edition. Initially, *amniotic band syndrome* changed to *amniotic band anomalads,* then to *early amnion rupture spectrum,* and finally to *early amnion rupture sequence.* These changes arose from the attempt to add a pathogenetic implication to the identification of the entity.

Social sensitivity demands discretion in terminology. Terms that are divisive, derogatory, negative, or degrading should be abandoned. *Happy puppet syndrome* has been replaced by *Angelman syndrome, fetal face syndrome* by *Robinow syndrome,* and *elfin facies syndrome* by *Williams syndrome.* A term in common use in the middle of this century, *mongolism,* or *mongoloid idiot,* as assigned by Langdon Down for a specific mental retardation syndrome, is discouraged in favor of *trisomy 21 syndrome* or *Down syndrome.*[40]

The designation *funny-looking kid* (FLK) may be viewed as derogatory by an affected child, family members, and caretakers. The term *dwarfism* to identify persons with disproportionate skeletal dysplasias has been discouraged for the same reason. *Special child* or *special needs child* has been used to indicate children with handicaps. Since all children are special, the use of this term for a child with a malformation appears inappropriate and patronizing.

The designation of syndromes by the initial of the proband (G syndrome, BBB syndrome) has been advocated by Opitz et al.[18] While intended to be neutral, this naming schema offers nothing to assist the user in remembering the syndrome, is liable for duplication, and has not found wide acceptance.

Anomalad was suggested by Fraser and advocated by Smith[17] to indicate a cascade of structural anomalies that derived from a single preceding anomaly or mechanical force. The term was debated for several years and has now disappeared, being replaced by some users with *sequence. Polyanomaly* has also been suggested to indicate multiple anomalies, specifically those that arise from the same pathogenesis. There is nothing to recommend this term over *multiple congenital anomalies,* and the term does not flow well.

Classification and coding

Classification

The systematic arrangement of structural anomalies on the basis of morphologic, anatomic, etiologic, or other criteria has been attempted by many observers. The number of classification schemas attests to the likelihood that no system has been entirely satisfactory. Nonetheless, finding some order among human congenital anomalies has utility in assisting human memory and in giving insights into the range and nature of human anomalies. A growing utility is now being found for computer retrieval of information. Some admixture between the classification schemas is to be expected in a brief accounting of the types of classifications used in the past.

1. Classification by cause. One of the oldest classification schemas, that set forth by Empedocles,[41] was based on causation. Five causes for human anomalies were recognized: excess semen, deficiency of semen, slowness of movement of semen, abnormal movement of semen, and division of semen into separate parts. Paré's classification[42] had 13 causes, including abnormalities of semen as well as mechanical injury, uterine compression, maternal impressions, and the supernatural. Cleland's system, published in 1889, had six causation categories, three leading to anomalies with morphologic deficiencies and three leading to anomalies of excess.[43]

2. Classification by morphologic alteration. Eight types of morphologic alterations were the major entries in the system of St. Isidore in AD 600:[44] large size, small size, transformation of a part, transformation of the whole body, transposition of a part, adhesion of parts, mixture of sexes, and the coexistence of multiple anomalies. These types were supplemented by two entries based on the precocious or delayed appearance of features. To this type of classification, Huber[45] added union of parts usually separated and closed state of canals usually open. Isidore and Etienne St. Hilaire set forth an extensive classification schema based on alterations of morphology.[46] All anomalies were assigned to a kingdom, the kingdom was subdivided into four divisions, each of which was further subdivided into classes, orders, tribes, families, and genera.

3. Classification by regional anatomy. Use of regional anatomy to arrange anomalies first appeared in the 1600s.[47,48] The systems used by Taruffi,[49] Lowne,[50] and Ballantyne[51] at the end of the nineteenth century utilized regional anatomy as well. These systems often incorporated subclassifications based on morphologic alteration (excess or deficiency of parts, and so forth).

4. Classification by system. Closely related to schemas based on regional anatomy is the use of anatomic systems to organize human anomalies. This variation is the basis of classifications used by Warkany[52] in the classic *Congenital Malformations,* in the *International Classification of Diseases* (ICD), in the Cardiff and Centers for Disease Control modifications of the ICD, and in the Systematized Nomenclature of Medicine (SNOMED).[53-56]

5. Other classifications. Several additional schemas are of historical interest. The earliest known system separated malformations into those that affected ordinary citizens and those that affected royal families. This was the only arrangement of anomalies to be found in the enumerations of human anomalies in the teratologic records of the Chaldeans.[57] Other systems have used viability of affected individuals, time of occurrence during embryogenesis, and various mixtures of the several foregoing schemas.[53,55,58,59]

The ICD is now in its ninth revision.[53] The clinical modification (ICD-9-CM) as published by the U.S. Government allots 20 categories with accompanying numerical codes for congenital anomalies. Considerable inconsistency has crept into this schema. Initially oriented to systems, there occur drifts into regional anatomy, and major divergence into causation (chromosome anomalies) in the nineteenth category. An admixture of systems, specific diseases, specific syndromes, and processes appears in the twentieth category. The system, although having lost its consistency, is widely used because of its acceptance for epidemiologic studies and for insurance categorization, but it does not accommodate a listing of rare but specific anomalies.

The British Pediatric Classification modifies the ICD system for anomalies by adding two additional numbers to the code, permitting a further specific subdivision of an ICD category.[54] The Centers for Disease Control (CDC) has further modified the ICD and British systems by adding a sixth digit to the code.[55] The addition of digits in the British and CDC modifications allows categories of defects to be subdivided into individual anomalies but fails to correct the admixing of causation, pathogenesis, regional anatomy, organ system, syndromes, and diseases in the original ICD system.

The Systematized Nomenclature of Medicine has been produced by the American College of Pathologists[56] based on their *Systematized Nomenclature of Pathology.* This schema utilizes seven sections to permit access from numerous perspectives: topography, morphology, etiology, function, disease, procedure, and occupation. Most useful in relation to structural anomalies are the topographic, morphologic, and etiologic fields.

Other systems that deal with certain individual anomalies and syndromes include McKusick's alphabetical listing of single gene disorders[60] and Shepard's alphabetical enumeration of environmental agents.[61] Several computerized data bases have been developed to assist the clinician in recalling information about entities having one or more morphologic characteristic. The three major systems—London Dysmorphology Database,[62] POSSUM (Pictures of Standard Syndromes and Undiagnosed Malformations)[63] and BDIS (Birth Defects Information Services[64]—all require coded entry of the anatomic description (topography and morphology) of individual features and search for entities in which the feature(s) occur.

Coding

At present there is no comprehensive coding system that is specific for structural anomalies that occur in humans. A five-digit system would be required to assign a unique number to each of the numerous structural variants and anomalies. To add an indicator of the major etiologies would require an additional digit. A further multidigit hindcode would be necessary to link individual anomalies to the various syndromes, diseases, or associations of which they might be a feature. Development of a uniform coding system for human anomalies will undoubtedly be encouraged by the increasing reliance on electronic systems for storage, retrieval, and manipulation of data.

References

1. International Anatomical Nomenclature Committee: Nomina Anatomica, ed 5. Williams & Wilkins, Baltimore, 1983.
2. Malacarne V: Memoires della societes itali, vol IX. 1798, p 49.
3. Robbins SL, Cotran RS: Pathologic Basis of Disease, ed 2. WB Saunders, Co, Philadelphia, 1979.
4. Gilbert SF: Developmental Biology, ed 2. Sinauer Associates, Sunderland, MA, 1988, p 597.
5. Rimoin DL, Hall J, Maroteaux P: International nomenclature of constitutional diseases of bone with bibliography. BDOAS, XV (10):1, 1979.
6. Horton WA: Histochemistry, a valuable tool in connective tissue research. Coll Rel Res 4:231, 1984.
7. Spranger J, Benirschke K, Hall JG, et al.: Errors of morphogenesis: concepts and terms. J Pediatr 100:160, 1982.
8. Mehes K: Minor Malformations in the Neonate. Akademiai Kiado, Budapest, 1983.
9. Myrianthopoulos NC, Chung CS: Congenital malformation in singletons: epidemiologic survey. BDOAS X(11):1, 1974.
10. Marden PM, Smith DW, McDonald MJ: Congenital anomalies in the newborn infant, including minor variations. J Pediatr 64:357, 1964.
11. Leppig KA, Werler MM, Cann CI, et al.: Predictive value of minor anomalies. I. Association with major malformations. J Pediatr 110:531, 1987.
12. van Regemorter N, Dodion J, Druart C, et al.: Congenital malformations in 10,000 consecutive births in a university hospital: need for genetic counseling and prenatal diagnosis. J Pediatr 104:386, 1984.
13. Blackburn W, Curtiss JR, Cooley NRJ: The role of dysmorphogenesis in perinatal morbidity and mortality: a perinatal pathologist's view. Proc Greenwood Genet Center 9:89, 1990.
14. Mattos TC, Giugliani R, Haase HB: Congenital malformations detected in 731 autopsies of children aged 0 to 14 years. Teratology 35:305, 1987.
15. Chavez GF, Cordero JF, Becerra JE: Leading major congenital malformations among minority groups in the United States. MMWR 37:17, 1988.
16. Holmes LB: Congenital malformations. N Engl J Med 295:204, 1976.
17. Smith DW: Classification, nomenclature, and naming of morphologic defects. J Pediatr 87:162, 1975.
18. Opitz JM, Herrmann J, Pettersen JC, et al.: Terminological, diagnostic, nosological, and anatomical–developmental aspects of developmental defects in man. Adv Hum Genet 9:71, 1979.
19. Pinsky L: The polythetic (phenotypic community) system of classifying human malformation syndromes. BDOAS XIII(3A):13, 1977.
20. Gilbert-Barness E, Opitz JM, Barness LA: The pathologist's perspective of genetic disease: malformations and dysmorphology. Pediatr Clin North Am 36:163, 1989.
21. McKusick VA: On lumpers and splitters, or the nosology of genetic disease. BDOAS V(1):23, 1969.
22. Christiansen RL: Classification and nomenclature of malformation. Lancet 1:798, 1974.
23. Spranger J, Smith DW: Pro and con the term "anomalad." J Pediatr 93:159, 1978.
24. Bartsocas CS, Smith DW, Fraser FC: "Anomalad" versus "polyanomaly." J Pediatr 88:899, 1976.
25. Benirschke K, Lowry RB, Opitz JM, et al.: Developmental terms—some proposals: first report of an international working group. Am J Med Genet 3:297, 1979.
26. Fiedler L: Freaks, Myths and Images of the Secret Self. Simon and Schuster, New York, 1978, p. 15.
27. Johannsen W: Elemente der exakten Erblichkeitslehre. Jena: Fischer, 1909, p 143.
28. de Lange C: Sur un type nouveau de degeneration (Typus Amstelodamensis). Arch Med Enf 36:713, 1933.
29. Rubinstein JH, Taybi H: Broad thumbs and toes and facial abnormalities: a possible mental retardation syndrome. Am J Dis Child 105:588, 1963.
30. Jones KL: Smith's Recognizable Patterns of Human Malformation, ed 4. WB Saunders, Philadelphia, 1988.
31. Opitz JM, Reynolds JF, Spano LM: The Developmental Field Concept. Alan R Liss, New York, 1986.
32. Mall FP: On stages in the development of human embryos from 2 to 25 mm long. Anat Anz 46:78, 1914.
33. Streeter GL: Developmental horizons in human embryos: description of age group XI, 13 to 20 somites, and age group XII, 21 to 29 somites. Contrib Embryol 30:211, 1942.
34. O'Rahilly R: Developmental Stages in Human Embryos, Part A: Embryos of the First Three Weeks (Stages 1 to 9). Carnegie Institute, Washington, DC, Publication 631, 1973.
35. Streeter GL: Developmental horizons in human embryos: description of age groups XIX, XX, XXI, XXII, and XXIII, being the fifth issue of a survey of the Carnegie Collection. Contrib Embryol 34:165, 1951.
36. Friedman JM: Teratogens and growth. Growth Gen Horm 3(4):6, 1987.
37. Smithells RW: The demonstration of teratogenic effects of drugs in humans. In: Drugs and Pregnancy: Human Teratogenesis and Related Problems. DF Hawkins, ed. Churchill Livingstone, Edinburgh, 1983.
38. van Etten AM: Dwarfs Don't Live in Doll Houses. Adaptive Living, Rochester, 1988, p 216.
39. Smith DW: Recognizable Patterns of Human Malformations, eds 1–3. WB Saunders, Philadelphia, 1970, 1976, 1982.
40. Allen G, Benda CE, Book JA, et al.: Mongolism. Lancet 1:775, 1961.
41. Empedocles: The Fragments of Empedocles. Translated by WE Leonard. Open Court Publishing, Chicago, 1908.
42. Pare A: On Monsters and Marvels. Translated by JL Pallister. University of Chicago Press, Chicago, 1982.
43. Cleland J: Memoirs and Memoranda in Anatomy, vol 1. Williams & Norgate, London, 1899.
44. St. Isidore: Etymologies. Wolff and Kerver, Paris, 1499.
45. Huber JJ: Observationes atque cogitationes non nullae de monstris. Hüteri and Harmes, Cassellis, 1748.
46. Geoffroy Saint-Hilaire I: Historie des Anomalies. vols. 1–3. JB Baillière, Paris, 1832–1837.
47. Schenck J: Observationum Medicarum, Rararum, Novarum, Admirabilium, et Monstrosarum Volumen. N Hoffmannum, Frankfurt, 1609.
48. Aldrovandus U: Monstrorum Historia. N Tebaldinus, Bononiae, 1642.
49. Taruffi: Storia della teratologia, vols. 1–VIII. Regia Tipografia, Bologna, 1881–1894.

50. Lowne BT: Descriptive Catalogue of the Teratological Series in the Museum of the Royal College of Surgeons of England. Taylor and Francis, London, 1893.

51. Ballantyne JW: Manual of Antenatal Pathology and Hygiene. The Embryo. William Green and Sons, Edinburgh, 1904.

52. Warkany J: Congenital Malformations: Notes and Comments. Year Book, Chicago, 1971.

53. International Classification of Diseases, Rev 9, Clinical Modification (ICD.9.CM), ed 3. U.S. Department of Health and Human Services, Washington, DC, Publication 1:639, 1989.

54. British Paediatric Association: Classification of Diseases, ed 2. British Paediatric Association, London, 1987.

55. Centers for Disease Control: 6-Digit Code for Reportable Congenital Anomalies, Version 6/89. U.S. Department of Health and Human Services, Atlanta, 1989.

56. Cote RA: Systematized Nomenclature of Medicine, ed 2, vol 1. College of American Pathologists, Skokie, IL, 1979.

57. Leichty E: The Omen Series Summa Izbu. JJ Augustin Publisher, Locust Valley, New York, 1970.

58. Billard CM: A Treatise on the Diseases of Infants, ed 3. (translated by J Stewart), G Adlard, New York, 1839.

59. Forster A: Handbuch der Pathologischen Anatomie, vol. II. Leipzig, 1862–1865.

60. McKusick VA: Mendelian Inheritance in Man, ed 8. Johns Hopkins University Press, Baltimore, 1988.

61. Shepard TH: Catalog of Teratogenic Agents, ed 6. Johns Hopkins University Press, Baltimore, 1989.

62. Winter RM, Baraitser M, Douglas JM: A computerised data base for the diagnosis of rare dysmorphic syndromes. J Med Gen 21:121, 1984.

63. Murdoch Institute: POSSUM Newsletter. September 1987.

64. Buyse M: Center for Birth Defects Information Services. BDOAS XVI(5):83, 1980.

3

Understanding Human Embryonic Development

MALCOLM C. JOHNSTON

Understanding the mechanisms of normal and abnormal human embryonic development is based on detailed observations of human embryos and human malformations as well as insights gained through studies of normal and abnormal subhuman embryos. It has long been recognized that higher vertebrate embryos have very similar appearances (Fig. 3-1), suggesting that underlying developmental mechanisms are essentially the same.[1] Also, detailed experimental studies of normal development in a wide range of vertebrate embryos, including mammals, have demonstrated very close similarities in mechanisms, even when the superficial morphologies (e.g., of amphibian embryos) appear quite different. Technical advances have improved our ability to compare the development of humans and experimental animals. For example, the three-dimensional configuration of embryonic cells as shown by scanning electron microscopy often provides clues as to their behavior (e.g., the bipolar configuration of migrating cells). Insights into the mechanisms of abnormal development and, by inference, normal developmental mechanisms have also come from the accidental exposures of human embryos to teratogens—e.g., thalidomide in the 1950s and, more recently, Accutane (13-*cis*-retinoic acid)—that have produced malformations similar to those produced in experimental embryos.

The mechanisms underlying the following developmental phenomena are considered in this chapter: differential gene activation, cell migrations, morphogenetic movements, cell and tissue interactions (including induction and differentiation), growth regulation, fields, fusion of embryonic primordia, and programmed cell death. Examples of abnormal perturbations of these phenomena are also provided.

A brief overview of normal embryonic development is first presented. The discussion is limited almost entirely to those aspects of normal development for which information is well established through both descriptive and experimental studies. Then the rapidly accumulating, sometimes controversial evidence on the regulation of development is presented, especially those aspects most relevant to human malformations. Examples of abnormal development are then given, beginning with those that occur earliest in development (e.g., the holoprosencephalies and cyclopia, neural tube defects, the retinoic acid syndrome, clefts of the lip and/or palate, limb defects, and renal malformations). Many examples involve head and neck development, the area with which the author is most familiar. Finally, some general considerations relating to normal and abnormal development, including developmental weakpoints, are presented.

A detailed description of normal human embryonic development is not provided in this chapter because a number of excellent texts on the subject are available.[2–5] However, these texts provide limited discussion of abnormal development. Sadler's embryology text[2] provides a number of examples of developmental mechanisms as derived from studies of experimental embryos. Although a little dated, the text by Hamilton and Mossman[4] provides extensive detail in descriptive human embryology. Normal developmental mechanisms are presented in some detail in Gilbert's *Developmental Biology.*[6]

Fig. 3-1. Embryos of man, pig, reptile, and bird at corresponding developmental stages. The striking resemblance of the embryos to one another is indicative of the fundamental similarity of the processes involved in their development. From Patten.[1]

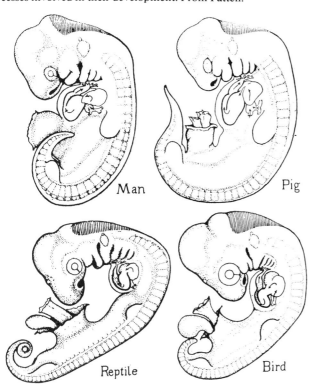

Overview of normal development

The surface morphology of the developing human embryo is presented in Figure 3–2.[7] By day 19 (stage 8), the three germ layers have formed and development of the anterior neural plate has been initiated. By day 22 (stage 10), the neural plate has rolled up to form the neural tube, and blocks of mesoderm, the somites, cause raised areas by the embryo's surface. Visceral arches are seen in the stage 11 embryo (day 25), and surface elevations indicate the presence of optic vesicles. By

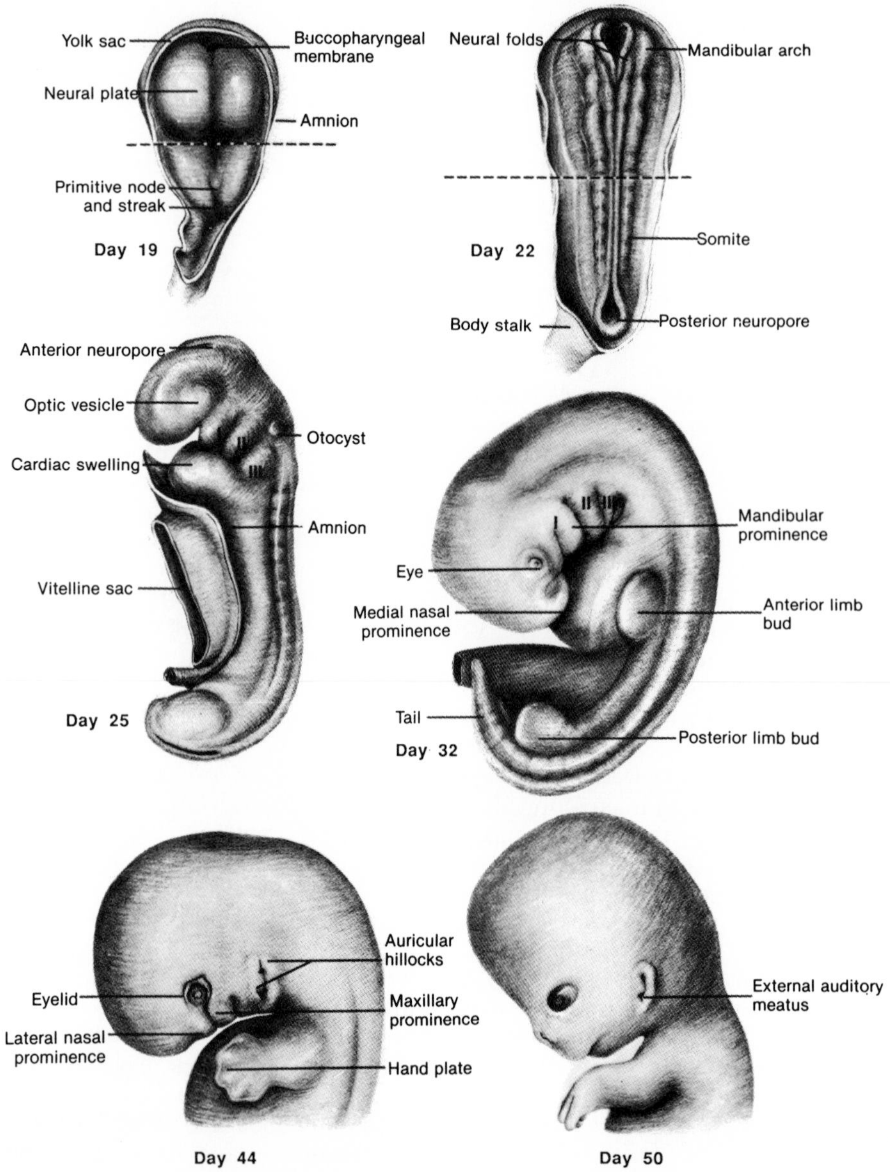

Fig. 3–2. Development of the human embryo from the germ layer stage (day 19) to near the end of the embryonic period (day 50). The visceral arches are numbered with Roman numerals. Up to day 32, surface features of the human embryo are very similar to those of other higher vertebrates, indicating similar developmental mechanisms. Most major malformations have occurred by day 50. From Johnston and Sulik.[7]

day 32 (stage 14), the size of the facial prominences demonstrates the degree of development of the primary palate, lip, and midface. Upper and lower limb buds are present by this stage as well. External ear development has been initiated by day 44 (stage 18), and by day 50 (stage 20) the embryo is easily distinguished as being human (cf. day 32 embryo in Fig. 3–2 to those in Fig. 3–1). Although most malformations are already present by day 50, many systems (e.g., the skeletal system) are still largely underdeveloped, with little to distinguish them except, for example, mesenchymal condensations.

Fertilization through establishment of the initial "body plan" (days 1–27)

Development through day 27 is depicted schematically for the human in Figure 3–3. Repeated divisions of the fertilized egg give rise to the morula (Fig. 3–3C). Fluid accumulation within the morula transforms the developing organism into a blastocyst (Fig. 3–3D), only a portion of which (the inner cell mass) will participate in formation of the embryo, with the remaining cells developing into support structures such as part of the placenta. The inner cell mass develops into two layers, the epiblast and the hypoblast (Fig. 3–3E). It now appears that only the epiblast will participate in embryo formation, as shown by recent studies using cell-marking procedures in the chick[8,9] and mouse.[10] As is discussed in the section on the regulation of development, cell differentiation begins before germ layer formation (Fig. 3–4). For example, there is now some evidence that an interaction between the hypoblast and the epiblast is responsible for a portion of the epiblast differentiating into mesodermal cells. The exact manner in which the endodermal and mesodermal layers are formed from the epiblast, however, is still not clear. It ap-

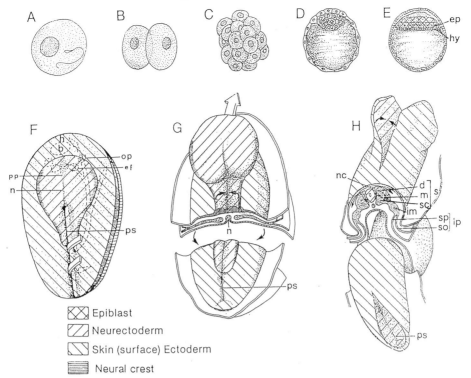

Epiblast
Neurectoderm
Skin (surface) Ectoderm
Neural crest

Fig. 3–3. Sketches summarizing development of embryos from fertilization through neural tube formation. It now appears that all three germ layers are formed from the epiblast (ep in E). In F, the notochord (n) and its rostral (anterior) extension, the prechordal plate (pp), as well as associated pharyngeal endoderm, form as a single layer (G), principally from the anterior end of the primitive streak (ps), the primitive node. Prospective mesodermal cells migrate (arrows in F) through the primitive streak and insert themselves between the epiblast and hypoblast. Epiblast cells remaining on the surface constitute the ectoderm. Cells of the notochord (and prechordal plate?) and adjacent mesoderm (collectively termed the *chorda-meso-* induce overlying cells to form the neural plate (neuroectoderm). Only later does the notochord separate from the endoderm (H), while folding movements and differential growth (arrows in G and H) continue to shape the embryo. The components of the mesoderm are illustrated in H: The somite (s) consists of three layers, the dermatome (d), myotome (m), and sclerotome (sc); the intermediate mesoderm (im); and the lateral plate (lp), which is split into the somatic (so) and splanchnic (sp) mesoderm. h, heart; b, buccal plate; op, olfactory placode; ef, eye field; and nc, neural crest. Modified from Johnston and Sulik.[7]

pears that the prospective endodermal cells and the notochordal and prechordal plate cells (Figs. 3–3F,G and 3–5B) are formed from the more anterior (rostral) end of the primitive streak (Fig. 3–3F) and remain as a continuous layer that is inserted into the hypoblast. The hypoblast is displaced laterally. Eventually, it forms the extraembryonic endoderm that lines the yolk sac and allantois (Fig. 3–5D). Other cells migrating through the primitive streak form the middle germ layer (mesoderm; arrows in Fig. 3–3F). Cells remaining in the upper layer form the ectoderm. Collectively, the movements of prospective endodermal and mesodermal cells are often referred to as *gastrulation*. Gastrulation continues until the closure of the posterior neuropore, which occurs at about gestational day 27 in the human embryo.

The epiblast and its derived ectoderm form compact layers of cells, firmly connected together with little intercellular substance. Such compactly arranged cell populations are termed *epithelia*. In contrast, when epiblast cells migrate away from the primitive streak to form mesoderm they form loosely arranged cell populations with few intercellular contacts. Such tissues are termed *mesenchyme*. These are histologic terms for many embryonic tissues that tell nothing about the origins of cells and should not be confused with the names of the germ layers (Fig. 3–4).

Gastrulation sets up new associations between cell popu-

lations that often interact with one another to alter their differentiated state. These interactions are discussed further in the following section on the regulation of development and thus are only briefly described at this time. The notochord, presumably along with the prechordal plate and adjacent strips of mesoderm (collectively termed the *chorda-meso-*

Fig. 3–4. The terms *epithelia* and *mesenchyme* are descriptive and are used by embryologists to describe compactly and loosely organized embryonic tissues, respectively. Neither germ layer origins nor derivatives are considered. From Johnston and Sulik.[17]

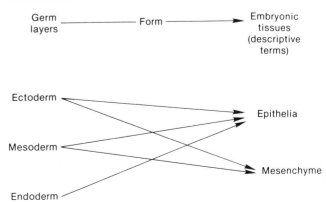

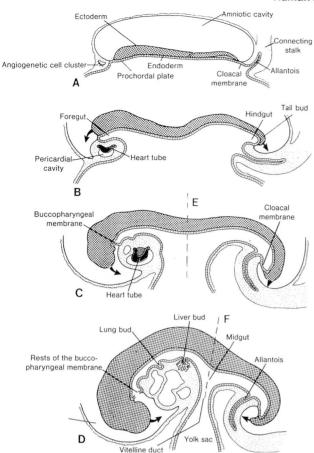

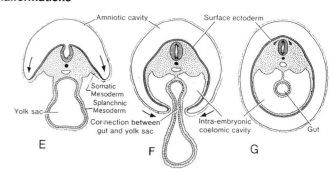

Fig. 3–5. Folding movements and differential growth involved in formation of the GI tract. A–D. Schematic drawings representing the sagittal sections through human embryos from approximately gestational day 17 (A) to day 36 (D). Neural overgrowth (arrows) at the cephalic and caudal ends and dorsal flexion radically change the outline of the embryo. E–G. Cross sections of human embryos from approximately day 37 (E) to day 40 (G). The planes for E and F are illustrated on C and D. The lateral body walls fold downward (arrows), eventually fusing with the yolk sac. Later, the gut tube separates from the ventral body wall (G). Modified from Sadler.[2]

derm), induce the overlying ectoderm to differentiate into the neural plate (neuroectoderm, Fig. 3–3F), which is the forerunner of the central nervous system and other cell populations. As with all inductive interactions, once the poorly understood inductive stimulus has passed, the induced neural plate is able to undergo independent development if removed to culture without the continued presence of the inducing tissue. New associations between embryonic cell populations with subsequent inductive interactions occur repeatedly in development and constitute an exclusively embryonic phenomenon. In such inductive interactions, much of the specificity lies in the responding tissue, which is said to be *competent*. For example, abnormal environmental influences, including heat shock, will elicit the neural plate response in competent ectoderm.[11] Once a responding tissue becomes committed to form a certain component, such as the neural plate, it is said to be *determined*.

Although ectoderm removed to culture shortly after contact with the underlying chorda-mesoderm will form a neural plate, its organization is haphazard in respect to both the numbers of derived neural plate structures (e.g., excessive numbers of olfactory placodes) and their positions. If separated from underlying chorda-mesoderm at progressively later stages and raised in culture, the developing neural plate becomes progressively better organized. Because of this function, the prospective chorda-mesoderm is sometimes referred to as the *organizer*.[11]

Experimental separation of the prospective mesoderm and endoderm from the prospective ectoderm shows that the me-

soderm and endoderm are capable of self-organization into derivatives such as notochord, somites, and muscle.[32] The ectoderm is not capable of such organization and remains undifferentiated.

Tubulation: the formation of the neural and gastrointestinal tubes

Folding movements and differential growth lead to formation of two embryonic tubes: the ectodermally derived neural tube and the endodermally lined gastrointestinal tube. Neural tube closure represents the first clear example of a morphogenetic ("form-producing") movement. Much of the force generation for neural tube closure lies within the neural plate epithelium, as experimental embryology students learn when they first excise neural plates in salamander and other embryos. The forces involved in ventral folding of the lateral body wall are probably similar. In both cases, fusion and separation of different components are involved.

Differential growth further complicates the formation of the neural and gastrointestinal tubes. Rapid growth of the neural tube, primarily in the forebrain region (Figs. 3–3G and 3–5), alters the relative position of the prospective heart and buccopharyngeal membrane and leads to the formation of the pharynx with its lateral and ventral walls separating into the visceral arches. Visceral arch formation (Fig. 3–2, day 32) is associated with segmentation of mesoderm with intervening indentations of surface ectoderm and evaginations of pharyngeal endoderm that contact each other in the proximal regions of the arches. This contact ruptures in fish and amphibian larvae to form gill slits. Rapid growth of the caudal portion of the embryos results in tail bud formation and alters the position of the cloacal membrane (Fig. 3–5C,D).

In most regions, the lateral portion of the mesoderm (the lateral plate mesoderm) forms as two distinct layers, the somatic mesoderm associated with the surface ectoderm and the splanchnic mesoderm associated with endoderm (Figs. 3–3H and 3–5 E–G). With closure of the ventral body wall, a cavity is formed between these layers and is termed the *intraembryonic* coelomic cavity (Fig. 3–5G). Eventually, the organs resulting from endodermal ingrowth into splanchnic mesoderm, such as the liver and lung buds (Fig. 3–5D), project into this space. The developing heart also projects into the coelom. Primarily due to the formation of septa from the splanchnic mesoderm, the coelom becomes separated into the pleuropericardial and peritoneal cavities. Septum formation also leads to separation of the pleural and pericardial cavities.

Origins of tissues, organs, and systems

At the completion of germ layer formation, many cell types are already determined. Figure 3–6 illustrates the derivatives of the different germ layers. Some general comments are in order.

The origin of many cell types is rather straightforward. Myoblasts of skeletal muscles are almost entirely derived from the myotomes of somites (Fig. 3–3H) or from comparable structures rostral to the otic placode. Endothelial cells apparently arise from the splanchnic mesoderm (Fig. 3–3H). The peripheral nervous system (PNS) derives largely from the neural crest (Fig. 3–3F) and the central nervous system (CNS) from the remaining neural plate. Epithelial components of the skin and associated glands are formed from surface ectoderm and the epithelia and glands of the digestive tract largely from endoderm.

The origins of skeletal and connective tissues are more complicated. These tissues have many origins including the cranial neural crest and all portions of the initial mesoderm except the myotome. All sources appear to be capable of forming certain types of cells, especially those of the general connective tissues. For example, cranial neural crest and most mesodermal cells appear to be equally capable of forming the fibroblasts and smooth muscle cells of the blood vessel walls when they find themselves adjacent to developing capillaries. Certain cells, however, appear to have specific derivation. Odontoblasts, for example, are derived only from neural crest.

The vascular system

The key cell in the vascular system is the endothelial cell, which is derived entirely, or almost entirely, from the splanchnic mesoderm (Figs. 3–3H, 3–7, and 3–8). Endothelial cells are first observed forming the walls of blood islands that contain developing blood cells. From these blood islands develop capillaries that may be present as solid cords and that invade almost all tissues of the body. These embryonic vessels recruit cells from local mesenchyme to form the remainder of the vessel wall (e.g., fibroblasts and smooth muscle cells). The heart is essentially a modified blood vessel (Fig. 3–7) except that its connective tissue mesenchyme is entirely derived from lining endothelial cells for all but the conotruncus, which derives much of its mesenchyme from cranial neural crest cells (vide infra). Other aspects of vascular development, including those of the yolk sac and the chorioallantoic placenta, are illustrated in Figure 3–8.

Voluntary (skeletal) musculature

The key cell of voluntary muscles is the myoblast, which is derived from the myotomes of somites or comparable structures in the preotic somitomeres. These myoblasts migrate extensively throughout the embryo (Figs. 3–9; see also Fig. 3–19, below) and are followed by motor nerve axons that enter the myotome immediately as the myoblasts leave the myotome. Myoblasts that contribute contractile cells to limb muscles demonstrate a primary migration into the cores of the limbs (Fig. 3–9) and, after breaking into groups, demonstrate secondary migrations to their final locations. When they reach their final destinations, the myoblasts fuse together, forming multinucleated muscle fibers. Some myoblasts form specialized cells (muscle spindles) that monitor muscle stretch and are innervated by sensory fibers. The connective tissue of muscles develops from local mesenchyme.

Nervous system

Almost the entire nervous system develops from the neural plate and specialized ectodermal placodes that develop as thickenings in the surface ectoderm (Figs. 3–3, 3–6, and 3–17, below). Most of the neural plate develops into elements of the CNS. Exceptions are the neural crest, which forms most of the PNS, and the eye vesicles which develop from "eye fields" in the anterior neural plate. Much of the neural plate is segmented into neuromeres, which appear to be of considerable significance for both normal and abnormal development.

During much of the CNS development, mitosis occurs at the luminal surface of the neural tube (including the cerebral and cerebellar hemispheres), with daughter cells either remaining in the proliferation pool or differentiating into neurons and supporting cells. Neurons then migrate toward their final destinations such as in brain stem nuclei or the surface layers of the hemispheres.

Neural crest cells form along almost the entire margins of the neural plate except the most anterior portion (Fig. 3–3F). As indicated in Figure 3–6, they migrate extensively and form a wide variety of cells and tissues, including cells that form most of the PNS. These include cells forming neurons in the sensory and autonomic ganglia, as well as those forming the supporting cells (the satellite cells on the surface of neuronal cell bodies), and, except for the olfactory nerve ganglion, all the sheath cells. Neurons of the sympathetic nervous system are from trunk crest cells and depend on interactions with somite mesoderm for their differentiation. In contrast, parasympathetic neurons form almost entirely from cranial crest cells and depend mostly on interactions with endoderm for their differentiation. Some of these cells undergo very long migrations along the gastrointestinal tract and are innervated by preganglionic fibers of the vagal nerve. Many neurons in the cranial sensory ganglia are derived from placodes in the surface ectoderm (see Fig. 3–17).

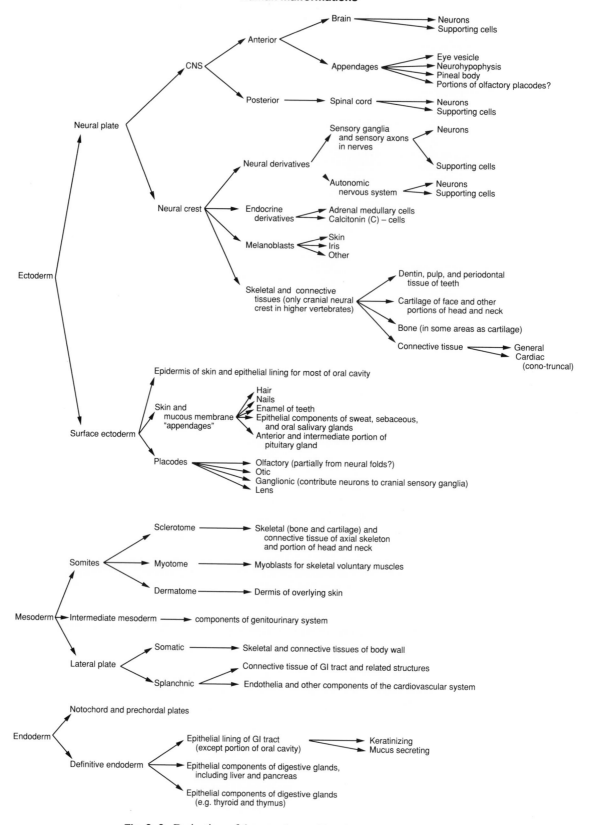

Fig. 3–6. Derivatives of the germ layers. For discussion, see text.

Development of the sense organs is complex. The eye vesicles develop from the eye fields of the neural plate as evaginations of the forebrain (Figs. 3–3F and 3–10).[12] The lens forms as an invaginating placode in the surface ectoderm, and the connective tissues are formed from local mesen-chyme, principally from the neural crest cells. Sensory cells (rods and cones) develop in the retinal layer of the vesicle, and impulses are relayed centrally by neurons also developing in this layer. The corneal stroma and almost all of the sclera are of neural crest origin. The inner ear is derived from

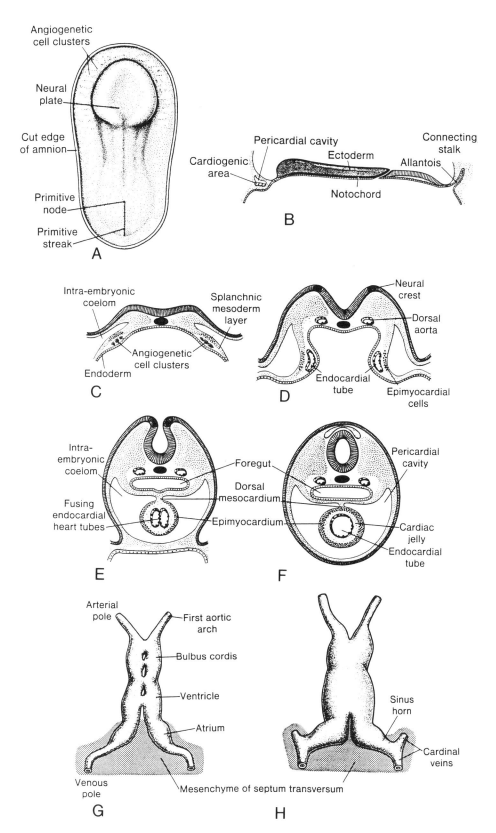

Fig. 3–7. Formation of the heart. Angiogenic clusters of prospective endothelial and blood cells form in the splanchnic mesoderm as indicated in the dorsal view of the embryo in A and in the sections in B and C. Eventually, the endothelial cells link up to form bilateral tubes (D) that contact (E) and fuse in the midline F–H. The different portions of the embryonic heart are labeled in G and H. Myoblasts differentiate in the epimyocardium, which is derived from the outerlayers of the splanchnic mesoderm (D–F). The acellular cardiac jelly is shown in F. Later, mesenchyme cells will migrate from the endothelial cells to populate the cardiac jelly. Modified from Sadler.[2]

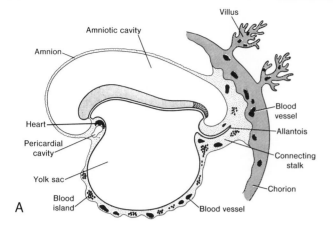

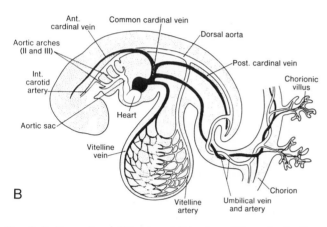

Fig. 3–8. Formation of blood vessels in the yolk sac, chorioallantoic placenta, and embryo. A. Angiogenic cell clusters form blood islands (endothelial sacs containing blood cells) that will later link up to form blood vessels in the yolk sac and placenta. Angiogenic clusters also form in the embryo's splanchnic mesoderm (not shown). B. The principal intra- and extraembryonic vessels of an embryo of approximately 36 days gestational age. From Sadler.[2]

the invaginating otic placode (Figs. 3–6, 3–11), which gives rise not only to the sensory apparatus but also to the neurons of the eighth nerve ganglion. The middle and external ears become associated with the inner ear and are derived principally from neural crest mesenchyme. The olfactory apparatus develops from the olfactory placode (Fig. 3–3F), which also plays a major role in primary palate development (see Fig. 3–21, below). Receptors and neurons, including those found in the olfactory nerve, are also derived from the placode.

Skeletal and connective tissues

The multiple origins of skeletal and connective tissues have already been noted. Most of these tissues are derived from the mesoderm, with skeletal and connective tissues of neural crest origin being largely limited to the head and neck (see Fig. 3–18). Regardless of their initial location, most of the primordial cells are appparently able to differentiate into certain derivatives such as general connective tissues, while only a small number may be able to form certain skeletal derivatives. Odontoblasts, for example, are derived only from neural crest cells. As is discussed later, the specific morphology of the skeletal elements may be programmed into a small number of primordial cells (e.g., crest cells at a particular location in the neural folds). All cell populations giving rise to skeletal and connective tissues, therefore, are not equivalent.

The fates of different populations of mesodermal progenitor cells is variable. Sclerotome cells give rise to the axial skeleton (spinal column and so forth) and to large portions of the cranial skeleton. On the other hand, the dermatome forms only limited portions of the dermis overlying the somites. Intermediate mesoderm forms the connective tissue of the urogenital system. Splanchnic mesoderm forms the connective tissue of other viscera, including the mesothelium. Somatic mesoderm froms both skeletal and connective tissues of the body wall and limbs and portions of the neck.

Cranial neural crest cells form almost all of the skeletal and connective tissues of the face and anterior neck and a considerable portion of the cranial base and vault (see Figs. 3–6, 3–18). This population of cells has been studied extensively

Fig. 3–9. The myotomes of somites give rise to the contractile cells in skeletal voluntary muscle. Those in the forelimb migrate as a condensed mesenchymal mass (A) into the core of the limb bud (see text). Later, they split into extensor and flexor groups, and the core

becomes occupied by mesenchyme that forms skeletal elements (B). The origins and migrations of the visceral arch and extrinsic ocular myoblasts is more complex (see Fig. 3–19 and related text). Modified from Sadler.[2]

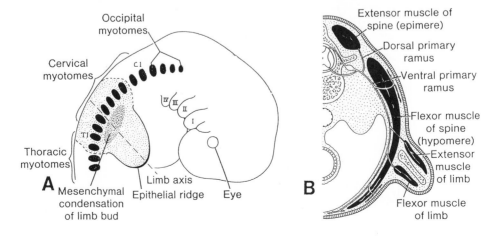

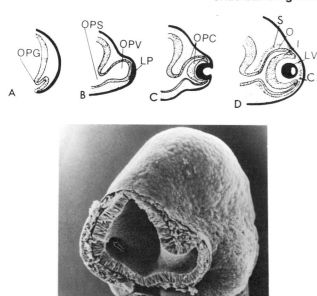

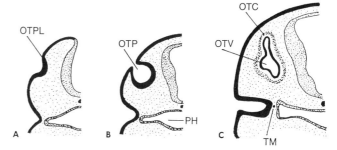

Fig. 3–11. Development of the inner ear. The otic placode (OTPL) invaginates to form the otic pit (OTP). The otic epithelium separates from the surface to form the otic vesicle (OTV) and becomes surrounded by the otic capsule (OTC). The tympanic membrane (TM) and pharynx (PH) are also shown. Modified from Waterman and Meller.[12]

Fig. 3–10. Development of the eye as seen in frontal sections. The optic groove (OPG) in A is the initial outpouching of the forebrain that forms the optic vesicle (OPV in B), which remains connected to the forebrain by the optic stalk (OPS in B). On contact of the optic vesicle with the overlying epithelium, the vesicle induces the epithelium to differentiate into the thickened lens placode (LP in B). The lens placode invaginates with the invaginating optic cup (OPC in C). Finally, the lens vesicle (LV in D) pinches off from the overlying ectoderm and separates from the optic cup. The inner layer of the optic vesicle (I in D) forms the neural retina, while the outer layer (O in D) forms the pigmented retina. Almost all of the sclera and all of the corneal stroma (CS) are of neural crest origin. The scanning EM specimen in E is slightly less advanced than the frontal section in B. The section is asymmetric, cutting in front of the eye vesicle on the embryo's right side. A solid arrow indicates the opening into the cavity of the optic stock. The open arrow indicates the tip of the developing mandibular process. A–D modified from Waterman and Meller.[12] E from Johnston and Sulik.[17]

with respect to both normal and abnormal development, and further details are provided below.

Urogenital development

The intermediate mesoderm (Fig. 3–3H), or the urogenital ridge, gives rise to the urinary and genital systems. Urinary development repeats phylogenetic development by first forming a vestigial pronephros, then a temporarily functional mesonephros, and, finally, the definitive metanephros (Fig. 3–12). The collecting ducts for the mesonephros and metanephros (Fig. 3–13) develop as invaginations from the peritoneal surface cells. Other tubules form from condensation in the mesenchyme, the terminal portions of which form Bowman's capsule at one end and connect with the collecting ducts at the other (Fig. 3–13). Vascular networks within the cavity encompassed by Bowman's capsules form the glomeruli.

Development of the genital system is closely related to the mesonephros (Fig. 3–14). Primordial germ cells migrate

from the yolk sac into the genital ridge. Also, during the sexually indifferent stage, a new paramesonephric (Müllerian) duct (Fig. 3–14) develops from a mesothelial invagination. In the male, the developing testis produces a Müllerian-inhibiting substance and testosterone. Testosterone stabilizes the mesonephric duct, and the testosterone derivative dihydrotestosterone is responsible for development of the external male genitalia. Sperm are collected by a modified mesonephric duct system (Fig. 3–15), while the paramesonephric duct regresses. Since testosterone is absent in the female, the mesonephric duct regresses. Estrogen may be involved in development of the uterine tubes and uterus (Fig. 3–16). Development of external genitalia and part of the vagina is stimulated by estrogen.

Fig. 3–12. Early development of the urinary system. A. Evolution of the urinary system is recapitulated in the human embryo. All components develop from the intermediate mesoderm. B. The pronephros was the earliest to evolve and is only vestigial in the human embryo. The mesonephric system is functional for a period but eventually regresses, apart from the persisting mesonephric duct in the male, which forms the ductus deferens in the male embryos (see Fig. 3–15). The metanephros forms the definitive urinary system. From Sadler.[2]

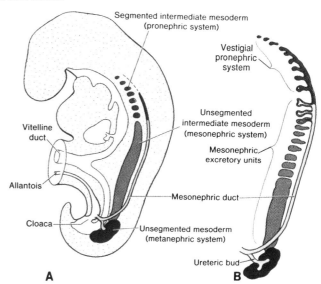

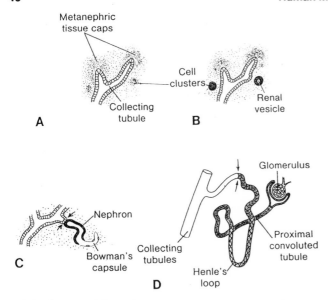

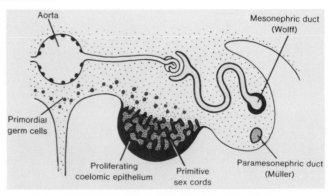

Fig. 3–14. At this early stage, the development of the gonad has not yet begun to diverge into the male testis and female ovary. The primitive sex cords are extensions from the celomic epithelium, and the primordial germ cells are migrating from the yolk sac. The mesonephric system is still functioning at this stage in development. From Sadler.[2]

Fig. 3–13. Development of the permanent kidney involves two developing systems. The collecting tubules are extensions of the ureteric bud (see Fig. 12B), which invades the metanephric mesenchyme. The excretory unit develops from this mesenchyme, first appearing as cell clusters (in A and B) that form vesicles (in B), which then form tubules that connect with the collecting ducts at one end (arrows in C and D) and form Bowman's capsules at the other end (C). The indentation in the capsules becomes invaded by blood vessels that form the glomeruli (D). From Sadler.[2]

Covering and lining epithelia and their derivatives—general comments on epithelial–mesenchymal interactions

Interactions between epithelia and mesenchyme dominate development of the digestive and respiratory systems, the integument, and the limbs. For this reason a few general comments are in order. Epithelial–mesenchymal interactions are dominated by the mesenchymal component. For example, experimentally abnormal epithelial–mesenchymal combinations show that resulting structures differentiate according to the mesenchymal source. Combinations of tooth papilla mesenchyme and leg epithelium result in the production of enamel matrix by the leg epithelia. Thus the fact that the anterior two-thirds of the oral cavity is lined with epithelia of ectodermal origin while that of the posterior one-third (oropharynx) is lined with epithelia of endodermal origin may have little developmental relevance. It is possible that the epithelia may exert some form of growth control, but the nature of such control is uncertain and the source of the epithelium may matter little. While there is morphologic evidence of epithelial–mesenchymal interactions (e.g., the mesenchymal cell process meshwork to be described later), the mechanisms of such interactions remain unclear.

Digestive and respiratory systems

Some aspects of the digestive and respiratory systems were considered in the section dealing with the development of body cavities. Development of the head and neck components of these systems (the naso-oro-pharyngeal complex) is complicated and is emphasized in this section.

Part of the complexity of naso-oro-pharyngeal development is related to evolutionary changes. Much speculation has been devoted to this topic, particularly the role of neural crest cells.[13–15] Only brief reference to the problem is made in this review. In chordates, such as the amphioxus, the anterior end of the animal consists of a series of visceral arches through which fluid is moved by ciliary motion controlled by an extensive neuronal network. This fluid movement permits both gas exchange and the acquisition of food. With the evolution of the jawless fishes (cyclostomes, of which the lamprey is an existing example), development of cartilage and muscle in the visceral arches permitted the movement of fluid by a pumping action, a system used by other contemporary fish (all of which have jaws): teleosts (bony fishes, such as the salmon) and elasmobranchs (cartilagenous fishes, such as the shark). The skeletal elements of the visceral arches, as well as the jaws and middle ear ossicles, are of neural crest origin. It has been argued that cells of the pharyngeal neuronal net of the chordates have been modified to form cartilage. Also of possible relevance are the odontoblasts and similar cells in the denticles of shark skin and other "bony" plates that may have some neural function as well as a skeletal/connective tissue–forming function. The neural crest origin of other skeletal and connective tissues (Figs. 3–6 and 3–18), including similar skeletal and connective tissue elements in cyclostomes, is more difficult to explain. The "lung" developed as an air bladder (used in controlling depth) in higher fishes and as a conventional lung (for respiratory function) in the contemporary lung fish. The nasal (olfactory) system remained separate from the digestive and respiratory systems in fish but became an integral component of these systems in amphibia.

Development of the naso-oro-pharyngeal complex begins with formation of the olfactory placode (Fig. 3–3F). The next major event is the migration of neural crest cells into the frontonasal and visceral arch regions (Fig. 3–17). Also illustrated in Figure 3–17 is the initial establishment of the cranial sensory ganglion, which, unlike their counterparts in the trunk, have some of their neurons originating from surface ectodermal placodes. Most of the neural crest cells eventually differentiate into skeletal and connective tissues, the distribution of which is illustrated in Figure 3–18. Crest cells surround the mesoderm already present in the visceral arch. These mesodermal cells form only components of the vascular system, and, once these components are formed, the remaining mesodermal cells die.[16] They are eventually re-

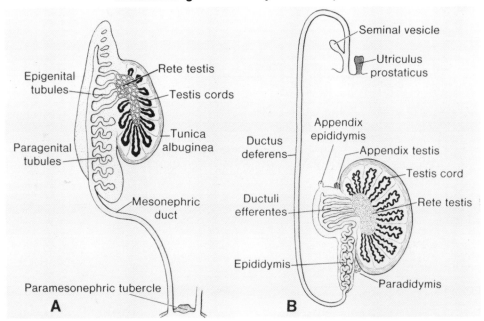

Fig. 3–15. Genital ducts and testis of the male embryo before (A) and after (B) the descent of the testis. The germinal epithelium (testis cords) develops primarily from the sex cords shown in Figure 3–14.

They are connected via the rete testis to the ductule efferentes, epididymis, and ductus deferens, all of which are derived from the mesonephric duct. From Sadler.[2]

placed by myoblasts migrating in from somites and somitomeres (Fig. 3–19).[17,18] The endodermal origin of epithelial components of the pharyngeal glands is illustrated in Figure 3–20. Their connective tissue components are derived from neural crest. The anterior pituitary arises from oral ectoderm and also has connective tissues of crest origin.

Development of the primary palate is illustrated in Figure 3–21. It forms the initial separation between nasal and oral cavities and eventually gives rise to portions of the nose, upper lip, and anterior maxilla. Palatal shelves extending

from the inner portion of the maxillary prominences form the secondary palate. The secondary palate gives rise to most of the bony palate and to all of the soft palate.

The integument

The integument consists of the epidermis, dermis, and skin appendages, such as hair, nails, and sweat, sebaceous, and mammary glands. The sebaceous glands are often associated with hair follicles. Melanoblasts invade the epidermal basal

Fig. 3–16. The ovary and genital ducts of the female embryo. The uterine tube (in A) is derived from the paramesonephric duct and forms the Fallopian tube and the uterus and a small portion of the

vagina as in B (transition not shown). Only vestigial elements of the mesonephros are found in the older embryo (B). From Sadler.[2]

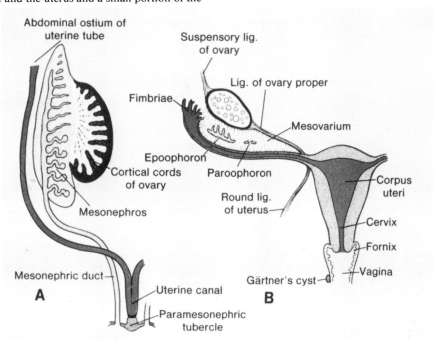

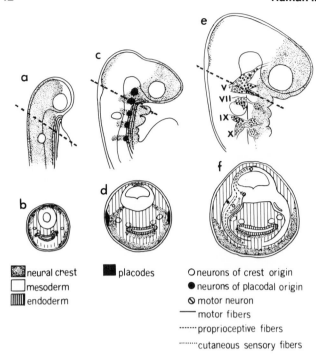

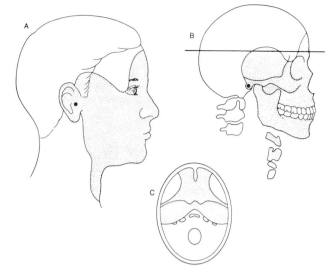

Fig. 3–17. Pattern of cranial neural crest migration (a,b) and formation of the cranial sensory ganglia. At the completion of crest cell (stipple) migration, cords of these cells have maintained contact with the neural tube, and these cords will form the initial primordia of the cranial sensory ganglia (c,d). Ganglionic placodal cells migrate into the distal portions of the ganglia, and these placodal cells will form the earliest differentiating neurons (e,f). Other neurons (e,f) and supporting cells in the ganglia are derived from the neural crest cells. From Johnston and Hazelton.[176]

Fig. 3–18. Apparent distribution (stipple) of connective (A) and skeletal (B,C) tissues of crest origin in the head and neck. Of the skeletal tissues in the face, only the enamel of the teeth is not of crest origin. The distribution of crest-derived connective tissues (dermis and subcutaneous tissues, voluntary muscle, glands, eyes, meninges, blood vessels, and so forth) roughly coincides with the skeletal tissues. The distribution is roughly coincident with crest cell distribution at the end of migration; see Fig. 3–17c,d. Modified from Johnston MC, Bhakdinaronk A, Reid YC: An expanded role for the neural crest in oral and pharyngeal development, in *Fourth Symposium on Oral Sensation and Perception,* JF Bosma, ed, U.S. Govt. Printing Office, Washington, D.C., 1974, p 37.

layer and differentiate into pigment-packed melanocytes. Naked nerve fibers are also present in the epidermis and are sensitive to noxious (painful) stimuli. The dermis and subcutaneous layers are derived from mesenchyme of many sources, including the dermatome, sclerotome, and somatic portions of the mesoderm, and from the neural crest (Fig. 3–18). While the surface ectoderm is probably responsible for the initial induction of dermis and subcutaneous tissue, considerations outlined earlier indicate that regional patterns such as dermatoglyphic ridging and the amount and distribution of hair and glands are probably under mesenchymal control. Abnormalities, however, could result from the inability of the ectodermal epithelium to respond to the regulating influences of the mesenchyme.

Limb development

Although limb development has been a popular subject for study for many years, some very important aspects are only recently beginning to be understood. This includes the origins of two major types of progenitor cell populations, that is, the skeletal and connective tissue cells that are derived from the lateral plate mesoderm and the myoblasts that are derived from the myotome (Fig. 3–9).[19,20] As in the case of the visceral arches, the myoblasts first migrate into the core of the developing limb and secondarily split up into groups that move peripherally to form the limb muscles. Limb bud development is initiated through an interaction between the

surface ectoderm and underlying somatic mesoderm. The result is the formation of the apical ectodermal ridge (AER; Fig. 3–22), which together with the underlying mesoderm progressively lays down the primordia of skeletal and other components, beginning with the scapula.[19,20] The proximodistal organization of the limb bud (e.g., the thumb to small finger sequence of the hand) is determined by the zone of polarizing activity (ZPA; sometimes termed the *posterior necrotic zone* [PNZ], a name based on the fact that its cells eventually degenerate). As is discussed below, the ZPA may exert its effects by producing a morphogen that diffuses to form a distoproximal gradient across the limb bud. Programmed cell death leads to the elimination of tissue between the developing digits.

Recent findings on the regulation of development

Although information has accumulated steadily on the more descriptive aspects of development such as the origins of cells, the migrations of cells, the interactions between cell populations (as in induction), and the consequences of cell interactions (such as cell differentiation), many of the central questions of development (e.g., the molecular basis of induction and differentiation) remained unresolved. However, the methods of molecular biology show great promise in answering some of these questions. To a large degree, the methodology is catching up with the problems. As might be expected from the rapid increase in information in this area, there is a

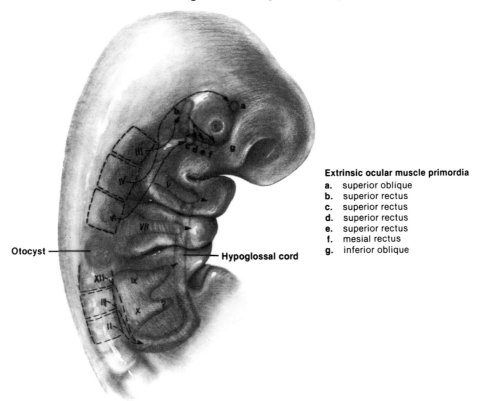

Otocyst ——

—— Hypoglossal cord

Extrinsic ocular muscle primordia
a. superior oblique
b. superior rectus
c. superior rectus
d. superior rectus
e. superior rectus
f. mesial rectus
g. inferior oblique

Fig. 3–19. Almost all of the voluntary (skeletal) musculature in the head and anterior neck is first organized in the visceral arches. Cells of the original mesodermal cores in the visceral arches (see Figs. 17c,d and 21A) undergo cell death once they have vascularized the surrounding neural crest mesenchyme. They are then replaced by myoblasts that migrate from the preotic somitomeres and postotic somites (V, VII, IX, and X). After having reached the visceral arches, many of the myoblasts undergo extensive secondary migra-tions (not shown), such as those from the first arch that will form the temporalis muscle. The first three postotic somites give rise to the hypoglossal cord, which in turn forms the myoblasts of the tongue muscle, and other muscles innervated by the hypoglossal (twelfth) nerve. Finally, the extrinsic ocular muscles arise either from the pre-chordal plate or somitomeric mesoderm (see text) and are inner-vated by cranial nerves III, IV, and VI. From Johnston and Sulik.[7]

considerable amount of confusion and controversy. A brief review of some of the molecular methods and findings pre-cedes an examination of their utilization in understanding abnormal development. Some aspects of their roles in nor-mal development are reviewed by Gilbert[6] and Alberts et al.[20]

Gene function in development

Some relevant aspects of gene structure and function are out-lined in Figure 3–23. Promoters are segments of DNA lo-cated immediately "upstream" that are capable of causing the gene to transcribe a premessenger RNA, which is then processed further into definitive mRNA molecules that through translation form specific proteins. Enhancers, which are often at some distance from the gene, also play a poorly understood role in regulation of gene function. During de-velopment, gene activity can be maintained by a permanent demethylation of its DNA, feedback from cytoplasmic com-ponents, or feedback from extracellular materials. A large number of molecules interact with promoters and enhancers, and the mechanisms by which they alter gene activity is be-ginning to be understood.[6]

It now appears that much of the control of cell differenti-ation is at the level of mRNA processing (Fig. 3–23). In most instances mRNA processing involves only removal of those portions of pre-mRNA that were transcribed by the intron portions of genes. There is increasing evidence that specific portions of the pre-mRNA may be removed and the remain-ing portions recombined through a phenomenon termed *al-ternate gene splicing,* an example of which is illustrated in Figure 3–23. In combination with different promoters being located between exons, alternative gene splicing is presum-ably responsible for the generation of different isoforms of compounds such as RARβs and TGFαs, as will be discussed below. The regulation of alternative gene splicing in differ-entiating cells is unknown. An excellent contemporary re-view of this problem is found in Gilbert.[6]

Through the use of restriction enzymes that cleave DNA at specific points, it is possible to break down DNA into frag-ments that contain genes or parts of genes.[20] These fragments are termed *restriction fragment length polymorphisms* (RFLPs). A fragment can be spliced into bacterial DNA through the use of viruses and large amounts of mRNA pro-duced. It is then possible to make DNA that is complemen-tary to the mRNA, which is termed a DNA *probe.* Such probes are usually radiolabeled so that they can be used to detect the presence of specific RFLPs by Southern blot hy-bridization or to locate specific mRNAs in tissue sections through in situ hybridization. As is discussed below, there is now a tremendous amount of research being conducted on

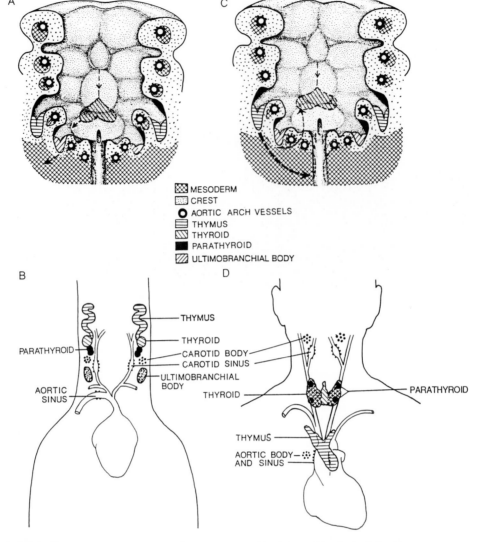

Fig. 3–20. Comparative development of the pharyngeal glands and chemoreceptors (carotid body) and baroreceptors in avian and human embryos. In A and B, the primordia of the glands in the two classes are virually identical. Movements of the primordia in later development (B and D) display a tendency to displace the primordia laterally in avians and medially in humans. Note the fusion of the ultimobranchial body with the thyroid in the human, which is responsible for bringing the neural crest calitonian cells into the thyroid. Modified from Johnston et al.[177]

embryos using in situ hybridization. Immunohistochemical procedures to determine the locations of embryonic proteins and other molecules are also widely used.

Another method for studying the roles of genes in development is to splice genes with active promoters into fertilized eggs or other embryonic cells of mice, which are then incorporated into the embryonic cell masses by injecting them into the blastula cavity (Fig. 3–3D).[21] Frequently, a "reporter" gene is also attached to the spliced gene so that the engineered cells can be identified by color reactions or immunohistochemistry in the resulting chimeric mice. In this way, it is possible to study the effects of the mRNA in cells that do not normally contain it. A related technique that is technically more difficult but potentially more powerful is "gene targeting," in which a specific gene is hybridized with a probe which renders it nonfunctional. Through inbreeding it is possible to obtain mouse embryos that are homozygous for the deleted gene and to examine the effects of the absence of the gene product.

The role of regulatory molecules

Another very active area involves the study of the roles of growth factors and hormones of the steroid–thyroxin–retinoic acid "superfamily."[22,23] Transport into cells and the mechanism of gene activation for these two groups of control molecules are illustrated in Figure 3–24.

Growth factors are usually peptides that, although originally studied for their effects on cell proliferation in culture, now appear to have many diverse effects on embryonic development. An example is the apparent role of members of the transforming growth factor (TGFβ) family in the induction of mesodermal cells as the first inductive interaction in development. Although most of the studies have been conducted on amphibian embryos,[24] work on the chick embryo, which is morphologically similar to the human embryo, indicates that the inducing cells (responsible for production of the substance) are in the caudal region of the hypoblast.[25,26] The peptide's (sometimes termed *activin* or *vitellin*) mRNA

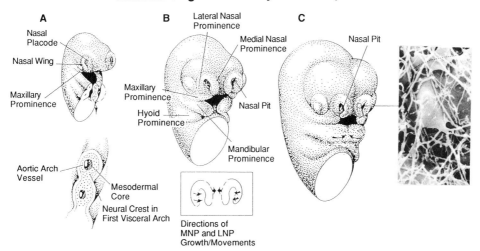

Fig. 3–21. At the completion of their migrations, crest cells surround the mesodermal cores in the visceral arches (A) and form all the mesenchyme between the covering epithelium and underlying brain and eye in portions of the face above the oral cavity. Maintenance of high proliferation rates (possibly mediated by cell process meshwork underlying the epithelium, which has been removed in the scanning EM in C) and major morphogenetic movements (summarized in the inset in B) are responsible for facial prominence formation, and their contact initiates separation between the developing oral and nasal cavities. Failure of this contact leads to cleft lip. Modified from Johnston and Sulik.[7]

is present in the appropriate cells at the appropriate time and when added to media used for epiblast culture (or comparable structures from amphibian embryos) the peptide is able to induce a mesodermal "organizer" that then leads to the development of a primitive embryo.

This is only one example of a growth factor involved in regulating one aspect of embryonic development. Others are TGFα (an embryonic epidermal growth factor [EGF], variants of which are associated with some types of human cleft lip and palate), nerve growth factor (NGF), fibroblast growth factor (FGF), and platelet-derived growth factor (PDGF).

Evans[23] has reviewed the evolution and functions of the steroid–thyroxin–retoinic acid "superfamily," and Melton[24] and others[25,26] have reviewed their role in development. Particular attention has been focused on retinoic acid with respect to limb development and many other aspects of development.[27–30] At least three groups of retinoic acid receptors have been identified (RARα, β, and γ). They appear to have specific functions in development, e.g., RARβ for regulating programmed cell death (probably not its only function), and RARγ for cartilage development. As is discussed below, many retinoids are teratogens. Interest has been greatly stimulated by the human malformations resulting from the use of 13-*cis*-retinoic acid (isotretinoin, Accutane; an isomer of the all-*trans*-RA normally present).

Homeobox and related genes

Numerous studies, conducted primarily on *Drosophila* (the fruit fly) but with apparent major human relevance, have shed considerable light on the roles of gradients in segmental and field development and the coordination of development in complex structures such as limbs. In the *Drosophila* embryo, initial cephalocaudal segmentation is regulated by a maternally synthesized glycoprotein that falls in concentration from the head to the tail. Further divisions within the segments are controlled by other regulatory genes. Finally, "homeotic" genes are responsible for coordinating the development of structures such as legs and antennas from specific segments and subsegments. Most of these regulatory genes have a common or very similar segment or "box" that appears to be involved in binding the regulatory molecules to specific DNA segments. These molecules have been highly conserved during evolution, and comparable genes have been identified in mammals, including humans. Their possible roles in normal and abnormal human development are considered in the next section.

Fig. 3–22. Limb bud development. A. Early limb bud development is largely regulated by the apical ectodermal ridge, along with underlying mesenchyme and the zone of polarizing activity. B. Late limb bud development is characterized by cell death (stipple) between the developing digits, leading to their separation. The function of the interior cell death is unknown. The broken lines indicate the locations of condensing cartilage primordia. Modified from Tabin.[19]

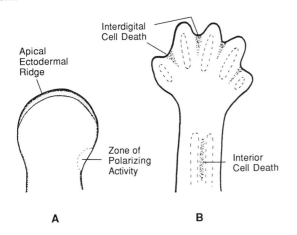

Abnormal development

Human developmental abnormalities often provide information relevant to normal developmental mechanisms. Par-

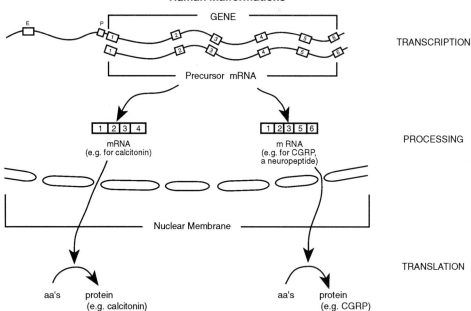

Fig. 3–23. Gene regulation and RNA processing. Promotors (P) are segments of DNA that initiate transcription of the gene located immediately downstream. The promotor can be activated in many ways, such as by growth factors (see Fig. 3–24). Enhancers (E), which may be located at some distance from the gene, also influence gene transcription when they are brought into proximity of the gene by looping of the chromosome. The entire DNA segment of the gene is transcribed to form premessenger RNA, which is then processed in the nucleus to remove the segments transcribed by the introns shown as lines connecting the numbered exons. Only then can the messenger RNA be moved through the nuclear pores into the cy-toplasm. Usually all RNA transcribed by the exons is perserved to form the definitive mRNA. However, it now appears that through a process termed *alternate gene splicing,* different portions of the precursor RNA may be eliminated and the remaining portions spliced together to form distinctly different mRNAs that give rise to distinctly different proteins through translation. The example used above is the calcitonin-CGRP gene, which is responsible for the formation of calcitonin in the C cells of the thyroid and a neuropeptide (CGRP) in the brain. The translated protein may undergo further modification, as in the transformation of procollagen to collagen.

Fetal alcohol syndrome (FAS) and the holoprosencephalies

It now appears that the full FAS (Fig. 3–25) results from developmental alterations occurring at the time of germ layer formation. This occurs at about gestational day 17 (stage 8), so early in pregnancy that the mother is usually not yet aware that she is pregnant. Information about the interactions between the chorda-mesoderm and the developing neural plate may be of considerable importance with respect to the pathogenesis of the FAS and a number of other human malformations such as the holoprosencephalies (apparently including the FAS) and cyclopia (Figs. 3–26, 3–27).[31–33] Many years ago, Adelmann[31] showed that it was possible to create cyclopia (single large median eye) by removing the prechordal plate (Fig. 3–3F), while Holtfreter[11,32] showed that cyclopia could be produced by interfering with gastrulation movements.

Ethanol administration to pregnant mice at about this stage of development produces a somewhat different series of malformations,[34–38] which are similar to most human holoprosencephalies (Figs. 3–25, 3–26, 3–27).[39–41] The term *holoprosencephaly* relates to diminished forebrain size, which frequently results in a single ventricle in place of the first three ventricles, i.e., a "single cavity forebrain" holoprosen-cephaly. While eye size is diminished, a single midline eye is not found in the mouse fetuses (see below).

Although mesoderm is severely depleted in the ethanol mouse model, it is not clear whether this leads to the midline deficiency in the anterior neural plate or whether the neural plate problem is a direct effect of the ethanol. In less severely affected specimens, facial and brain malformations are very similar to those seen in the FAS (Fig. 3–25).[34–38] Starting with the clearly defined deficiency of the midline portion of the anterior neural plate, the sequence of developmental changes leads to closer approximation of the olfactory placodes, deficient medial nasal prominences, and loss of midline facial structures (Fig. 3–26). The midline loss may be very precise in single gene human holoprosencephalies with apparent loss of the mesial halves of upper central incisors leading to formation of a symmetric midline tooth.[39–41] More severely affected mouse embryos show placodal contact (Fig. 3–26E) and malformations similar to arhinencephaly (Fig. 3–27B), another variant of the holoprosencephalies.[38] We have not observed the intermediate cleft lip and palate seen in human holoprosencephalies.[36,37] This may be because the mouse strain used (C57Bl/6J) is cleft lip resistant.

In both the mouse and human holoprosencephalies (Fig. 3–27), the eyes, while progressively reduced in size, never form a single large midline eye.[37,39,40] For this reason, the formation of a single large eye or of large "fused" eyes (cyclopia and synophthalmia) do not appear to be part of the series and may result from specific elimination or failure of formation of the prechordal plate leading to midline fusion of the bilateral eye fields as in Adelmann's experiments.[31] He reasoned

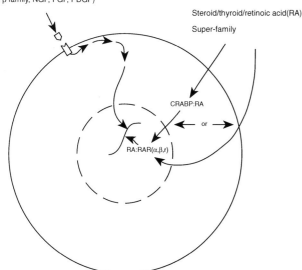

Growth factors

(e.g. TGFα family (similar to EGF),

TGFβ family, NGF, FGF, PDGF)

Steroid/thyroid/retinoic acid(RA)

Super-family

CRABP:RA

or

RA:RAR(α,β,r)

Fig. 3–24. Schematic diagram representing the interactions of two main groups of regulatory substances with embryonic cells. The growth factors are usually peptides that are soluble in blood and tissue fluids but require specific membrane components to get them into the cell. Further interactions with membrane-bound and cytoplasmic compounds are required for the alterations in gene function. The second major group is made up of hormones of the steroid–thyroxin–retinoic acid (RA) "superfamily." The hormones are insoluble and are transported in blood and tissue fluids by carrier proteins. Unlike the growth factors, they easily pass through cell membranes and complex with intracellular receptors. The resulting complexes alter gene function. The role of intracellular binding proteins for RA (CRABPs) is unclear. It was initially thought that they "presented" the RA to the receptors, but the finding that some cells responsive to RA do not have binding proteins has complicated this interpretation (for further discussion, see text).

that the prechordal plate is necessary for the formation of the thinned floor plate, which normally separates the eye fields in a manner similar to the effect of the notochord on the development of the neural tube.[32] The bilateral eye fields would then fuse in the midline, giving the large medial eye found in cyclopia or the large "fused" eyes found in synophthalmia. It

should be noted that in a recent study on a mutant fish embryo with cyclopia/synophthalmia, the floor plate never forms and the authors conclude that it is the neural plate's inability to respond to the notochord and prechordal plate that leads to cyclopia/synophthalmia.[33] In contrast, parachordal mesoderm has a stimulatory effect on neural tube and neural plate development.[32,42] Deficiency in this mesoderm could lead to the bilateral smaller eyes seen in the most common holoprosencephalies. As observed in Sulik's laboratory (K. K. Sulik, personal communication) and in the author's laboratory, C57Bl/6J mice have a low incidence of similar malformations, and there may be a basic mesodermal defect in this strain, as is discussed later in relation to otocephaly.

Otocephaly

The dominant features of human otocephaly are agnathia (or, occasionally, micrognathia), microstomia, and external ears that are separated by a major "cleft" and are sometimes close to the midline (Fig. 3–28).[40,43] Some of the features of holoprosencephaly are found in many cases, such as absence of the philtrum (cf. Fig. 3–28B and 3–27A) or even apparent failure of medial nasal prominences (Fig. 3–21) to form (cf. Fig. 3–28C and 3–27B) as in arhinecephaly (premaxillary agenesis) formation. Severe forebrain reductions (holoprosencephaly type) are sometimes found, and this combination is termed *agnathia-holoprosencephaly*.[39,43]

Two animal models with spontaneous otocephaly have been studied extensively.[45,46] In both cases, holoprosencephaly is part of the spectrum. In the mouse model,[46] a balanced Robertsonian translocation in C57Bl/6J mice, the mandibular loss is associated with premature cell death in the mesodermal core of the mandibular arch, prior to vascularization of the surrounding crest cells. As noted earlier, these core cells are involved in vascularization of the surrounding crest cell mesenchyme, and normally undergo cell death once the mesenchyme is vascularized.[16] In the mouse otocephaly model,[46] the crest mesenchyme cells are apparently lost secondarily and the mandibular arch degenerates. Thus the crest cell involvement is secondary rather than primary, as had been postulated earlier.[45,47] More extensive (and/or earlier) mesodermal involvement presumably accounts for the more severely affected specimens.

Fig. 3–25. Children (A,B) with the fetal alcohol syndrome (FAS) compared with FAS (C) and control (D) mouse embryos. Affected structures are indicated. These changes are very consistent. From Sulik et al.[34]

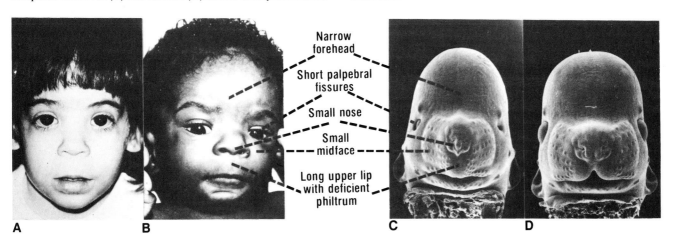

Narrow forehead

Short palpebral fissures

Small nose

Small midface

Long upper lip with deficient philtrum

A B C D

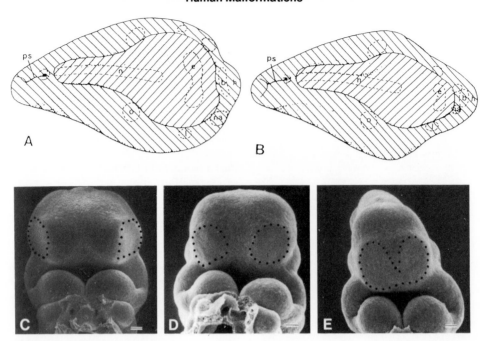

Fig. 3–26. Maternal ethanol treatment narrows the anterior neural plate (compare B with control embryos in A), apparently due to developmental failure of the midline portion. The olfactory placodes are moved toward the midline to a moderate to severe degree (compare dotted outlines in D and E to control embryo in C; see also B). Also, the eye fields (e) are reduced (B). Other structures are na, nasal (olfactory) placode; b, buccopharyngeal membrane; h, heart; l, lens placode; o, otic placode; n, notochord; ps, primitive streak. A and B modified from Johnston and Sulik.[7] C–E modified from Sulik.[178]

FAS features, usually associated with micrognathia, have been observed to occur spontaneously in a small number (less than 1%) of C57Bl/6J embryos, both in Sulik's laboratory (K. K. Sulik, personal communication) and in our laboratory. The possibility that the Robertsonian translocation in the Juriloff et al.[46] study is merely permitting greater expression of an inherent defect is thoroughly discussed in their report. Thus the C57Bl/6J mouse model for the ethanol-induced FAS described above is already genetically predisposed for this defect. The absence of mandibular effects in the FAS model may be a matter of timing. This predisposition to FAS presumably also accounts for the FAS features observed in C57Bl/6J mice following administration of very low doses of 13-*cis*-retinoic acid (see below) at the time of germ layer formation. Such features have not been reported for humans exposed to this compound at the same stage in pregnancy.

Neural tube defects (NTDs)

Most NTDs appear to result from partial or complete failure of closure of the neural tube. While normal closure was briefly described in the normal overview section, a consideration of closure defects warrants a more complete description of the mechanisms involved.

The force leading to neural tube closure appears to be generated by a terminal web apparatus (Fig. 3–29), which is probably universal to many epithelial foldings and other epithelial shape changes that occur throughout embryonic development. At this stage of development, the neural plate is a simple columnar epithelium with cells extending from the basal to the future luminal surface of the neuroepithelium. The web consists of circumferential rings of actin filament that encircle the cells at their luminal ends. The filaments are anchored at one end into the membranes of the cells. Interactions of the filaments with myosin in the cell cytoplasm causes the ring to contract, thereby decreasing the diameter of this end of the cell (Fig. 3–29). Since the cells are all connected together at their luminal ends, concerted contraction of all the cells throughout a portion of the neural plate has the effect of decreasing the surface area and warping the epithelium. Microtubules running longitudinally through the cells appear to maintain cell length. Restriction of possible movements, presumably by the notochord and the surrounding tissues, appears to limit the neural plate shape change largely to a folding movement. In rodent embryos the morphogenetic movement is very complex, and Sadler et al.[49] have shown a very nice correlation between the sites of morphogenetic change and the concentration of polymerized actin and myosin. Other factors, such as matrix synthesis beneath the neural folds, apparently promote neural tube closure.[50] The relation between dietary folate and NTDs also indicates that (differential) cell proliferation is a factor.

Even before the neural folds make contact, the epithelium is undergoing changes that apparently mediate contact and adhesion. The epithelial cells in the area of future contact send out long processes in the direction of the opposite neural fold.[51] Once contact is made the neural folds fuse with each other, as does the overlying surface epithelium. Penetration of mesenchymal cells between the neural tube and the surface epithelium further consolidates the fusion.

It is probable that most NTDs (partial or complete failure to close, as in anencephaly and spina bifida) arise because of failure of neural fold elevation and contact. Experimentally, this can be achieved through the use of cytochalasin D, a substance that interferes with actin polymerization.[52–54] Further

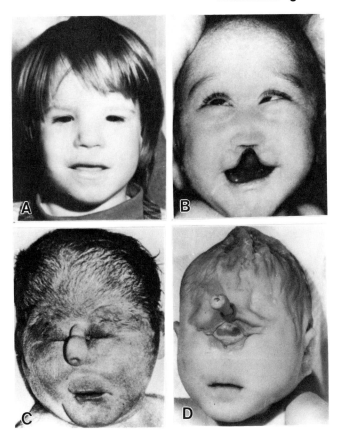

Reducing the recurrence rates for NTDs by maternal vitamin supplementation during pregnancy is somewhat controversial.[57-60] Convincing evidence has recently been found that folate supplementation by itself is effective,[59,60] suggesting that cell proliferation is also important in neural tube closure.

Experimentally, NTDs can be produced after neural tube closure.[61] In this case, drug-induced cell death in tissues dorsal to the neural tube resulted in postclosure opening. It seems unlikely that many human NTDs are produced by the mechanism.

Malformations with major (primary) involvement of the cranial neural crest (retinoic acid syndrome and related malformations)

Studies of the malformations of the human retinoic acid syndrome (RAS; retinoic acid embryopathy; Fig. 3–30) and animal models designed to determine its pathogenesis provide one of the best examples of how an abnormality of human development provides indirect evidence about normal developmental mechanisms. Other teratogens and altered homeobox gene activity produce similar malformations. The relevance of these studies to the human DiGeorge syndrome, hemifacial microsomia, and other malformations will also be discussed. An understanding of these malformations is dependent on information about the mechanisms of crest cell differentiation and migration and on the axial organization of the neural crest and head segmentation. A brief review of this material is in order.

Fig. 3–27. A–C represent holoprosencephalies of increasing severity. The child with the fetal alcohol syndrome (A) has a mild form; arhinencephaly or premaxillary agenesis (B) is of intermediate severity; ethmocephaly (C) is the most severe expression. Eye size apparently decreases with increasing severity. The single large eye seen in cyclopia perfecta (D) probably arises by a somewhat different mechanism (see text). A courtesy Dr. Sterling Clarren; B from Ross and Johnston[179]; C from Taysi and Tinaztepe[180]; D from Gorlin et al.[40]

The differentiation and migration of neural crest cells

Crest cells differentiate as the most lateral portion of the neural plate (Fig. 3–3) and are presumably under the same inductive influences as the neural plate in general, although little definitive information is available on this point. However, the early loss of cell adhesion molecules (CAMs), which bind neural crest cells to each other and to other neural plate cells, and the formation of cell surface fibronectin receptors, have been described in some detail.[62] Also, components in the matrix through which crest cells migrate and how these cells make attachments to matrix molecules (e.g., fibonectin) have also been described.[62] The changing morphology of crest cells

evidence that neural tube closure is usually the problem is the fact that mouse embryos in a glucose-deficient culture medium have delayed neural tube closure.[55] Approximately 95% of the ATP generated by the embryo at this stage of development is derived from anaerobic glucose metabolism[56]

Fig. 3–28. Otocephaly. A, B: Typical malformation with severe microstomia and small philtrum. The defect between the ears (also seen in C) apparently results from degeneration of the mandibular arch (see text). C: The lack of median nasal prominence derivatives in this specimen is also seen in arhinencephaly (Fig. 3–27B). From Gorlin et al., 1990.[40]

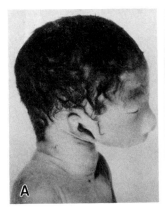 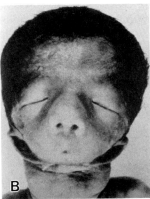 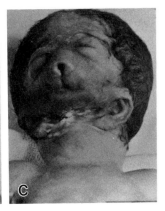

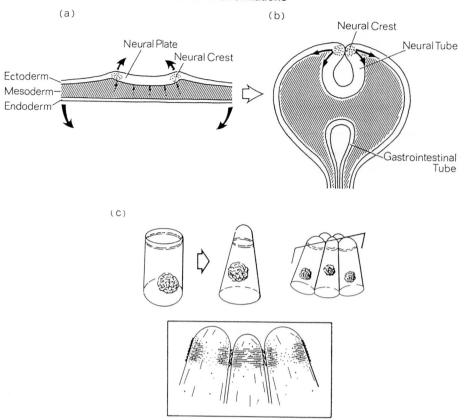

Fig. 3–29. a. Cross section through three germ layer embryo. The neural plate has been induced by an inductive stimulus passing from underlying mesoderm (broken arrows). The initiation of neural plate and lateral wall folding processes is indicated by solid arrows. b. Following fusion of approximating surfaces the neural tube and gastrointestinal tubes will separate from the embryo's surface. The directions of neural crest migration are indicated by arrows. The po-

sition of the terminal web, the actinomyosin network that provides the force for neural tube closure, is just below the luminal surface. c. Changes in the shape of columnar neuroepithelial cells shown in the ventral portion of the neural tube in (b). The terminal web encircles the luminal ends of the neuroepithelial cells as shown in three-dimensional sketches and section (box). a and c from Johnston and Pratt.[181]

migrating into the corneal stroma has been studied by time lapse photomicroscopy[63] and is similar to that of the crest cells illustrated in Figure 3–31.

Head segmentation and the neural crest

Figure 3–32 is from a recent review on head development by Noden.[64] It schematically presents the segmental relations of different components in the embryonic head and neck, ignoring for clarity the fact that all structures are not present at the same time. For example, by the time the fourth aortic arch vessel has developed, the first aortic arch vessel has already regressed.

Several observations have highlighted the importance of head segmentation. While all cranial neural crest cell populations have the ability to respond to environmental cues from the pharyngeal arch endoderm to form cartilage, the morphology of these skeletal elements depends on the initial axial position of the crest cells. If, prior to their migration, second arch crest cells are replaced with first arch crest cells, they migrate into the second arch but still form first arch skeletal elements in response to the second arch environment.[65] Also, if crest cells that normally form a major portion of the septal mesenchyme of the conotruncus are replaced by other cranial neural crest cells, the substituted cells are unable to form this mesenchyme.[93]

Expression of different homeobox genes is often confined to particular neuromeres, as indicated in Figure 3–33. The *Hox 2* family shows a peculiar distribution of activity. *Hox 2.9* is only expressed in neuromere 4, while the remainder show an overlapping distribution, with only *Hox 2.8* expressed in neuromere 3. *Hox 2.7* is added in neuromere 5, *Hox 2.6* in neuromere 7, and *Hox 2.1* in neuromere 9. Of considerable relevance to the axial specificity of crest cells is the very recent observation that *Hox 2* gene expression is found in crest derived from the same neuromeres and that this pattern of expression is eventually found in the ectoderm overlying the arches.[66] It is conceivable that the *Hox 2* genes play a critical role in directing the formation of the visceral arch skeletal elements. These crest cells could conceivably also contribute to the specificity of the second arch ganglionic placode. It has been shown experimentally that when trigeminal placodes are used to replace other ganglionic placodes, the derived neurons still make the appropriate fifth nerve synapses in the brain stem nuclei.[67]

The RAS and related malformations

Because of the wide range of resulting malformations and high degree of reproducibility, retinoids (vitamin A and related compounds) have long been popular as experimental teratogens. It was on the basis of this information that the ret-

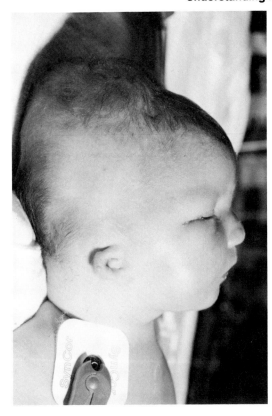

Fig. 3–30. Child with retinoic acid syndrome showing hypoplasia of the external ear and the mandible. These malformations may be largely confined to one side. Courtesy Dr. Paul M. Fernhoff, Emory University School of Medicine, Atlanta, GA.

inoid 13-*cis*-retinoic acid (13-*cis*-RA, isotretinoin, Accutane), used for the treatment of severe cystic acne, was marketed in 1982 as a category X drug (not to be taken if there is any risk of pregnancy). The therapeutic effectiveness of 13-*cis*-RA led to widespread use, and within 1 yr severely malformed children (Fig. 3–30) were born to mothers who were accidentally exposed.[68,69]

The incidence and severity of the resulting malformations were much higher than predicted.[68] The reason is apparently related to differences in the metabolism of the drug[70] in humans and in experimental animals, particularly the attain-

ment of high blood levels of the 4-oxo-metabolite in the human, about three to five times higher than that of the parent compound.[71] When tested in whole embryo culture, the two compounds are equally teratogenic.[72-74] At the concentration found in human blood, 13-*cis*-RA had only very mild growth effects, but with the addition of an equal amount of 4-oxo-13-*cis* RA developmental alterations resulted that were identical to those occurring in an in vivo mouse model for the RAS.[73]

One of the main targets for 13-*cis*-RA is the neural crest. Particularly affected are the second arch crest cells, most of which are killed before leaving the neural plate.[75] This is a portion of the neural plate where there is normally a large amount of cell death at a slightly later stage, and Morriss[76] and Morriss and Thorogood[77] provided evidence many years ago that its development was inhibited by retinol. This is also the portion of the neural tube where the *Hox-2.9* gene is expressed (see above), and there is a particularly high level of the RA-binding protein CRABP in this portion of the neural tube.[78,79] Expression of the RARβ gene also extends forward into the anterior hind brain region.[80] There is some evidence that, among other functions, RARβ may be involved in regulating normal (programmed) cell death. Also, there is a very high correlation between CRABP and the effects of RA. Certainly CRABP is highest in the dorsal portions of rhombomere 4, coinciding exactly with the area of greatest RA-induced cell death.[75,79]

RA also has effects on migrating crest cells both in vivo[73] and in vitro.[81,82] The peak period of sensitivity to the effects of 13-*cis*-RA on thymus and conotruncal development in the mouse is well after the onset of the crest cells migrating to this region.[73] During migration, crest cells have high levels of CRABP[78,79,84] and also demonstrate high levels of ^{14}C-RA uptake.[83,84] Although not as well documented, migrating crest cells also appear to have at least some RARβ mRNA.[85]

Consistent with the greatest effect being on second arch crest was the finding of only rudimentary development of the second visceral arch, with a missing portion at what would have been the dorsal portion of the arch.[73] The gap would presumably block incoming myoblasts and may account for the facial "paresis" frequently observed in RAS patients.[68]

RAS malformations are frequently unilateral.[68] This may be related to the ability of crest cells to make up for large deficits by additional proliferation.[86,87] Unpublished observations in our laboratory indicate that reductions of the original

Fig. 3–31. Neural crest cells (diamond pattern) before (A) and during (B) the early stages of crest cell migration. They follow two major routes of migration (arrows in B). In the scanning EM shown in C, the surface ectoderm has been peeled back (as indicated in B) to show the three-dimensional morphology of crest cells. The crest cells are frequently bipolar and oriented in the direction of migration (arrow in C). From Johnston and Sulik.[7]

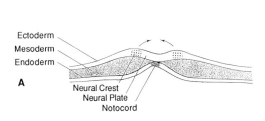

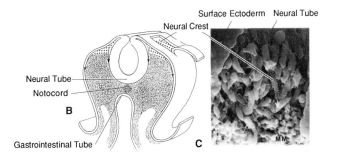

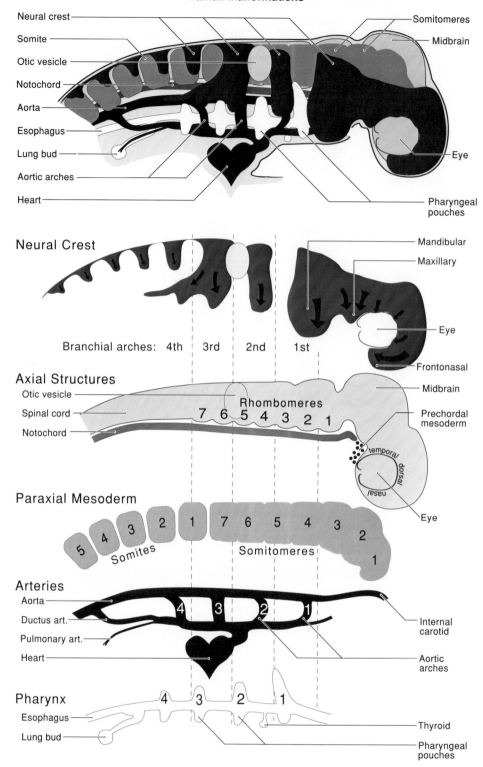

Fig. 3–32. Schematic presentation of different components in the embryonic head and neck emphasizing their segmental relationships. In the upper diagram the surface ectoderm has been removed, illustrating the relationships of the different components, and the remaining diagrams illustrate the components individually. Modified from Noden.[64]

crest cell population by less than 80% lead to almost normal development. Thus a deficit of 75% on one side and 85% on the other could lead to a unilateral malformation.

A dominant feature of the RAS are major effects on the cerebellum in both the human[68,88] and animal models.[73,89] The anterior midline portion (including the vermis) is most affected. The affected portions of the cerebellum are consistent with the greatest concentration of dead cells in mouse embryos from RA-treated mothers.[75]

13-*cis*-RA also has effects on many other cells. These include cells that will form the primary palate, vertebrae, and the limb, as is discussed in later sections.

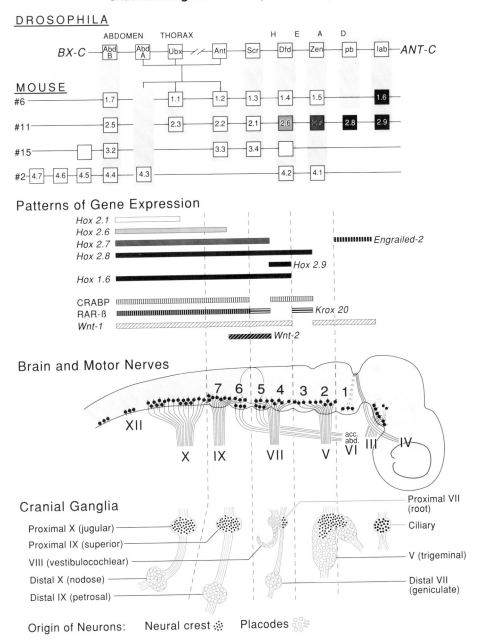

Fig. 3–33. Homeobox gene expression in *Drosophila* and in the head and neck of mouse and chick embryos. The sequential arrangements in the genes of *Drosophila* and mouse are also illustrated. The sequences are also found in human chromosomes. Neuromeres 1–7 are indicated in the diagram of the chick embryo brain. Modified from Noden.[64]

Syndromes with features overlapping those of the RAS

There are a number of human syndromes with malformations similar to the RAS. These include DiGeorge syndrome, hemifacial microsomia, CHARGE association, and Down syndrome. All of these conditions have cardiovascular malformations of the conotruncal type, and in this respect the studies of Kirby and her coinvestigators[90–93] have been particularly helpful. Not only have they shown that postotic cranial neural crest cells make very substantial contributions to the conotruncal septum, but also they have identified the spectrum of cardiovascular malformations resulting from their experimental removal of this neural crest. For example, in addition to the expected abnormalities of the great vessels, the incidence of interventricular septal defects rises, presum-

ably secondary to defects in the conotruncal septum with which the interventricular septum lines up and fuses in normal development. In fact, in the least affected cases interventricular septal defects are often the only cardiovascular defects. Much less consistent are defects of pharyngeal glands, which occur secondarily to removal of postotic cranial neural crest[91] and are found only in RAS and DiGeorge syndrome. This could be explained if the human malformations relate at least partially to problems of crest cell migration, since the distances involved are much greater for crest cells contributing to the conotruncal septum, particularly to that portion closest to the interventricular septum.

The human syndrome that most closely resembles RAS is DiGeorge syndrome (Fig. 3–34).[94–96] Pharyngeal gland and cardiovascular defects are almost identical in the two. How-

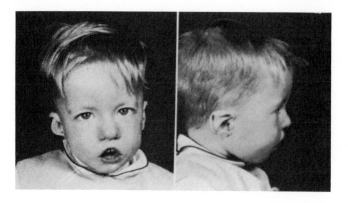

Fig. 3–34. The malformations found in the DiGeorge syndrome are very similar to those found in the retinoic acid syndrome (RAS; see Fig. 3–30). Principle differences are the milder abnormalities of the external and middle ear and the characteristic short medial segment of the upper lip. From Kretschmer et al.[94]

ever, in DiGeorge syndrome, ear and cerebellar malformations are much less severe, and there is a fairly consistent effect on the upper lip, which is vertically short in the midline (Fig. 3–34). The syndrome is sometimes associated with maternal alcoholism.[96]

There are two apparently useful animal models for DiGeorge syndrome. In the first model, ethanol was administered to pregnant mice at a time when preotic crest cells are entering the visceral arches and postotic crest cells have just begun their migrations.[97] This treatment is lethal for a large percentage of the crest cells, even for those entering the frontonasal region, which appear to be virtually unaffected by RA. This may account for the effects on the upper lip in humans (short median portion) and also for a possibly increased incidence of cleft lip with or without cleft palate.[95] Ethanol appears to produce many of its biologic effects through membrane destabilization,[98] which may make migrating cells particularly vulnerable because of their high level of membrane turnover.

Very recently, a particularly interesting model for DiGeorge syndrome was developed.[99] This was a gene "knockout" experiment in mice that rendered one of the homeobox genes *(Hox 1.5)* nonfunctional. The resulting malformations included cardiovascular defects of the conotruncal variety, thymus deficiencies, and a short mandible. The squamous (temporal) bone was deficient, and there was also a "submaxillary" deficiency. Limited studies on pathogenesis indicated that the third and fourth visceral arches were the most severely affected.

Several aspects of Down syndrome (trisomy 21) are similar to DiGeorge syndrome (which maps to chromosome 22). These include very similar upper lip and external ear defects. There is also a high incidence of conotruncal defects. A trisomy 16 mouse model shows many characteristics of Down syndrome.[100] The mouse chromosome 16 is partially homologous with human chromosome 21. Abnormalities are found in the migration of neuronal cells[100] and the cardiac endothelial cells that are migrating to form mesenchyme.[101] Migrating crest cells have not been examined in this model.

Hemifacial microsomia (Fig. 3–35)[102–105] is in many ways similar to RAS (Fig. 3–30). The key features in hemifacial

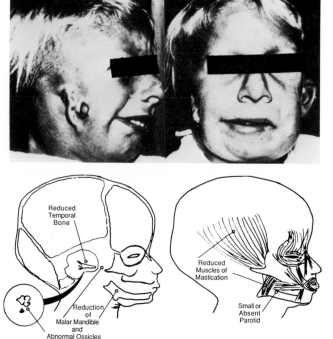

Fig. 3–35. Hemifacial microsomia. In addition to the malformation of the external ear, as seen in this patient, many regional structures are usually deficient (patient and diagram). These include the middle ear ossicles, squamous portion of the temporal bone, mandible, muscles of mastication, and the parotid gland. The malformations are often largely limited to one side, as in the patient illustrated. From Poswillo.[114]

microsomia are abnormalities of the external and middle ears and of other structures in this region. Usually the defects are primarily limited to one side. Most cases have abnormalities of other structures that are often at some distance, such as epibulbar dermoids (connective tissue protuberances on the sclera of the eye, found in approximately 20% of cases), vertebral defects (e.g., hemivertebrae in about 30%), cleft lip and/or palate (5%–22%), and cardiovascular abnormalities (55%–60%), almost always of the conotruncal variety. Attempts have been made to establish heterogeneity. For example, a combination of the ear abnormalities with epibulbar dermoids and vertebral defects are sometimes considered to be oculo-auriculo-vertebral (OAV) syndrome. However, there are many cases with epibular dermoids and no vertebral abnormalities and vice versa.

Hemifacial microsomia illustrates similarities to, and differences from, RAS. External and middle ear defects are similar, and there is a high incidence of conotruncal malformations in both. Although brain malformations may occur in hemifacial microsomia,[105] they rarely involve the cerebellum. There are other important differences. Although the incidence of conotruncal defects is high, no cases of pharyngeal gland deficiencies have been reported in hemifacial microsomia. There is a relatively high incidence of cleft lip, a malformation not reported for RAS. Also, there is a high incidence of vertebral defects,[40,104] in contrast to a paucity of these defects in RAS (E. Lammer, personal communication). RA administered to mice at certain stages (e.g., gastrulation) cause very similar vertebral defects (e.g., hemivertebrae).[106]

Interestingly, mesodermal cells migrating from the primitive streak, some of which will form vertebrae, have high levels of RARβ expression.[80]

A number of other syndromes have very high incidences of conotruncal abnormalities associated with abnormal craniofacial development. The CHARGE association probably has major crest cell involvement,[107] although many other embryonic cell types must be developing abnormally. In the velocardiofacial (Shprintzen) syndrome, there may be minor (secondary?) involvement of cranial crest, in addition to cardiac crest.[108]

Treacher Collins syndrome

An apparently good example of secondary involvement of crest cells are the abnormalities resulting from a primary RA-induced alteration in other cells that leads to malformations closely resembling Treacher Collins syndrome (Fig. 3–36).[111–114] Treatment at the time that ganglionic placodal cells are forming the early differentiating neurons in the distal portions of the trigeminal ganglion (Fig. 3–17E) causes widespread death among these cells.[112] Since these cells are already in position, the cell death appears not to be related to their migration. Normally, a large percentage of neurons in the trigeminal ganglion undergo cell death at a later stage, and this treatment may simply cause the cells to die earlier. Although sensory ganglia, including cranial sensory ganglia, have high levels of CRABP[78,79] and concentrate radiolabeled RA,[83,84] their content of RARβ messenger RNA is unknown. Large amounts of debris from dead cells are phagocytosed by crest cells in the area, and this appears to affect secondarily the development of derived skeletal elements such as the zygomatic bone. Death of other placodally derived ganglionic neuroblasts may account for minor pharyngeal abnormalities[109] and the high incidence of inner ear abnormalities associated with this syndrome. Using thalidomide in the monkey at the same developmental stages as the above RA studies, Poswillo[114] produced developmental alterations that were very similar. However, he concluded that the malformations were

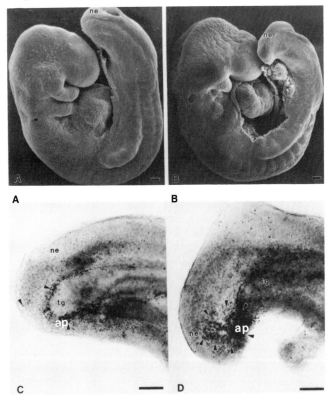

A   **B**

Fig. 3–37. Developmental abnormalities in mouse embryos following maternal retinoic acid administration initiated 36 (B) and 12 (D) h earlier. A,B. Scanning EMs of embryos from control (A) and treated (B) mothers. Abnormalities of the visceral arches and caudal regions are observed, including abnormalities of the neural ectoderm (ne) that lead to spina bifida. C,D. Whole mounts of embryos from control (C) and treated (D) mothers stained with Nile blue sulphate to demonstrate patterns of cell death. Note the cell death associated with tail gut (tg) in the control embryo which is greatly increased in the embryo from the treated mother. The approximate position of the anal plates (ap) is illustrated. Modified from Alles and Sulik.[163]

Fig. 3–36. One of the key features of the Treacher Collins syndrome is the severe depression in the region of the zygomatic bone. This bone is frequently hypoplastic or absent. Other structures in this area (e.g., mandibular condyle and ramus) are also deficient. An animal model for this malformation strongly suggests that the regional deficiencies are secondary to cell death in the developing trigeminal ganglion (see text). From Ross and Johnston.[179]

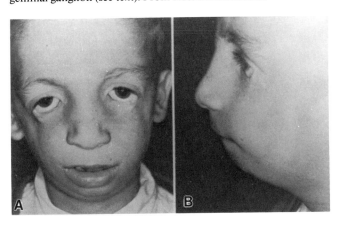

those of hemifacial microsomia. Newman and Hendrickx[115] repeated Poswillo's studies and concluded that the resulting malformations more closely resembled the Treacher Collins syndrome than hemifacial microscomia, contrary to the conclusion of Poswillo.[114] The high incidence of cleft palate (usually wide clefts of the soft palate only) apparently results from interference with the development of the proximal portion of the maxillary prominence, which, in normal development, gives rise to the soft palate.[113]

Cleft lip with or without cleft palate

As noted earlier, primary palate development (Fig. 3–21) is complex, involving high rates of cell proliferation and matrix production, morphogenetic movements, and epithelial adhesion and breakdown with mesenchymal consolidation. This sequence can be experimentally disrupted in many ways, all of which lead to superficially similar cleft lip and palate (or comparable clefts in birds). Examples include reduction of crest cells before they migrate[86,87,116,117] or possibly during migration as in the ethanol/DiGeorge model above, and reduction of ATP formation[118-122] which may in turn interfere with cell proliferation[119] and/or morphogenetic movement. Although somewhat controversial, it appears that cigarette smoking substantially raises the incidence of cleft lip with or without cleft palate (CL[P]).[123-128] The most extensive prospective study[128] indicates that the increase is in the order of 25% and that there are often other malformations, with the combinations not representing known syndromes. This latter finding indicates that if the cigarette smoking is sufficient to cause CL(P), it is likely to cause other malformations as well. Presumably, hypoxia and ATP reduction are involved.[129] By this stage in development, about one-half of the ATP is generated by oxidative metabolism.[56]

Recent studies on the genetic aspects of human CL(P) are of considerable interest, providing evidence of two major types of CL(P) in whites.[130-133] One type appears to be under the control of a single major gene,[130] which may code for a TGFα variant,[131] while the other has a multifactorial etiology.[130] There is little evidence for major gene etiology in most Oriental populations,[130-134] although this may not be true for at least one Chinese population (M. Melnick, personal communication). Nasal cavity width is presumably determined largely by the point at which the medial nasal prominence stops the medial growth and/or movement of the lateral nasal and maxillary prominences. Studying nasal cavity widths in CL(P) subjects is complicated by growth distortions secondary to the cleft but monozygotic (MZ) noncleft co-twins would not have this problem. Studies of 23 such noncleft co-twins showed an apparently bimodal distribution of nasal cavity widths, with two-thirds having moderately to severely reduced nasal cavity widths and the other one-third having average to moderately increased nasal cavity widths.[132,133] Many developmental alterations could lead to narrow nasal cavity widths, including a growth direction of the medial nasal prominences that keeps them too close to the midline,[135] medial nasal prominences that are small, as in the Japanese embryo,[136] or nasal placodes that are set too close to the midline (see discussion of FAS, holoprosencephaly, and cyclopia, above).

Rare TGFα variants have been associated with CL(P).[131] Since TGFα is thought to be the embryonic form of epidermal growth factor (EGF) it is tempting to speculate that the clefting results from failure of the epithelial seam between the facial prominences to break down. Such an effect on the epithelial seams of palate shelves in culture is produced by EGF.[137] However, TFGα also is known to have many other effects.[22]

There is some evidence that prenatal vitamin supplements may be effective in reducing the incidence of human CL(P).[138-141] Unfortunately, the numbers have been insufficient for statistical significance. Little has been done with animal models, although it has been known for many years that folate-deficient diets in combinations with antifolates are effective in inducing CL(P) in rats.[142] Preliminary results indicate that it is also possible to increase the incidence of CL(P) in genetically sensitive A/WySn mice if the prospective mother is placed on a folate-free diet for 50 or more days prior to fertilization, by which time the blood levels are brought to less than 10% of controls.[143] This level (approximately 6 μg folate per ml of serum) is thought to be a level sufficiently low to be effective for NTD induction in humans.[58] Although studies on the pathogenesis have not been conducted, the high level of cell proliferation would probably make the primary palate particularly sensitive to folate deficiency.

Cleft palate (CP)

Forty years have elapsed since Fraser and Fainstat[144] first showed that it is possible to produce a high incidence of CP in genetically susceptible mice by the administration of cortisone to the mother. As discussed earlier, steroids have major effects on developing systems, and much is now known about the mechanisms involved in the pathogenesis of CP in animals treated with steroids and other teratogens. The etiology and pathogenesis of the common nonsyndromic forms of human CP, however, remain largely unknown.

It appears that a number of teratogens may increase the incidence of CP in humans, each to a mild degree. These include cigarette smoke[145] and ethanol.[146] The facial morphology of eight unaffected co-twins of MZ pairs discordant for CP was examined and compared with a large number of controls. The differences were large and consistent and indicate that large tongue size may be a factor.[132,133]

Caudal dysplasias

There are numerous malformations involving the caudal region of the embryo. Emphasis here is on the caudal regression/sirenomelia malformations and the VATER association. Although development of the "tail bud" is probably of critical importance, little is known about either its normal or abnormal development.

Tail buds are found in all vertebrate embryos (Fig. 3–1) and consist of epithelially covered mesenchymal blastemas that form caudal to the posterior neuropore, which is roughly between somites 31 and 34 in birds and mammals. The caudal neuropore closes at about stage 12 (day 27) in the human embryo. Use of the ^{3}H-thymidine cell marker[147] and the quail nuclear chromatin marker[148] has shown that the tail bud mesenchyme gives rise to a neural tube (by "secondary neurulation"), as well as neural crest cells and somites in the avian tail. The notochord and gut epithelium are formed by invasion (extension) from the host. In studies of human embryos, Müller and O'Rahilly[149-151] placed the posterior neuropore at the junction of somites 31 and 32, which indicates that the last three of the five sacral vertebrae and the coccyx would be derived from the tail bud, together with the corresponding spinal cord, sensory ganglia, nerve, and muscle. The human tail bud is unusually well developed,[149-151] with little apparent cell death. Much of the human tail bud must therefore eventually be incorporated into the embryo. The muscles innervated by the nerve plexus to which the last three sacral and the coccygeal nerves contribute are mostly related to the anus. Also, the dermatomes (cutaneous innervation fields) for these nerves are arranged in concentric circles around the anus, with the coccygeal dermatomes being the most central.

Meanwhile, the last mesoderm to form by gastrulation immediately cranial to the tail bud forms the caudalmost intermediate mesoderm (which forms the definitive urogenital system, including the metanephros) and the lateral plate (which forms the skeletal and connective tissues of the hind limb and the connective tissue of the caudal viscera). The limb buds form at the level of somites 25–31 and are thus in the area formed by "conventional" gastrulation. The ureteric bud is derived from the mesonephric duct and invades the metanephric mesenchyme to induce the formation of other renal components (Figs. 3–12 and 3–13).[2] The kidney forms at the level of the upper sacral somites, and it also would be barely in the area formed by conventional gastrulation. Initially, the ureteric collecting tubules empty directly into the lower portion of the GI tube (the cloaca; see Fig. 3–12A). Eventually, a mesodermally derived urogenital septum separates the two systems. Neural crest cells from the caudal-most neural folds form the parasympathetic innervation of the most caudal portion of the gut and the urogenital system. Cell marking experiments show that for a brief period crest cells are found in the metanephrogenic mesenchyme, but their function and final fates are unknown.

Although an attempt has been made to separate sirenomelia and caudal regression,[152] it seems more likely that they are variants of the same general problem since they appear to form a continuous series of defect combinations. However, a word of caution is in order, since in animal models two different treatment times with retinoic acid are required to produce sirenomelia and caudal regression (see below). In humans, some associated malformations are found at distant sites, but most involve only caudal structures.[152–154] Urogenital structures are frequently absent, and there is a high incidence of imperforate anus and rectal agenesis, as well as abnormalities of the sacral vertebrae. The sirenomelic abnormalities consist of fused (unseparated) or single hindlimbs. There are peculiar vascular changes, such as large single umbilical arteries that originate high on the dorsal aorta in many, if not all, cases of sirenomelia.[154] Other than an increased incidence in twins and in infants of diabetic women, little is known about their etiology.

There are a number of apparently relevant animal models. Similar malformations are found in the genetically determined (dominant) rumpless chicken. The abnormal embryos can be identified very early by increased cell death in the ventral side of the developing tail bud, a region that has considerable cell death in controls.[155] All tail bud structures are affected, including the invading gut epithelium and notochord. Similar malformations can be induced by injecting insulin,[156] trypan blue,[157] or RA[157] into the egg.

In mammals, RA has been used to produce similar malformations. In a very comprehensive study of teratogenicity in the hamster, Shenefelt[158] found that maternal administration at about somites 5–9 (about day 21 in the human) resulted in sirenomelia (sympodia) and other caudal malformations. The incidence of sympodia was probably fairly low, since Wiley (personal communication) found less than 1% sympodia using a similar regimen in the hamster, and Yasuda and colleagues[159] produced only one case of sympodia out of 105 abnormal embryos from a high dose of maternally administered RA at the same developmental age. As noted earlier, the hindlimb buds are positioned lateral to somites 23–30, and Wiley[160] found that the vertebrae formed from these somites were the most affected at this administration time. Presumably, sympodia would only result from elimination of all structures between the limb buds, and extirpation of these structures has been shown to be effective in producing sympodia in chick embryo.[161] Other features of caudal regression have been produced at this and later stages with RA in hamsters and in mice.[162–164] Only Shenefelt[158] examined the umbilical vessels, finding a number of abnormalities, including malpositions, that may be similar to the

vascular alterations noted in human sirenomelia by Stevenson et al.[154] Vascular hemorrhages and hematomas were observed in the tail bud area by Wiley,[160] although a later study[165] in his laboratory indicated that the vascular alterations were not the major problem. In the studies of Alles and Sulik,[163,164] prolonged exposures covering both periods were used. Although they did not observe sirenomelia, they observed most of the other malformations. Using both whole mounts stained for cell death (Fig. 3–37) and histologic sections, they found patterns of cell death in embryos from treated mothers and from controls very similar to those observed in rumpless and control chick embryos by Zwilling.[155]

It is difficult to be sure whether the umbilical artery changes observed by Stevenson et al.[154] were primary or secondary. The umbilical artery in the human initially forms as a branch of the dorsal aorta at about the level of the somite 17 (second thoracic vertebra), but, with growth of the more caudal region, the umbilical artery continues to move caudally through anastomosis with more caudal blood vessels of the dorsal aorta.[4] Finally, the definitive anastomosis is with the fifth lumbar somatic artery, and the more rostral connections with the dorsal aorta are lost. Midline fusion of the dorsal aortas does not extend this far caudally, and the still separate aortas become the iliac arteries, with the umbilical arteries as branches. As noted above, experimental teratogens often lead to vascular problems, such as hemorrhage and hematomas in the caudal region, which would be expected to interfere with the umbilical arteries. If the embryo is to survive, a functional vascular connection with the placenta must be maintained. The yolk sac and its blood vessels also migrate caudally. The yolk sac is adjacent to the body stalk, which carries the umbilical vessels (Fig. 3–8), and the two structures eventually fuse. One would expect vascular anastomoses between the developing umbilical and vitelline arterial systems which could account for the connection between the aberrantly placed umbilical artery and the vitelline artery observed by Shenefelt.[158] It would also support the conclusion of Stevenson et al.[154] that the single umbilical artery in sirenomelics is, in fact, a vitelline vessel. Alternatively, problems in the caudal region could lead to a persistence of the earlier, more rostral connections of the umbilical artery to the aortas at a position where the aortas fuse in the midline. Occlusion of the umbilical artery was also observed by Shenefelt,[158] which could account for the loss of one of the umbilical arteries observed by Stevenson et al.[154]

Other anomalies overlap with sirenomelia and caudal regression. These include the VATER association, in which most of the subjects demonstrate caudal defects, including anal atresia, renal anomalies, and vertebral defects including spina bifida. About one-third have single umbilical arteries. There are a large number of defects not related to caudal development, including tracheoesophageal fistulas (TEFs), ventricular septal and other cardiac defects, and forelimb defects.[154,166,167] Hindlimb defects are absent or very rare. Since the TEFs are often associated with vertebral defects, in the same area it seems probable that the TEFs may result secondarily to mesodermal abnormalities similar to those noted above.[166]

Urinary system anomalies

Malformations of the urinary system occur with other caudal defects as noted above, as isolated defects, and with other abnormalities that appear to be secondary. In Potter syndrome, the secondary anomalies appear to result from compression caused by a paucity of amniotic fluid (oligohydramnios), which is produced predominantly by the kidneys. Kidneys are absent in Potter syndrome. Although there appear to be no satisfactory animal models, the classic in vitro studies of Grobstein[168] have shown that renal agenesis could result from failure of the ureteric bud to induce formation of other components from the metanephrogenic mesenchyme (Fig. 3–13).

A recent study by Gage and Sulik[169] has shown that it is possible to produce hydronephrosis and hydroureter by a blockage of the ureter through excessive cell death caused by the maternal administration of ethanol fairly late in the development of the urinary system. The cell death occurred at the junction of the ureteric bud with the mesonephric duct (Fig. 3–12).

Limb abnormalities

In recent years, there has been dramatic progress in the understanding of normal and abnormal limb development. The limb bud is progressively organized by the AER and associated mesenchyme, beginning with the humerus and finishing with the terminal digits and nails. Through administration of RA, Sulik and Dehart[170] were able to induce preaxial and postaxial reduction defects very similar to those seen in the thalidomide syndrome. Increased cell death under the AER may lead to these malformations. A more localized physical blockage of digital formation appears to be caused by hematomas in the AER region. Petter et al.[171] found that anomalies of the digits ("lobster claw" defects) induced by maternal hypoxia in the rat were associated with hematomas under the AER. They also showed[172] that a very similar spontaneous defect in the rabbit could be prevented by maternal hyperoxia and that the prevention was associated with elimination of the hematoma. In both of these examples, development of the central digits was suppressed or distorted, apparently by the physical presence of the hematoma.

Limb reduction malformations very similar to those resulting from thalidomide can also be produced by RA. Administering RA to pregnant mice at a later time, Alles and Sulik[173] found that the limb reductions were associated with expanded cell death in the center of the limb bud, between the mesenchymal condensations that will form the radius and ulna (Fig. 3–32). Chambon and coworkers (unpublished data) have shown that the normal cell death in this region is associated with the presence of the RARβ promoter, as detected by linkage of the RARβ to Lac C. This activity is greatly increased by administration of RA to the mother, an example of the characteristic upregulation of the RARβ gene by RA, an upregulation not observed for other RAR genes.

Apparent "amputation" of the limb in the forearm region is fairly often observed in infants. Hemorrhage[174,175] and amniotic bands in these regions have been postulated as the pathogenic mechanisms.

Concluding remarks

An understanding of human embryonic development is based on information derived from a number of sources. Much can still be learned from direct studies of normal and abnormal human embryos, sometimes with the utilization of newer techniques (e.g., scanning electron microscopy). Careful documentation of abnormal development in human subjects is of critical importance in the development of animal models, which then provide the opportunity for studying the pathogenesis and other aspects of developmental abnormalities. Particularly useful are instances in which it is possible to compare the developmental alterations caused by human teratogens, such as RA and ethanol, in humans and in experimental animals. Utilization of new techniques such as in situ hybridization and transgenic mice is becoming increasingly helpful.

Normal development

Reference has frequently been made throughout this chapter to observations on human embryos. A number of collections of human embryos are still available, such as the very large series of electively aborted embryos at Kyoto University. As noted in the introductory comments, the application of newer techniques such as scanning electron microscopy to the study of the human embryo not only provides more detailed information but also may indicate function, such as the characteristic three-dimensional configuration of migrating cells.

While most studies on the mechanisms of normal development have been conducted on subhuman embryos, there is ample evidence that the findings are also relevant to humans. For example, regulatory genes that coordinate the development of complex structures are found not only in experimental embryos but also in the human embryos. New cell marking procedures have permitted accurate descriptions of the fates of both cell populations and individual cells, determining, for example, the pluripotentiality of cranial neural crest cells. Progress has been made regarding the central problems of development, such as the nature of inductive interactions and the establishment of segmentation and fields. The roles of hormones and growth factors are being studied through the use of in situ hybridization and other procedures. The means by which homeotic genes coordinate the three-dimensional configuration of complex structures should be of particular interest to dysmorphologists, and considerable progress has been made in this area also. Use of transgenic mice holds great promise for the future in that both overexpression and underexpression of genes can be studied. For example, gene targeting of Hox 1.5 "knocks out" this gene by substituting a nonfunctional transgene, and its absence results in abnormalities of development much like DiGeorge syndrome. Studies of the pathogenesis of these malformations should provide insight into the normal function of Hox 1.5.

Abnormal development

Key to an understanding of abnormal human development is the accurate description of human malformations, including evaluations of possible heterogeneity. Such descriptions permit the establishment of the relevance of animal models for human malformations. This includes the potentially significant increased incidence of rare TGFα variants in some subjects with cleft lip with or without cleft palate. Another example presented in this chapter was the use of MZ twins

SUSCEPTIBILITY TO TERATOGENESIS FOR ORGAN SYSTEMS
(SOLID BAR DENOTES HIGHLY SENSITIVE PERIODS)

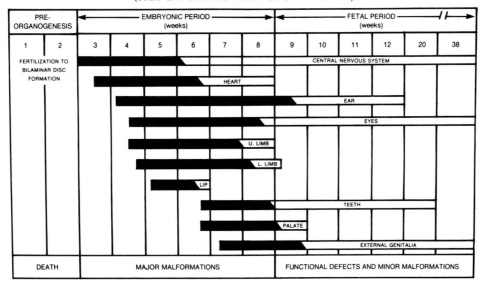

Fig. 3–38. The approximate developmental ages of human embryos for which different organ systems show greater (solid bars) or lesser (open bars) sensitivity to teratogenic influences. From Sadler.[2]

discordant for facial clefts to provide clues as to the nature of the abnormal craniofacial development in the embryo. Many of the 60,000 electively aborted human embryos in the Kyoto collection have malformations, and several studies of these embryos were described in the chapter.

Particularly useful are the rare instances when a large number of human embryos are malformed by maternal use of drugs such as thalidomide, ethanol, and RA. The development of suitable animal models permits studies of the sequence of developmental alterations leading to particular malformations. Particularly interesting are the studies related to retinoids, since it now appears that one of these compounds, all-*trans*-RA, is involved in many aspects of normal development. Accumulating evidence indicates that RA turns on regulatory genes such as those involved in the zone of polarizing activity (ZPA) in the limb bud, and it may also function as a diffusible morphogen produced by the ZPA. In situ hybridization and other studies are establishing the locations of RA receptors and providing clues as to the roles of these receptors and RA-binding proteins. Many activities of RA are mimicked by thalidomide, including effects on craniofacial and limb development. Possibly, it does so by binding to RARs or otherwise altering their effects on gene function. There is also very close comparability in terms of sensitive species, suggesting that thalidomide metabolism may be very similar to that of RA (e.g., the possible production of a 4-oxo-metabolite).

Use of animal models is the most efficient manner for obtaining evidence concerning the pathogenesis of malformations. Various aspects of development show differential susceptibility. Sensitive aspects include normal (programmed) cell death, cell migrations, morphogenetic movements, growth regulation, and fluid balance. Other aspects of development, such as inductive interactions, seem to be much less vulnerable.

Low-level gene activity may signal the partial commit-

ment of cells in different developmental fields. Examples used were homeobox genes showing low-level specific activities of crest cells in different neuromeres, which is maintained during their migrations and which may be involved in the direction of arch-specific complex structures such as the mandibular arch cartilages. Such low-level activities also appear to exist in particular fields that are to be involved in programmed cell death, which may be mediated by the RARβ that is upregulated by the presence of excessive amounts of RA, as for example, in the production of limb reduction defects.

Other teratogenic effects may be more specific for other aspects of development. Teratogens that destabilize membranes, such as ethanol, may be particularly damaging to cells with a high level of membrane turnover, such as migratory neural crest cells in an animal model for DiGeorge syndrome. Morphogenetic movements, such as those involved in neural tube closure and primary palate formation, may be particularly vulnerable to environmental factors such as altered glucose availability or to maternal and embryo hypoxia caused by cigarette smoking. Hypoxia also appears to have other effects, such as on vascular function, that are poorly understood. Altered levels of cell proliferation would be expected to result from altered dietary folate levels.

Formation of different structures may be particularly vulnerable at specific times in their development (Fig. 3–38). Examples used in this chapter included development of the anterior neural plate in FAS and the holoprosencephalies, neural crest formation and migration in the RA syndrome, and primary palate development in cleft lip with or without cleft palate. Many different alterations can lead to CL(P), including those affecting olfactory placode position, neural crest development, or late development of the facial prominences. In general, the earlier the initial developmental disturbance, the greater the likelihood of associated malformations.

Acknowledgment—We are grateful for the assistance and advice of Kathleen Sulik, Ajit Alles, and Peter Bronsky.

References

1. Patten W: Evolution. Dartmouth College Press, Dartmouth 1905.
2. Sadler TW: Langman's Medical Embryology, ed 6. Williams & Wilkins, Baltimore, 1990.
3. Moore KL: The Developing Human, ed 4. WB Saunders, Philadelphia, 1989.
4. Hamilton WJ, Mossman HW: Hamilton, Boyd and Mossman's Human Embryology. Williams & Wilkins, London, 1978.
5. O'Rahilly R, Müller F: Developmental Stages in Human Embryos. Carnegie Institution of Washington Publication 637, Washington, DC, 1987.
6. Gilbert SF: Developmental Biology, ed 3. Sinauer Associates, Sunderland, MA, 1991.
7. Johnston MC, Sulik KK: Development of the face and oral cavity. In: Orban's Oral Histology and Embryology, ed 9. SN Bhaskar, ed. CV Mosby, St Louis, 1980, p 1.
8. Nicolet G: Analyse autoradiographique de la localisation des differentes ebauches presomptives dans la ligne primitive de l'embryon de Poulet. J Embryol Exp Morphol 23:79, 1970.
9. Stern CO: The marginal zone and its contribution to the hypoblast and primitive streak of the chick embryo. Development 109:667, 1990.
10. Tam PPL, Beddington RSP: The formation of mesodermal tissues in the mouse embryo during gastrulation and early organogenesis. Development 99:109, 1987.
11. Holtfreter JE: A new look at Spemann's Organizer. In: Developmental Biology, vol 5. LW Browder, ed. Plenum, New York, 1988, p 127.
12. Waterman RE, Meller SM: Normal facial development in the human embryo. In: Textbook of Oral Biology. JH Shaw, EA Sweeny, CC Cappuccino, SM Meller, eds. WB Saunders, Philadelphia, 1978, p 24.
13. Gans C, Northcutt RG: Neural crest and the origin of vertebrates: a new head. Science 220:268, 1983.
14. Maderson PFA: Developmental and Evolutionary Aspects of the Neural Crest. John Wiley, New York, 1987.
15. Hall BK, Horstadius S: The Neural Crest. Oxford University Press, London, 1988.
16. Johnston MC, Listgarten MA: the migration interaction and early differentiation of oro-facial tissues. In: Developmental Aspects of Oral Biology. HS Slavkin, LA Bavetta, eds. Academic Press, New York, 1972, p 55.
17. Johnston MC, Sulik KK: Embryology of the head and neck. In: Pediatric Plastic Surgery. D Serafin, NG Georgiade, eds. CV Mosby, St. Louis, 1984, p 184.
18. Noden DM: The embryonic origins of avian craniofacial muscles and associated connective tissues. Am J Anat 186:257, 1983.
19. Tabin CJ: Retinoids, homeoboxes, and growth factors: toward molecular models for limb development. Cell 66:199, 1991.
20. Alberts B, Bray D, Lewis J, et al.: Molecular Biology of the Cell, ed 2. Garland Press, New York, 1989.
21. Smithies O: Altering genes in animals and humans. In: Etiology of Human Disease at the DNA level. J Lindsten, U Petterson, eds. Raven Press, New York, 1991, p 221.
22. Lee DC, Han KM: Expression of growth factors and their receptors in development. In: Peptide Growth Factors and Their Receptors, MB Sporn, AB Roberts, eds. Springer-Verlag, Berlin, 1990, p 611.
23. Evans RM: The steroid and thyroid hormone receptor superfamily. Science 240:889, 1988.
24. Melton DA: Pattern formation during animal development. Science 252:234, 1991.
25. Mitrani E, Ziv T, Thomsen G, et al.: Activin can induce the formation of axial structures and is expressed in the hypoblast of the chick. Cell 63:495, 1990.
26. Cooke J, Wong A: Growth-factor–related proteins that are inducers in early amphibian development may mediate similar steps in amniote (bird) embryogenesis. Development 111:197, 1991.
27. Eichele G: Retinoids and vertebrate limb pattern formation. Trends Genet 5:246, 1989.
28. Wanek N, Gardiner DM, Muneoka K, et al.: Conversion by retinoic acid of anterior cells into ZPA cells in the chick wing bud. Nature 350:81, 1991.
29. Noji S, Nohno T, Koyama E, et al.: Retinoic acid induces polarizing activity but is unlikely to a morphogen in the chick limb bud. Nature 350:83, 1991.
30. Zelent A, Mendelsohn C, Kastner P, et al.: Differentially expressed isoforms of the mouse retinoic acid receptor are generated by usage of two promoters and alternative splicing. EMBO J 10:71, 1991.
31. Adelmann HB: The problem of cyclopia. Q Rev Biophys 11:61, 284, 1937.
32. Holtfreter J, Hamburger V: Amphibians. In: Analysis of Development. DH Willier, PA Weiss, B Hamburger, eds. WB Saunders, Philadelphia, 1955, p 230.
33. Hatta K, Kimmel CB, Ho RK, et al.: The cyclops mutation blocks specification of the floor plate of the zebrafish central nervous system. Nature 350:339, 1991.
34. Sulik KK, Johnston MC, Webb MA: Fetal alcohol syndrome: embryogenesis in a mouse model. Science 214:936, 1981.
35. Nakatsuji N, Johnson KE: Effects of ethanol on the primitive streak stage mouse embryo. Teratology 29:369, 1984.
36. Sulik KK, Johnston MC: Embryonic origin of holoprosencephaly: interrelationship of the developing brain and face. Scan Electron Microsc 1:309, 1982.
37. Sulik KK, Johnston MC: Sequence of developmental changes following ethanol exposure in mice: craniofacial features of the fetal alcohol syndrome (FAS). Am J Anat 166:257, 1983.
38. Sulik KK, Lauder JM, Dehart DB: Brain malformations in prenatal mice following acute maternal ethanol administration. Int J Dev Neurosci 2:203, 1984.
39. Siebert JR, Cohen MM Jr, Sulik KK, et al.: Holoprosencephaly: an Overview and Atlas of Cases. Wiley-Liss, New York, 1990.
40. Gorlin RJ, Cohen MM Jr, Levin S: Syndromes of the Head and Neck, ed 3. Oxford University Press, New York, 1990.
41. Ardinger HH, Bartley JA: Microcephaly in familial holoprosencephaly. J Craniofac Genet Dev Biol 8:53, 1988.
42. Kallen B: Contribution to the knowledge of the regulation of the proliferation processes in the vertebrate brain during ontogenesis. Acta Anat (Basel) 27:351, 1956.
43. Pauli RM, Pettersen JC, Arya S, et al.: Familial agnathia-holoprosencephaly. Am J Med Genet 14:677, 1983.
44. Cohen M, Jr: Perspectives on holoprosencephaly: part III, spectra, distinctions, continuities, and discontinuities. Am J Med Genet 34:271, 1989.
45. Wright S, Wagner K: Types of subnormal development of the head from inbred strains of guinea pigs and their bearing on the classification and interpretation of vertebrate monsters. Am J Anat 54:383, 1934.
46. Juriloff DM, Sulik KK, Roderick TH, et al.: Genetic and developmental studies of a new mouse mutation that produces otocephaly. J Craniofac Genet Dev Biol 5:121, 1985.
47. Johnston MC: The neural crest in abnormalities of the face and brain. BDOAS 1X(7):1, 1975.
48. Wei SH, Alles AJ, DeHart DB, et al.: Cell death patterns associated with ochratoxin A–induced craniofacial malformations. Teratology 43:430, 1991.
49. Sadler TW, Lessard JL, Greenberg D, et al.: Actin distribution patterns in the mouse neural tube during neurulation. Science 215:172, 1982.
50. Solursh M, Morriss GM: Glycosaminoglycan synthesis in rat embryos during the formation of the primary mesenchyme and neural folds. Dev Biol 57:75, 1977.
51. Waterman RE: Topographic changes along the neural fold associated with neurulation in the hamster and mouse. Am J Anat 146:151, 1976.
52. Burnside B: Microtubules and microfilaments in newt neurulation. Dev Biol 26:416, 1971.
53. Karfunkel P: The activity of microtubules of microfilaments in neurulation in the chick, J Exp Zool 181:289, 1972.
54. Schroeder TE: Cell constriction: contractile role of microfilaments in division and development. Am Zool 13:949, 1973.
55. Smoak IW: Embryopathic Effects of Hypoglycemia in Mouse Embryos in Vitro. PhD dissertation, UNC, 1991.
56. Hunter ES III, Sadler TW: Embryonic metabolism of foetal fuels in whole embryo culture. Toxicol In Vitro 2:163, 1988.
57. Smithells RW, Sheppard S, Shorah CJ, et al.: Possible prevention of neural tube defects by periconceptional vitamin supplementation. Lancet 1:339, 1980.
58. Lawrence KM: Causes of neural tube malformations and their prevention by dietary improvement and preconceptional supplemen-

tation with folic acid and multivitamins. In: Recent Vitamin Research. MM Briggs, ed. CRC, Boca Raton, FL, 1986.

59. Mulinare J, Cordero HF, Erickson J: Periconceptional use of multivitamins and the occurrence of neural tube defects. JAMA 260:3141, 1988.

60. MRC Vitamin Study Research Group: Prevention of neural tube defects: results of the medical research council vitamin study. Lancet 338:131, 1991.

61. Kokos J, Cekanova E, Kithierova E: Pathogenesis of trypan-blue–induced spina bifida. J Pathol 118:253, 1976.

62. Tucker GC, Duband JL, Dufour S, et al.: Cell-adhesion and substrate-adhesion molecules: their instructive roles in neural crest cell migration. Development 103(Suppl):82, 1988.

63. Bard JBL, Hay ED: The behavior of fibroblasts from the developing avian cornea: their morphology and movement in situ and in vitro. J Cell Biol 67:400, 1975.

64. Noden DM: Vertebrate craniofacial development: the relation between ontogenetic process and morphological outcome. Brain Behav Evol 38:190, 1991.

65. Noden DM: The role of the neural crest in patterning of avian cranial skeletal, connective, and muscle tissues. Dev Biol 96:144, 1983.

66. Hunt P, Wilkinson D, Krumlauf R: Patterning the vertebrate head: murine *Hox 2* genes mark distinct subpopulatins of premigratory and migrating cranial neural crest. Development 112:43, 1991.

67. Szekley G: Functional specificity of cranial sensory neuroblasts in urodela. Acta Biol Acad Sci Hung 10:107, 1959.

68. Lammer EJ, Chen DT, Hoar RM, et al.: Retinoic acid embryopathy. N Engl J Med 313:837, 1985.

69. Rosa FW, Wilk AL, Kelsey FO: Teratogen update: vitamin A congeners. Teratology 33:355, 1986.

70. Ward A, Brogden RN, Heel RC: Isotretinoin. A review of its pharmacological properties and therapeutic efficacy in acne and other skin disorders. Drugs 28:6, 1984.

71. Brazzell RK, Vane FM, Ehmann CW, Colburn WA: Pharmacokinetics of isotretinoin during repetitive dosing to patients. Eur J Pharmacol 24:695, 1983.

72. Webster WS: Isotretinoin embryopathy: the effects of isotretinoin and 4-oxo-isotretinoin on postimplantation rat embryos in vitro. Teratology 31:59A, 1985.

73. Webster WS, Johnston MC, Lammer EJ, et al.: Isotretinoin embryopathy and the cranial neural crest: an in vivo and in vitro study. J Craniofacial Genet Dev Biol 6:211, 1986.

74. Goulding EH, Pratt RM: Isotretinoin teratogenicity in mouse whole embryo culture. J Craniofac Genet Biol 6:99, 1986.

75. Sulik KK, Cook CS, Webster WS: Teratogens and craniofacial malformations: relationships to cell death. Development 103(Suppl):213, 1988.

76. Morriss G: Morphogenesis of the malformation induced in rat embryo by maternal hypervitaminosis A. J Anat (Lond) 113:241, 1972.

77. Morriss GM, Thorogood PV: An approach to cranial neural crest cell migration and differentiation in mammalian embryos. In: Development in Mammals, vol 3. MH Johnson, ed. North Holland, Amsterdam, 1978, p 363.

78. Dencker L, Annewall E, Bush C, Eriksson E: Localization of specific retinoid-binding sites and expression of cellular retinoic-acid–binding protein (CRABP) in the early mouse embryo. Development 110:343, 1990.

79. Dencker L, Annerwall E, Bush C, Eriksson U: Retinoid-binding proteins in craniofacial development. J Craniofac Genet Dev Biol 11(Suppl):303, 1991.

80. Ruberte E, Dolle P, Chambon P: Retinoic acid receptors and cellular retinoid binding proteins. II. Their differential pattern of transcription during early morphogenesis in mouse embryos. Development 111:60, 1991.

81. Thorogood P, Smith L, Nicol A, et al.: Effects of vitamin A on the behaviour of migratory neural crest cells in vitro. J Cell Sci 57:331, 1982.

82. Thomas-Smith L, Lott I, Bronner-Fraser M: Effects of isotretinoin on the behavior of neural crest cells in vitro. Dev Biol 123:276, 1987.

83. Dencker L: Embryonic–fetal localization of drugs and nutrients. In: Advances in the Study of Birth Defects, vol 1: Teratogenic Mechanisms. TVN Persaud, ed. MTP Press, Lancaster, England, 1979, p 1.

84. Dencker L, D'Argy R, Danielsson RH, et al.: Saturable accumulation of retinoic acid in neural and neural crest derived cells in early embryonic development. Dev Pharmacol Ther 10:212, 1987.

85. Rowe A, Richman JM, Brickell PM: Distribution of RAR-β transcripts in the neural crest-derived mesenchyme of the developing chick facial primordia. In preparation.

86. Johnston MC: The Neural Crest in Vertebrate Cephalogenesis. Ph.D. dissertation. University of Rochester, Rochester, NY, 1965.

87. McKee GJ, Ferguson MW: The effects of mesencephalic neural crest cell extirpation on the development of chicken embryos. J Anat 139:491, 1984.

88. Lammer EJ, Armstrong DL: Malformations of hindbrain structures among human exposed to isotretinoin (13-*cis*-retinoic acid) during early embryogenesis. In: Retinoids in Normal Development and Teratogenesis. G Morriss-Kay, ed. Oxford University Press, New York, 1991.

89. Willhite CC, Hill RM, Irving DW: Isotretinoin-induced craniofacial malformations in humans and hamsters. J Craniofac Genet Dev Biol 2(Suppl):193, 1986.

90. Kirby ML, Gale TF, Stewart DE: Neural crest cells contribute to normal aorticopulmonary septation. Science 220:1059, 1983.

91. Bockman DF, Kirby ML: Dependence of thymus development on derivatives of the neural crest. Science 223:498, 1984.

92. Bockman DE, Redmond ME, Kirby ML: Alteration of early vascular development after ablation of cranial neural crest. Anat Rec 225:209, 1989.

93. Kirby ML: Plasticity and predetermination of mesencephalic and trunk neural crest transplanted into the region of the cardiac neural crest. Dev Biol 134:402, 1989.

94. Kretschmer R, Say B, Brown D, et al.: Congenital aplasia of the thymus gland (DiGeorge's syndrome). N Engl J Med 279:1295, 1968.

95. Conley ME, Beckwith JB, Mancer JF, Tenchoff L: The spectrum of the DiGeorge syndrome. J Pediatr 94:883, 1979.

96. Ammann AJ, Wara DW, Cowan AJ, et al.: The DiGeorge syndrome and the fetal alcohol syndrome. Am J Dis Child 136:906, 1982.

97. Daft PA, Johnston MC, Sulik KK: Abnormal heart and great vessel development following acute ethanol exposure in mice. Teratology 33:93, 1986.

98. Chin JH, Goldstein DA, Parsons LM: Fluidity and lipid composition of mouse biomembranes during adaptation to ethanol. Alcoholism Clin Exp Res 3:47, 1979.

99. Chisaka O, Capecchi MR: Regionally restricted developmental defects resulting from targeted disruption of the mouse homeobox gene *hox-1.5.* Nature 350:473, 1991.

100. Grausz H, Richtsmeier JT, Oster-Granite ML: Morphogenesis of the brain and craniofacial complex in trisomy 16 mice. In: The Morphogenesis of Down Syndrome. CE Epstein, ed. Wiley-Liss, New York, 1991, p 169.

101. Funderburg FM, Langford JK, Hiltgen GG: Chondroitin sulfate proteoglycans: do they play a role during cardiac morphogenesis? In: The Morphogenesis of Down Syndrome. CE Epstein, ed. Wiley-Liss, New York, 1991, p 227.

102. Tenconi R, Hall BD: Hemifacial microsomia: phenotypic classification, clinical implications and genetic aspects. In: Treatment of Hemifacial Microsomia. EP Harvold, ed. Alan R Liss, New York, 1983, p 39.

103. Rollnick BR, Kaye CL: Hemifacial microsomia and variants: pedigree data. Am J Med Genet 15:233, 1983.

104. Shokeir MHK: The Goldenhar syndrome: a natural history. BDOAS XIII (3C):67, 1977.

105. Aeksic S, Budzilovich G, Greco MA: Intracranial lipomas, hydrocephalus and other CNS anomalies on oculoauriculo-vertebral dysplasia (Goldenhar-Gorlin syndrome). Childs Brain 11:285, 1984.

106. Jarvis BL, Sulik KK, Johnston MC: Congenital malformations of the external, middle and inner ear produced by isotretinoin exposure in fetal mice. Otol Head Neck Surg 102:391, 1990.

107. Siebert JR, Graham JM, MacDonald C: Pathological features of the "CHARGE" association: support for involvement of the neural crest. Teratology 31:331, 1985.

108. Shprintzen RJ, Goldberg RB, Lewin HL: A new syndrome involving cleft palate, cardiac anomalies, typical facies, and learning disabilities: vel-cardio-facial syndrome. Cleft Palate J 15:56, 1978.

109. Shprintzen RJ: Palatal and pharyngeal anomalies in craniofacial syndromes. BDOAS XVIII(1):53, 1982.

110. Livingstone G: Congenital ear abnormalities due to thalidomide. Proc R Soc Med 58:493, 1965.

111. Phelps PD, Poswillo D, Lloyd GAS: The ear deformities in mandibulofacial dysostosis (Treacher-Collins syndrome). Clin Otolaryngol 6:15, 1981.

112. Sulik KK, Johnston MC, Smiley SJ, et al.: Mandibulofacial dysostosis (Treacher Collins syndrome): a new proposal for its pathogenesis. Am J Med Genet 27:359, 1987.

113. Sulik KK, Smiley SJ, Turvey TA, et al.: Pathogenesis involving the secondary palate and mandibulofacial dysostosis and related syndromes. Cleft Palate J 26:209, 1989.

114. Poswillo D: The pathogenesis of the first and second branchial arch syndrome. Oral Surg 35:302, 1973.

115. Newman LM, Hendrickx AG: Fetal ear malformations induced by maternal ingestion of thalidomide in the bonnet monkey *(Macaca radiata)*. Teratology 23:351, 1981.

116. Eto K, King CTG, Johnston MC: Developmental effects of teratogens influencing the incidence of cleft lip. J Dent Res 55(Spec Iss):203, 1976.

117. Johnston MC, Morris CM, Kushner D, et al.: Abnormal organogenesis of facial structures. In: Handbook of Teratology, vol 2, JG Wilson, FC Fraser, eds. Plenum, New York, 1977.

118. Trasler DG, Reardon CA, Rajchgot H: A selection experiment for distinct types of 6-aminonicatinamide-induced cleft lip in mice. Teratology 18:49, 1978.

119. Millicovsky G, Johnston MC: Hyperoxia and hypoxia in pregnancy: simple experimental manipulation alters the incidence of cleft lip and palate in CL/Fr mice. Proc Natl Acad Sci USA 9:4723, 1981.

120. Landauer WJ, Sopher D: Succinate, glycerophosphate and ascorbate as sources of cellular energy as antiteratogens. J Embryol Exp Morphol 24:282, 1970.

121. Bronsky PT, Johnston MC, Sulik KK: Morphogenesis of hypoxia-induced cleft lip in CL/Fr mice. J Craniofac Genet Dev Biol 2(Suppl):113, 1986.

122. Bronsky PT, Johnston MC, Moore NB, et al.: Lateral nasal placodal morphogenesis in mice: normal developing alterations leading to hypoxia-induced cleft lip. In preparation.

123. Erikson A, Kallen B, Westerholm P: Cigarette smoking as an etiologic factor in cleft lip and palate. Am J Obstet Gynecol 135:343, 1979.

124. Christianson RE: The relationship between maternal smoking and the incidence of congenital anomalies. Am J Epidemiol 112:684, 1980.

125. Shiono PH, Klebanoff MA, Berendes HAW: Congenital malformations and maternal smoking during pregnancy. Teratology 34:65, 1986.

126. Werler MM, Lammer EJ, Rosenberg L, et al.: Maternal cigarette smoking during pregnancy in relation to oral clefts. Am J Epidemiol 132:926, 1990.

127. Khoury MK, Weinstein A, Parry S, et al.: Maternal cigarette smoking and oral clefts: a population based study. Am J Public Health 77:623, 1987.

128. Keels MA: The Role of Maternal Cigarette Smoking in the Etiology of Cleft Lip With or Without Cleft Palate. Ph.D. Dissertation, University of North Carolina, Chapel Hill, 1991.

129. Longo LD: Environmental pollution and pregnancy: risks and uncertainties for the fetus and infant. Am J Obstet Gynecol 137:162, 1980.

130. Chung CS, Bixler D, Watanabe T, et al.: Segregation analysis of cleft lip with or without cleft palate: a comparison of Danish and Japanese data. Am J Hum Genet 39:603, 1986.

131. Ardinger HH, Buetow KH, Bell GI, et al.: Association of genetic variation of the transforming growth factor-alpha gene with cleft lip and palate. Am J Hum Genet 45:348, 1989.

132. Johnston MC, Hunter WS: Cleft lip and/or palate in twins: evidence for two major cleft lip groups. Teratology 39:461, 1989.

133. Johnston MC, Hunter WS, Niswander DJ: Facial morphology in twins discordant for clefts of the lip and palate: a pilot study. In preparation.

134. Chung CS, Mi MP, Beechert AM: Genetic epidemiology of cleft lip with or without cleft palate in the population of Hawaii. Genet Epidemiol 4:415, 1987.

135. Trasler DG: Pathogenesis of cleft lip and its relation to embryonic face shape in A/J and C57Bl mice. Teratology 1:33, 1968.

136. Diewert VM, Shiota K: Morphological observations in normal primary palate and cleft lip embryos in the Kyoto collection. Teratology 41:663, 1990.

137. Pratt RM, Yoneda T, Silver MH, et al.: Involvement of glucocorticoids and epidermal growth factor in secondary palate development. In: Current Trends in Prenatal Craniofacial Development. RM Pratt, RL Christiansen, eds. Elsevier/North Holland, New York, p 235, 1980.

138. Briggs RM: Vitamin supplementation as a possible factor in the incidence of cleft lip/palate deformities in humans. Clin Plastic Surg 3:647, 1976.

139. Tolarova M: Periconceptional supplementation with vitamins and folic acid to prevent recurrence of cleft lip. Lancet 2:217, 1982.

140. Tolarova M: Orofacial clefts in Czechoslovakia. Scand J Plast Reconstr Surg 21:19, 1987.

141. Tolarova M: Genetics, gene carriers, and environment. In: Proceedings of Conference of Risk Assessmet in Dentistry. J Bader, ed. University of North Carolina Department of Dental Ecology, Chapel Hill, 1990.

142. Asling CW: Congenital defects of the face and palate following maternal deficiency of pteroylglutamic acid. In: Congenital Anomalies of the Face and Associated Structures. S Pruzansky, ed. Charles C Thomas, Springfield, IL. 1961, p 173.

143. Lidral AC, Johnston MC, Switzer B: The Relationship Between Vitamins and the Prevalence of Cleft Lip in Mice. J Dental Research 70 (special issue):407, 1991.

144. Fraser FC, Fainstat TD: The production of congenital defects in the offspring of pregnant mice treated with cortisone: a program report. Pediatrics 8:527, 1951.

145. Keels MA, Savitz DA, Stamm JW: An etiologic study of cleft palate in humans. J Dental Research 70 (special issue): 431, 1991.

146. Clarren SK, Smith DW: The fetal alcohol syndrome: a review of the world literature. N Engl J Med 298:1063, 1978.

147. Schoenwolf GC: Tail (end) bud contributions to the posterior region of the chick embryo. J Exp Zool 201:227, 1977.

148. Schoenwolf GC, Chandler NB, Smith JL: Analysis of the origins and early fates of neural crest cells in caudal regions of avian embryos. Dev Biol 110:467, 1985.

149. Müller F, O'Rahilly R: The development of the human brain and closure of the rostral neuropore at stage 11. Anat Embryol 175:205, 1986.

150. Müller F, O'Rahilly R: The development of the human brain. The closure of the caudal neuropore, and the beginning of secondary neurulation at stage 12. Anat Embryol 176:413, 1987.

151. Müller F, O'Rahilly R: The development of the human brain from a closed neural tube at stage 13. Anat Embryol 177:203, 1988.

152. Jones KL: Smith's Recognizable Patterns of Human Malformation. ed 4. WB Saunders, Philadelphia, 1988.

153. Duhamel B: From mermaid to anal imperforation: the syndrome of caudal regression. Arch Dis Child 36:152, 1961.

154. Stevenson RE, Jones KL, Phelan MC, et al.: Vascular steal: the pathogenetic mechanism producing sirenomelia and associated defects of the viscera and soft tissues. Pediatrcs 78:451, 1986.

155. Zwilling E: The development of dominant rumplessness in chick embryos. Genetics 27:641, 1942.

156. Zwilling E: The effects of some hormones on development. Ann NY Acad Sci 55:196, 1952.

157. Jelinek R, Rychter Z, Seichert V: Syndrome of caudal regression in the chick embryo. Folia Morphol 18:125, 1970.

158. Shenefelt RE: Morphogenesis of malformations in hamsters caused by retinoic acid: relation to dose and stage of treatment. Teratology 5:103, 1972.

159. Yasuda Y, Okamoto M, Konishi H, et al.: Developmental anomalies induced by all-*trans* retinoic acid in fetal mice: I. Macroscopic findings. Teratology 34:37, 1986.

160. Wiley MJ: The pathogenesis of retinoic acid–induced vertebral abnormalities in golden Syrian hamster foetuses. Teratology 28:341, 1983.

161. Wolff E: La Science des Monstres. Gallimard, Paris, 1948.

162. Tibbles L, Wiley MJ: A comparative study of the effects of retinoic acid given during the critical period for inducing spina bifida in mice and hamsters. Teratology 37:113, 1988.

163. Alles AJ, Sulik KK: Pathogenesis of retinoic acid–induced spina bifida. Development 108:73, 1990.

164. Alles AJ, Sulik KK: A review of caudal dysgenesis and an experimental model of its pathogenesis. In preparation.

165. Griffith CM, Wiley MJ: Direct effects of retinoic acid on the de-

velopment of the tail bud in chick embryos. Teratology 39:261, 1989.

166. Stevenson RE: Extra vertebrae associated with esophageal atresias and tracheoesophageal fistulas. J Pediatr 81:1123, 1972.

167. Carey JC, Greenbaum B, Hall BD: The OEIS complex (omphalocele, exstrophy, imperforate anus, spinal defects). BDOAS XIV(6B):253, 1978.

168. Grobstein C: Inductive interaction in the development of the mouse metanephros. J Exp Zool 130:319, 1955.

169. Gage JC, Sulik KK: Pathogenesis of ethanol-induced hydronephrosis and hydroureter as demonstrated in a mouse model. Teratology 44:299, 1991.

170. Sulik KK, Dehart DB: Retinoic acid–induced limb malformations resulting from apical ectodermal ridge cell death. Teratology 37:527, 1988.

171. Petter C, Bourban J, Maltier JP, et al.: Production d'Hemorrages des Extremities chez la foetus de rat Sous a une Hypoxie in Utero. CR Acad Sci Paris 277:2488, 1971.

172. Petter C, Bourban J, Maltier JD, et al.: Prevention des Amputations Congenitales Hereditaives due Lapin par une Hyperoxia Maternelle. CR Acad Sci 277:801, 1971.

173. Alles A, Sulik KK: Retinoic-acid–induced limb-reduction defects: perturbation of zones of programmed cell death as a pathogenetic mechanism. Teratology 40:163, 1989.

174. Van Allen MI: Fetal vascular disruptions: mechanisms and some resulting birth defects. Pediatr Ann 10:219, 1981.

175. Jones KL, Smith DW, Hall BD: A pattern of craniofacial and limb defects secondary to aberrant tissue bands. J Pediatr 84:90, 1974.

176. Johnston MC, Hazelton RD: Embryonic origins of facial structures related to oral sensory and motor function. In: Oral Sensory Perception: the Mouth of the Infant. JF Bosma, ed. Charles C. Thomas, Springfield, IL, 1972.

177. Johnston MC, Bhakdinaronk A, Reid YC: An expanded role for the neural crest in oral and pharyngeal development. In: Fourth Symposium on Oral Sensation and Perception. JF Bosma, ed. U.S. Government Printing Office, Washington, DC, 1974, p 37.

178. Sulik KK: Critical Periods for Alcohol Teratogenesis in Mice, With Special Reference to the Gastrulation Stage of Embryogenesis. Ciba Foundation Symposium no. 105, Pitman Books Ltd, London, 1984, p 124.

179. Ross RB, Johnston MC: Cleft Lip and Palate. Williams & Wilkins, Baltimore, 1971.

180. Taysi K, Tinaztepe K; Trisomy D and the cyclops malformation. Am J Dis Child 124:710, 1972.

181. Johnston MC, Pratt RM: A developmental approach to teratology. In: Applied Teratology. Ed Poswillo, CL Berry, eds. Springer-Verlag, Berlin, 1975, p 2.

4

The Contribution of Epidemiologic Studies to Understanding Human Malformations

IAN LECK

The concerns of epidemiologic studies have been defined as "the distribution and determinants of health-related states or events in defined populations."[1] Such studies can contribute to all the main approaches to the control of human malformations: prevention, prenatal diagnosis, and effective treatment and care. To prevention they contribute by providing evidence of etiology; to prenatal diagnosis, by showing which groups of pregnancies are at high enough risk of malformations to warrant screening; and to treatment and care, by determining the numbers of affected children for whom services should be provided and by comparing the efficacy of different clinical procedures.

Three kinds of epidemiologic studies—descriptive, analytic, and experimental—are commonly distinguished. *Descriptive studies* of malformations seek to describe how frequently they occur and how their frequencies vary with three kinds of factors: time, place, and personal characteristics of the affected children and their relatives (e.g., child's gender and mother's age). These studies do not set out to test etiologic hypotheses, and the factors with which they are concerned cannot of themselves cause malformations. However, the chances of being exposed to teratogens can vary with such factors, and therefore the finding of an association between one of these factors and the frequency of a malformation in a descriptive study can often generate etiologic hypotheses. For example, an increase over time in the frequency of a type or types of malformations may suggest that pregnant women are being exposed to a new teratogen. One function of descriptive studies is therefore to monitor the frequencies of malformations so that increases can be detected quickly. Descriptive studies are also used to determine which pregnancies merit screening and how many children need services. Many descriptive studies do not involve gathering new data, since all the information required can be obtained from routine records.

The testing of etiologic hypotheses, and also of control measures, is the function of *analytic* and *experimental studies* of malformations. Each of these approaches involves looking for associations between exposure variables and outcome variables. In studies of etiology and prevention, the exposure variables are typically potential teratogens or protective factors, and the outcome variables are malformations. In studies of treatment and care, the exposure variables may be clinical procedures and the outcome variables may be improved duration and quality of life. The distinction between analytic and experimental studies hinges on whether the exposure status of the subjects being studied (i.e., whether and/or to what extent they are exposed to the exposure variable under investigation) is deliberately determined as part of the

study. An experimental study is one in which this happens; an analytic study is one in which the exposure status has been acquired in other ways, e.g., by fortuitous contact with a source of infection if the exposure variable under study is maternal rubella, toxoplasmosis, or influenza, or by the personal preferences of cardiac surgeons if the exposure variable is a method of repairing a heart defect. Unlike many descriptive studies, most analytic and experimental ones involve collecting new data.

In the first section of this chapter the methods used in descriptive studies are introduced and the findings as to the frequencies of malformations that these methods have yielded are illustrated. In the second section the use of analytic and experimental studies to elucidate the etiology of malformations is introduced with two main examples—defects due to thalidomide and neural tube defects.

Descriptive studies of the frequencies of malformations

The frequency of a malformation is generally expressed as the number of affected children per 100, per 1000, or per 10,000 births. There is, however, diversity of practice in that some workers call this figure *incidence* and others *prevalence;* some favor including late fetal deaths (stillbirths) in the figure while others do not;[2,3] and the gestational age at which delivery must occur for a fetal death to count as late is 20 weeks or more from onset of the last menstrual period in some jurisdictions (e.g., most of the United States) and 28 weeks in others (e.g., the United Kingdom).

Against including stillbirths in the figure, it is argued that their pathologic features tend to be underreported; and the extent of this underreporting varies between populations and between defects, which can make it misleading to compare the resulting statistics. A counterargument is that including stillbirths gives a more complete picture of the impact of the more obvious malformations (especially anencephaly, which is associated with late fetal death much more often than with live birth) on fetuses who survive beyond midpregnancy. If the focus of interest is the impact that malformations would make on such fetuses in the absence of prenatal diagnosis and induced abortion, cases in which abortion is induced for abnormality should also be included.

The terms *incidence* and *prevalence* should not be used indiscriminately. The simplest meanings of these terms are that the *incidence* of any disorder is the number of members of a defined population in whom the disorder arises (generally during a specified period of time) and that the *prevalence* is the number affected by the disorder (generally at a point in time).[1] These numbers are usually multiplied by 10^n (where n is a whole number) and divided by the number in the population concerned to give what are generally known as incidence/10^n and prevalence/10^n, respectively, although it would be more correct to call them the *incidence rate* and *prevalence ratio*/10^n.

It follows that if a type of malformation arises in, for example, the third week after conception, its incidence/100 will be the percentage of all third-week embryos in whom it arises. If the miscarriage rate is high among the affected embryos (as it is in embryos and fetuses with severe malformations in general) the incidence/100 will be higher than the percentage of fetuses born in late pregnancy in whom the malformation is present. The correct term to use for the latter percentage is the *prevalence at birth* or *birth prevalence*/100. It is important to include the word *birth* in this term to avoid confusion with the overall prevalence of the malformation per 100, which is the percentage of people alive at all ages who are affected by the malformation. The percentage of fetuses who would be born with malformations if all pregnancies in which abortion is induced because of fetal abnormality were to continue until birth can be termed the *termination-adjusted birth prevalence*/100. This figure will of course tend to be somewhat higher than the birth prevalence would be if no abortions were induced for abnormality, since in the latter case the malformed children in the pregnancies that would otherwise have been terminated would not necessarily all survive long enough to be counted as births.

In the present account, the methods used in studies of birth prevalence and some of the results obtained by these methods are considered first, followed by methods, results, and implications of studies of incidence.

Methods of studying birth prevalence

In any study of the birth prevalence of malformations, one must determine both the numbers affected by the defects under investigation and the total number of births in a defined population. Evidence of how the population and the affected children are distributed in respect to time, place, and personal characteristics will also be needed if the relationship of these variables to birth prevalence is to be explored. Some of the problems involved in gathering the necessary data are considered below, as are some on-going malformation databases and techniques used in monitoring birth prevalence.

Ascertainment and classification of malformations

Malformations can be ascertained from a wide variety of routine sources. These include government records in several European and North American jurisdictions, where physicians (and in some cases midwives) are asked to report malformations diagnosed at birth; statutory registers of deaths and stillbirths; clinical records, including those of births and of hospital admissions and attendances; and reports of necropsies and of disabilities that are affecting or may affect children's education. Data on malformations for epidemiologic studies are almost always gathered from one or more of these sources, since this is very much less costly than it would be to set up special examinations of every child in a population of the size required to ascertain adequate numbers of cases. It is therefore important to be aware of the incompleteness and

inaccuracy to which diagnostic difficulties, inadequate reporting, and imperfect coverage of the population can give rise in routine data sets. The need for care in classifying malformations should also be noted.

Diagnostic difficulties. The completeness and accuracy with which malformations are diagnosed are affected by how infants are examined (e.g., by the frequency and thoroughness with which those who die are necropsied), by what diagnostic criteria are used (e.g., by how the normal ranges of measurements such as head circumference are defined), and by age. As evidence of the importance of age, it should be noted that when neonates are examined, some abnormalities are seriously underdiagnosed (e.g., certain cardiac anomalies[4]), and others may be overdiagnosed (e.g., congenital hip dislocation[5]). The prevalences of some types of malformations that are underdiagnosed at birth can of course be estimated from routine sources such as hospital admission records which cover contacts with medical or other relevant services throughout the first few months or years of life; but care must then be taken that conditions such as hydrocephaly of intranatal or postnatal origin are not counted as congenital malformations.

Inadequate reporting. Incomplete and inaccurate reporting of diagnosed malformations are especially widespread in some of the schemes for notifying government departments of cases diagnosed at birth. England and the United States have schemes of this kind. In these countries, space for reporting malformations is generally provided on the statutory birth certificates or notification forms used by physicians and midwives. There is evidence that less than one-half the malformations mentioned in the hospital records of newborn children in the United States are reported on their birth certificates.[6,7] In England, data on malformations of the types for which birth notification statistics are routinely published suggest that one in five cases of these defects diagnosed within 1 week of birth is not notified and that one in six reports of these defects is spurious.[8]

Inadequate reporting is, however, not confined to government notification schemes. It can for example arise in local studies based directly on hospital birth records. Before the advent of computerization, studies of this type in which hundreds of thousands of records were reviewed tended to yield much lower estimates of prevalence than those based on populations of 10,000 or 20,000.[9] This was presumably because of incomplete reporting in the larger studies. It must have been more difficult in these studies than in the smaller ones to select only hospitals with good records and to search each record thoroughly for any mention of a malformation.

Imperfect coverage of the population. A study of the birth prevalence of a malformation should if possible cover all the births in a defined time period to residents of a defined geographic area. Studies that cover only births in hospitals can be less satisfactory. In communities where infants are often born at home, disproportionately large numbers of those born in hospital are likely to be malformed, since some malformations produce obstetric problems such as hydramnios that can lead to women being delivered in hospital who otherwise would have stayed at home. Even in places where virtually all births occur in hospitals, women with particular problems may tend to go to one hospital rather than another. For these reasons hospital births are not always representative of all births to local residents, and their representativeness can be expected to vary between different hospitals and periods. Comparisons of hospital-based statistics therefore cannot be totally relied on to show how the prevalence of malformations among all births is related to time and place.

Unfortunately there are large tracts of the world where most births occur at home but data are only available for hospital births. In these circumstances the prevalences of some defects in hospital births may be 50% higher than among all births.[10] Although such a bias would be serious in some contexts, it is small in relation to the extent to which the birth prevalence of some defects, e.g., anencephaly and cleft lip, varies between different countries. It therefore seems reasonable to use data for hospital births to explore these variations in places where data for all births are not available. In such studies, scheduled confinements and emergency hospital confinements should if possible be analyzed separately, since malformations tend to be overrepresented mainly among emergency admissions (to which anencephaly, for example, may lead by causing obstetric problems).

Classification. The instrument that epidemiologists most commonly use to classify disorders is the *International Classification of Diseases, Injuries and Causes of Death* (ICD), published by the World Health Organization. Section XIV ("Congenital Anomalies") of this classification includes almost all malformations. Among these defects, epidemiologists tend to focus on the ones that cause death or substantial handicap or that would do so in the absence of treatment. Even these defects are not always classified in the same way, which can simulate or obscure variations in prevalence between populations. One difficulty is that rarely diagnosed conditions are sometimes classified with one supposedly related condition and sometimes with another (e.g., encephalocele has been classified as anencephaly in some studies and as spina bifida in others).

A more complex problem is the classification of cases of multiple malformations. Some workers have assigned all such cases to a single separate category, while others have enumerated them all under every relevant defect. Others have analyzed multiple defects in one or another of these two ways after making certain exceptions: cases of well-established syndromes (which have been counted separately) and sequences such as hydrocephaly and talipes secondary to spina bifida (which have been classified under their primary defects). It would be helpful if published data on each type of defect always included separate totals for cases with and without nonsecondary malformations of other types, both to facilitate comparisons with previous studies and because the etiologies of at least some common types probably vary between cases of these two kinds.[11-13]

Conclusions. Studies of birth prevalence in which several databases have been linked indicate that there is no one source from which all types of malformations may be ascertained adequately. This point may be illustrated from a study in which summaries of the clinical records of almost all newborn infants (including stillbirths) in Birmingham, England, were linked to stillbirth and death certificates and to records of necropsies, hospital inpatient treatment, and disabilities that were affecting or might affect children's education.[14] The most complete sources of data as to which children were malformed were the neonatal clinical summaries and the inpatient records, which reported malformations in about two-thirds and one-half, respectively, of the cases ascertained from all sources combined. As Table 4–1 illustrates, more than 90% of cases of anencephaly, spina bifida, and cleft lip were reported in records made within 2 weeks of birth (mainly neonatal clinical summaries), but even these and inpatient records combined only identified 83% of the cardiac defects and 72% of the cases of Down syndrome that were ascertained from all sources. Furthermore, even with the full range of sources used it appears that many cases of cardiac defects were not ascertained. The birth prevalence of the ascertained cases (4.2/1000) was no more than two-thirds as high as the results obtained in several studies in which cases were ascertained from outpatient as well as inpatient records or from special examinations of all children several months or years after birth.[15]

The quality of some sources, including neonatal records, may of course have improved as a result of advances in diagnostic methodology since the Birmingham data were collected. However, it remains true that defects like congenital heart disease cannot be adequately ascertained from routine sources except by the use of multiple databases extending well beyond the neonatal period. Good neonatal records may on the other hand suffice for the ascertainment of obvious major defects such as open neural tube defects and cleft lip.

When cases of malformations have been ascertained from two or more sources, attempts are sometimes made to use the numbers ascertained from these sources to estimate the number missed.[16,17] A *capture–recapture* approach of this kind

Table 4–1. Completeness of records of neonatal findings and hospital admissions relative to all available sources of data on malformations: Birmingham, England, 1950–1954

Type of malformation	Birth prevalence per 1000 total births	Percentage ascertained	
		From records for ages 0–2 weeks	From records for ages 0–2 weeks and/or hospital admission data for ages 2 weeks to 6 yr
Anencephaly	2.01	100	100
Spina bifida aperta (without anencephaly), encephalocele	2.49	94	98
Malformations of heart and great vessels	4.23	50	83
Cleft lip (± cleft palate)	1.38	92	98
Talipes	5.72	74	92
Down syndrome	1.61	53	72

Data are from Leck et al.[14] and from Leck.[15]

was for example used in an analysis of 283 Hungarian patients with hypospadias in which the sources of ascertainment were notifications at birth and records of surgical operations for this defect.[17] Surgical operations were recorded in 157 cases, of which 85 (54%) had been reported at birth. The remaining 126 cases had no recorded surgical treatment and were ascertained from birth notifications alone. It was assumed that the surgically treated cases were representative of all cases in respect to completeness of notification at birth. In these circumstances there would have been 391 cases in all (since 211, the total number of cases notified at birth, is 54% of 391), implying that 72% (283/391) were ascertained. The problem with this and related methods of assessing the completeness of data from multiple sources is that the approach assumes that the sources are independent (e.g., that cases reported at birth are neither more nor less likely than others to be treated surgically). Such assumptions are not generally true.[18] It follows that this approach should not generally be used except to obtain a very general impression of the completeness of ascertainment.

Ascertainment of time, place, and personal characteristics

As has been indicated, descriptive studies often enquire into how the birth prevalence of a malformation is related to time, place, and routinely recorded personal characteristics. The status of each malformed child in respect to these variables can generally be ascertained from the document on which the malformation is recorded or by linking this document with entries about the child in a separate routine database (e.g., hospital birth records or the records often kept by statutory health departments). The total numbers of births in each period and place and with each associated personal characteristic under study can often be obtained from the same database. These numbers can then be used to convert the numbers of malformed children to birth prevalence ratios for the times, places, or groups under consideration.

If total numbers of births are not readily available, the relationship of birth prevalence to personal characteristics is often explored by comparing cases of malformations with nonmalformed control infants. These infants are usually *individually matched controls*, i.e., each control is picked so as to match an individual case with respect to variables such as birth date, gender, and hospital of birth. If several nonmalformed infants are found to resemble a case with respect to the matched variables, the study protocol may require that the matched control should be picked from these infants randomly or that the one born immediately before or immediately after the case should be chosen. The personal characteristics of the cases and controls (and/or of their parents) are next determined, often by interviewing the mothers and/or reviewing hospital records. It is assumed that the controls are representative of nonmalformed children. The question whether they differ materially from the cases with respect to the characteristics under study is explored below (pages 80–81 and 89–90) using the standard methods of analyzing case–control studies.

Ongoing malformation databases

Many of the above-mentioned methods of ascertaining malformations and relating them to other factors are widely used to maintain ongoing databases. Many of these databases were set up primarily to monitor birth prevalence in the hope that if pregnant women were to be exposed to a new teratogen its effects on prevalence would be recognized without the amount of delay that occurred after the introduction of thalidomide. These databases are also being used increasingly in epidemiologic work generally, since when they exist it is often much more economical to use them than to collect data specially. When carrying out or appraising such studies one must of course remember that the databases rely on sources such as birth certificates, which are subject to incomplete and inaccurate ascertainment.

The databases can be divided into those that only attempt to ascertain malformations identified during the first few days after birth and those that also include data on cases diagnosed later. Some of the databases in the former group cover births to residents in geographic areas (e.g., England and Wales, Norway) while others relate to births in groups of hospitals (e.g., groups in the United States and South America that contribute, respectively, to the Birth Defects Monitoring Program of the Centers for Disease Control and the Latin American Collaborative Study of Congenital Malformations [ECLAMC]).[19] The data that these databases contain always originate from the physicians and/or nurse-midwives who examine newborn infants, but the databases differ in how these data reach them.

For example, England and Wales have a voluntary scheme under which the physicians and midwives are asked to report malformations to their local public health departments on the forms that they are required to use to report all births. The malformation data are passed to the Office of Population Censuses and Surveys (the agency that processes vital statistics at a national level).[20,21] The Birth Defects Monitoring Program in the United States, by contrast, obtains its data from two data-processing organizations to which thousands of the country's hospitals send abstracts of diagnostic and other details of their inpatients (including newborn infants) for analysis.[13,22]

The second group of databases comprises those that include malformations diagnosed later than a few days after birth. These databases gather together information on malformations not only from reports of examinations of the newborn but also from sources such as records of deaths, hospital admissions, and cytogenetic examinations throughout at least the whole of the first year after birth. In Finland and Hungary there are national databases of this type, and it is at least theoretically compulsory for physicians to report their malformed patients;[23,24] there is evidence of incomplete reporting in both countries.[17,25] Databases that aim to include malformations diagnosed at any time in at least the first year of life are also located in the Canadian province of British Columbia, the metropolitan area of Atlanta in the United States, and numerous areas in Western Europe.[26]

Both types of databases include the total numbers of births in the specified areas or hospitals. They can therefore provide overall birth prevalence ratios for the malformations they record. They differ, however, in the data they contain regarding the personal characteristics of malformed infants and the distribution of all births with respect to these characteristics. Some databases (e.g., those for Finland, Hungary, Atlanta, and the South American hospitals) include personal data on matched controls as well as on cases for the whole or part of the period they cover. The extent of these data varies widely between databases, but some cover not only demographic characteristics but also potential teratogens. For example, the Atlanta database includes data on occupation, disease, and drug use for both the mothers and the fathers of cases and controls born in 1968–1980. These data, which were collected by interview, have been made accessible to workers elsewhere.[27]

There are two international agencies that between them collate data from all the databases mentioned. One is the European Registration on Congenital Anomalies and Twins (Eurocat) Project. This links about 25 predominantly Western European databases through a central registry at the Catholic University of Louvain in Brussels (EPID 30.34, Catholic University of Louvain, Clos-Chapelle-aux-Champs 30, 1200 Brussels), where tabulations covering all the participating centers are produced regularly.[28] Combined data are also being used to explore special issues such as the impact of prenatal diagnosis and termination on the birth prevalence of malformations.[29,30]

The agency that links the other databases is the International Clearinghouse for Birth Defects Monitoring Systems in Norway (International Center for Birth Defects, University of Bergen, N-5021 Bergen, Norway). Four databases participate in both this and the Eurocat project, but most of the 21 other Clearinghouse participants cover considerably more births than most of the Eurocat databases, which makes them more likely to reveal quickly any increase in prevalence. Being restricted (as many of them are) to malformations diagnosed soon after birth is no disadvantage when the aim is to detect possible increases quickly, since this would in any case rule out delaying data analysis until malformations diagnosed long after birth could be included.

Appropriately therefore, the International Clearinghouse places more stress than the Eurocat project on the expeditious monitoring of prevalence and less on other epidemiologic approaches. It produces reports collating quarterly statistics from the participating databases for an agreed list of significant types of defects.[19] From time to time it has also asked its databases for information about the local use of certain suspected or established teratogens (e.g., isotretinoin[31]) and about malformations in users of these products.

Techniques used in monitoring birth prevalence

The aim of monitoring is to detect any increases in birth prevalence that reflect greater exposure to causal factors while dismissing changes due to random variation. An increase is more likely to be of the former type if it is highly significant statistically and if increases have also occurred during adjacent periods in the same locality and/or simultaneously in adjacent localities. Two methods, one based on the Poisson distribution and one on the cusum (cumulative sum) technique, are routinely used to identify statistically significant increases. Both techniques involve calculating the number of cases to be expected in a predetermined unit of time (e.g., a quarter) according to past experience, and then dividing the time during which monitoring is in operation into periods of this length. When an increase is examined by the method based on the Poisson distribution, the number of cases of the defect observed among births in the relevant period is compared with the expected number. The increase may be considered to merit further attention if the expected figure is below the lower 99% confidence interval of the observed figure according to the Poisson distribution.[32]

The cusum technique involves subtracting the expected number of cases from the number born in each period during which monitoring is in operation. The resulting differences for successive periods (i.e., the amounts by which the numbers born during these periods exceed the expected figure) are then cumulated. An increase that merits further attention is considered to have occurred if the cumulated excess (cusum) ever reaches a predetermined significance level. This technique is especially sensitive to runs of high numbers of cases in successive periods. Such runs may be overlooked if the significance of each number is only tested separately, as it is if the previous method based on the Poisson distribution is used.

The databases that use the Poisson distribution in monitoring include some in the United States[22] and the national program for England and Wales. The latter uses the cusum technique as well.[20]

Neither technique has thus far identified a new teratogen. This is strong evidence that no agent as highly teratogenic and widely used as thalidomide has been introduced into the areas with monitoring programs during the period since these programs were launched. However, monitoring would be most unlikely to pick up the effects of drugs like valproic acid and isotretinoin. Each of these drugs is thought to be taken by no more than 1/1000 pregnant women and to cause increases of the order of 20-fold in the birth prevalence of certain malformations among those exposed;[33] and if 1/1000 infants suffered a 20-fold increase in the birth prevalence of a malformation and the other 999 experienced no increase, the increase experienced by all infants would only be $\{[(20 \times 0.001) + (1 \times 0.999)] - 1\}$ or 1.9% of the initial birth prevalence. Thalidomide by contrast brought about an increase of many thousand percent in the birth prevalence of certain limb and ear defects among all infants in West Germany.

Results of studying birth prevalence

The size of the problem posed by potentially lethal or handicapping malformations is considered in this section. How etiologic hypotheses can be generated and how groups of pregnancies that merit screening can be identified by studying variations in birth prevalence with time, place, and personal characteristics are then illustrated.

The size of the problem

Some relatively reliable estimates of birth prevalence based on data from the United States, the United Kingdom, and Japan are given in Table 4–2. The estimates relate to potentially lethal or handicapping malformations that have been reliably reported to occur in at least 1/1000 births (including stillbirths) in one or more of these countries. The American and Japanese figures are derived from special studies carried out many years ago. These results are cited here in preference to more recent figures from routine sources because they appear less likely to have been distorted by incomplete and inaccurate ascertainment.

The Japanese figures are based on follow-up of more than 60,000 nonconsanguineous pregnancies that were registered in three cities in 1948–1954, primarily to serve as controls in an Atomic Bomb Casualty Commission study in which the cases were pregnancies involving a parent with a history of substantial radiation exposure in the nuclear attacks of 1945.

Table 4–2. Estimated birth prevalence of common potentially lethal or handicapping malformations

| Type of malformation | Prevalence per 1000 births[a] | | | |
| | Japan[b] | United States (single births)[c] | | United Kingdom (White)[d] |
		Black	White	
Anencephaly	0.6	0.2	1.0	1.6
Spina bifida aperta (without anencephaly)	0.2	0.7	0.7	2.0
Malformations of heart and great vessels	7.0	7.5[e]	8.2[e]	6.9[f]
Cleft lip ($\pm$ cleft palate)	2.2	0.7	1.4	1.2
Infantile hypertrophic pyloric stenosis	Not included	0.8	3.2	3 to 4[h]
Clubfoot	1.4[g]	4.2[e]	3.6[e]	6.2[g]
Dislocation of hip	7.1	0.8	4.0	3.2
Down syndrome	0.9	1.0	1.2	1.6

[a]Including stillbirths of 28 or more weeks gestation in the United Kingdom and 20 or more weeks elsewhere.
[b]Data are from Neel.[4]
[c]Data are from Myrianthopoulos and Chung.[34]
[d]Data are from Knox and Lancashire.[36]
[e]Data are from Heinonen et al.[35]
[f]Data are from Kenna et al.[37]
[g]Clubfoot not secondary to other malformations.
[h]Data are from Knox et al.,[38] Walsworth-Bell,[39] and Webb et al.[40]

Infants from both sets of pregnancies were examined by physicians employed by the Commission. Initially this was normally done within 10 days of birth. Random samples of nearly 30% of the infants from two of the three cities were reexamined between 8 and 10 months later.[4]

The American figures[34] come from the Collaborative Perinatal Project. In this study the influence of a wide range of prenatal factors on development was explored in more than 50,000 pregnancies booked in 1959–1965 for delivery at 12 university-affiliated medical centers in cities where hospital delivery was almost universal. Data on exposure variables were collected during pregnancy, and outcome was assessed by examining infants on the first 7 days after delivery and again at 1 yr and/or at death and by interviewing the mothers at other times.[35]

Most of the British figures were yielded by the study in Birmingham, England, which was described on page 67. They relate to white infants born in 1964–1981, data for the next few years having been excluded because of doubts about their quality.[36] Estimates from other studies that covered observations made after the neonatal period are given for congenital heart disease[37] and infantile hypertrophic pyloric stenosis.[38–40] The Birmingham study did not cover infantile hypertrophic pyloric stenosis, and its apparent failure to ascertain a significant proportion of cases of congenital heart disease has already been noted.

Among the malformations listed in Table 4–2, congenital heart disease (a very heterogeneous category) and Down syndrome varied in prevalence by a factor of less than 2, while the highest figure for each of the other conditions was more than three times as high as the lowest. However, the figures for talipes and hip dislocation should be treated with considerable reserve, since they may include many neonatal cases of positional foot deformities and hip joint instability that

even if untreated would have resolved spontaneously. In white populations, much lower figures have been reported for established hip dislocation in the absence of neonatal screening and treatment (0.8–1.6/1000)[5] and for persistent nonpostural talipes equinovarus requiring orthopedic treatment in infants without other defects (1.2/1000).[41] The evidence provided in Table 4–2 that hip dislocation is relatively common in Japan and uncommon in black populations is, however, supported by data for children who have not been screened and treated at birth.[42–44] Cleft lip showed a similar trend among Japanese, white, and black children.

For anencephaly and pyloric stenosis, the highest figures shown in Table 4–2 are for whites and the lowest are for blacks. There is no difference between the black and white American figures shown for spina bifida, but statistics based on more births, e.g., those covered by the Atlanta database and by the Birth Defects Monitoring Program (page 68), suggest that spina bifida and anencephaly are both two or three times more common among whites than among blacks in the United States.[11,45] The Japanese series yielded a lower figure than the others for spina bifida, while its figure for anencephaly lay between those for blacks and whites. It did not include data for pyloric stenosis; however, in Hawaii surgically treated cases of this condition were reported to be less than one-third as prevalent in Japanese infants as in whites.[46]

One further point about the figures in Table 4–2 is that some of those relating to pyloric stenosis and to the neural tube defects (NTD) would have been significantly different if data for other years had been used. The range given for pyloric stenosis in the United Kingdom (3–4/1000) is based on figures for the late 1970s that appeared in three reports that hospital admission rates for this condition were higher then than in the immediately preceding period.[38–40] At least part of this trend may have been due to a tendency to admit more cases to hospital for surgery as opposed to treating them by drugs at home.

The birth prevalence of NTD in many countries (including the United States and the United Kingdom) is lower now than in the years covered by the figures in Table 4–2.[21,45] In England and Wales, for example, the proportions of infants (including stillbirths) in whom anencephaly and spina bifida were recorded at birth in 1989 were only 4% and 12%, respectively, of the corresponding figures for 1964–1981 (the period covered by the British data in Table 4–2). These reductions are part of a decline that started early in the 1970s. Over the whole period of this decline, birth prevalence fell by 97% for anencephaly and by 90% for spina bifida. About one-half of each of these two reductions appears to have been brought about by antenatal screening and induced abortion for NTD.[47] The reductions reported from the United States (e.g., 70% for anencephaly and 60% for spina bifida in Atlanta between 1970–1971 and 1988–1989)[45] have been more modest, perhaps because fewer affected pregnancies are terminated there.

Before leaving the topic of overall birth prevalence, mention should be made of the birth prevalence of potentially lethal and handicapping malformations of all kinds in the series on which Table 4–2 is based. This figure was not published for the 1964–1981 birth cohort of Birmingham infants to which most of the United Kingdom figures relate, but earlier data from the same source suggest a figure of 2.5%.[15] The Japanese series also yields a figure of 2.5% if one excludes conditions that are minor or not generally regarded as malformations.

Precisely comparable figures for the United States study are not available. About 3.3% of white and 2.3% of black children were reported to have "major malformations."[35] This category consisted mainly of the same potentially lethal and handicapping malformations as were included in the other two series, but there were a few discrepancies. For example, syndactyly was included and talipes equinovarus was not, and the limits of normal head circumference seem to have been less broadly defined than in the other studies.

The problem of deciding where to draw the line between normal and abnormal that is illustrated by the last example arises more widely when attempts are made to estimate the birth prevalence of defects that do not usually cause death or severe handicap even if untreated. The above British and United States studies included attempts of this kind. Another line that can be particularly difficult to draw in studies of minor defects is one between malformations and other disorders. For example, inguinal and umbilical hernia in infancy were counted as malformations in the United States study although not classified as congenital anomalies in the ICD, whereas the reverse is true of pigmented nevi. A further problem is the impossibility of estimating accurately the overall frequency of nonlethal, nonhandicapping malformations, given that those that are internal are only likely to be found in cases that come to surgery or necropsy for other reasons.

Among the external conditions that are generally recognized as anomalies but have little effect on the health of most of those affected, the most common in the West seem to be polydactyly, syndactyly, hypospadias, and the neonatal positional foot deformities and hip joint instability mentioned already (page 70). In the above studies of British and American whites, polydactyly was reported in 1.3 and 1.5/1000

total births, respectively, syndactyly in 1.5 and 4.1/1000 total births, and hypospadias in 3.6 and 8.1/1000 male births. Variations between the two studies in the thoroughness with which children were examined for minor defects may have contributed to the differences in reported prevalence. However, support for a real difference in the prevalence of hypospadias is provided by a comparison of two reports including data on severity, one from each country.[48,49] In this comparison, not only was the American prevalence the higher overall, but its ratio to the British prevalence was almost as high for the more severe—penile and perineal—cases as for the milder, whereas one would have expected the contrast to apply mainly to the milder cases had it been due only to the American data being the more complete.

Etiologic hypothesis generation

Comparisons between populations like those just described are one of two main approaches to the analysis of descriptive data that have been used to generate etiologic hypotheses. The other approach is to study the relationship of prevalence to time and to personal characteristics within individual populations. Both approaches are illustrated below with data on NTD and cleft lip. In these data, cranial meningocele and encephalocele have been grouped with spina bifida, craniorachischisis (anencephaly and spina bifida combined) with simple anencephaly, and cleft lip alone with cleft lip and palate—partly because this was done in some of the series quoted and partly because the distributions seen when the more detailed categories are examined separately[50] are in agreement with familial and embryologic studies in suggesting that the conditions grouped together are etiologically similar.

Comparisons between populations. A major reason for using cleft lip and NTD as examples at this point is that far more extensive comparisons of birth prevalences in different populations can usefully be carried out for these malformations than for any others. This is because it seems justifiable, for reasons given earlier (page 67), to use maternity hospital data in comparisons relating to cleft lip and NTD; and such data have been published from many centers. Far fewer useful data sets are available for the other types of major defects, since these are less common and/or less readily diagnosed at birth.

Estimates of the birth prevalence of cleft lip and NTD from a large number of studies (some hospital-based and some area-based) are plotted in Figure 4–1. The reason for selecting these particular estimates was that each was based on a denominator of more than 10,000 liveborn and stillborn infants (15,000 for each estimate for cleft lip) who could all or almost all be inferred to belong to one broad ethnic group and who had been examined by methods that should have ascertained all or nearly all cases, including those associated with stillbirth or other malformations.[51] To avoid confusion between differences in the prevalence of NTDs that could be of etiologic significance and differences due to antenatal screening and induced abortion, none of the NTD estimates in Figure 4–1 relates to the period since the introduction of screening.

The figures can be criticized for including cases in which cleft lip or NTD were accompanied by other malformations not secondary to them, since such cases may differ in their epidemiology from cases of NTD or cleft lip alone (page

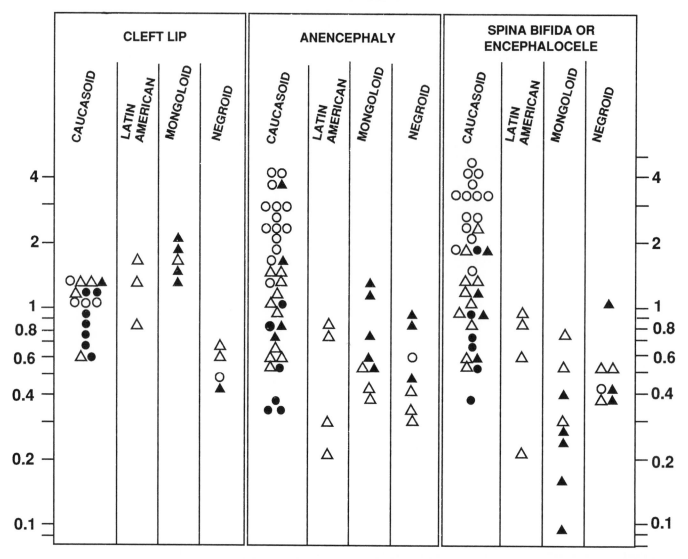

Fig. 4–1. Birth prevalence of cleft lip and neural tube defects per 1000 total births (log scale) in series of relatively uniform racial origin. The alignment of the point plotted for each estimate of prevalence shows the predominant primary race of the population concerned, and the type of point shows its location (open circles, Great Britain and Ireland; open triangles, the Americas, including Hawaii; closed circles, mainland Europe; closed triangles, other continents).

67). However, the reports of some of the studies did not distinguish between cases with and without other defects, and it would have destroyed the comparability of the figures if some but not all had excluded the former.

The starting point when considering any difference in birth prevalence between populations is generally to consider whether race or place appears to be the main source of variation. If the difference is primarily between infants of different racial groups and persists even between members of these groups who reside in the same place, it may well be genetically determined (although one should not forget that racial groups may also differ with respect to life-style even when they live near each other). If on the other hand the difference is primarily between infants from different places and there is little or no variation between infants of different racial groups living in the same place, the source of the difference is more likely to be environmental. In Figure 4–1 the type of point plotted for each estimate gives a broad indication of

place, and its vertical alignment shows predominant primary race. Latin Americans described as Mestizo or European have been aligned separately since they are of mixed Caucasoid and American Indian ancestry.

The birth prevalence of cleft lip varies relatively little between places with populations of the same racial group and much more between races. The low, moderate, and high figures given in Table 4–2 for black, white, and Japanese infants, respectively, are seen in Figure 4–1 to be typical of Negroid, Caucasoid, and Mongoloid populations. The range for Latin Americans, whose ancestors on the American Indian side were probably of Mongoloid origin, lies between the Caucasoid and Mongoloid ranges. Live birth statistics indicate that cleft lip is even more common in some North American Indian populations[52,53] than in the Mongoloid populations represented in Figure 4–1, which were of Western Pacific origin. The Negroid–Caucasoid–Mongoloid gradient tends to persist even among those living in the same place, as is exemplified by various figures for black and white communities in England and the United States (including those in Table 4–2) and for white infants and those of Western Pacific origin in Hawaii and California.[51] All these findings can be interpreted as evidence that the birth prevalence of cleft lip is strongly affected by the genotype but little if at all by the environment.

The pattern for NTD is much more complex. Before antenatal screening and induced abortion for them became widespread, both anencephaly and spina bifida varied in prevalence by a factor of more than 10 between places with Caucasoid populations. The lowest birth prevalence ratios shown in Figure 4–1 for this racial group came from mainland Europe and the highest from Great Britain and Ireland (especially around the Irish sea). There is also some evidence that India and the Eastern Mediterranean (excluding the Jewish population of Israel) are covered by a belt of high birth prevalence and that in this belt, unlike in the West, anencephaly is substantially more common than spina bifida. In Caucasoid populations that have migrated from one place to another (e.g., people of South Asian and Irish origin in England and the descendents of migrants from mainland Europe and Ireland to North America), the birth prevalence of NTD tends to be closer than it is in the countries of origin to the norm for the place to which they have come.[36,51] This finding suggests that the variation in birth prevalence between Caucasoids in different places is due at least in part to environmental differences (although the migrants could theoretically have been selected in some way that affected their genetic predisposition to bear offspring with NTD).

The non-Caucasoid birth prevalence ratios shown in Figure 4–1 are comparable to the lower Caucasoid ratios except that spina bifida (but not anencephaly) is much less common in Mongoloids. However, since this material was assembled, our knowledge about prevalence in Mongoloids has been substantially augmented by the publication of data for mainland China and in particular its northeast, which includes areas where the prevalence of NTD is among the highest known and where anencephaly and spina bifida occur almost equally often.[54,55] From experience in places in England and the United States to which Mongoloid and/or Negroid populations have migrated, it appears that in the descendents of these migrants NTD tend to be less common than in the white population and not consistently more common than in their countries of origin. However, spina bifida was more common relative to anencephaly in these migrant groups and in their white neighbors than it was in series from the latter countries.[36,51] These findings suggest that genetic factors are largely responsible for NTD being less common in Mongoloids and Negroids than in English and U.S. Caucasoids but that environmental factors may influence whether affected children have anencephaly or spina bifida.

Comparisons between populations thus reveal markedly different patterns for cleft lip and NTD. The pattern for cleft lip is largely one of differences between primary racial groups that invite a genetic explanation. The birth prevalence of NTD, by contrast, varies markedly within as well as between these groups, and both environmental and genetic factors appear likely to be involved in this pattern of variation.

Studies within individual populations. Studies within populations can be illustrated by the study in Birmingham, England, for which details of the sources of data on malfor-

mations have been given above (page 67). City Health Department data for 632,096 infants (including stillbirths) born to residents of the city in 1950–1984 have been used to explore the birth prevalence of these malformations by time, place, and personal characteristics.[36,56] Figure 4–2 shows how the birth prevalence of cleft lip and NTD in 1950–1969 (when 406,507 of these infants were born) varied with month and year of birth, sex and birth rank of child, mother's age, and parental socioeconomic status according to the "Social Class" system used in official United Kingdom statistics. This system classifies each occupation on a scale of I (e.g., physician) to V (e.g., unskilled laborer). The reason for restricting Figure 4–2 to the first 20 years' births[56] is that the later material (which yielded broadly similar findings) was published in a different format.[36] The social class figures shown are further restricted by the exclusion of infants born before 1960 and those whose parents both were Afro-Caribbean. Social class was not recorded for births before 1960, and as Afro-Caribbeans are at relatively low risk of cleft lip and NTD their inclusion would have tended to depress birth prevalence in the less privileged social classes where they are concentrated.

Each birth prevalence ratio shown in Figure 4–2 was compared with the ratio for the remainder of the population and was plotted as significantly increased or decreased if the χ^2 test with Yates's correction gave a positive result when applied to these figures.[56] This approach has the disadvantage of not taking account of the sequence in which high and low rates occurred, which may also affect the interpretation of such variations. For example, the monthly variations in the birth prevalence of spina bifida should be taken more seriously than those for cleft lip not only because they are more extreme but also because of the sequence of the monthly figures: the highest for spina bifida occurred in adjacent months (December and January) and so did the lowest (in June and July), whereas the extreme ratios for cleft lip occurred in widely separate months (the highest in April and December and the lowest in January and July). There are ways of estimating statistical probability that take account of sequence, but to introduce them might unduly complicate this account.

The influence of the genotype on birth prevalence is evidenced in Figure 4–2 by significant excesses of females with anencephaly and spina bifida and of males with cleft lip. Such findings are usual in Caucasoid populations. The only other association between the prevalence of cleft lip and the variables listed in Figure 4–2 that was shown to be significant at the 1% level in the Birmingham series was an increase among third and later births to mothers aged 35 yr or more. This increase may well have been a function of maternal age alone, since there were so few first and second births to mothers over 35 yr that the differences in birth prevalence between these and the third and later births could readily have arisen by chance. Other studies also indicate that the birth prevalence of cleft lip increases with parental age, but there is some evidence that the increase is confined to cases with multiple defects.[57,58] Such cases can be caused by chromosomal or genic mutations that are more common at high parental ages.[59,60] Here as in the comparisons of different populations illustrated above, there is thus no evidence that environmental as opposed to genetic factors play a major role in the etiology of cleft lip, although analytic studies have indicated

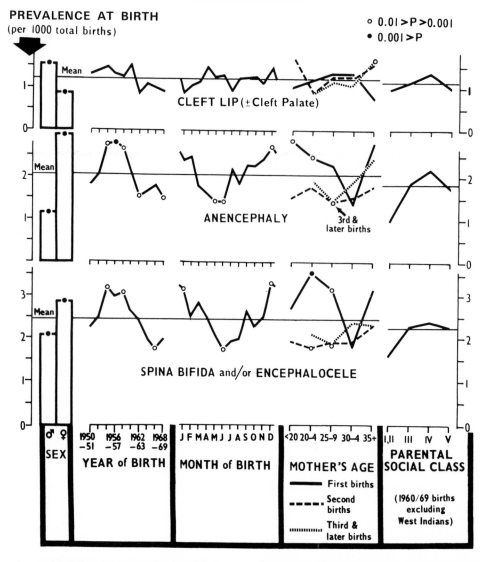

Fig. 4–2. Birth prevalence of cleft lip and neural tube defects in various groups of infants born in Birmingham, England, in 1950–69.[56] Groups that differed significantly from the rest of the population were identified by the χ^2 test with Yates's correction. (From Leck[56] by permission of Butterworth Heinemann)

that a few cases are caused by maternal anticonvulsant therapy.[61]

In contrast to cleft lip, both anencephaly and spina bifida exhibited significant variations in birth prevalence with several factors—season and year of birth, birth order, and social class—that are likely to be correlated more closely with environmental influences than with genetic background. Among the 1950–1969 Birmingham births on which Figure 4–2 is based, the birth prevalence of each of the NTD was higher in winter than in summer, peaked in the mid-1950s, and was high among first births (except to mothers in their early thirties) and low among second births. The infants of parents in Social Classes I and II (professional and managerial workers) were also at low risk, although the difference between these and other infants only became significant at the 1% level when the data for the two NTD were combined.

The analysis of more recent Birmingham births[36] revealed similar trends with season, birth order, and social class and demonstrated that if every birth had occurred on its expected

date of delivery the winter peak in birth prevalence would have been nearly 2 months earlier for anencephaly than for spina bifida. As elsewhere in England, the secular trend (pattern of long-term change in frequency over time) during the 1970s and 1980s was dominated by the decline following the introduction of antenatal screening for NTD (page 71). The possibility that NTD exhibit clustering (the occurrence of more cases in close proximity of space and time than would be likely to happen at random) was also explored in the more recent analysis, but with largely negative results.

Variations with time, birth order, and social class have also been observed elsewhere in the United Kingdom and appear from nationwide studies to be largely independent of each other.[62,63] Associations with these factors have also been observed in many other countries, although the pattern of variation appears to be far from stable at an international level.[64,65]

Comparisons between populations and studies within individual populations thus agree in suggesting that the environment plays a substantially greater part in the etiology of NTD than of cleft lip. This view is also supported by family studies, which have yielded estimates of heritability (the contribution of genetic factors to liability) ranging from 63% to 85% for NTD[65] compared with 90% for cleft lip.[66]

The results of the above descriptive studies have also helped to generate and support more specific etiologic hypotheses. For example, the Mongoloid–Caucasoid–Negroid gradient in the birth prevalence of cleft lip has suggested a link between this condition and the race-related genetic factors that influence face shape (which apparently tends to be less convex in the parents of children with cleft lip than in others of the same race[67]). Various dietary constituents (e.g., blighted potatoes, tea, and several electrolytes) have come under suspicion as teratogens on the grounds that their intake appears to have varied in space and time in parallel with the birth prevalence of NTD, although the evidence for any of these items being of etiologic importance is tenuous.[65] The hypothesis that one or more nutritional deficiencies may predispose to NTD in humans (discussed below in the context of analytic and experimental studies) included among its main sources the epidemiologic evidence that birth prevalence is high in the less privileged social classes and in infants conceived in spring, when the body's reserves of some nutrients may be minimal.

Screening policy development

Although prenatal diagnosis (including screening) is considered in a later chapter, the present discussion of descriptive studies would be incomplete if it did not mention their contributions in this field. Despite our ability to diagnose some types of malformations by routine procedures such as ultrasonography, there are of course many antenatal diagnostic procedures, e.g., those carried out on amniotic fluid and chorionic villus samples, that are only appropriate when the risk of malformation is high since they may harm the fetus or are too costly in resource terms to use routinely. In such circumstances, birth prevalence ratios derived from descriptive studies have been used in three ways, first, in assessing when it is worth using clinical and laboratory-based screening tests to select fetuses for diagnostic procedures; second, in identifying substitutes for such screening tests; and third, in monitoring the effectiveness of screening.

The use of birth prevalence ratios to assess when screening is justified. An example of a problem that should be approached in this way is the diagnosis of NTD. The most widely used laboratory-based screening test for these conditions is of course the measurement of maternal serum α-fetoprotein (MSAFP). When carried out at 16–18 weeks gestation, this test is commonly regarded as positive if it yields a figure at least 2.5 times the median for all pregnancies of the same gestation length. The diagnostic procedure mainly used in these circumstances is ultrasonography, followed if negative by amniocentesis and measurement of amniotic fluid α-fetoprotein. At 16–18 weeks gestation, the MSAFP test was found to be positive in 88% of singleton pregnancies with anencephaly, 69% with spina bifida, and 3.3% with no NTD.[68] In other words, its sensitivity (the proportion of cases in which the test is positive) was 88% for anencephaly and 69% for spina bifida, and its specificity (the proportion of non-cases in which the test is negative) was 96.7% (i.e., $100 - 3.3$).

The birth prevalence of NTD in any population for which MSAFP screening is being considered needs to be examined in conjunction with the above information before an informed decision can be made on whether screening is justified. In England and Wales, anencephaly and spina bifida each had a birth prevalence of the order of 1.5/1000 at the time when the MSAFP screening test became available. If one screened 1 million pregnancies in these circumstances, one would expect to obtain false-positive results in 32,901 (i.e., 3.3% of 997,000) and true-positive results in 2355 (i.e., 88% of 1500 anencephalics and 69% of 1500 fetuses with spina bifida). The predictive power of a positive test would thus be 6.7% (i.e., 2355/[32,901 + 2355]). In other words, 6.7% or 1 in 15 of the fetuses whose mothers were referred for diagnostic tests (ultrasonography with or without amniocentesis) because of a positive screening test would be found to be affected.

Bearing in mind that NTD posed a major problem for the population and for those affected and that the 6.7% of amniocenteses estimated to result in the diagnosis of an NTD was considerably greater than the proportion causing the death of a normal fetus (probably 1% or less),[69] most British authorities concluded that MSAFP screening was justified. They might very reasonably have reached the opposite conclusion had anencephaly and spina bifida been as rare there as in Finland (where each affects only about 0.35/1000 births):[70] in these circumstances 1 million pregnancies would be expected to yield false-positive results in 32,977 (i.e., 3.3% of 999,300) and true-positive results in 550 (i.e., 88% of 350 anencephalics and 69% of 350 fetuses with spina bifida), so that only 1.6% (i.e., 550/[32,977 + 550]) of those referred for diagnostic tests would be affected.

The use of birth prevalence ratios to identify substitutes for screening tests. This application is illustrated by the use of age-specific birth prevalence ratios of Down syndrome at different maternal ages to define which pregnancies should be selected for diagnostic tests.

The upward trend in the birth prevalence of Down syndrome with maternal age was recognized by Penrose[71] in 1934 and is by far the strongest of the associations that have been identified between common birth defects and the variables examined in descriptive studies. Over most if not all of the maternal age range, the trend can be described as an exponential increase from a baseline value: i.e., it appears to satisfy the equation $y = a + \exp(bx - c)$, where y is prevalence at age x, a is the baseline value, and b and c are other constants.[72] In Figure 4–3, a curve satisfying this equation has been fitted to data from a Swedish series that appears to be more complete than any other of comparable size for which separate figures for each year of maternal age have been published.[73] Prevalence increased by only about one-half between maternal ages 20 and 30 yr, but by almost 100-fold between ages 30 and 48 yr (the highest figure shown).

Observations such as these have been used to identify a specific lower maternal age limit (usually 35 yr) to serve as a substitute for a screening test in determining which pregnant women should be offered a diagnostic test (fetal cell culture and karyotyping following amniocentesis or chorionic villus sampling) for Down syndrome. In other words, couples who are not known to be chromosomally abnormal or to have already had a chromosomally abnormal child are commonly offered a diagnostic test if the woman's age is at least 35 yr.

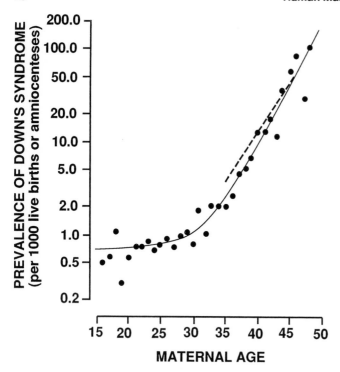

Fig. 4–3. Trends in the prevalence of Down syndrome with maternal age. Points show observed live birth prevalence (y) at each single year of age (x) in Sweden.[73] Solid line is fitted to these points using the equation y = 0.000710047 + exp (0.31070x − 17.17133). Dashed line shows trend of prevalence at amniocentesis predicted by logistic regression analysis of figures for single years of age in Collaborative European Study on 52,965 cases.[74]

At this age the risk of bearing an affected infant is one in 400 according to Figure 4–3. The prevalence of Down syndrome at the stage in pregnancy at which amniocentesis is carried out is rather higher—about one in 250 according to the international series of more than 50,000 amniocenteses which yielded the interrupted regression line shown in Figure 4–3.[74] The difference between these two figures reflects the fact that some affected pregnancies would abort spontaneously between the time of amniocentesis and birth if abortion was not included deliberately.

An amniocentesis at age 35 yr (although not at over age 40 yr) has therefore a lower chance of detecting an affected child than the chance of up to 1% that it will cause the death of a normal fetus.[69] Chorionic villus sampling causes fetal death more often,[75] but has the advantages of being feasible earlier in pregnancy and allowing faster karyotyping than amniocentesis.

The sensitivity and specificity of using maternal age in this way to screen for Down syndrome depend heavily on the maternal age distribution of all births. In Birmingham in 1964–1984, 33,179 stillbirths and live births, including 189 cases of Down syndrome (5.70/1000 total births), were reported among mothers aged 35 yr and over, and 317,912 stillbirths and live births, including 293 with Down syndrome (0.92/1000), were reported among younger mothers.[36] Sensitivity was therefore 39.2% (i.e., 189/[189 + 293]) and specificity was 90.6% (i.e., [317,912 − 293]/[317,912 + 33,179 − 293 − 189]) in this population. In populations with fewer elderly mothers, specificity is higher but sensitivity is even lower.

Numerous suggestions have recently been made for improving sensitivity by using various laboratory tests that tend to give higher or lower values in pregnancies in which the fetus has Down syndrome, e.g., maternal serum concentrations of α-fetoprotein, unconjugated estriol, and human chorionic gonadotropin.[76] It has not been proposed that such tests should take the place of maternal age in screening but that the result of each test should be translated into the probability of the pregnancy concerned being affected if only this one result was known, after which the overall risk is calculated from the probabilities yielded by all these tests (including the probability of being affected given the mother's age). It has been estimated that a sensitivity of 60% combined with a specificity of 95.3% could have been achieved if the above three tests and maternal age had been used in this way to screen the 1981–1985 population of England and Wales.[76]

The use of birth prevalence ratios to monitor the effectiveness of screening. Mention has already been made (page 71) of the evidence that about half the dramatic decline in the birth prevalence of NTD in England and Wales since the early 1970s was due to screening. Statistics for this population, which allow for the incomplete ascertainment of NTD among abortions, indicate that in 1985 anencephaly and spina bifida were only present in 1/10,000 and 6/10,000 births, respectively. These figures would have been 9/10,000 and 13/10,000 if all pregnancies that were terminated because of NTD had continued until birth.[47]

Birth prevalence statistics suggest that the use of maternal age to screen for Down syndrome has been less effective. In women aged 35 yr or more (the age group for whom antenatal diagnosis is advocated), at least as many affected pregnancies ended in birth as were terminated among those reported in 1980–1988 in each of 11 European populations in which amniocentesis and induced abortion for Down syndrome are available.[77] Indeed, there were two British cities (Belfast and Liverpool) where births outnumbered terminations by over four to one; but this may reflect cultural factors rather than the availability of screening.

The study of incidence

Two kinds of methods, which may be called the *direct* and the *indirect* approaches, have been used to estimate the incidence of major malformations (i.e., the proportion of embryos in which they occur). The direct approach is to examine their frequency in embryos and early fetuses removed at medically induced abortion. It is assumed that these products of conception are representative of all embryos in the uterus at the time when the malformations arise, in which case the proportion affected by malformations would be the same as the incidence. The indirect approach is to collect data on malformations in fetuses that have been miscarried as well as in births and (if numbers warrant) induced abortions. Often in studies of this kind, the data on miscarriages, induced abortions, and births do not all relate to precisely the same population. In this case the formula to use for estimating incidence is $(r_m p_m + r_a p_a + r_b p_b)$, where r_m, r_a, and r_b are the prevalence ratios for malformations among miscarriages, induced abortions, and births, respectively, and p_m, p_a, and p_b are the proportions of all recognized pregnancies that end in these three ways, respectively.

Neither method is entirely accurate, for various reasons. By considering only induced abortions, the direct approach misses cases in which miscarriage occurs before the time at which abortion would have been induced, and its database is also unlikely to be representative of all pregnant women with respect to age, social circumstances, or even health (although the reasons for most induced abortions are not strictly medical). The indirect approach also misses early losses, since it can only take note of miscarriages for which the products of conception have been available for examination (generally hospital cases). In both approaches the available fetal material is often insufficiently well preserved to determine whether malformations are present. The best that the investigator may then be able to do is to estimate the frequency of malformations some time after their inception, after making the somewhat dangerous assumption that the materials from miscarriages at each stage of gestation that were fit to study were representative of all the miscarriages that occurred at that stage.

Despite the limitations of these approaches, the figures that they yield for malformations that are visible in late embryos and early fetuses are likely to give a clearer picture of incidence than can be inferred from birth prevalence statistics. In what follows, the results of studies of early induced abortions in Kyoto, Japan, and spontaneous abortions in London, England, are mainly cited to illustrate the direct and indirect approaches, respectively. The incidence of all obviously abnormal embryos is considered first, followed by the findings for specific defects.

Incidence of abnormal embryos

In the Japanese series of induced abortions, chromosomal anomalies were detected in 1.9% of 4–8-week-old embryos, while localized external malformations were observed in 4.2% of undamaged embryos aged 6–8 weeks after conception.[78] Chorionic sacs that had contained no embryo appear to have been observed even more often.[79] By contrast, the birth prevalence of chromosomal aberrations is about 0.7%,[80,81] and only about 0.5% of Japanese neonates (including stillbirths) exhibit external malformations of types that might be detected by examination during the embryonic period.[4]

The spontaneous abortions in the London series had occurred at gestational ages of 8–28 weeks. Among the cases in which a complete embryo or fetus or a sac that had apparently contained no embryo was recovered, focal malformations were reported in 4.7%, more extensively disorganized embryos were reported in 4.9%, and empty sacs were reported in 31.9%. Among the successfully karyotyped cases in the series, chromosomal anomalies were present in 55% of empty sacs, 69% of extensively disorganized embryos, 36% of embryos with focal malformations, 12% of those who appeared normal, and 42% of products of conception that were too fragmentary to be evaluated morphologically.[82] Fetuses aborted before 16 weeks (among which chromosomal anomalies tend to be concentrated) were underrepresented in this series. Standardization to the age distribution of miscarriages given by French and Bierman[83] yields a figure of 42.6% for the prevalence of chromosomal anomalies among all spontaneous abortions at 8–28 weeks gestation. In other countries also, more than two-fifths of spontaneous abortions seem to be associated with chromosomal anomalies.[84]

Like the Japanese statistics, these figures suggest that only a minority of embryos with chromosomal or major anatomic

defects survive until birth. Before medically induced abortions were widely performed, external malformations that might have been detected in a spontaneously aborted embryo or early fetus were present in about 0.8% of total (i.e., live and still) births in England,[14] and the corresponding figure for chromosomal anomalies was 0.7%.[81] Assuming that spontaneous abortion is the outcome of 13.4% of pregnancies that reach 8 weeks gestation (6 weeks from conception),[83] the figures from England suggest that at this stage the anomalies mentioned above are present in the following proportions of pregnancies. Externally obvious localized malformations:

$$(0.134 \times 4.7) + (0.866 \times 0.8) = 1.3\%$$

extensively disorganized embryos:

$$0.134 \times 4.9 = 0.7\%$$

empty chorionic sacs:

$$0.134 \times 31.9 = 4.3\%$$

chromosomal anomalies:

$$(0.134 \times 42.6) + (0.866 \times 0.7) = 6.3\%$$

Estimates of this nature do not show the total impact of maldevelopment, because they do not take account of very early miscarriages and because the later abortions on which they are based are unlikely to be representative of all such abortions. In addition, these figures only cover malformations that can be diagnosed by external inspection and are based on embryos and fetuses many of which were too young for some defects to be apparent. When spontaneous abortions that occurred from 4 weeks gestation onward in Seattle, Washington, were examined by methods including the dissecting microscope, defects were found in 19.0% of cases in which an embryo or fetus not affected by severe disorganization was recovered.[85]

Of particular interest is the frequency with which maldevelopment might be expected to ensue in pregnancies that reach 4 weeks gestation if the last-mentioned proportion occurred in conjunction with the spontaneous abortion rate of 23% reported for pregnancies that reach 4 weeks gestation,[83] and with the English prevalence ratios for empty sacs and extensively disorganized embryos among spontaneous abortions (31.9% and 4.9%) and for all potentially lethal and handicapping malformations among births (2.5%). These figures suggest that the proportion of pregnancies reaching 4 weeks gestation in which maldevelopment of at least this degree of severity would ensue is 13% (i.e., 0.23[31.9 + 4.9 + {19.0(100 − 31.9 − 4.9)/100}] + [0.77 × 2.5]). This estimate that maldevelopment occurs in more than one in eight such pregnancies is of course open to criticism, not least because it assumes that empty sacs and severe disorganization are associated with the same proportions of 4–8-week-old abortions as of those occurring later. Nevertheless, it may be as close as we can get to the true risk of severe maldevelopment once a pregnancy has reached the point at which the embryo normally becomes distinguishable from the rest of the conceptus. Among all conceptions, including those that never reach this stage, the proportion that fail to develop normally is probably even higher: in a series of 34 zygotes from women who underwent hysterectomy 2–17 days after conception, 40% were abnormal.[86]

Incidence of specific defects

The data for induced abortions in Kyoto[87] and spontaneous abortions in London[82,88] have been used elsewhere[15] to estimate the frequency of specific types of malformations in late embryos or early fetuses. The results are compared in Figure 4–4 with birth prevalence statistics from the same countries.[15] This comparison suggests that the malformations shown, except for spina bifida in London, are at least two times as common in early pregnancy as at birth. In three more recent series from predominantly white populations,[85,89,90] spina bifida was reported in at least three times as high a proportion of spontaneous abortions as in the London series, which suggests that some cases in the latter series may have been overlooked.

The studies on which Figure 4–4 is based also suggest that various anomalies such as cyclopia, polydactyly, and abnormal karyotypes other than Down syndrome, which do not pose enough of a problem among infants to be included in this figure, are at least 10 times as common in embryos as in fetuses that survive to the last trimester. Indeed, most of the anomalies seen in early conceptuses are of types seldom or never seen at birth. Even those that are morphologically like malformations observed in the newborn may often differ in etiology: for example, most spontaneously aborted embryos (as opposed to fetuses) with NTD have chromosomal anomalies,[90] which is true of very few infants (including stillbirths) with these defects. However, the frequency of spontaneously aborted malformations that are etiologically similar to those seen in infants may still be substantial enough in relation to the numbers of affected infants to imply that spontaneous abortion accounts for a high proportion of cases of the etiologic types seen in infants. Certainly this is true for Down syndrome, which has the same immediate cause (triplication

of most or all of autosome 21) in aborted and born cases alike.

It follows that when the birth prevalence of a type of malformation is high in a particular group of pregnancies, it cannot be taken for granted that incidence also is relatively high; it may be rather that fewer affected individuals are lost by spontaneous abortion in this group than in others. There are at least two generally applicable ways of exploring which of these possible explanations for a high birth prevalence is more likely to be correct. The more direct approach is to use data either for spontaneous abortions and births or for induced abortions to estimate the incidence of malformations in different groups of embryos and to compare the results, as Figure 4–4 enables us to do for anencephaly in Japan and England. The conclusion in this example is that the differences in birth prevalences between these two countries reflect a difference in incidence. The other main approach is to look for variations in the proportion of *all* pregnancies ending in spontaneous abortion, on the assumption that in groups in which this proportion is lowest the impact of spontaneous abortions on malformation frequency is likely to be lightest. If this proportion therefore is found to be particularly low in a group of pregnancies among which the birth prevalence of a type of malformation is high, the reason for the high birth prevalence is postulated to be that relatively few cases have been lost by spontaneous abortion.[91]

Both of these approaches have been used mainly to explore the variations in the birth prevalences of NTD observed in descriptive studies (pages 71–75). The results suggest that some (but not all) of the associations of birth prevalence with locality and birth rank are secondary to variations in the frequency of spontaneous abortion but that the high prevalence ratios seen in infants born in winter or to parents of low so-

Fig. 4–4. Estimated frequency of common malformations per 1000 total births (solid blocks) and embryos (total blocks).[15] (From Leck,[147] by permission of Hemisphere Publishing Corporation) Estimates for embryos are based on births and miscarriages in England (dashed lines, a), and births and induced abortions in Japan (solid lines, b).

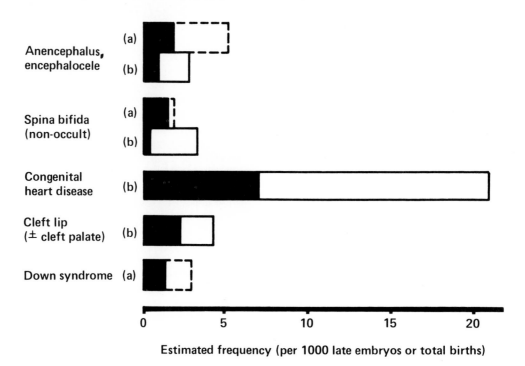

Estimated frequency (per 1000 late embryos or total births)

cioeconomic status are more likely to reflect trends in incidence.[15]

It has also been suggested[92] that variations in the frequency of spontaneous abortion may be responsible for the increase in birth prevalence of Down syndrome with maternal age (pages 75–76). This suggestion was not based on evidence from the two approaches just described, but on two lines of enquiry that are only applicable to chromosomal anomalies: one, a study of disomy in sperm (the precursor of trisomy in conceptuses); and two, a comparison between the maternal age distributions of maternal and paternal cases of Down syndrome (i.e., those found by chromosome banding studies to owe their trisomy-21 to disomic ova and sperms, respectively).

In the study of disomy in sperms, 3 in 1000 were found to be disomic for autosome 21. It was concluded that the incidence of Down syndrome at conception was much higher than its frequency 6 weeks later, as estimated from data on spontaneous abortions and births. An incidence ratio of 12:1000 (3:1000 of paternal origin and 9:1000 of maternal) was suggested, based on the fact that three times as many liveborn cases are maternal as are paternal. If this ratio is correct, 90% of cases must be lost before birth.

The maternal age distributions of maternal and paternal cases suggested that these two groups were associated almost equally with maternal age. This seemed to imply that the association did not date from conception. An association with maternal age arising at this time would be likely to be due to an age-related increase in the frequency of disomy in women's ova, which would only cause an association between maternal age and the incidence at conception of *maternal* cases of Down syndrome. If men as well as women produced more disomic gametes as they aged, this would of course cause a paternal age–related increase in the incidence of paternal cases, which would be reflected in an association with maternal age because paternal and maternal ages are positively correlated; but in these circumstances Down syndrome would tend to be more common at high paternal ages irrespective of maternal age, which seems not to be the case.[74]

Although the involvement of paternal as well as maternal cases of Down syndrome in the association with maternal age suggests that this association is due to variation in the frequency with which cases are eliminated during pregnancy rather than in incidence at conception, the evidence that the incidence ratio is about 1.2% is flawed as support for this hypothesis. If incidence did not rise above this level with advancing maternal age, it would be lower than prevalence at amniocentesis (Fig. 4–3) from age 40 yr upward, which could only happen if the spontaneous abortion rate in this age group was higher for normal pregnancies than for those with Down syndrome. Two other arguments for attributing the maternal age effect to variation in incidence rather than in prenatal survival should also be noted. First, this effect is seen in spontaneous abortions[93] as well as in live births. Second, any variation in prenatal survival with maternal age might be expected to affect cases in which the source of the extra chromosome is a lifelong abnormality in one parent's karyotype (regular or mosaic trisomy-21 or a translocation-21) as well as those due to new mutations, whereas in fact the inherited cases show little or no variation in prevalence with maternal age.[94,95]

The impact that prenatal losses of malformed embryos and fetuses can have on epidemiologic data has thus far been illustrated largely by examples of how variations in prenatal mortality may cause prevalence at birth to vary in the opposite direction. If prenatal mortality is influenced both by whether a malformation is present and by exposure to a factor such as a possible teratogen, a further problem is that the prevalences ratios of the malformation in liveborn and aborted conceptuses may for statistical reasons vary in the same direction with exposure even if its overall frequency is the same in exposed and unexposed. For example, if one-third of recognized pregnancies were associated with smoking, 15% with prenatal death, and 0.283% with cases of Down syndrome (30% of them liveborn), and if smoking increased the probability of prenatal death by 30%, it has been calculated that the prevalence ratio of Down syndrome in the offspring of smokers as a percentage of its ratio in nonsmokers' offspring might be 100% in all pregnancies at the same time as being 70% in the pregnancies that ended in live birth and 90% in the remainder.[96] There are also other circumstances in which real associations between risk factors and malformations of above-average prenatal mortality may be missed or simulated for statistical reasons when only birth prevalence ratios are available, especially when these ratios differ by a factor of three or less.[97] All of these findings illustrate the need for caution when interpreting variations in the birth prevalence ratios of malformations, especially when these variations are relatively small.

Analytic and experimental studies of the etiology of malformations

Epidemiology was initially the study of epidemics. Since its scope broadened to cover disease frequency in general, one of its most obvious achievements has continued to be to provide information on the causes of various epidemics—information that has enabled the epidemics to be ended. This section begins with an example of such an epidemic: the dramatic increase in the birth prevalence of deficiencies of the limbs and ears in various countries around the year 1960 that was eventually shown to be due to the drug thalidomide. Next, the use of analytic and experimental studies to explore the etiology of endemic malformations is illustrated by describing how the hypothesis that one or more nutritional deficiencies may predispose to NTD (page 75) has been tested. Finally, an attempt is made to generalize from these examples of analytic and experimental studies.

Studies of thalidomide-associated defects

During 1961, various clinicians in Germany[98] and one in Australia[99] became concerned because each had recently seen several infants with limb defects of certain types (notably amelia, phocomelia, and radial agenesis) that had previously been very rare. Informal inquiries by the German clinicians at that time established that their cases were part of an epidemic involving hundreds or thousands of infants with these defects or ear anomalies who had been born within the past 1–2 years in West Germany. Many of these infants were also affected by internal malformations.

The obvious causal hypothesis suggested by this, as by any

epidemic, was that some extrinsic factor that had recently become more widespread must be the cause. Three classic types of analytic studies—case study, case–control study, and cohort study—were carried out to refine this hypothesis. All findings incriminated thalidomide, a recently introduced hypnotic drug, which had become very popular and had been available without prescription for a time in West Germany. Also, once thalidomide came under suspicion, correlations between its use and the prevalence of limb and ear defects at different times and places were demonstrated in ecologic studies ("studies in which the units of analysis are populations or groups of people, rather than individuals"[1]).

A case study

The most influential case study was carried out by Lenz and Knapp,[98,100] who obtained detailed antenatal histories from the mothers of 46 affected children, mainly by interviewing the mothers (often repeatedly) and their physicians, although records of prescriptions were also consulted when available. Lenz, a human geneticist, initiated these inquiries without suspecting any particular type of extrinsic factor. His suspicions, however, were aroused when two or three interviewees volunteered that during early pregnancy they had taken the hypnotic drug thalidomide, which they speculated might be to blame for their children's defects. In light of these speculations and the fact that thalidomide had become very popular around 1960, specific inquiries about the taking of thalidomide were made in all the other cases. The results suggested that 41 of the 46 affected children could have been exposed to the drug early in prenatal life. Being a case study, this investigation provided no information about the frequency of thalidomide use by the mothers of normal children and therefore could not formally prove that the relevant defects were more common after thalidomide use, let alone that thalidomide was a teratogen; but its results were highly suggestive.

A case–control study

Very soon after Lenz's suspicions of thalidomide were aroused, he mentioned them to Weicker, another German physician. Weicker too had carried out a case study of affected children, but had not seriously considered thalidomide as a possible cause of the epidemic because he had understood, wrongly, that the drug had also been widely used in the United States (which had not experienced the epidemic).[98] In view of Lenz's suspicions, Weicker and his colleagues returned to 50 of the mothers of affected children in

his case study and asked them directly about thalidomide use during early pregnancy; these investigators also questioned two other series of parents—one a control group with normal children, the other a small group whose children had limb deficiencies of types that had not become more common (e.g., absent hands and digits). All three groups were also asked about use of drugs of various other types.[101]

Table 4–3 shows how often thalidomide and drugs of two other types—antiemetics and hormonal preparations—were said to have been taken by the 50 mothers of affected children and by 90 normal controls. Also shown for each type of drug is the *odds ratio*—the index most often used in case–control studies to measure the strength of the association between exposure variables such as use of thalidomide and outcome variables such as occurrence of the defects under investigation. The odds ratio is the ratio between the numbers of affected and control subjects who were exposed divided by the corresponding ratio for the unexposed subjects: $e_a u_c / e_c u_a$, where e_a and e_c are the numbers of affected and control subjects who were exposed and u_a and u_c are the numbers who were unexposed.

In case–control studies such as this, in which the size of the population from which the cases were drawn is unknown, the odds ratio is computed because it is the best estimate available of the number of times by which the exposure under study increases the prevalence of the outcome under study. The latter number can be defined as the ratio of the prevalence in the exposed to the prevalence in the unexposed and is generally known as the *relative risk* or *risk ratio*: $e_a u_p / e_p u_a$, where e_a and u_a again are the numbers of exposed and unexposed affected subjects and e_p and u_p are the numbers exposed and unexposed in the population from which the affected subjects are drawn. For the odds ratio to be an accurate estimate of the relative risk, the same proportion of the controls as of the population must have been exposed, and the information about each subject's exposure must be accurate. To some extent, the case–control study of Weicker et al.,[101] like those of many others, probably failed to meet these conditions. It can therefore be used to illustrate the effects that such failures can have.

First, the very fact that exposure in the Weicker et al.[101] study was more common in affected than in unaffected children makes it likely that a larger proportion of the population than of the controls was exposed, in which case the odds ratio yielded by this study would be higher than the relative risk. If, for example, the 50 cases and 90 controls had come from a population of 10,000 infants (which prevalence estimates from other sources suggest is of the right order), the controls would if perfectly selected have been representative of the 9950 unaffected infants rather than of the whole population.

Table 4–3. Reported drug use in a case–control study of infants with limb defects of types that increased after the introduction of thalidomide[a]

	No. of cases		No. of controls		
Type of drug	Drug mentioned (e_a)	Drug not mentioned (u_a)	Drug mentioned (e_c)	Drug not mentioned (u_c)	Odds ratio ($e_a u_c / e_c u_a$)
Antiemetics	18	32	20	70	2.0
Hormonal preparations	15	35	9	81	3.9
Thalidomide	34	16	2	88	93.5

[a]Data are from Weicker et al.[101]

Table 4–4. Birth prevalence of skeletal limb defects in a cohort of infants classified by whether their mothers were prescribed thalidomide[a]

| | No. of infants[b] | | Birth prevalence (%) of skeletal limb defects |
History	With skeletal limb defects	Total	
Thalidomide prescribed 0–8 weeks after conception	10	24	41.67
Thalidomide not prescribed in early pregnancy	51	21,485	0.24

[a]Data are from McBride.[103]

[b]Includes stillbirths.

If so, and if the exposure data were accurate, the total number of infants exposed would have been 255 (i.e., [9950 × 2/90] + 34), and the relative risk would have been 81.2 (i.e., [34{10,000 − 255}]/[255{50 − 34}]). The odds ratio of 93.5 (Table 4–3) overestimates this by 15%.

The second and more important source of inaccuracy in case–control studies that the Weicker et al. study appears to illustrate is poor recall of exposure. It is noteworthy, as shown in Table 4–3, that odds ratios of two or more were associated with exposure to drugs other than thalidomide and also that the proportion of mothers of affected infants who recalled having taken thalidomide (68%) is considerably lower than the 89% of cases in which Lenz (who examined medical records as well as questioned mothers) obtained evidence of thalidomide use. One reason why more mothers of cases than of controls recalled taking drugs other than thalidomide was probably because occurrences in pregnancy are likely to be remembered—or imagined—much more clearly than usual, by both patients and their physicians, if the outcome is abnormal (an example of *recall bias*). The failure of many patients' mothers to recall taking thalidomide highlights the fact that even the memories of parents of malformed infants cannot be relied on. The guilt feelings that some parents have may even lead them to suppress memories of anything that they suspect has caused the malformation—a source of memory bias of the reverse kind to that mentioned above.

Despite this evidence of the limited reliability of exposure data in case–control studies, the elevated odds ratio for thalidomide exposure appeared much too high to be attributed to recall bias, especially as no associations of anything like the strength of that between thalidomide and the defects involved in the epidemic were found between these defects and drugs other than thalidomide or between this drug and the types of limb deficiencies that had not become more common.

A cohort study

The suspicions in Australia that thalidomide might be teratogenic originated with McBride,[102] an obstetrician. He knew nothing about the German epidemic of limb defects but observed similar defects in six children whose mothers had been included in a clinical trial carried out between early 1960 and mid-1961 to evaluate the effectiveness of thalidomide for treating morning sickness.[102] This observation later prompted him to carry out an analysis of hospital records of births in 1957–1962 in the obstetric department where this clinical trial had been carried out.[103] His source of informa-

tion about exposure was records of the thalidomide prescribed to each woman at the time of the trial. The investigation was therefore a cohort study—a study in which members of a population ("cohort") are classified according to their experience of an exposure variable into groups that are then compared with respect to the frequency of an outcome.

McBride's study had two advantages over that of Weicker et al. that cohort studies typically have over case–control studies. First, the data on the exposure variable (thalidomide use or nonuse in early pregnancy) were relatively accurate and not biased by the outcome (condition of child at birth), since they were recorded at the time the exposure occurred and several months before the outcome was known. Second, as the numbers exposed and unexposed in the population (e_p and u_p) were known, the relative risk associated with thalidomide use could be computed.

Table 4–4 shows the data required to calculate the relative risk for the infants of mothers for whom thalidomide was reported to have been prescribed within 8 weeks of conception. In addition, there were a few cases of the characteristic limb defects in which prescribing was first recorded 8–16 weeks after the estimated data of conception; but it seems likely that conception occurred later than estimated in these cases, since subsequent work indicates that thalidomide is only teratogenic during the embryonic period (which ends 8 weeks after conception). For infants reported to have been exposed during the latter period, the birth prevalence of skeletal limb defects of all kinds was 41.67%, as opposed to 0.24% for the unexposed. The relative risk of these defects was therefore 174 (i.e., 41.67/0.24). The specific types of skeletal limb defects that were involved in the epidemic must have had a much lower prevalence in unexposed children and a correspondingly higher relative risk. This suggests that the estimate of relative risk yielded by the Weicker et al. case–control study of defects of these types (about 80) was far too low—further evidence that some of the mothers of affected infants in their series who did not recall taking thalidomide had in reality done so.

It is sometimes desirable to know not only the extent to which a particular exposure increases the risk of a malformation or other outcome of pregnancy (the relative risk) but also the impact it has on the total prevalence of the outcome. Several indices of this impact may be encountered. Each of them is sometimes loosely called the "attributable risk" and requires data of the kind shown in Table 4–4 for its calculation. The names of these indices, their values for skeletal limb defects following exposure to thalidomide, and the formulae by which these values were calculated are as follows.

Risk difference (exposed)—the amount by which the risk to the exposed exceeds the risk to the unexposed:

$$41.4\% \qquad (e_a/e_p) - (u_a/u_p)$$

Attributable fraction (exposed)—the proportion of the risk to the exposed that may be attributable to the exposure:

$$99.4\% \qquad [(e_a/e_p) - (u_a/u_p)]/(e_a/e_p)$$

Risk difference (population) or *population excess risk*—the amount by which the risk to the whole population exceeds the risk to the unexposed:

$$0.462/1000 \qquad [(e_a + u_a)/(e_p + u_p)] - [u_a/u_p]$$

Attributable fraction (population)—the proportion of the risk to the population that may be attributable to the exposure:

$$16.3\% \qquad \frac{[(e_a + u_a)/(e_p + u_p)] - [u_a/u_p]}{(e_a + u_a)/(e_p + u_p)}$$

An example of a question about a teratogen that one of these indices might be useful in answering would be whether a nation should launch a program to eliminate a teratogenic infection—a decision that might turn on the magnitude of the population excess risk of malformation associated with the infection. These indices, however, are seldom used in etiologic studies. The relative risk is of more use when deciding whether an association between an exposure and an outcome is likely to be one of cause and effect. It is much easier to believe that such an association may only be indirect—due, that is, to factors that predispose independently to both exposure and outcome—if it has a relative risk of only two or three than if this risk is into double or (as in the case of thalidomide) triple figures.

Ecologic studies

Although the strength of the association with thalidomide revealed by the above studies was strong evidence that this drug was responsible for the epidemic of limb and ear deficiencies, there were still some investigators who suggested that use of the drug and occurrence of the defects might be linked only indirectly, e.g., by a common cause such as one of the disorders treated by thalidomide. This hypothesis, however, was quickly rejected, first because of animal experiments in which defects were observed in litters whose mothers had been given thalidomide in pregnancy[104] and second because of ecologic studies in which the prevalence of limb and ear deficiencies in groups of infants born at different times and in different places was examined for correlations with the levels of exposure to thalidomide that these groups were likely to have experienced. These ecologic studies were needed (as studies of groups often are when an association between an outcome and an exposure that may be causal has been demonstrated in individuals) because it was to be expected that the prevalence of the defects and levels of exposure would be closely correlated if the association seen in individuals was causal but not if it was secondary to a causal relationship between the defects and another exposure, e.g., a maternal condition that was commonly treated by thalidomide.

Weicker, Lenz, and associates supported the case for regarding the association as causal by means of ecologic studies of data for different places and different times, respectively.

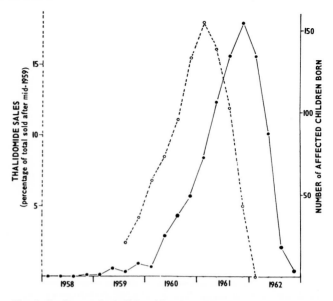

Fig. 4–5. Quarterly thalidomide sales (dashed line) and numbers of infants born with defects of types characteristically seen after thalidomide exposure (solid line) ascertained by Lenz[106] for West Germany, excluding Hamburg. (From Leck[56] by permission of Butterworth Heinemann)

Weicker and Hungerland[105] assembled data showing that the relevant defects had become more common in countries where thalidomide had been used and not elsewhere. Lenz[106] showed that the numbers of affected infants known to him who were born each quarter in West Germany were correlated very closely with thalidomide sales 9 months earlier (Fig. 4–5). The period covered by these data includes the time late in 1961 when, in response to the results of the studies of individuals, thalidomide was withdrawn from use. Consequently, not only the initial increase in prevalence of the defects but also a decline almost to zero 9 months after the drug was withdrawn can be shown (Fig. 4–5). The decline started in early 1962, no doubt because the drug's popularity had already fallen in mid-1961 after it had been found to cause neuropathy in some users. Once its teratogenic effects became known, some women who had taken it during early pregnancy sought induced abortions, which probably explains why the numbers of affected births in mid-1962 were low in proportion to the uptake of thalidomide 9 months earlier.

Studies relating NTD to nutritional deficiencies

The hypothesis that nutritional deficiencies might be involved in causing human NTD arose out of studies of three kinds—animal experiments, a case study, and descriptive epidemiologic work. The animal experiments were those of Hale,[107] Warkany,[108] Giroud,[109] and their successors, who produced NTD and other defects in several species by inducing maternal vitamin deficiencies during pregnancy. In the case study, two fetuses with NTD (anencephaly in one case and meningocele in the other) were observed in a series of 24 pregnancies—16 of them aborted—in which aminopterin (a folic acid antagonist) had been given in order to test its efficacy as an abortifacient.[110,111] As was indicated earlier (page 75), the descriptive epidemiologic work showed that the risk factors for a high birth prevalence of NTD included low socioeconomic status and conception in spring, when the body's reserves of some nutrients may be minimal.

The first analytic and experimental studies testing the resulting "nutritional deficiency hypothesis" took place mainly in the United Kingdom during the 1970s. Although not entirely conclusive, the results of this work suggested that a high intake of one or more vitamins around the time of conception might reduce the risk of NTD and stimulated a "second generation" of investigations in the 1980s. Prominent among these were several analytic studies in Australia and the United States and an international experimental study. In the following account, the studies are grouped by methodology rather than by whether they belonged to the first or second generation.

Ecologic studies

The possibility that groups of women at high risk of bearing infants with NTD (as opposed to high-risk individuals) tend to be relatively poorly nourished has been explored in relation to the two NTD risk factors last mentioned—socioeconomic status and spring conception—by studying groups in the first trimester of pregnancy in two English cities, Leeds and London. Nutrition was investigated in two ways. First, intake of calories, protein, carbohydrate, fat, and some vitamins (vitamin A in both studies, folic acid in the London study only, and several other vitamins in the Leeds study only) was estimated from diaries recording weighed food intake over 1 week. Second, blood levels of certain vitamins (including erythrocyte and serum folates and serum vitamin A in both studies) were measured.

With one exception (carbohydrate intake in the London study), the intake of every nutrient measured was positively associated with socioeconomic status in both studies. An analysis of the London data, which took account of the quality of recording of food intake, suggested that this association was in part an artifact brought about by more complete recordkeeping by the more privileged women; but the association of socioeconomic status with vitamin intake appeared to be real. Blood vitamin levels were also consistently higher in women of high socioeconomic status than in the remainder.[112-114]

Dietary diaries are unreliable as a source of data on seasonal variation because some foods may vary in vitamin content by season, and even the seasonal data on blood vitamin levels that these studies collected were inconclusive. Seasonal peaks in serum folate occurred in London in the July–September quarter and in Leeds in October–December, which are the two quarters when infants with NTD are least often conceived. Mean erythrocyte folate, however, showed no seasonal change in Leeds and was high from October through March in London.[114,115]

Case–control studies

The results of nine case–control studies of the relation of maternal nutrition to NTD are summarized in Table 4–5. The five studies that are listed first[116-120] are comparable to the Weicker et al. case–control study of children with limb defects (Table 4–3) in that they involved gathering particulars about the behavior of mothers of malformed and other chil-

dren. The remaining studies[121-124] were concerned with biochemical measures.

The cases were ascertained from health service records or from registers based on them. The controls in most of the studies were sampled by matching each individual case with one or two control infants from the same population who resembled the case in one or more respects (e.g., locality,[117,120] maternal age,[121,124] or date of mother's last menstrual period[119,121]). Three studies had other kinds of control groups. In one of these three studies[118] the control group was "frequency matched" by race and by quarter and hospital of birth, i.e., although not individually matched to cases, its members were sampled in such a way that their distribution by these variables was similar to that of the cases. The other two studies were concerned with women who were not pregnant. Instead of the cases and controls in these studies being infants, the cases were mothers who had borne offspring with NTD and the controls were other women: in one study[116] sisters of these women who had borne only nonmalformed children and in the other[122] blood donors and mothers of nonmalformed children who were taking part in another study. In commenting further on these case–control studies, it is convenient to distinguish between those analyzing the mothers' behavior and those examining their biochemistry.

Studies of maternal behavior. Unlike most case–control studies (including that of Weicker et al.), these were concerned with exposures that the hypothesis under test envisaged as protective factors rather than as teratogens. The five were, however, typical of case–control studies in that most of them were dependent on mothers for information about exposure. The one exception was the study in which the exposure was prescription of folic acid.[117] In this study the exposure data were abstracted from the family physicians' records of all the mothers in the study. These records dated from the time of exposure and therefore could not have been biased by knowledge of the outcome of pregnancy, unlike the exposure data in the other studies.

Among the three memory-dependent studies in which exposure was defined in terms of vitamin intake before and after conception, the first[118] was based on interviews carried out between 30 mo and 16 yr after the relevant birth, but most of the interviews in the other two studies of this kind[119,120] took place within 6 mo of birth. These three studies were also based on different exposure criteria: in the first, multivitamin use at least 3 days per week throughout the half year that had as its midpoint the onset of the last menstrual period; in the second, relatively high figures for folate intake, estimated from a questionnaire about diet during the year centered on the end of the first trimester; and in the third, intake of enough vitamin tablets and/or vitamin-enriched cereals to reach the U.S. Recommended Daily Allowances of folate and of combinations of vitamins on at least 6 days per week during the 75 days starting 1 mo before onset of the last menstrual period.

Four of the five case–control studies of maternal behavior yielded odds ratios of 0.5 or less, and three of these low ratios differed significantly from unity. However, there was virtually no difference in exposure between the cases and controls in the fifth of these studies. In seeking an explanation for such a discrepancy, one must first consider the possibility that some findings may have been distorted by the problem of recall bias (page 81).

Table 4–5. Results of case–control studies of the relationship of maternal nutrition to NTD

Definition of exposure (refers to mother)[a]	No. of cases		No. of controls		Odds ratio
	Exposed	Unexposed	Exposed	Unexposed	
Nonpregnant diet not "poor"[116]	144	100	91	32	0.51[b]
Folic acid prescribed between 3 mo before and 4 weeks after OLMP[117]	6[c]	758[c]	13	751	0.46
Multivitamins taken regularly from 3 mo before to 3 mo after OLMP[118]	24	157	405	1075	0.41[b]
Above median intake (from 3 mo before to 9 mo after OLMP) of:					
Free folate	26	49	83	67	0.43[b]
Total folate[119]	30	45	79	71	0.60
Recommended daily allowances taken (from 30 days before to 45 days after OLMP) of:					
4+ Vitamins	89	476	90	477	0.99
Folate[120]	69	496	69	498	1.00
Formiminoglutamic acid excretion test for folate deficiency positive around birth date[121]	24[c]	11[c]	6	29	10.55[b]
Nonpregnant erythrocyte folate ≤5th percentile[122]	16	52	7	93	4.09[b]
Nonpregnant leukocyte ascorbic acid ≤5th percentile[122]	14	53	3	67	5.90[b]

Maternal hematologic variable	Mean value for mothers of cases (No. of subjects)		Mean value for mothers of controls (No. of subjects)		Ratio between means
Nonpregnant erythrocyte folate (ng/ml):					
England[122]	200	(68)	222	(100)	0.90
Netherlands[123]	260	(16)	217	(15)	1.20
Scotland[124]	178[d]	(20)	269	(20)	0.66[b]
Nonpregnant leukocyte ascorbic acid (μg/ml of blood)[122]	2.08	(67)	2.19	(70)	0.95

[a]OLMP, onset of last menstrual period.

[b]$P < 0.05$.

[c]Cases of any malformation of central nervous system.

[d]Women with *two* offspring with NTD.

As has already been noted, three of the five studies relied on mothers' recall of circumstances during and before pregnancy. Recall may well have been far from accurate, especially among the mothers who were not interviewed until several years after the relevant birth, but all three reports included evidence that the accuracy of recall was not much affected by whether the offspring was malformed. In each study, this evidence was in the form of data from a second control group (not shown in Table 4–5) that consisted of infants born with abnormalities other than NTD. The proportions of mothers recalling exposure to high levels of vitamins were almost the same for these groups as for the other controls. It may be concluded that pregnancy outcome has little effect on the accuracy with which mothers remember their vitamin intake and that the differences found in some studies between the reported vitamin intakes of mothers of cases and nonmalformed infants cannot be explained in this way.

Apart from recall bias, the most important issues to consider when interpreting the results of a case–control study are perhaps the complementary problems of *confounding* and *overcontrolling*. Confounding would be a problem if NTD were not caused by low vitamin intake but by some other effect of low socioeconomic status. In these circumstances one would still expect NTD to be relatively common in the off-spring of women whose vitamin intake is low, because vitamin intake and socioeconomic status are confounded—they both tend to be low in the same women. It is possible to allow for such confounding either by matching each case with a control of similar socioeconomic status or by using methods such as multiple logistic regression to standardize for socioeconomic status during the analysis of the data. If, however, low vitamin intake was teratogenic, and if this was why the offspring of women of low socioeconomic status was at high risk of NTD, any attempt to neutralize the effect of socioeconomic status would run the risk of obscuring the association of NTD with vitamin intake. If this happened it would be an example of overcontrolling.

Despite the risk of overcontrolling, the data from all three memory-based studies of periconceptional vitamin intake[118–120] were analyzed by methods designed to neutralize the effects of socioeconomic status or related variables (educational attainment, family income) and other risk factors. The odds ratios yielded by these methods differed very little from those shown in Table 4–5, which were calculated by the simple formula stated in Table 4–3. It therefore seems unlikely that the latter odds ratios were distorted by confounding. Indeed, given the precautions against recall bias and confounding that were taken in all three studies, the discrepancy

Table 4-6. Results of cohort studies of the relationship of maternal nutrition to NTD

| Definition of exposure (refers to mother)[a] | No. of fetuses/infants | | | | Relative risk |
| | Exposed | | Unexposed | | |
	Affected	Total	Affected	Total	
First trimester diet not "poor" in previous pregnancies[b,125]	82	168	92	129	0.68[c]
First trimester diet not "poor" in current pregnancy:					
First Welsh cohort[b,125]	0	138	8	30	0.00[c]
Second Welsh cohort[b,116]	0	144	5	32	0.00[c]
Intake at least weekly during early pregnancy (starting before or ≤6 weeks after OLMP) of multivitamins:					
Containing folate	10	10,713	39	11,944	0.29[c]
Not containing folate[128]	3	926	46	21,731	1.53

Maternal hematologic variable	Mean value for mothers of cases (No. of subjects)		Mean value for mothers of unaffected (No. of subjects)		Ratio between means
First trimester erythrocyte folate (ng/ml):					
England[112]	149	(5)	228	(959)	0.65[c]
Wales[b,116]	229	(6)	265	(60)	0.86
First trimester leukocyte ascorbic acid (μg/ml of blood)[112]	1.67	(4)	2.42	(1098)	0.69[c]

[a]OLMP, onset of last menstrual period.

[b]Mothers studied had already borne at least one offspring with NTD.

[c]$P < 0.05$.

between the negative results of one and the evidence of a protective effect in the other two seems a highly surprising finding, which is further discussed later in this review.

Studies of maternal biochemistry. Two general points are illustrated by the results of these studies. On the one hand, one appropriate way to examine the relationship of quantitative variables to outcomes such as NTD is to compare the mean values of these variables in affected and unaffected subjects. On the other hand, comparisons of the proportions of cases and controls with extreme readings can sometimes reveal significant variations that are not reflected in differences between means. Thus Table 4-5 includes data from one study of various blood vitamin levels in nonpregnant women[122] in which the mean values for erythrocyte folic acid (EFA) and leukocyte ascorbic acid (vitamin C) were almost the same for mothers of NTD cases and controls, whereas the mothers of cases were more than four times as likely as the mothers of controls to have very low values for these variables.

Table 4-5 shows two other significant biochemical differences: a reduction in the mean nonpregnant EFA level in mothers of *two* offspring with NTD[124] and a marked difference between mothers of children with malformations of the central nervous system and other mothers in the proportion excreting abnormally large amounts of formiminoglutamic acid (a marker of folic acid deficiency) at around the time of delivery.[121] Compared with studies in which the data on exposure are gathered at interview when the outcome is known, these and other biochemical studies have of course the advantage that their results cannot be affected by recall bias.

Cohort studies

It is generally true of epidemiologic research that cohort studies require more resources than do case-control studies, with the result that fewer are undertaken. Studies of the relationship of nutrition to NTD are not an exception to this generalization. There appear to be only three groups of workers who have reported analytic studies of nutrition and NTD in cohorts of women and their offspring. Their findings are summarized in Table 4-6.

The first three and the penultimate rows of figures in Table 4-6 are based on one of two cohorts of South Wales women who had borne offspring with NTD before being studied.[116,125] After ascertainment through health service records and registers in which their malformed offspring had been recorded, these women were questioned about both their nonpregnant diet and their diet during the first trimester of each of their pregnancies. Some of those who planned to have further children were invited to become subjects in two experimental studies. If they agreed they were asked to notify the investigators if they became pregnant. If this happened they were interviewed again, this time about diet early in the new pregnancy.

Some of the results of these studies were concerned with the effects of the experimental interventions, which will be considered later in this chapter; but the investigators also provided four sets of data relating pregnancy outcome to their assessments of diet as recorded at interview. One of these data sets involved the comparison between the mothers of offspring with NTD and their sisters, which was summarized as a case-control study in the first row of Table 4-5. The other three sets were concerned exclusively with cohorts of pregnancies in mothers of affected offspring and are therefore summarized in Table 4–6. The first of these three sets (in the first row of Table 4–6) was based on the pregnancies that the mothers had already undergone when first interviewed. It is therefore atypical of cohort studies (but typical of case–control studies) in that the data on exposure (in this instance diet in pregnancy) were collected *retrospectively,* i.e., not at the time of exposure but subsequently, when outcome was known and could have biased the mothers' recall. More typically for cohort studies, the remaining two Welsh data sets were based on the pregnancies that were studied *prospectively* (i.e., while they were happening instead of only later), of which there were two cohorts. The published exposure data for these two cohorts cannot have been biased by an effect of outcome on maternal recall. However, it has been suggested that the worker who finally assigned each mother's diet to a category such as "poor" may not always have been unaware ("blind") as to the outcome, which could in this case have biased the category assigned.[126,127]

One of the two Welsh prospective studies also yielded some data on maternal biochemistry in early pregnancy,[116] including EFA readings. The mean levels of the readings for pregnancies in which supplementary folic acid was not being given are shown in the penultimate line of Table 4–6. In pregnancies in which the offspring were later found to have an NTD, the mean EFA level was lower than in other pregnancies; and although this difference was not statistically significant, significant differences of this kind in both EFA and leukocyte ascorbic acid levels were found by one of the two other teams who have reported cohort studies of nutrition and NTD.[112] This team was based in Leeds, England. Its study cohort was not restricted to pregnancies in mothers of affected children, as were those studied in Wales, but included all pregnancies in Leeds residents who booked between certain dates for obstetric care, were in the first trimester, and had consented to be studied.

The third team was based in Boston, MA, and collected data on vitamin use and other exposures at about 16 weeks gestation for two cohorts of pregnancies.[128] At this time the pregnancies in the larger cohort—69% of the total—had just been assayed for maternal serum α-fetoprotein level at one hospital in Boston, whereas those in the smaller cohort had just undergone amniocentesis either there or at a variety of other genetic centers. In Table 4–6, this study is represented by two analyses of both cohorts combined. The data are broken down in the first of these analyses by whether multivitamin preparations including folic acid had been taken in early pregnancy and in the second by whether other combinations of vitamins had been used. The first but not the second of these exposures appeared to be protective.

In this study, the mothers' recall of vitamin use could have been biased in relation to outcome both because some of them (7% of the cohort that had undergone amniocentesis) knew the results of the amniocentesis at the time of interview and because the risk of bearing a malformed child appeared at that time to be increased for many more (the rest of those in the cohort that had undergone amniocentesis, together with any in the other cohort whose maternal serum α-fetoprotein level had been reported to be abnormal before they were interviewed). However, the relative risks of NTD that the study yielded for exposure to multivitamins containing folic acid were much less extreme for those who knew the results of amniocentesis (0.54) than for those who had not had

amniocentesis (0.07) or who were still awaiting its results (0.08), which suggests that there is an association between folic acid intake and outcome that knowledge of outcome tends to weaken rather than to exaggerate.

The results of these cohort studies, as of the case–control ones reviewed earlier, should not be accepted as evidence that folic acid or any other aspect of nutrition protects against NTD without considering the possibility of confounding between diet and other possible effects of low socioeconomic status. In the Boston study, multivariate logistic regression methods were used to control for the effects of some correlates of socioeconomic status (maternal education and number of previous children) and other risk factors. As when similar methods were used in case–control studies (page 84), the adjusted estimate of risk was virtually identical to the uncorrected one shown in Table 4–6.

Experimental/intervention studies

In an intervention study, subjects who are at risk of an adverse outcome such as the occurrence of an NTD are deliberately subjected to an intervention—a procedure designed to protect against exposure to a suspected cause such as vitamin deficiency—after which the frequencies of the outcomes in this group and those in unprotected subjects are compared. Some intervention studies have an intervention group consisting of all members of a population at risk who were available to undergo the intervention and a non-intervention group made up of the other members of this population. Others are true experimental studies, i.e., the intervention and nonintervention groups are both made up of subjects available to undergo the intervention, each of whom is allocated to one or the other group according to a scheme controlled by the investigators.

Generally, in experimental studies allocation is random, which results in the two groups being comparable except in regard to whether they undergo the intervention. In other intervention studies, the fact that the groups differ in availability for intervention may mean that they also differ in respects such as socioeconomic status, which may lead to bias. Experimental studies are therefore the more reliable. However, when investigations other than intervention studies yield very strong evidence linking exposure and outcome (as was the case for thalidomide and limb defects), the only kind of intervention study considered ethical may be a nonexperimental one such as the comparison between the frequency with which infants with limb defects were born before and after the intervention of withdrawing thalidomide. (Fig. 4–5).

Table 4–7 summarizes the results obtained by three teams of workers who have carried out experiments and two who have used other intervention study designs to explore the relationship of nutrition to NTD. The first three rows of figures relate to the two experimental studies on South Wales women mentioned above (page 85). These two studies were based on a single cohort of women who were planning to have further children after bearing offspring with NTD. For the study listed first in Table 4–7, the members of the cohort were selected to receive dietary advice or not on the basis of where they lived. For the other study, they were invited to enter a randomized double-blind trial in which each woman was given tablets of folic acid or placebo to take twice daily, starting when she discontinued contraception and finishing

Table 4–7. Results of experimental/intervention studies of the relationship of maternal nutrition to NTD[a]

Intervention applied to mother	No. of fetuses/infants				Relative risk
	Intervention group		Nonintervention group		
	Affected	Total	Affected	Total	
Allocation of intervention controlled by investigators					
Preconceptional dietary advice[b,125]	3	99	5	69	0.42
Folic acid 4 mg/day, analyzed by:					
Treatment allocated[b]	2	60	4	51	0.43
Treatment received[b,129]	0	44	6	67	0.00
Multivitamins, including folic acid 0.8 mg/day[130]	0	599	3	703	0.00
Folic acid 4 mg/day (± other vitamins)[b,131]	6	593	21	602	0.29[d]
Multivitamins ± folic acid[b,131]	12	597	15	598	0.80
Allocation of intervention not controlled by investigators					
Multivitamins, including folic acid 0.36 mg/day[c]:					
Multiple U.K. centers[b,132,133]	3	459	24	529	0.14[d]
Yorkshire, England[b,134]	1	150	18	320	0.12[d]
Northern Ireland[b,135]	4	511	17	353	0.16[d]
Folic acid 5 mg/day[b,136]	0	80	4	118	0.00

[a]In all vitamin supplementation studies, subjects were recommended to take the supplement from at or before discontinuation of contraception until second missed period or later.

[b]Mothers studied had already borne at least one offspring with NTD.

[c]There was some overlap between these series.

[d]$P < 0.05$.

at 12 weeks gestation.[116,125,129] Analysis of the cohort by outcome according to whether dietary advice had been given yielded a relative risk of 0.4. A similar figure was obtained when the members of the cohort who entered the double-blind trial were analyzed by outcome according to whether folic acid had been allocated. The entrants to this trial were also analyzed by whether blood folic acid assay indicated that those allocated folic acid had taken it as instructed. None of the mothers of affected infants had done so. This last analysis (the third in Table 4–7) can, however, be criticized on the ground that it involved comparing groups of women who were not identical in all respects except for the intervention: those who took folic acid were all compliant, while those who did not were a mixture of compliers and noncompliers.

Each of the other two teams who undertook experimental studies used double-blind designs that involved giving other vitamins as well as folate and placebo to women who were hoping to conceive. For one of these experiments, based in Hungary, only interim figures appear thus far to have been published.[130] This experiment is unique among the studies listed in Table 4–7 in including women who have not previously had an affected child. The reason for the other studies being restricted to mothers of offspring with NTD is these women's increased risk of producing further affected offspring. If the frequency of NTD was to change by any given percentage, fewer of these women's pregnancies than of all pregnancies would need to be studied in order to demonstrate the change.

The most recently reported experiment was an international project in which most of the study pregnancies were British or Hungarian.[131] A unique feature of this study was

that it dealt with folic acid and a selection of other vitamins as separate interventions: women with affected offspring who wished to conceive again were randomly allocated to receive folic acid and other vitamins, folic acid alone, other vitamins alone, or placebo, from the time of entry into the study until 12 weeks after onset of the last menstrual period. In Table 4–7 the results are analyzed in two ways—first, by whether folic acid was allocated, and, second, by whether other vitamins were. The figures are consistent with the results of the Boston cohort study (Table 4–6) in pointing to a significant protective effect for folic acid but not for other vitamins.

The latter two experiments were undertaken in response to the positive results yielded by the South Wales trial of folic acid and by the first of the four nonexperimental intervention studies listed in Table 4–7. In all four nonexperimental studies, women with affected offspring who wished to conceive again were advised to take vitamin supplements from 1 month before unprotected intercourse until 2 months or more after onset of the last menstrual period. The pregnancy outcomes in the women who accepted this advice were compared with those in mothers who presented after conception with a history of having previously borne affected offspring. The first of the four studies was a collaborative project involving pregnant women cared for at several medical centers in the United Kingdom.[132,133] Subsequently the investigators in two of these centers, Northern Ireland and Yorkshire, published separate reports for their areas, covering many later cases as well as those they had contributed to the multicenter study.[134,135] The intervention in these studies was a multivitamin preparation including folic acid. The fourth and final study was from Cuba. There, the only intervention was a folic acid supplement.[136] The relative risks yielded by all four studies suggest that vitamin supplementation has an even stronger protective effect than that demonstrated for folic acid by the recent international trial. However, this difference between the results of the latter study and the earlier results could well be due to chance or to the relative risks yielded by the nonexperimental studies being exaggerated by bias.

Conclusions

The research on NTD and nutrition provides an excellent example of the way in which etiologic hypotheses can be developed and tested with increasing rigor by ecologic, case–control, cohort, and experimental studies. However, all that the recent international trial can be claimed to prove is that folic acid intake influences the risk of *recurrence* of NTD. It does not show how many of the cases of NTD that occur in previously unaffected families—as most do—might be prevented by folic acid. The answer to this question may depend on whether the recurrence risk is elevated to a modest extent (of the order of tenfold) in most affected families or is low in the majority but greatly elevated in a few (including most of those in which recurrences occur). One would expect familial and other cases to be similar in etiology (and thus to respond similarly to folic acid) if the former model applied but not if the latter was true.

Some support for the view that familial cases are etiologically distinct is given by the biochemical data in Table 4–5. These data suggest that, among nonpregnant women, EFA levels tend to be low in those who have had more than one offspring with NTD,[124] but not in those with only one affected offspring (except for a minority who may be women at high risk of producing more cases).[122] However, the view that a relative lack of folic acid plays some part in the etiology of more than a small subgroup of NTD is supported by other findings—first, the strength of the associations between multivitamin or folic acid intake and NTD observed in most case–control and cohort studies (Tables 4–5 and 4–6), and, second, the low EFA levels seen during early NTD pregnancies (Table 4–6) and the evidence of folic acid deficiency at the end of such pregnancies provided by the formiminoglutamic acid test (Table 4–5), which were common to most cases in the two studies cited.[112,121] Folic acid supplementation might therefore be expected to confer worthwhile protection against NTD on pregnancies in general rather than exclusively on those with a positive family history. However, some uncertainty will remain until this possibility has been tested in one or more large trials. When it includes enough subjects, the Hungarian trial of vitamin supplementation in pregnancies not selected for positive family history,[130] for which interim figures are given in Table 4–7, should help to meet this need.

Two other findings in Tables 4–5 and 4–6 call for comment in light of the results from the international trial given in Table 4–7. The first is the occurrence of low levels of leukocyte ascorbic acid as well as EFA in all women with affected offspring who were tested in early pregnancy (Table 4–6)[112] and in a minority of those tested in the nonpregnant state (Table 4–5).[122] This finding seems more likely to be due to confounding between folic acid and ascorbic acid levels than to any direct relationship between ascorbic acid and NTD, given that ascorbic acid was one of the combination of vitamins other than folic acid that had no significant effect on the risk of NTD in the trial.

The second noteworthy finding is that, despite the evidence of a protective effect of folic acid provided by the trial, no association between folic acid intake and risk of NTD was detected in one of the three memory-based case–control studies of periconceptional vitamin intake (Table 4–5).[120] It has been suggested[137] that this finding indicates that the effect of folic acid is most pronounced in areas where NTD are relatively common, since their frequencies in California (the main base of the study with negative results) are considerably lower than in the areas where associations between vitamin intake and NTD were observed (Atlanta[118] and Boston[128] in the United States and centers in Australia,[119] Hungary, and the United Kingdom.[116,117,125,129–135]).

The hypothesis that folic acid confers most protection in high-risk areas is also supported by evidence that the recurrence rate following periconceptional vitamin supplementation is lower in the region of the United Kingdom where NTD are most common (Northern Ireland) than in the region where they are least common (southeastern England).[135] It could be that folic acid or a related compound plays a critical part in neural tube closure and that areas at high risk of NTD owe their high risk to genetic and/or environmental factors that tend to render inadequate the supply of this compound to the embryo. If this were so, it would not be surprising if increased folic acid intake reduced the risk disproportionately in high-risk areas.

General comments on analytic and experimental studies of etiology

It may be helpful to conclude by returning to certain general points that are illustrated by the above examples of how analytic and experimental studies may clarify the etiology of malformations.

The origins of hypotheses

The first question to be considered is how suspicions that a particular exposure is teratogenic or protective in humans may first arise. Except when prompted by animal experiments, such suspicions usually stem originally from an impression that malformations (often those of a specific type or types) are especially common in a particular category of infants. This category may consist of infants born in a certain place or period (e.g., the recent past, as was the case in the early 1960s in Germany for the thalidomide-related defects) or of infants whose parents have characteristics that are plausible causes of maldevelopment (e.g., diabetes mellitus)[138] or that might be correlated with exposure to such causes (e.g., low socioeconomic status in the case of NTD). Although the first hint that such a category is at high risk has sometimes come from descriptive epidemiologic studies, as in the last-mentioned example, what has more often happened is that the suspicions of an alert clinician or clinicians (e.g., Lenz, McBride, and Weicker in the case of thalidomide) have been aroused by seeing several cases of some type of defect in a short period or in the offspring of a particular group of women. A common initial response in these circumstances is for the clinician to carry out a case study covering both the clinicopathologic findings in the infants and the circumstances of the parents (including exposure to any factors that might be causally related to the defects) during and before the pregnancy, as Lenz and Knapp did in response to the epidemic of limb defects caused by thalidomide (page 80).

Limitations of case studies

The most that a case study can show is that a proportion of cases of a type of defect have occurred after exposure to some factor such as a disease or medication of the mother during early pregnancy. It does not show that the exposure has occurred in a higher proportion of cases than of all pregnancies and therefore cannot be regarded as proof that this exposure is even a risk factor for the defect, let alone a cause. This may seem too obvious to need saying; but the mass media have sometimes encouraged the public to believe that some widely used drug or other is teratogenic for no better reason than that a substantial number of mothers of malformed children have taken it in pregnancy, instead of recognizing that this number is only large because the drug has been used in a high proportion of all pregnancies. For example, the medication marketed in the United States as Bendectin and in the United Kingdom as Debendox—a preparation of doxylamine, pyridoxine, and (when first used) dicyclomine, which was used to treat nausea of pregnancy—was widely accused of being a teratogen because many mothers of malformed children recalled using it; but case–control and cohort studies alike suggested that it did not increase the risk of malformations,[139] from which one can conclude that the number of affected children of users was large only because the total number of pregnancies in which it was used was extremely large—perhaps about 33 million.[140]

Case studies in which an exposure that could be teratogenic or protective is reported in a suggestive number of cases therefore need to be followed by case–control or cohort studies to determine whether the odds ratio or relative risk is significantly different from unity.

Relative merits of case–control and cohort studies

As was illustrated when the McBride and the Weicker et al. studies of thalidomide and malformations were compared (page 81), cohort studies typically have the advantage over case–control studies of being able to determine the relative risk and the various measures of the impact of the exposure under investigation that can be subsumed by the term "attributable risk." Also, the data on exposure are generally recorded prospectively in cohort studies but retrospectively in case–control studies, and retrospectively collected exposure data can often be affected by recall bias (page 81) if they consist of what the mothers of subjects can remember about exposure.

In most of the memory-dependent case–control studies that were cited above, attempts were made to allow for the impact that having abnormal offspring might have had on recall by comparing the cases with abnormal as well as normal controls, with results that suggested that not much recall bias had occurred in these particular studies. However, the results of memory-dependent case–control studies of defects are sometimes far from unbiased. For example, a study of this kind in Finland suggested that antipyretic and related drugs such as aspirin had been used in early pregnancy in nearly four times as high a proportion of cases of central nervous system defects as of controls,[141] whereas no association between this exposure and outcome was found in an American cohort study in which the data were gathered prospectively.[35] Each of these studies was based on subjects who were born mainly during the 1960s, and each included about 80 cases whose mothers were classified as exposed. The most probable explanation for the discrepancy between the results is that in the Finnish series the mothers of controls had forgotten and/or the mothers of cases imagined events such as drug use that the latter could blame for their misfortune.

Differences in recall between the mothers of cases and the mothers of controls are not the only source of bias in case–control studies.[142] The most important other source is selection bias, which arises when the controls are selected in ways that impair their comparability to the cases. Among the case–control studies described in this chapter, the one most open to this criticism was probably the study of blood vitamin levels in which the controls with whom mothers of offspring with NTD were compared were blood donors and mothers of nonmalformed children who were taking part in another study (page 83). A more closely comparable and therefore preferable group to use as controls would have been a sample of women who lived in the same locality as the cases' mothers and bore normal children during the period when the cases were born.

Selection bias can also arise from self-selection, when some subjects who have been selected as cases or controls refuse to participate. The more refusers there are, the less representative of the study population are the participants likely to be.

Against all these disadvantages of case–control studies must be set the advantage that they tend to take less time and use fewer resources than cohort studies in which the data are collected prospectively. It is much cheaper and quicker to ask 100 mothers of offspring with NTD and 100 control mothers to reminisce than it is to interview and follow-up a cohort of over 10,000 pregnant women, which one might need to do to get prospective data covering even 50 affected pregnancies. The cohort size required increases with the rarity of the type of defect to be studied, which virtually rules out studying the less common types in this way. Even when exploring the etiology of a relatively common condition, it is generally best not to embark on a prospective cohort study unless case–control studies strongly suggest that a particular exposure is causal. This last piece of advice would not, however, apply if prospectively recorded exposure data for a cohort were already available, as they were to McBride when his case study of children with limb defects led him to suspect that thalidomide was teratogenic (page 81).

It should also be noted that not all case–control studies are prone to recall bias. For example, this problem did not arise when mothers of offspring with NTD and of normal children were compared with respect either to prescriptions recorded before and during early pregnancy (page 83) or to biochemical findings at around the time of delivery or later (page 85). Recall bias is also avoided when case–control studies are "nested" in cohort studies, as they were in an enquiry in which the possibility of maternal viral infections causing NTD was explored (with negative results) by comparing maternal antibody titers for the NTD pregnancies in the Collaborative Perinatal Project (page 70) with titers for a control group sampled from the other pregnancies covered by this project.[143] Blood for measuring the titers was available because specimens from virtually all the pregnancies in the study had been banked.

Another modified case–control design that carries relatively little risk of recall bias is that used by the Central-East France Register of Congenital Malformations. There, data on drug use (and other matters) are collected only from women with malformed offspring. To detect associations between drugs and defects, the proportion of exposures to each drug of interest among cases of each major type of defect is compared with the corresponding proportion for cases of all other defects, so that the latter cases serve as controls for the former. Valproic acid first came under suspicion as a teratogen when its use in early pregnancy was found to have been reported in 6% of the Register's cases of spina bifida as against 0.3% of its cases of other defects.[144]

Confounding and its control

Irrespective of which type of study design, case–control or cohort, one uses to test for an association between an exposure and a malformation, the problems of confounding and overcontrolling (page 84) must be borne in mind. Multivariate regression methods are being used increasingly often, as they were in several of the case–control and cohort studies of nutrition and NTD (pages 83 and 85), as a means of attempting to neutralize the effects of confounding variables; but these methods should not be applied by the statistically naïve without expert help.[145]

In case–control studies, confounding is liable to be aggravated by selection bias and is commonly addressed (as it was in most of the case–control studies of nutrition and NTD [page 83]) by individual or frequency matching of cases and controls as well as or instead of by an analytic procedure such as multiple logistic regression. To achieve any control of confounding variables, the matching must of course be by variables that are of this kind, as socioeconomic status or (at least in the United Kingdom) region might be in a study of NTD and nutrition. If each case is individually paired with one control on this basis, there is a strong argument for retaining the pairing when the data are analyzed.[146] This means that the odds ratio is calculated by dividing the number of pairs in which the case but not the control was exposed by the number for which the reverse was true. The distinction between this approach and the method used in Tables 4–3 and 4–5 (analysis of data for individuals as opposed to pairs) is illustrated in Table 4–8 by figures from the case–control study relating folic acid prescription to the birth of children with central nervous system defects (page 83), which was based in England and Wales. In this example the cases and controls were matched for physician and therefore for locality, and the pairwise analysis suggests more strongly than the analysis of individuals that folic acid prescription during the first trimester was protective (although the results were not statistically significant). It may be concluded that in the analysis of individuals, any association between nonprescription of folic acid and malformations was weakened by confounding between prescription and physician or locality.

Ecologic studies can provide a further means of testing whether an association between a malformation and exposure to a possible teratogen is due to confounding, provided that the exposure and the variable that is confounded with it in individuals are not confounded at the level of the populations that are to be compared. For example, when it was

Table 4–8. Results of analyses of unpaired and paired data on whether folic acid was prescribed during the first trimester of pregnancy in cases (fetuses/infants with central nervous system defects) and controls (normal infants)[a]

Distribution of individuals			
	Cases	Controls	Total
Folate prescribed	241	266	507
Folate not prescribed	523	498	1,021
Total	764	764	1,528

$$\text{Odds ratio} = \frac{241 \times 498}{266 \times 523} = 0.86$$

$$\chi^2 = \frac{[(241 \times 498) - (266 \times 523)]^2 \times 1528}{764 \times 764 \times 507 \times 1021} = 1.84$$

Distribution of case–control pairs			
	Controls		
Cases	Folate prescribed	Folate not prescribed	Total
Folate prescribed	168	73	241
Folate not prescribed	98	425	523
Total	266	498	764

Odds ratio = 73/98 = 0.74. $\chi^2 = (98 - 73)^2/(98 + 73) = 3.65$

[a]Data are from Winship et al.[117]

suggested that the association of limb defects with thalidomide might be due to confounding between thalidomide use and a hypothetic teratogenic disease of pregnancy that the drug had been used to treat, this suggestion could be dismissed because the birth prevalence of the defects varied with thalidomide use between periods and places for which no parallel variation in the frequency of any such disease could be demonstrated (page 82).

Conclusion

The evidence of teratogenesis or protection that all of these case–control, cohort, and ecologic study methods provide cannot of course match the level of proof that can be achieved by a well-planned and well-executed intervention study, like the most recent randomized double-blind trial of vitamin supplementation in women with NTD offspring (Table 4–7). However, with the exception of the still ill-defined problem that is corrected by folic acid supplementation, all the known human teratogens have been incriminated by methods that have stopped short of experimental studies in humans. What has often happened is that suspicions aroused by a case study have been supported or refuted by the use of purely analytic epidemiologic methods (case–control, cohort, and/or ecologic). Diseases, medicaments, and other factors to which parents or their offspring may be exposed have generally been accepted as teratogenic if epidemiologic research of this kind has shown that pregnancies in which there is a history of exposure are substantially more likely than others to yield malformed offspring, provided that certain other conditions have also been satisfied:

1. That the association appears unlikely to be caused by bias or confounding (e.g., because the odds ratio or relative risk is very high—perhaps in double figures—or because several analytic studies using different methods and databases have yielded similar risk estimates)

2. That the malformations responsible for the excess of cases among exposed offspring are largely of one or a few specific types, as opposed to being distributed by type in the same way as the cases seen in the general population

3. That the time during pregnancy at which the cases involved in the excess have been exposed is no later than the time at which their defects would have originated

4. That experience in fields other than epidemiology (e.g., animal experiments or, in the case of microorganisms, laboratory evidence of fetal infection in humans) makes it plausible that the exposure and malformations under consideration should be causally related.

It is recommended that students of malformations should continue to use the above methods and criteria when evaluating possible teratogens. If a strong association between an exposure and a defect does not satisfy the last three criteria, the possibility that the exposure is reducing prenatal mortality among malformed fetuses rather than causing malformations may merit consideration.

References

1. Last JM: A Dictionary of Epidemiology, ed 2. Oxford University Press, New York, 1988.
2. Hook EB: Incidence and prevalence as measures of the frequency of birth defects. Am J Epidemiol 116:743, 1982.
3. Czeizel A: Re: "incidence and prevalence as measures of the frequency of birth defects." Am J Epidemiol 119:141, 1984.
4. Neel JV: A study of major congenital defects in Japanese infants. Am J Hum Genet 10:398, 1958.
5. Leck I: An epidemiological assessment of neonatal screening for dislocation of the hip. J R Coll Phys Lond 20:56, 1986.
6. Mackeprang M, Hay S, Lunde AS: Completeness and accuracy of reporting of malformations on birth certificates. HSMHA Health Rep 87:43, 1972.
7. Frost F, Starzyk P, George S, et al.: Birth complication reporting: the effect of birth certificate design. Am J Public Health 74:505, 1984.
8. Knox EG, Armstrong EH, Lancashire RJ: The quality of notification of congenital malformations. J Epidemiol Community Health 38:296, 1984.
9. Leck I, Record RG: Sources of variation in the reporting of malformations. Dev Med Child Neurol 5:364, 1963.
10. Master-Notani P, Kolah PJ, Sanghvi LD: Congenital malformations in the newborn in Bombay. Part I. Acta Genet 18:97, 1968.
11. Erickson JD: Racial variations in the incidence of congenital malformations. Ann Hum Genet 39:315, 1976.
12. Khouri MJ, Erickson JD, James LM: Etiologic heterogeneity of neural tube defects: clues from epidemiology. Am J Epidemiol 115:538, 1982.
13. Khoury MJ, Waters GD, Erickson JD: Patterns and trends of multiple congenital anomalies in birth defects surveillance systems. Teratology 44:57, 1991.
14. Leck I, Record RG, McKeown T, et al.: The incidence of malformations in Birmingham, England, 1950–1959. Teratology 1:263, 1968.
15. Leck I: Fetal malformations. In: Obstetrical Epidemiology. SL Barron, AM Thomson, eds. Academic Press, London, 1983, p 263.
16. Morton NE, Chung CS, Mi M-P: Genetics of Inter-Racial Crosses in Hawaii. Karger, Basel, 1967.
17. Kallén B, Bertollini R, Castilla E, et al.: A joint international study on the epidemiology of hypospadias. Acta Paediatr Scand Suppl 324, 1986.
18. Little J, Carr-Hill RA: Problems of ascertainment of congenital malformations. Acta Genet Med Gemellol 33:97, 1984.
19. International Clearinghouse for Birth Defects Monitoring Systems: Congenital Malformations Worldwide: A Report from The International Clearinghouse for Birth Defects Monitoring Systems. Elsevier, Amsterdam, 1991.
20. Weatherall JAC, Haskey JC: Surveillance of malformations. Br Med Bull 32:39, 1976.
21. Office of Population Censuses and Surveys: Congenital Malformation Statistics: Notifications (Series MB3 Nos. 1–5). Her Majesty's Stationery Office, London, 1983–91.
22. Edmonds LD, Layde PM, James LM, et al.: Congenital malformations surveillance: two American systems. Int J Epidemiol 10:247, 1981.
23. Klemetti A, Saxén L: The Finnish Register of Congenital Malformations: Organization and Six Years of Experience (Paper 9), Health Services Research of the National Board of Health in Finland, Helsinki, 1970.
24. Czeizel A, Rácz J: Evaluation of drug intake during pregnancy in the Hungarian case–control surveillance of congenital anomalies. Teratology 42:505, 1990.
25. Tikkanen J, Heinonen OP: Maternal exposure to chemical and physical factors during pregnancy and cardiovascular malformations in the offspring. Teratology 43:591, 1991.
26. Weatherall JAC, de Wals P, Lechat MF: Evaluation of information systems for the surveillance of congenital malformations. Int J Epidemiol 13:193, 1984.
27. Erickson JD: Risk factors for birth defects: data from the Atlanta Birth Defects Case–Control Study. Teratology 43:41, 1991.
28. Dolk H, Goyens S, Lechat MF: Eurocat Registry Descriptions 1979–90: Final Report (EUR 13615). Commission of the European Communities, Luxembourg, 1991.
29. Ten Cate LP, Dolk H, Cornel MC, et al.: Frequency of births with potentially avoidable serious chromosomal anomalies in EEC countries, 1979–1982. J Epidemiol Community Health 42:266, 1988.
30. EUROCAT Working Group: Prevalence of neural tube defects in 20 regions of Europe and the impact of prenatal diagnosis, 1980–1986. J Epidemiol Community Health 45:52, 1991.
31. Lancaster PAL: Teratogenicity of isotretinoin. Lancet 2:1254, 1988.
32. Hook EB: Timely monthly surveillance of birth prevalence rates of congenital malformations and genetic disorders ascertained by registers or other systematic data bases. Teratology 41:177, 1990.
33. Khoury MJ, Holtzman NA: On the ability of birth defects monitoring to detect new teratogens. Am J Epidemiol 126:136, 1987.
34. Myrianthopoulos NC, Chung CS: Congenital malformations in singletons: epidemiologic survey. Report from the Collaborative Perinatal Project. BDOAS X(11):1, 1974.
35. Heinonen OP, Slone D, Shapiro S: Birth Defects and Drugs in Pregnancy. Publishing Sciences Group, Littleton, MA, 1977.
36. Knox EG, Lancashire RJ: Epidemiology of Congenital Malformations. Her Majesty's Stationery Office, London, 1991.
37. Kenna AP, Smithells RW, Fielding DW: Congenital heart disease in Liverpool: 1960–69. Q J Med 44:17, 1975.
38. Knox EG, Armstrong E, Haynes R: Changing incidence of infantile hypertrophic pyloric stenosis. Arch Dis Child 58:582, 1983.
39. Walsworth-Bell JP: Infantile hypertrophic pyloric stenosis in Greater Manchester. J Epidemiol Community Health 37:149, 1983.
40. Webb AR, Lari J, Dodge JA: Infantile hypertrophic pyloric stenosis in South Glamorgan 1970–9: effects of change in feeding practice. Arch Dis Child 58:586, 1983.
41. Wynne-Davis R: Family studies and the cause of congenital club foot. Talipes equinovarus, talipes calcaneovalgus and metatarsus varus. J Bone Joint Surg 46-B:445, 1964.
42. Robinson GW: Birth characteristics of children with congenital dislocation of the hip. Am J Epidemiol 87:275, 1968.
43. Salter RB: Etiology, pathogenesis and possible prevention of congenital dislocation of the hip. Can Med Assoc J 98:933, 1968.
44. Yamamuro T, Ishida K: Recent advances in the prevention, early diagnosis, and treatment of congenital dislocation of the hip in Japan, Clin Orth Rel Res 184:34, 1984.
45. Yen IH, Khoury MJ, Erickson JD, et al.: The changing epidemiology of neural tube defects: United States, 1968–1989. In press, 1991.
46. Shim WKT, Campbell A, Wright SW: Pyloric stenosis in the racial groups of Hawaii. J Pediatr 76:89, 1970.
47. Cuckle HS, Wald NJ, Cuckle PM: Prenatal screening and diagnosis of neural tube defects in England and Wales in 1985. Prenat Diagn 9:393, 1989.
48. Roberts CJ, Lloyd S: Observations on the epidemiology of simple hypospadias. Br Med J 1:768, 1973.
49. Sweet RA, Schrott HG, Kurland R, et al.: Study of the incidence of hypospadias in Rochester, Minnesota, 1940–1970, and a case–

control comparison of possible etiologic factors. Mayo Clin Proc 49:52, 1974.

50. Leck I: The etiology of human malformations: insights from epidemiology. Teratology 5:303, 1972.

51. Leck I: The geographical distribution of neural tube defects and oral clefts. Br Med Bull 40:390, 1984.

52. Niswander JD, Adams MS: Oral clefts in the American Indian. US Public Health Rep 82:807, 1967.

53. Lowry RB, Trimble BK: Incidence rates for cleft lip and palate in British Columbia 1952–71 for North American Indian, Japanese, Chinese and total populations: secular trends over twenty years. Teratology 16:277, 1977.

54. Lian Z-H, Yang H-Y, Li Z: Neural tube defects in Beijing–Tianjin area of China: urban–rural distribution and some other epidemiological characteristics. J Epidemiol Community Health 41:259, 1987.

55. Chinese Birth Defects Monitoring Program: Central nervous system congenital malformations, especially neural tube defects in 29 provinces, metropolitan cities and autonomous regions of China. Int J Epidemiol 19:978, 1990.

56. Leck I: Epidemiological aspects of paediatrics: insights into the causation of disorders of early life. In: Scientific Foundations of Paediatrics ed 2. JA Davis, J Dobbing, eds. Heinemann Medical, London, 1981, p 947.

57. Hay S: Incidence of clefts and parental age. Cleft Palate J 4:205, 1967.

58. Emanuel I, Culver BH, Erickson JD, et al.: The further epidemiological differentiation of cleft lip and palate: a population study of clefts in King County, Washington, 1956–65. Teratology 7:271, 1973.

59. Polani PE: Autosomal imbalance and its syndromes, including Down's. Br Med Bull 25:81, 1969.

60. Jones KL, Smith DW, Harvey MAS, et al.: Older parental age and fresh gene mutation: data on additional disorders. J Pediatr 86:84, 1975.

61. Smithells RW: Environmental teratogens of man. Br Med Bull 32:27, 1976.

62. Record RG: Anencephalus in Scotland. Br J Prev Soc Med 15:93, 1961.

63. Fedrick J: Anencephalus: variation with maternal age, parity, social class and region in England, Scotland and Wales. Ann Hum Genet 34:31, 1970.

64. Elwood JM, Elwood JH: Epidemiology of Anencephalus and Spina Bifida. Oxford University Press, Oxford, 1980.

65. Leck I: Epidemiological clues to the causation of neural tube defects. In: Prevention of Spina Bifida and Other Neural Tube Defects. J Dobbing, ed. Academic Press, London, 1983, p 155.

66. Carter CO: Genetics of common single malformations. Br Med Bull 32:21, 1976.

67. Kurisu K, Niswander JD, Johnston MC, et al.: Facial morphology as an indicator of genetic predisposition to cleft lip and palate. Am J Hum Genet 26:702, 1974.

68. Report of UK Collaborative Study on Alpha-Fetoprotein in Relation to Neural-Tube Defects. Maternal serum alpha-fetoprotein measurement in antenatal screening for anencephaly and spina bifida in early pregnancy. Lancet 1:1323, 1977.

69. Turnbull AC: Amniocentesis. In: Antenatal and Neonatal Screening. NJ Wald, ed. Oxford University Press, Oxford, 1984, p 445.

70. Granroth G, Hakama M, Saxén L: Defects of the central nervous system in Finland. I. Variations in time and space, sex distribution, and parental age. Br J Prev Soc Med 31:164, 1977.

71. Penrose LS: The relative etiological importance of birth order and maternal age in mongolism. Proc R Soc B 115:795, 1934.

72. Lamson SH, Hook EB: A simple function for maternal age specific rates of Down's syndrome in the 20–49 age interval and its biological implications. Am J Hum Genet 32:743, 1980.

73. Hook EB, Lindsjö A: Down's syndrome in livebirths by single year maternal age interval in a Swedish study: comparison with results from a New York State study. Am J Hum Genet 30:19, 1978.

74. Ferguson-Smith MA, Yates JRW: Maternal age specific rates for chromosome aberrations and factors influencing them: report of a collaborative European study on 52,965 amniocenteses. Prenat Diagn 4:5, 1984.

75. MRC Working Party on the Evaluation of Chorionic Villus Sampling: Medical Research Council European Trial of chorionic villus sampling. Lancet 337:1491, 1991.

76. Wald NJ, Cuckle HS, Densem JW, et al.: Maternal serum screening for Down's syndrome in early pregnancy. Br Med J 297:883, 1988.

77. EUROCAT Working Group: EUROCAT Report 4: Surveillance of Congenital Anomalies 1980–88. EUROCAT Central Registry, Brussels, 1991.

78. Nishimura H: Incidence of malformations in abortions. In: Congenital Malformations: Proceedings of the Third International Conference (International Congress Series No 204). FC Fraser, VA McKusick, eds. Excerpta Medica, Amsterdam, 1970, p 275.

79. Shiota K: Maternal fertility, reproductive loss, and defective human embryos. J Epidemiol Community Health 43:261, 1989.

80. Redding A, Hirschhorn K: Guide to human chromosome defects. BDOAS IV(4):1, 1968.

81. Alberman ED, Creasy MR: Frequency of chromosomal abnormalities in miscarriages and perinatal deaths. J Med Genet 14:313, 1977.

82. Creasy MR, Crolla JA, Alberman ED: A cytogenetic study of spontaneous abortions using banding techniques. Hum Genet 31:177, 1976.

83. French FE, Bierman JM: Probabilities of fetal mortality. US Public Health Rep 77:835, 1962.

84. Hassold T, Chen N, Funkhouser J, et al.: A cytogenetic study of 1000 spontaneous abortions. Ann Hum Genet 44:151, 1980.

85. Shepard TH, Fantel AG, Fitzsimmons J: Congenital defect rates among spontaneous abortuses: Twenty years of monitoring. Teratology 39:325, 1989.

86. Hertig AT, Rock J, Adams EC: Description of 34 human ova within first 17 days of development. Am J Anat 98:435, 1956.

87. Nishimura H: Prenatal versus postnatal malformations based on the Japanese experience on induced abortions in the human being. In: Aging Gametes: Their Biology and Pathology. Proceedings of the International Symposium on Aging Gametes, Seattle, Washington, June 13–16, 1973. RJ Blandau, ed. Karger, Basel, 1975, p 349.

88. Creasy MR, Alberman ED: Congenital malformations of the central nervous system in spontaneous abortions. J Med Genet 13:9, 1976.

89. MacHenry JCRM, Nevin NC, Merrett JD: Comparison of central nervous system malformations in spontaneous abortions in Northern Ireland and south-east England. Br Med J 1:1395, 1979.

90. McFadden DE, Kalousek DK: Survey of neural tube defects in spontaneously aborted embryos. Am J Med Genet 32:356, 1989.

91. Stein Z, Susser S, Warburton D, et al.: Spontaneous abortion as a screening device: the effect of fetal survival on the incidence of birth defects. Am J Epidemiol 102:275, 1975.

92. Stein Z, Stein W, Susser M: Attrition of trisomies as a maternal screening device: an explanation of the association of trisomy 21 with maternal age. Lancet 1:944, 1986.

93. Boué J, Boué A, Lazar P: Retrospective and prospective epidemiological studies of 1500 karyotyped spontaneous human abortions. Teratology 12:11, 1975.

94. Hook EB: Down syndrome rates and relaxed selection at older maternal ages. Am J Hum Genet 35:1307, 1983.

95. Peters GB, Ford JH, Nicholl JK: Trisomy 21 mosaicism and maternal age effect. Lancet 1:1202, 1987.

96. Hook EB, Regal RR: Conceptus viability, malformation, and suspect mutagens or teratogens in humans: the Yule-Simpson paradox and implications for inferences of causality in studies of mutagenicity or teratogenicity limited to human livebirths. Teratology 43:53, 1991.

97. Khoury MJ, Flanders WD, James LM, et al.: Human teratogens, prenatal mortality, and selection bias. Am J Epidemiol 130:361, 1989.

98. Lenz W: Thalidomide embryopathy in Germany, 1959–1961. In: Prevention of Physical and Mental Congenital Defects. Part C: Basic and Medical Science, Education, and Future Strategies. M Marois, ed. Alan R Liss, New York, 1985, p 9.

99. McBride WG: Thalidomide and congenital abnormalities. Lancet 2:1358, 1961.

100. Lenz W, Knapp K: Die Thalidomid-Embryopathie. Dtsch Med Wochenschr 87:1232, 1962.

101. Weicker H, Bachmann KD, Pfeiffer RA, et al.: Thalidomid-Embryopathie: II. Ergebnisse individueller anamnestischer Erhebungen in den Einzugsgebieten der Universitäts-Kinderkliniken Bonn, Köln, Münster und Düsseldorf. Dtsch Med Wochenschr 87:1597, 1962.

102. McBride WG: Personal communication cited by Ingalls TH, Klingberg MA in Congenital malformations: clinical and community considerations. Am J Med Sci 249:316, 1965.

103. McBride WG: The teratogenic action of drugs. Med J Aust 2:689, 1963.

104. Somers GF: Thalidomide and congenital abnormalities. Lancet 1:912, 1962.

105. Weicker H, Hungerland H: Thalidomid-Embryopathie: I. Vorkommen inner- und ausserhalb Deutschlands. Dtsch Med Wochenschr 87:992, 1962.

106. Lenz W: Discussion (Session 5). In: A Symposium on Embryopathic Activity of Drugs. JM Robson, FM Sullivan, RL Smith, eds. Churchill, London, 1965, p 182.

107. Hale F, The relation of vitamin A to anophthalmos in pigs. Am J Ophthalmol 18:1087, 1935.

108. Warkany J: Etiology of congenital malformations. Adv Pediatr 2:1, 1947.

109. Giroud A: Les malformations congénitales et leur causes. Biol Méd 44:1, 1955.

110. Thiersch JB: Therapeutic abortions with a folic acid antagonist, 4-aminopteroyl-glutamic acid (4-amino P.G.A.) administered by the oral route. Am J Obstet Gynecol 63:1298, 1952.

111. Thiersch JB: The control of reproduction in rats with the aid of antimetabolites and early experiences with antimetabolites as abortifacient agents in man. Acta Endocrinol 23(suppl 28):37, 1956.

112. Smithells RW, Sheppard S, Schorah CJ: Vitamin deficiencies and neural tube defects. Arch Dis Child 51:944, 1976.

113. Smithells RW, Ankers C, Carver ME, et al.: Maternal nutrition in early pregnancy. Br J Nutr 38:497, 1977.

114. Leck I, Iles CA, Sharman IM, et al.: Maternal diet and nutrition during early pregnancy and after delivery in North London. In: Prevention of Spina Bifida and Other Neural Tube Defects. J Dobbing, ed. Academic Press, London, 1983, p 197.

115. Schorah CJ: Commentary on "Maternal diet and nutrition during early pregnancy and after delivery in North London." In: Prevention of Spina Bifida and Other Neural Tube Defects. J Dobbing, ed. Academic Press, London, 1983, p 215.

116. Laurence KM, Campbell H, James NE: The role of improvement in the maternal diet and preconceptional folic acid supplementation in the prevention of neural tube defects. In: Prevention of Spina Bifida and Other Neural Tube Defects. J Dobbing, ed. Academic Press, London, 1983, p 85.

117. Winship KA, Cahal DA, Weber JCP, et al.: Maternal drug histories and central nervous system anomalies. Arch Dis Child 59:1052, 1984.

118. Mulinare J, Cordero JF, Erickson JD, et al.: Periconceptional use of multivitamins and the occurrence of anencephaly and spina bifida. JAMA 260:3141, 1988.

119. Bower C, Stanley FJ: Dietary folate as a risk factor for neural-tube defects: evidence from a case–control study in Western Australia. Med J Aust 150:613, 1989.

120. Mills JL, Rhoads GG, Simpson JL, et al.: The absence of a relation between the periconceptional use of vitamins and neural-tube defects. N Engl J Med 321:430, 1989.

121. Hibbard ED, Smithells RW: Folic acid metabolism and human embryopathy. Lancet 1:1254, 1965.

122. Schorah CJ, Wild J, Hartley R, et al.: The effect of periconceptional supplementation on blood vitamin concentrations in women at recurrence risk for neural tube defect. Br J Nutr 49:203, 1983.

123. Steegers-Theunissen RP, Boers GHJ, Trijbels FJM, et al.: Neural-tube defects and derangement of homocysteine metabolism. N Engl J Med 324:199, 1991.

124. Yates JR, Ferguson-Smith MA, Shenkin A, et al.: Is disordered folate metabolism the basis for the genetic predisposition to neural tube defects? Clin Genet 31:279, 1987.

125. Laurence KM, James N, Miller M, et al.: Increased risk of recurrence of pregnancies complicated by fetal neural tube defects in mothers receiving poor diets, and possible benefit of dietary counselling. Br Med J 281:1592, 1980.

126. Kirke P: Commentary on "The role of improvement in the maternal diet and periconceptional folic acid supplementation in the prevention of neural tube defects." In: Prevention of Spina Bifida and Other Neural Tube Defects. J Dobbing, ed. Academic Press, London, 1983, p 115.

127. Leck I: Commentary on "The role of improvement in the maternal diet and periconceptional folic acid supplementation in the prevention of neural tube defects." In: Prevention of Spina Bifida and Other Neural Tube Defects. J Dobbing, ed. Academic Press, London, 1983, p 113.

128. Milunsky A, Jick H, Jick SS, et al.: Multivitamin/folic acid supplementation in early pregnancy reduces the prevalence of neural tube defects. JAMA 262:2847, 1989.

129. Laurence KM, James N, Miller MH, et al.: Double-blind randomised controlled trial of folate treatment before conception to prevent recurrence of neural-tube defects. Br Med J 282:1509, 1981.

130. Czeizel A, Fritz G: Ethics of a randomised trial of periconceptional vitamins. JAMA 262:1633, 1989.

131. MRC Vitamin Study Research Group: Prevention of neural tube defects: results of the Medical Research Council Vitamin Study. Lancet 338:131, 1991.

132. Smithells RW, Sheppard S, Schorah CJ, et al.: Apparent prevention of neural tube defects by vitamin supplementation. Arch Dis Child 56:911, 1981.

133. Smithells RW, Nevin NC, Seller MJ, et al.: Further experience of vitamin supplementation for prevention of neural tube defect recurrences. Lancet 1:1027, 1983.

134. Smithells RW, Sheppard S, Wild J, et al.: Prevention of neural tube defect recurrences in Yorkshire: final report. Lancet 2:498, 1989.

135. Nevin NC, Seller MJ: Prevention of neural-tube-defect recurrences. Lancet 335:178, 1990.

136. Vergel RG, Sanchez LR, Heredero BL, et al.: Primary prevention of neural tube defects with folic acid supplementation: Cuban experience. Prenat Diagn 10:149, 1990.

137. Seller MJ, Nevin NC: Vitamins during pregnancy and neural tube defects. JAMA 263:2749, 1990.

138. Kučera J: Rate and type of congenital anomalies among offspring of diabetic women. J Reprod Med 7:73, 1971.

139. Orme ML'E: The Debendox saga. Br Med J 291:918, 1985.

140. Anonymous: Debendox is not thalidomide. Lancet 2:205, 1984.

141. Granroth G: Defects of the central nervous system in Finland. III. Diseases and drugs in pregnancy. Early Hum Dev 2:147, 1978.

142. Kopek JA, Esdaile JM: Bias in case–control studies. A review. J Epidemiol Community Health 44:179, 1990.

143. Kurent JE, Sever JL: Perinatal infections and epidemiology of anencephaly and spina bifida. Teratology 8:359, 1973.

144. Bjerkedal T, Czeizel A, Goujard J, et al.: Valproic acid and spina bifida. Lancet 2:1096, 1982.

145. Evans SJW: Uses and abuses of multivariate methods in epidemiology. J Epidemiol Community Health 42:311, 1988.

146. Feinstein AR: Quantitative ambiguities in matched versus unmatched analysis of the 2×2 table for a case–control study. Int J Epidemiol 16:128, 1987.

147. Leck I: Frequency of malformations: clues to etiology. In: Occupational Hazards and Reproduction. K Hemminki, M Sorsa, H Vainio, eds. Hemisphere Publishing, Washington, D.C., 1985, p 249.

5

Contributions of Animal Studies to Understanding Human Congenital Anomalies

RICHARD H. FINNELL and MICHAEL VAN WAES

Understanding human congenital anomalies is complicated by the lack of available working material. Animal models—as substitutes for human embryos—have provided a body of knowledge that would otherwise be unattainable. In humans, individual malformations may occur infrequently, whereas an animal model can be bred until sufficient quantities are available for research. Furthermore, in human populations there is little control over the diet or social living conditions of the patients in question, but with animal models it is possible to control the environment and thus to focus on those factors that modify the phenotypic manifestation of the congenital abnormality. Moreover, in contrast to human studies, with animals one is not limited to investigating only the final manifestation of a developmental disorder but can examine in detail the pathogenesis of the malformations.

There is another reason to consider using animal models to study malformations. Laboratory rodents, particularly mice but in some cases rats as well, are remarkably similar to humans in their genetic constitution. Along with the ethical dilemmas that human studies entail, these considerations clearly indicate that our knowledge of human malformations would be distinctly limited were it not for the discovery of various animal models for these malformations.

Historical perspective

Study of normal development and mechanisms

Animals have been used to study both normal and abnormal development since the time of the ancient civilizations of Egypt, India, and China. Although all three cultures had the ability to incubate fowl eggs artificially, the primary embryologic focus was to determine when the immortal spirit took residence in the developing embryo[1] rather than to study embryologic development systematically.[2]

The first clear-cut embryologic knowledge comes from Hippocrates in the fifth century BC. It remains uncertain whether he or his son-in-law Polybus authored the three-volume work (Regimen, The Work on Generation, The Nature of the Infant) relating to embryology, but the author did know how to study embryology, which requires the observation of successive stages of development at regular intervals. In fact, the author recommended the following to his students: "Take 20 eggs or more and give them to 2 or 3 hens to incubate. Then each day from the second onwards til the time of hatching, take out an egg, break it, and examine it. You will find everything as I say in so far as a bird can resemble a man."[3] Regrettably, this advice was ignored for the next two thousand years.

Aristotle followed Hippocrates as the next great embryologic theorist. His multivolume treatise On the Generation of Animals,[4] firmly established his credentials as a comparative embryologist; he developed a classification system in volume II that separated vertebrates from invertebrates and viviparous species from oviparous species. Aristotle most certainly dissected the embryos of a variety of mammalian, bird, and amphibian species, because he described the fetal membranes and cotyledons of the ruminant uterus[5] and the yolk sac placenta of ovoviviparous species of shark.[6] There is some evidence to suggest that he also had experience with aborted human fetuses.[7] While Aristotle never described keeping daily observational records of chick development, or systematic observations of any other animal species he worked with, he divided chick development into three stages. The first stage included incubation days 1–5, the second stage continued variously until day 10 or 14, and the third stage extended until hatching. His descriptions of the day 10 chick embryo suggested that all of the organ systems had developed at this point, yet the head and the eyes were disproportionately large. Having failed to follow the advice of Hippocrates and perform daily observations on developing systems, Aristotle's impact on future embryologists rests more on his theoretical constructs than on his body of actual descriptive work. His ideas on the primacy of cardiac development and his thoughts on the origin of diverse structures and differentiation (epigenesis) were complete departures from the Hippocratic school of thought.[8,9] Nonetheless, his fragmentary accounts were a most credible beginning that was unparalleled until the sixteenth century.

Galen the Pergamite's descriptions of fetal membranes made a considerable contribution to the understanding of embryogenesis. Having dissected several mammalian species, including human fetuses, Galen noted that the embryo is surrounded immediately by the amnion, over which lies the allantois, which opens into the bladder. These two fetal membranes are engulfed by the chorion, which attaches the fetus to the uterus. His other contribution concerns the sequence of organ formation; he believed that the liver develops before the heart, which develops before the brain. In fact, his four stages of embryonic development are based largely on the appearance of these three organs. In stage one, the conceptus is indistinct, while in stage two the primordia of the heart, liver, and brain can be distinguished. These organs are well defined in stage three, and by stage four all organ systems are clearly visible.[9,10]

Perhaps Galen's greatest contribution came not from what he accurately described, but from the mistakes he made. He habitually applied to humans physiologic features that were obviously observed in other species. For example, he described a large, sausage-like allantois and the presence of two veins in the umbilical cord. These are features, like that of the cotyledons in the uterus, not of humans, but of domesticated ruminants. Thus Galen fell victim to the most common of pitfalls when working in experimental animal systems, i.e., extrapolating incorrectly to the human situation. This problem recurs throughout the embryologic literature. No less than Leonardo da Vinci drew pictures of the human uterus with the cotyledons, chorionic villi, and uterine crypts of the ox.[9,11] Andreas Vesalius accurately described the annular placentation of the dog and similarly ascribed it to the human fetus. He did, however, perform comparative studies of the ruminant and human uterus and determined that cotyledons are found only in ruminant species.[9,12]

In the sixteenth century systematic experimental embryology was advanced through the work of Volcher Coiter. Finally heeding the advice of Hippocrates, Coiter examined chicken eggs on each successive day of incubation, and, in a clear, dispassionate account, he described the fetal anatomy of the developing chick. Unaided by lens or microscope, he accurately described the blastoderm on incubation days 1 and 2, along with such structures as the area pellucida, the area opaca, and the primitive streak. Coiter even described the yolk stalk and included it within the abdominal cavity, implying that he understood that the contraction of the amnion plays a part in this process.[9,13] This work was ultimately embellished by Fabricius,[14] who, in 1621, published his treatise *Formation of the Egg and of the Chick*. In this work, highly accurate, detailed illustrations of daily chick development are provided. Fabricius was the first to determine the function of the ovary and the oviduct and added to the basic understanding of different placental types.[9,14]

The controversy in embryology from the time of Hippocrates until the nineteenth century centered on the origin of diversity of form and structure. William Harvey, the brilliant student of Fabricius, was able to utilize a microscope to aid his studies on chick development. It was Harvey[15] who wrote that one organ system developed epigenetically before other organs. While Hartsoeker and others continued to propose that all the structures in an embryo were preformed, evidence was beginning to accumulate that favored the epigeneticists.[16] By 1828, Karl Ernst von Baer,[17] the foremost embryologist of the time, described the mammalian and the human ova for the first time and explained that—contrary to von Haeckel's hypothesis—ontogeny does not recapitulate phylogeny, thus giving further support to the epigeneticists' view that the embryo starts development as a formless mass and gains diversity through growth and differentiation. It was the early teratologists working in the latter half of the eighteenth century and the beginning of the nineteenth century who convincingly demonstrated that the preformist logic was inconsistent with the accumulated knowledge based on embryologic development.

Study of abnormal development

Credited with being the original teratologist, Etienne Geoffroy Saint-Hilaire not only coined the term "teratology," but advanced the field by exposing incubating chick eggs to various environmental hazards. In actuality, the credit for being the original teratologist may well belong to de Réaumur; at the turn of the eighteenth century, he was manipulating controlling temperature incubators to alter the development of chicken eggs.[18]

Isidore Geoffroy Saint-Hilaire, following the path laid down by his father, demonstrated that no defects could be induced in chicks when the teratogenic treatment was administered prior to the third day of incubation.[19] This work has its corollary in mammalian teratogenesis, a principle of which is that no structural malformations can be induced in the preimplantation period.[20]

Working at the end of the nineteenth century, Camille Dareste used a variety of teratogenic treatments to alter development at a specific time during gestation and found that they could all result in the same developmental endpoint. Dareste felt that the observed malformations were the result of altering amniotic conditions which somehow arrested embryonic development. This work, and subsequent studies by Charles Féré, demonstrated that the timing of exposure to the teratogen was more important for the type of malformation produced than was the specificity of the actual teratogen.[21] Féré injected alcohol, nicotine, and a variety of drugs into the albumin of eggs and concluded that the observed malformations resulted from an altered nutritional status in the embryo.

In the twentieth century, teratologists began to exploit several different animal species in their experimental designs. Stockard[22] used both fish and amphibians to demonstrate that the teratogen-induced structural defects are stage specific. He believed that the time when the adverse exposure took place during gestation could be determined by the type of defect(s) that resulted from the teratogen. While in many instances this can in fact be accomplished, when used in isolation it may easily lead to erroneous conclusions.

At that time the prevailing opinion was that all congenital malformations were the results of abnormal genes. By the onset of World War II, however, the varied contributions of Warkany, Nelson, and others left little doubt that environmental factors also have a significant impact on embryonic development. This was demonstrated in a variety of animal species, including rats, swine, and rabbits.[23-25] With the association of thalidomide exposure to the epidemic of limb reduction anomalies in the mid-1960s, teratology as a scientific discipline was fixed; its role in understanding and preventing human malformations has never been more important.

Animal models

The use of animal models to study malformations and morphogenesis has significantly furthered the understanding of congenital malformations. While such information, in all probability, will not immediately reduce the frequency of selected malformations in the human population, it is important to pursue such studies; by better understanding biologic systems, the likelihood of being able to avert some birth defects may be increased. Through animal studies, testable hypotheses can be generated to help clarify puzzling clinical situations. Years of work by dedicated teratologists such as Clarke Fraser and Daphne Trasler, for example, have resulted in an understanding of how the genetic background of the test animal can influence the response frequencies when it is exposed to a given teratogen, and, furthermore, just how morphologic features of the exposed embryos may put one genotype at an increased risk.[26-29]

Animal models can also be extremely useful in changing or clarifying current thought on the development of a particular malformation. For example, it has long been held that neural tube defects result from (1) improper elevation of the neural folds as a result of abnormal development of the paraxial mesoderm;[30] (2) nonfusion of the neural folds because of abnormal neurocytoarchitecture;[31,32] (3) nonfusion because of excessive cell death, caused in turn by vascular disruption[33] or (4) rupturing of a previously closed neural tube.[34] In support of the first hypothesis, experimental studies exposing mouse embryos to hyperthermic conditions have shown that the induction of the neural tube defect can occur prior to the elevation of the neural folds.[35] On the other hand, using the mouse mutant *splotch (Sp)*, Morris and O'Shea[36] demonstrated that embryos with neural tube defects also had neuroepithelial alterations in the cranial region, an increase in intracellular space, and other changes suggestive of the second proposed hypothesis (abnormal cytoarchitecture of the neural folds) for the pathogenesis of neural tube defects. Moreover, studies in the mouse by Edwards et al.[37,38] have shown the importance of cell death in the etiology of neural tube defects. Thus, through continued experimentation with animal models (see Multifactorial malformations: neural tube defects, below), it is possible to reshape current thinking on the etiology of human congenital malformations.

Finally, animal models may suggest, indirectly or as a direct result of an experimental observation, possible means by which to prevent malformations. One such example is the correction of a genetically determined ocular defect by cortisone treatment in mice. It has been demonstrated that administration of cortisone to mice bearing one of the many lid-gap mutations accelerates the process of eyelid flattening and the growth of the eyelid over the cornea, which results in the fusion of the eyelids in animals in which it would otherwise remain unfused.[39-41] Likewise, prenatal dietary manipulations have proved valuable in preventing the development of murine vestibular abnormalities.[42]

Society continues to reap the rewards from both the varied uses of genetic animal models and the inspired work of experimental teratologists. Whether the information on human malformations and morphogenesis generates new hypotheses or tests old ones, there are, in many cases, simply no substitutes for animal models in studying the pathogenesis of congenital malformations. In the discussion that follows, the cited examples show how the use of animal models has helped to further the understanding of various developmental defects. While not an all-inclusive catalog, the models represented are those in which a significant understanding of the genetics and the embryologic basis of the malformation has been worked out. This chapter therefore is focused on models that arise spontaneously, such as those for growth disorders, neural tube defects, and cytogenetic defects, and those that are induced, such as environmental insults to the developing embryo or the use of transgenic animal models for the study of malformations, and concludes with descriptions of some models that helped delineate a few of the mechanisms involved in normal and/or abnormal development, specifically, cell death and secondary induction.

Spontaneously occurring models

Single gene defects: growth disorders and skeletal dysplasias

A number of interesting animal models have been used to investigate abnormal skeletal development and growth. In reviewing these mutations, it is important to recognize that in many cases the phenotypically similar chondrodystrophies in mice have different morphologic, immunochemical, and ultrastructural characteristics. These differences are more often than not associated with, if not directly responsible for, the observed growth disorders.

Short limb dysplasias

Mouse mutations may serve as models of the molecular and developmental mechanisms involved in numerous growth disorder syndromes, particularly the short limb chondrodysplasias in humans. This largely heterogeneous group of defects of the endochondral skeleton includes over 80 genetically determined skeletal dysplasias.[43-45] When dealing with genetic models of skeletal defects, it is important to keep in mind that the defect is often just one of many pleiotropic effects of a given gene and that the primary effects may be quite removed from skeletal development.[46] It is also important to remember that there is often no molecular, biochemical, or morphologic similarity between an animal model and a human disorder bearing the same name.[47] Therefore it is essential to correlate the clinical disorder and the pattern of transmission, along with the other suggested criteria of Lalley and McKusick[48] before claiming homology between the animal mutant and the human disorder.

A sampling of the murine models for chondrodysplasias and somite-derived disorders is presented below. Although a number of chicken and rat models are also available, the advantage of a murine model is the ability to study the genetic disorder in a variety of inbred backgrounds. The general accessibility that these models provide is also advantageous.

The first of the chondrodysplasia mutants to be discussed is known as *cartilage matrix deficiency (cmd)*. Animals homozygous for this gene are born alive but succumb almost immediately postpartum.[49] Affected fetuses present with short snouts, cleft palates, and short extremities because of a reduction of long bone lengths to <50% of control lengths. These mice are unable to synthesize the core protein of proteoglycan.[50] The absence of this protein would readily account for the decreased size of the Golgi apparatus, the histologically observed compact arrangement of the cells, and the absence of any staining of proteoglycan when examined with either histochemical or immunofluorescent techniques.[51]

This lack of the core protein has also been determined to be the primary defect in the nanomelic chicken *(nm)* model of chondrodysplasia;[52] thus a similar molecular mechanism exists for mutations in two different animal species.[46] In the *cartilage matrix deficient* mouse homozygotes, there is also a severe reduction in the quantity of extracellular matrix produced.[51] This decreased extracellular matrix and the hypercellular growth plate found in this mutation most resembles the human disorder achondroplasia.

The *brachymorphic (bm)* recessive mutation in the mouse,

first described by Lane and Dickie[53] in 1968, represents a more or less typical chondrodysplasia that is first detectable 4–5 days postpartum, when newborn mice appear to have short-domed skulls, short, thick tails, and a pronounced reduction in the length of the long bones. There is no reduction in bone width. Histologically the epiphyseal plates appear thinner in the mutants than in heterozygotes or homozygous wild-type mice. The composition of the cartilage appears to be normal,[54] although it is not possible to rule out a cartilage-specific proteoglycan defect that is responsible for the observed mesomelic growth disturbance.[46] Finally, in this proposed model for human chondrodysplasia there is some joint thickening, especially in the knees, because of a failure of resorption of abnormally placed cartilage.[55]

The mouse mutant achondroplasia (cn), an autosomal recessive gene mapped to chromosome 4,[46] is quite similar to the previously described brachymorphic mutant.[53] The achondroplastic mouse is recognized at birth by the presence of a domed skull, limbs that are reduced to 70% of normal length, a shortened tail, and a reduced body weight. The animals frequently suffer from malocclusion because of a reduced mandible.[46] The affected animals have a shortened life span, with premature death usually the result of cyanosis secondary to a crowded thorax. Unlike the brachymorphic mouse, the pathogenetic defect in the achondroplasia mutation appears to reside in an abnormal maturation of the chondrocytes. After examining the cartilage of these animals, Bonucci et al.[56] reported histologic changes that they thought were representative of premature aging of the chondrocytes. The pathology of this mutation remains somewhat obscured by the fact that there appear to be two distinct phenotypes of animals bearing the same genetic mutation.[57–59] In the severely affected animals, the cartilage columns are very short and separated by large amounts of extracellular matrix. Within the columns the chondrocytes are very small, and they are irregularly arranged.[56,60]

The autosomal recessive mutation found in the mouse and known as chondrodystrophy (cho) was described by Seegmiller et al.[61] as a mutant defective in endochondral bone formation. Affected mice are first recognized as early as gestational day 15 by their disproportionately short limbs, shortened spine, short snout, and reduced mandible. The mice have a normal-sized tongue, resulting in macroglossia.[51] It is lethal immediately after birth, the neonates having a small thoracic cage that may result in pulmonary hypoplasia,[62] although it has also been suggested that the failure of the cartilage formed in the tracheal rings to support an open airway is the cause of the premature demise of the mutant mice.[61] Death may also result from the median cleft palate, a result of retarded growth of Meckel's cartilage that limits the growth of the mandible.[63]

The morphologic and histologic features of the cho mutation resemble a broad range of skeletal dysplasias found in humans. The remarkable morphologic feature of the chondrodystrophic mouse is the appearance of long bones with flared metaphyses and an irregular distribution of matrix collagen.[46] A loss in the structural integrity of the extracellular matrix has been proposed to explain the observed cellular disarray.[61,64] This is based on histologic investigations of the chondrodystrophic mutant matrix, which appears to have been abnormally produced by the chondrocytes.[51,61,64,65] As a result of the abnormal meshwork consisting of large-diameter collagen fibrils, along with the presence of a fluid-like matrix, the proliferating chondrocytes do not align themselves in a column. By not forming such alignments, bone elongation fails to occur and thereby leads to the dwarfing condition.[51]

The stumpy (stm) mutation was first discovered as a result of a mutagenicity study and features a profound defect in endochondral bone formation.[66] The mutant animals experience abnormal periods of bone development, with near-normal growth up to day 16 postpartum, at which time there is a noticeable slowing of long bone growth. Although a short period of catch-up growth is observed in weeks 3 and 4, the homozygous stm mice are decidedly growth retarded.[67] Histologic studies of the growth plate indicate an abnormality in the shape and organization of the chondrocytes. The disorganization of the cartilage worsens over time.[68] The stumpy defect appears to be related to abnormalities in cellular division, as there is evidence of dumbbell nuclei and pyknotic cells in the epiphyseal plates, suggestive of abortive mitotic events. While the stumpy mutation shares many features in common with the previously described chondrodystrophy mutant, it lacks the wide collagen fibrils that typify the chondrodystrophic mouse.

The Disproportionate micromelia mouse mutant (Dmm) differs from those previously described in that it is inherited as an autosomal dominant trait.[69] Heterozygotes have reduced long bone length and shortened skulls. They occasionally are only mildly affected and appear almost normal in size, whereas in other Dmm/+ animals the presence of orofacial clefts is associated with neonatal death.[46] The homozygotes are more severely affected than are the heterozygotes, invariably having cleft palates and dying shortly after birth. The pathogenetic mechanism of the Dmm mutation remains unknown. Histologic studies have produced evidence of cytoplasmic vacuolization, in addition to an overall lack of Golgi vacuoles and a dilation of the rough endoplasmic reticulum. The abnormal rough endoplasmic reticulum in a dwarfing disorder makes this mouse model highly reminiscent of Kniest syndrome in humans.[45] The cartilage matrix of the affected animals was similar to that found in the chondrodystrophic mutant in that all of the collagen fibers were significantly thicker than normal, adding to an overall coarseness of the matrix.[51] It has been suggested that the problem in the Disproportionate micromelia mouse mutation involves an abnormality in protein transport out of the chondrocytes.[51,69]

Axial skeleton defects

Unlike the aforementioned mutations of growth and bone development, the primary embryologic site of action of this group of axial skeletal mutants is the differentiating somites. The abnormal sclerotome formation invariably leads to problems in the vertebrae and throughout the axial skeleton. These models include those of spondylocostal dysplasia. In the mouse, these mutants are invariably reflected in defective development of the tail, making them readily recognizable.

The first of the axial skeletal mutants is Rib-fusion (Rf), a semidominant gene with a mild expression in the heterozygotes.[70] The kinked tail in these animals is usually recognizable after the first week of life. In the Rf homozygotes, the severity of the disorder is such that most embryos die in utero; those that are not resorbed are invariably stillborn. The bodies of the Rf homozygotes are shortened, particularly from the rostral portion of the sacrum. During development, the embryos are identified as early as day 9, when there is a noticeable absence of any somites being formed.[71] There are clumpings of mesenchymal cells, but they fail to organize into somites.

The mouse mutant *pudgy (pu)*, an autosomal recessive gene located on chromosome 7, represents another example of a disorder affecting the axial skeleton. The mutant can be identified by the shortened tail length, and, upon skeletal examination, the vertebrae appear decidedly irregular.[72] The vertebral arches remain open dorsally, the spines of the affected mice are abnormally curved, and the ribs and sternum are all abnormal.[73] In developmental studies of this mutant, the somites are irregularly formed, which is visible in embryos during gestational days 9–11. Toward the caudal end of the embryo, the mesoderm remains unsegmented, appearing as somitic fusions.

Other well-described murine mutants of the axial skeleton include *Malformed vertebrae (My)*,[74] *Crooked tail (Cd)*,[75] and *rachiterata (rh)*.[76] It is noteworthy that of the axial mutants in the mouse affecting sclerotome differentiation, at least three genes are transmitted as dominant or semidominant traits.

Models of growth disorders and axial skeletal development have problems that are readily apparent and therefore more likely to be identified by investigators. In these models of defective endochondral bone growth, the mutants were utilized to help identify the biochemical or morphologic bases for the disorders. In most instances, a defect in the extracellular matrix was detected. For the mutants in axial skeletal development, the unifying theme has to be related to defective somite differentiation. The clinical implications of this latter group are not limited to the skeleton proper, but can have important ramifications for neural tube development as well.

In the case of murine single gene models, it is important to keep in mind that most of them are caused by recessive genes, which is often not the situation with human malformations. Therefore, care needs to be taken to avoid the simplistic assumption that similar phenotype necessarily implies similar origin. Nevertheless, the models continue to provide useful and interesting approaches to understanding the mechanisms that lead to normal and abnormal development.

Multifactorial malformations: neural tube defects

Neural tube defects are among the most commonly observed congenital defects observed in humans. Thus it is somewhat surprising that so little is understood regarding their etiology. Neural tube defects include craniorachischisis, in which the entire neural system is exposed; anencephaly, in which the cephalic neural tissue is exposed; myelomeningocele, in which there is an exposed region of the spinal cord; and, finally, encephalocele, or skin-covered protrusion of cranial neural tissue and/or meninges.[77] These abnormalities may be part of a broader spectrum of congenital anomalies, or they may appear as isolated defects, clearly emphasizing the etiologic heterogeneity of neural tube defects.[78]

There is little doubt that genetic factors are integral to an embryo's susceptibility to neural tube defects; indeed, epidemiologic evidence demonstrates a greater prevalence of these disorders in selected ethnic groups.[79,80] Furthermore, in these studies there is a predominance of affected females compared with males.[79,81,82] This sex difference is more pronounced for selected neural tube defects, particularly anencephaly, and is less prominent for defects such as myelomeningocele.[79,81]

Neural tube defects have been demonstrated to be associated with cytogenetic defects, such as trisomies 13, 18, and 21.[83] These abnormalities have also been described as defects of mutant single genes with various patterns of transmission, including sex-linked recessive,[84] autosomal recessive[85,86] and autosomal dominant.[87] There have also been reports of families in which neural tube defects and multiple anomalies, including omphalocele, vertebral fusion defects,[88] and congenital heart defects[89] are associated. Some investigators have concluded that the inherited genetic susceptibility is not for a neural tube defect per se, but for all anomalies involving the embryonic midline.[90] This is similar to current thinking about malformations observed in murine embryos bearing one of the many T-locus mutations.[91,92] While no single model fits all of the available empiric and clinical data, it would appear safe to say that isolated neural tube defects in humans are multifactorial, having both a genetic and an environmental component to their development.[93–95]

Four major hypotheses have been proposed to explain the pathogenesis of neural tube defects:

1. In the first scenario, there is a failure in the elevation of the neural folds, resulting from a lack of growth of the paraxial mesoderm. This is most likely secondary to unscheduled cell death or to mitotic interference, which ultimately results in an insufficient tissue mass.[30]
2. The second hypothesis proposes that neural tube closure is dependent on changes in the cellular architecture, particularly that of the neuroectoderm. If the cell shape is not correct, then there will be no fusion of the neural folds, resulting in a neural tube defect.[31,32]
3. The third hypothesis suggests that vasculature to the neural folds is compromised during development, and the resulting inadequate nutrient supply starves the rapidly developing neuroectodermal cells, resulting in the failure of the neural tube to fuse.[33,96,97]
4. The final hypothesis proposes that neural tube defects are the result of reopening or rupturing of a previously closed neural tube.[34]

While it would appear from the vast number of pathologic studies that have been conducted in humans that the majority of neural tube defects are related to a failure in neural tube closure,[7] the actual morphogenetic events involved in neural tube defects remain unknown.

There are several animal models, single gene or multifactorial, available to pursue mechanistic and genetic studies on the etiology of neural tube defects. It is important to keep in mind that this is not an exhaustive tabulation of neural tube defect models: the models described represent only a small proportion of models found in the mouse. For additional information, the reader is referred to a recent review by Winter.[98]

Splotch (Sp) mutant

Homozygous *Splotch* embryos fail to complete neural tube closure and are born with spina bifida, with or without exencephaly.[99] The defect in these animals appears to be localized to a region in the dorsal neural tube. The defect itself is likely secondary to an abnormality in the neural crest cells, because, in addition to the aforementioned abnormalities, these embryos often have anomalous spinal ganglia and lack normal pigmentation.[100]

Developmental investigations into the morphogenesis of the *Splotch* neural tube defect suggest that affected embryos have an elevated mitotic index in those portions of the neural tube where fusion has not yet occurred. This enhanced mitotic index is thought to result from the increased length of the cell cycle of the affected neuroepithelium.[101]

Other studies have revealed the presence of abnormal cellular processes in the hindbrain of *Splotch* homozygotes, together with an increase in the extracellular space in the basal portion of the neural tube.[36] The enhanced areas of extracellular space surrounding the neural tube results in the ectoderm and the neuroepithelium being closely compressed around each other.[102]

Other evidence suggests an overall lack of mesodermal cells in the nonsomitic regions of the *Splotch* homozygotes, perhaps the result of a lack of extracellular space into which they could expand. If this were the case, then the lack of mesodermal support of the elevating neural folds could possibly explain the presence of the neural tube defects observed in this mutations.[102]

In addition to the neural tube defect, the *Splotch* mutation embryos have abnormalities in their spinal ganglion and a regional lack of pigmentation. These abnormalities in neural crest cell–derived structures suggest a problem in the initial migration of neural crest cells.[103] The lack of migration was thought to be a secondary effect of the lack of space between the ectoderm and the neuroepithelium. It is also possible that the lack of neural crest cell migration, which amounts to only ~5% of that measured on wild-type embryos, was due to an inability of the neural crest cells to interact with the extracellular matrix.[103] Therefore, it is possible that the *Sp* gene alters a component of the extracellular matrix surrounding the neural tube and, in so doing, is either directly or indirectly responsible for the failure of neural tube closure in these embryos.

Curly tail (ct) mutant

The *curly tail (ct)* mutant was first described by Gruneberg.[104] The majority of curly tail mice have tail lesions or spina bifida, suggesting a delayed closure of the posterior neuropore.[105,106] In the extreme phenotypic expression of this mutation, the embryos have exencephaly, with or without spina bifida. Less severely affected embryos have small neural tube lesions that may regress, resulting in newborn animals having tails with various degrees of curling or minor kinking.[107]

Only 52% of *curly tail* incross offspring have neural tube defects, indicating not only that the mildest expression of this phenotype is indistinguishable from wild-type controls but also the importance of other factors in the production of the defect. The genetic background upon which the *ct* gene is placed has a great deal to do with the ultimate expression of the abnormal phenotype, because, when the trait is outbred to either the A strain or the BALB/c strain, no fetuses develop neural tube defects.[107] Environmental interactions are also significant in terms of expressing the neural tube defect phenotype.[99,108]

Several distinct homologies exist between neural tube defects in the curly tail model and those in humans. For ex-

ample, there is an elevation of α-fetoprotein levels in the amniotic fluid of affected fetuses in both species,[109] and associated defects found in humans such as hydrocephaly and polyhydramnios have similarly been described in this model.[107] A developmental study on neurulation in curly tail embryos between gestational days 6 and 11 clearly demonstrated that the neural tube defects observed in these embryos are the result of a lack of neural tube closure because no fusion of the neural folds was observed. As both cephalic and spinal neural tube defects are found in this model, the developmental study supports a common etiology for both spina bifida and exencephaly in curly tail homozygotes.[107]

Curtailed mutant (T^Cu)

One of the older and more interesting murine models for neural tube defects is the *Curtailed mutant (T^Cu)*, which was discovered in a radiation mutagenesis study as a new allele at the T locus[110]—a complex genetic region located near the centromere of chromosome 17, near the H-2 loci.[91] Animals that are heterozygous for the dominant *Brachyury (T)* allele *(T/+)* have shortened tails because of the abnormal development of the notochord; the result is a spinal cord that is distorted and often accompanied by fused vertebrae.[111] Embryos that are homozygous for the *Brachyury* allele *(T/T)* die at approximately gestational day 10.75 because of improper formation of placental connections. In these embryos, there is also a failure of the primitive streak to differentiate, resulting in a notochord that rapidly degenerates, thus compromising somitic derivatives and skeletal structures.[111]

Animals that are homozygous for the *Curtailed* allele *(T^Cu/T^Cu)* have a more severe phenotype than that described for homozygous *Brachyury* embryos. The curtailed embryos lack both forelimb and hindlimb buds, a tail, and any visible external somites. The neural folds are highly irregular and remain widely separated in the trunk region. In this embryolethal condition embryos fail to survive beyond gestational day 11.[110] When animals with the *Curtailed* allele are mated to those bearing one of the recessive *t* alleles, specifically *t^{w75}*, a proportion of the resulting neonates have dorsal blood blisters in the lumbosacral midline.[112] These animals, with what is apparently spina bifida aperta, survive for ~2 weeks, although one individual mouse survived for over 2 months. In a detailed analysis of the developmental pathology of the *Curtailed* mutation, Park et al.[112] examined embryos at selected periods of postneurulation. On gestational day 10.5, the affected embryos were recognizable by the presence of a secondary neural tube-like structure appearing on the ventral aspect of the primary neural tube. It appears to replace the notochord at a level just caudal to the hindlimb buds.[112] It is thought that this auxiliary neural tube develops when the floor plate of the neural tube loses its outer limiting membrane and neuroepithelial cells migrate away from the neural tube into the surrounding mesenchyme. These migrating cells ultimately become a branch of the neural tube, forming a lumen; the cells eventually exist as a secondary neural tube in these embryos.[112]

As development proceeds, the *T^Cu/t^{w75}* embryos become ever more distinctive. The dorsal blister is visible by gestational day 12.5, and the embryos are clearly tailless. Accessory neural tubes form, break down, and reform four to five times. The caudalmost accessory neural tube persists to the caudal end of the embryo, where the primary and secondary neural tubes fuse together to form a single tube.[112] In slightly older embryos, the dorsal blister becomes cystic, fluid filled, and covered with skin. At the level where the accessory spinal cords initially develop, the vertebral arches are irregular, with the fissure between the neural arches so great that it prevents fusion. Thus the entire spinal cord in the lumbosacral region of affected embryos is unprotected by a vertebral column. This absence of the vertebral bodies, together with a thinning dermal layer and the existence of a dorsal cystic mass, suggest that this genetic mutant represents an animal model for spina bifida with meningomyelocele.

As has previously been described, there are at least two major hypotheses concerning the pathogenesis of spinal neural tube defects. While the majority of clinical studies and experimental models support the hypothesis that spina bifida is the result of failure of the neural tube to close normally during development,[77] an alternative hypothesis is that a previously closed neural tube reopens during gestation. Embryologic evidence provided by the *Curtailed* mutant lends support to this latter hypothesis. The neural tubes of the developing T^{Cu}/t^{w75} embryos close and later reopen when the necrotic roof plate of the spinal cord ruptures because of increased pressure of the cerebral spinal fluid within the neural tube. The roof plate abnormalities are visible histologically in the affected embryos by gestational day 10.5, with the rupturing occurring shortly thereafter.[112]

SELH/Bc stock

Perhaps the most interesting of all the murine models for studying neural tube defects is the recently described mutant stock known as SELH/Bc.[113] Of the previously described models, all were single gene mutations resulting in embryos that develop neural tube defects. While these models have been highly informative, and a great deal of the current understanding of the processes involved in neural tube closure has been gained through such single gene models, it is far from clear whether the defects arise by the same mechanisms as in neural tube defects resulting from the cumulative effects of several minor genetic mutations plus environmental factors.[114–116] The multifactorial etiology found in the SELH/Bc mutant is likely to be somewhat more relevant to the etiology of the majority of human neural tube defects.

Breeding experiments have been conducted to determine the mode of inheritance for the neural tube defect trait in the SELH/Bc stock. When animals known to produce exencephalic progeny are incrossed, approximately 17% of the offspring are born with neural tube defects.[116] Of these affected animals, a pronounced percentage is female (73%); this is similar to the situation found in both the *curly tail* murine mutant[117] and in human epidemiologic studies.[79]

Reciprocal crosses between the SELH/Bc stock and an ICR strain were conducted to rule out potential sex-linked recessive or autosomal dominant genes and the possibility of any maternal effects on the transmission of the neural tube defect trait. In fact, data on the frequency of neural tube defects were applied to a number of potential genetic models, including those of multiple genes with reduced penetrance and duplicate epistasis; the data best fit the predictions based on the multifactorial threshold model.[116] The one drawback to this model, however, is that it yields very little information

about the number of loci responsible for the difference in liability for the production of neural tube defects between the SELH/Bc stock and that of the ICR mice. It is still a possibility that an autosomal recessive mutant allele, fixed in the SELH/Bc stock with reduced penetrance and modified by one or more loci, is responsible for the exencephaly.[116]

The defective development of the neural tube in the SELH/Bc embryos was extensively examined by Macdonald et al.[113] and compared with the normal development of the neural tube in two other mouse strains (ICR and SWV). The sequence of morphologic events in the SWV and ICR strains was found to be consistent with other descriptions of murine neural tube closure;[118,119] that is, in contrast to the classic description of a continuous zipper-like process, the neural tube of the mouse actually closes in an intermittent process with four distinct initiation sites.[113,118–126] The first initiation site begins at the level of somites one to three and proceeds bidirectionally (closure I, see Fig. 5–1). The second initiation site begins at the prosencephalic–mesencephalic border, and it too closes bidirectionally (closure II). The third site is unidirectional, with closure proceeding from the region of the stomodeum caudally until it meets with closure II. The final closure takes place over the rhombencephalon, which also meets closure II to complete neural tube closure.

In the mutant SELH/Bc embryos, the early stages of neural tube closure are indistinguishable from those in the SWV and ICR inbred mouse strains. The first distinctive features of abnormal development are observed in the initial elevation of the neural folds, which is delayed in the prosencephalon relative to overall growth in the control strains.[113] When the neural folds should be making their initial contact in the posterior portion of the prosencephalon (closure II), the neural folds remained widely opposed in the affected embryos.

Unlike the other strains, the SELH/Bc mice had the initial site of neural fold contact in the ventral portion of the prosencephalon in the region of closure III. Thus, unlike normal embryos, the mutant SELH/Bc embryos close off the region of the anterior neuropore while leaving the neural folds over the mesencephalon widely flared open.[113] This failure to close off the mesencephalon results in exencephalic fetuses. Histologically, the increased number of pyknotic mesenchymal and neuroepithelial cells observed in the affected embryos could not satisfactorily explain the failure in neural fold fusion.[113]

A similar alteration in the pattern of neural tube closure has recently been observed in SWV embryos subjected in utero to valproic acid,[121] and in exencephalic embryos with trisomy 12 or 14 (Fig. 5–1).[122] In all instances, the alternate pattern of neural tube closure (closure III without closure II) is pursued with varying degrees of success. That is, only 17% of the SELH/Bc embryos have exencephaly, whereas the vast majority manage after some delay to complete neural tube closure.[113] With valproic acid treatment, 65% of the embryos complete the alternate pathway for neural tube closure,[121] and 50% of the trisomy 14 embryos are similarly successful.[122] The aforementioned examples illustrate that the primary defect in neural tube production is in the failure of the neural tube to close properly during embryogenesis.

Describing all of the mouse models of neural tube defects is beyond the scope of this review. Additional information on a number of different models, including those that adversely affect segmentation, those affecting the primitive streak

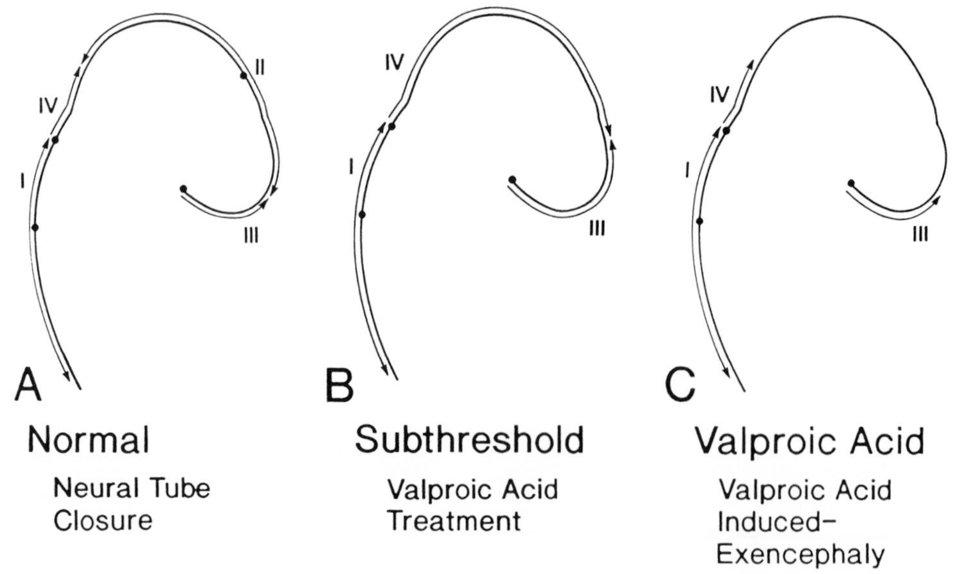

A
Normal
Neural Tube
Closure

B
Subthreshold
Valproic Acid
Treatment

C
Valproic Acid
Valproic Acid
Induced-
Exencephaly

Fig. 5–1. Altered sequence of neural tube closure in the mouse following valproic acid treatment. A. Normal pattern of neural tube closure. B. Altered pattern of neural tube closure following subteratogenic treatment (200 mg/kg) with valproic acid on gestational day 8.5. Note that closure III extends caudally beyond normal limits to meet closure IV, which extends more rostral than normal to compensate for the lack of closure II. C. Altered pattern of neural tube closure following teratogenic treatment (600 mg/kg) with valproic acid. Closure II fails to take place, and closures III and IV are unable to extend range to compensate. Open mesencephalon leads to exencephaly.

or notochord, and those primarily involved with alterations of the neural tube, can be found in the excellent review by Winter.[98]

Chromosome defects

Mouse trisomy 16

Several models of murine cytogenetic disorders have been developed to study the impact of trisomies on abnormal development. The first of the cytogenetic models to be well described was for mouse trisomy 16.[123] This was initially proposed as a possible model for human Down syndrome based on the fact that the genes coding for sensitivity to interferon (IfRec) and the soluble enzyme superoxide dismutase (SOD-1), which map to chromosome 21 band 21q22, were found to be syntenic on mouse chromosome 16.[123] Although the role of these genes in the production of the Down syndrome phenotype is not well understood, the presence of these genes on chromosome 16 suggested its utility as a model worthy of further investigation. Embryos carrying the additional chromosome develop only to the latter stages of gestation, at which point the disorder is lethal.[124]

To obtain trisomic mice, normal diploid females are mated to males doubly heterozygous for two different Robertsonian translocations involving arms of chromosome 16. The overall viability and the proportion of trisomic fetuses obtained will depend on the type of translocations used.[125] It is also possible to obtain adult trisomic tissue by constructing normal–trisomic chimeras using cells from the trisomic embryos (at the eight cell to early blastula stages).

The phenotype of murine trisomy 16 shares many features with that of Down syndrome. The mice have an overall decreased rate of growth and development, there is evidence of edema, facial dysmorphia, reduced brain weight, inner ear abnormalities, thymic hypoplasia, and various immunologic and hematologic anomalies comparable to those reported in humans.[125]

Mouse trisomy 19

Another potential murine model for human trisomy 21 is the mouse trisomy 19, which represents a homologous situation in the sense that the trisomic chromosome is the smallest one of the respective genomes and involves relatively similar amounts of DNA. The trisomic 19 mouse is one of the few murine trisomies that survives to birth, and, although no homology to any human chromosome has yet been determined, its value as a model rests on the assertion that the mental retardation aspect of human trisomies is probably not chromosome specific, but merely a function of the aneuploid status of the individual.

Trisomic 19 mice have survived a maximum of 20 weeks after birth, with the vast majority succumbing much earlier. Phenotypically, the affected fetuses displayed both prenatal and postnatal growth retardation, with subsequent delays in the onset of eye and pinnae opening of up to 3 days.[126] These developmental delays are strongly associated with both motor and sensory deficiencies that may be related to neurologic disorders. The neurologic implications of the affected mice suggest its potential value in studies of trisomy-induced developmental defects.

Of all the mouse trisomies examined to date, those for chromosomes 13, 14, 16, 19, and, perhaps, 18, are compatible with survival to term or into the immediate neonatal period.[127–132] Another group of trisomies involving the larger chromosomes 2–9, 11, 15, 18 usually are lethal by gestational day 12, and the embryos phenotypically abnormal.[133] For example, embryos that are trisomic for chromosome 15 have severe growth retardation and cardiac and hepatic malformations.

Artifically constructed models

Environmental insults

Animal models have proved to be extremely valuable in the study of environmentally induced congenital malformations. It is often difficult to establish causation between a prenatal exposure in humans and an adverse pregnancy outcome. Using experimental models, it is possible to administer the agent in question freely and to explore rigorously its potential for disrupting normal embryogenesis. In specific situations, animal studies may suggest that exposure to a compound, such as high doses of vitamin A, poses reproductive risks in humans.[134,135] In other situations, such as with alcohol or dilantin, animal models have helped to resolve the uncertainty as to whether an agent is teratogenic.[136-139] Although several different animal models have been highly successful in shedding light on teratogen-induced congenital anomalies, the discussion in this section will be limited to those involving ethanol, anticonvulsant drugs, retinoic acid, and hyperthermia.

Ethanol-induced teratogenicity

The potential teratogenicity of ethanol was first reported by Charles Féré around 1894 in chickens. After injecting various alcohols into the egg albumin, Féré found that a proportion of eggs either did not develop or generated a "monstrocity."[21] It was not until 1973 that the first widely accepted clinical descriptions of the prenatal alcohol syndrome in humans were published.[140-142] During the decade prior to recognition of the prenatal alcohol syndrome, experiments using a variety of species were reported. Investigators treated pregnant animals or exposed eggs to various quantities of ethanol at selected gestational stages, but the results produced either were unconvincing as a result of the methodology employed or were simply contradictory.[143,144]

While these studies reported the occurrence of selected malformations associated with ethanol exposure in human pregnancies, it was not until Chernoff[136] chronically administered ethanol in a liquid diet to pregnant mice prior to and throughout gestation that the resulting offspring bore the spectrum of defects observed in the human prenatal alcohol syndrome. That is, in a dose-related manner, the ethanol-exposed fetuses had a pattern of abnormalities including prenatal growth retardation, neural and cardiac defects, and abnormal skeletal ossification. By varying ethanol concentrations in the test diet, it was possible to determine the lowest maternal blood alcohol concentration (73 mg/100 ml) at which defects were induced. Furthermore, by utilizing different inbred mouse strains, it was possible to demonstrate a genetically determined difference in sensitivity to the adverse development effects of ethanol,[136] and that these differences were dependent on the detoxification rate of the alcohol based on the level of maternal alcohol dehydrogenase activity.[137]

By examining the effects of an acute administration of eth-

anol during the period of mouse neural tube formation, Sulik and Johnston[145,148] were able to demonstrate that the craniofacial changes induced in the animal model were the result of deficiencies in neural plate development. After examining scanning electron micrographs of ethanol-exposed embryos, it was apparent that the prosencephalic region was hypoplastic, tending to be more narrow and pointed than the corresponding region in control embryos.[145] Abnormal embryos were detected as early as gestational day 8, and by day 12 the entire craniofacial primordia were abnormal. What these animal models provide is a theoretic framework with which to consider how the exposure alters normal development. Studies by Chernoff and others showed clearly that chronic maternal alcohol consumption could be teratogenic, whereas from the animal model studies of Sulik and colleagues it was determined that disturbance of mesoderm formation during early embryogenesis could be one way in which ethanol induces structural changes in the developing murine embryo.

Anticonvulsant-induced malformations

Following the initial description of the prenatal hydantoin syndrome, an animal model was designed to follow a set of experimental criteria: use of animals that had a seizure disorder, oral administration of phenytoin to the dams prior to and throughout gestation in concentrations sufficient to reduce the frequency of seizures, and production of plasma drug concentrations similar to those found in humans.[138] This mouse model demonstrated that chronic maternal exposure to hydantoin anticonvulsants can result in fetuses with congenital defects bearing a remarkable similarity to those described in humans. The incidence of fetal abnormalities was shown to be dose related, with an increased risk for abnormal development associated with elevated plasma phenytoin concentrations. This animal model was effective in demonstrating that the observed malformations were not the result of the maternal seizure disorder, but rather were definitely drug induced.[147]

This mouse model has also been very beneficial in helping to elucidate a rationale for the variable expression observed in the human prenatal hydantoin syndrome. By examining the most frequently observed defects in the mouse prenatal hydantoin syndrome, it was possible to demonstrate significant differences in the pattern of malformations observed in the three inbred mouse strains that appeared to be related to genotypic differences in susceptibility to specific phenytoin-induced malformations.[139,148] Specifically, SWV females appeared to have two to three times as many affected fetuses with neural, renal, and sternebral defects than did the other two inbred mouse strains. Whether genetically determined differences in susceptibility to phenytoin-induced birth defects exist within the human population is currently unknown, although suggestive data have been reported in the literature.[121,149]

Animal models for the study of teratogen-induced neural tube defects have served as a helpful adjunct to the spontaneous genetic animal models. Maternal hyperthermia and various agents such as retinoic acid, valproic acid, and insulin have all been shown to induce cephalic neural tube defects in the mouse when exposure occurs during the period just prior to neural tube closure. As with other teratogen-induced malformations, susceptibility to neural tube defects appears to have a strong genetic component. Using either a brief, 10 min hyperthermic exposure gestational day 8.5 or an intraperitoneal injection of valproic acid (600 mg/kg/day), Finnell et al.[35,150] found the DBA/2J strain to be completely resistant to these teratogenic insults, the LM/Bc embryos to be moderately susceptible, and the SWV embryos to be very sensitive.

These findings have been supported by independent studies with valproic acid used to induce exencephaly in mice.[151] Subsequent studies to examine the underlying biochemical basis for the strain differences in susceptibility to both heat- and valproic acid–induced neural tube defects have been inconclusive, although significant strain differences in the heat shock response following the in vivo heat treatment have been reported.[152] In a developmental study of valproic acid–induced exencephaly, it was determined that the drug-exposed embryos underwent the same alternative pathway to closing the anterior neural tube as that described for the exencephaly-prone genetic mutant stock SELH/Bc.[113] Thus the embryos exposed to sufficiently high concentrations of valproic acid during the period of neural tube closure successfully complete closure III in the rostral portion of the developing facies, but fail to complete closure II in the area of the prosencephalon–mesencephalon.[153] Embryos that have been exposed to a subthreshold dose of valproic acid and are not as delayed developmentally are able to compensate for this alteration in the normal developmental sequence and close their anterior neural tube by extending the caudal limits of closure III and the rostral limits of closure IV (Fig. 5–1).[153]

Retinoic acid teratogenicity

A characteristic pattern of malformations has recently been described among infants exposed in utero to high concentrations of retinoic acid. The retinoic acid embryopathy consists of craniofacial, cardiac, and central nervous system malformations, including cleft palate, microtia, micrognathia, conotruncal and aortic arch heart defects, thymic disorders, and the neural tube defects hydrocephaly and microcephaly.[154] In many instances, nervous system, aular, and cardiac defects were observed in the same individual.

Many of these malformations had previously been described in animal retinoic acid models. Perhaps the earliest study was that of Cohlan,[155] who orally administered 35,000 IU of retinoic acid to pregnant Wistar rats on gestational days 4–16. This resulted in a frequency of neural tube defects that approached 52%. A similar result was obtained in rat pups administered 60,000 IU on gestational days 8–10.[156] Since that time, a vast experimental literature has evolved, further demonstrating the teratogenicity of vitamin A and its many analogs.[134,157–165]

From those studies in which the embryos were examined over a period of time following gestational exposure to retinoic acid, it was postulated that the neural tube defects were the result of abnormal cell migration and proliferation in the area of the cephalic mesoderm.[166] In this region, small defects resulting from the reduction in cell size and a subsequent enlargement of the intercellular spaces, together with an expansion of the subneural vasculature, were present within 6 hr posttreatment.[167] With time, this condition became more severe, with mesodermal cells rapidly becoming pyknotic and degenerating. The loss of this cell population resulted in the neuroepithelial folds not reaching their proper elevation, and

thus the neural tube was unable to close.[167–169] Sulik and colleagues[164,170,171] were able to answer selected mechanistic questions concerning the adverse effects of gestational retinoic acid on the development of the limbs and the craniofacies. From their experiments, it appears as if exposure to either the 13-*cis*-retinoic acid or the all-*trans*-retinoic acid results in an increased number of pyknotic cells in areas of programmed cell death. Thus, through the use of well-conceived animal models, known teratogenic agents can be utilized to better understand the developmental or pathogenetic principles involved in both spontaneous and iatrogenically induced congenital malformations in humans.

Transgenic mouse models of congenital abnormalities

Diploid organisms with long life cycles present decided problems for the geneticist trying to understand the morphogenetic and biochemical bases of malformations. While inbred mouse strains can be obtained that express a specific genotype, the number of genes that can be studied is limited to those that present an observable phenotype. The major disadvantage of this approach to the study of malformations is the lack of specificity and, with it, the inability to target specific cellular or developmental processes.

Recent advances in molecular biology make it possible to proceed with more direct approaches, including the introduction of foreign genes of interest into cells of higher organisms with the result of having foreign proteins synthesized by the transgenic organism. The first report of a stable integration of foreign DNA into a live mammalian species (mouse) was in 1980.[172] Since that time, a great deal of success has been attained in the production of transgenic mice.

The ability to introduce new genes, or extra copies of a gene already present, into the host embryo provides an excellent source of models for understanding molecular and cellular mechanisms fundamental to normal development. Transgenic animals are most commonly used for studies of gene interactions and dosage effects. One example involves a transgenic mouse line expressing the *pim-1* gene that was infected with the murine leukemia virus. This resulted in an enhanced production of tumors, concomitant with the expression of either *c-myc* or *N-myc*,[173] and evidence for some form of epigenetic interaction between the two genes. With respect to dosage effect analyses, mice were transfected with a construct containing the zinc/copper–superoxide dismutase *(Zu/Cu–SOD)* gene to study the effects of extra gene copies on developmental outcome.[125]

Transgenic mice are developed using the basic embryo transfer technology that has been refined over the past three decades. Modified protocols for this procedure result in a very high percentage (nearly 90%) of viable, transferred embryos in mice. Indeed, one of the very early approaches used to incorporate foreign DNA into mouse embryos was the generation of chimeric mice by embryo splitting at the two to eight cell stage and then fusing the embryos with similarly split embryos of different genotypes.[174] More recently, the pronuclear injection technique has become the primary means by which transgenic mice are created. In this procedure, linear DNA is microinjected into the most accessible of the pronuclei in a recently fertilized egg. The washed eggs are then planted in the oviduct of a pseudopregnant dam, and approximately 25% of the embryos incorporate the construct.[175]

Other techniques are also used to create transgenic mice. In most instances, there is no clear advantage of any of these procedures over the more standard pronuclear injection technique. For example, when foreign DNA is injected directly into the cytoplasm or the nuclei of a two cell embryo, incorporation rates of less than 1.5% are reported.[176] Additionally, multiple recombinative events between the molecules of the injected DNA may occur when incorporation is successful.

It is also possible to incorporate genetic information into early embryos using genetically engineered retroviruses. By removing the zona pellucida from eight cell mouse embryos and placing them in a medium containing retrovirus-infected fibroblasts, the viral particles are free to infect the embryo. This procedure has the advantage of limiting the number of gene copies incorporated into the embryo's genome to a single insert. However, the relatively late stage at which this procedure can be performed results in embryos that are mosaics that may lack the transgene in the germ line.[177] Finally, the size of the inserted DNA is limited using viral vectors, and in some cases very long constructs cannot be used with this type of procedure.

Although rather straightforward in principle, all of the aforementioned techniques involving embryo manipulation share the inherent problem of the embryo's extreme sensitivity to adverse environments, in addition to the difficulty of physically manipulating very small systems. Together, these problems result in the widely variable levels of efficiency reported by different laboratories using the same procedures but working with different equipment or levels of expertise. Finally, mention should be made of the problems that arise with transgenic mice secondary to the manner in which the foreign DNA is integrated into the host's genome. At present, the mechanism controlling integration is poorly understood and appears to be a random process. As a result, embryos that express the transgene may also exhibit developmental changes that are not abnormal products of the transgene but, rather, are due to a failure in normal gene expression caused by insertional mutagenesis.[175]

The potential for transgenic mouse technology to expand the understanding of congenital malformations is just beginning to be tapped. A few transgenic models are discussed to provide relevant examples of experiments currently being conducted. This brief review will certainly be supplanted by a more comprehensive collection of studies in a very short time.

Dosage-effect transgenic models

As described previously, most of the murine trisomies are, if not entirely inviable, limited in their capacity for long-term survival (see Chromosome defects, above); this renders many questions about the mechanisms of cytogenetic diseases difficult to approach. It has been hypothesized that the developmental defects caused by aneuploidies are due to dosage effects, i.e., having more (or less) of a certain protein synthesized according to the number of copies of the gene present; in particular, the phenotypic expression of Down syndrome may be the result of a 1.5-fold increase in the level of expression of the enzymes coded for by genes localized to human chromosome 21 band 21q22. Such is the case for the *Cu/Zn–SOD* gene, which maps to mouse chromosome 16.

A transgenic mouse strain was constructed by Epstein et al.[178] that contained extra copies of the human gene *(h-CuZnSOD)*. The resultant mouse–human heterodimer had a 1.6–6-fold increase in enzyme activity in the adult brain, although this was not related to any observed phenotypic abnormalities. The main advantage of working with the transgenic model is that it is possible to obtain adult tissue that expresses gene products coded on the manipulated chromosome. Moreover, a transgenic animal overexpressing a given gene may be considered as partially trisomic for the chromosome to which that gene maps; in this way, the liability for specific features of the phenotype can potentially be assigned to individual genes.

The legless mouse

The legless transgenic mouse model was initially described by McNeish et al.[179] at the University of Cincinnati School of Medicine. It represents an example of generating a new murine mutant by insertional inactivation or disruption of important regulatory sequences; thus the particular construct incorporated into the genome is apparently independent of the actual resulting phenotype. The investigators used a genetic construct containing the *Drosophila* heat shock 70 (hsp 70) promoter along with the herpes virus thymidine kinase gene and microinjected the construct into mouse oocytes. Three phenotypically normal mice were found to have incorporated the construct as determined by Southern hybridization analysis; however, when the progeny of these animals were interbred, one-fourth of the offspring expressed the abnormal legless phenotype.[179]

The legless mutation is characterized by the absence of hindlimb structures distal to the femur, aberrant forelimbs with ectrodactyly of the preaxial digits, and an occasional alteration in cranial development. Craniofacial abnormalities including orofacial clefting disorders were also observed in mice homozygous for the transgene. Neural defects such as aberrant or absent olfactory lobes and hemorrhagic protrusions from the cortex were commonly observed, as were hydrocephaly, thinning of the nasal septum, and an abnormal brain shape with a lack of distinction between the cerebral hemispheres. The affected animals all died within the first 24 hr postpartum.[179] By gross observation, the abnormal hindlimb bud can easily be detected on gestational day 11, and in fact, histologically, an abnormally high incidence of cell death can be observed in the anterior portion of the limb bud 1 day earlier.

In all instances, the mutant neonates are shown to be homozygous for the mutation, while those mice with normal phenotypes were either heterozygous or not transgenic, suggesting that it is a recessive mutation caused by the disruption of an endogenous gene.[179] There are several possible explanations for the abnormal phenotype observed in the legless mutation. It is possible that there is a loss or a disruption in the function of a gene that is directly involved in the differentiation or formation of the affected structures. It is also possible that some regulatory sequence or a gene that controls the expression of other developmental genes has been adversely affected by the inserted construct. Distinguishing between the effects of a specific gene or a regulatory sequence involved in development is not an easy task, since pleiotropic effects are to be expected from both developmental and regulatory genes.

Dominant facial malformation

Dominant facial malformation represents another animal model in which the relevant event was most likely not the incorporation of a specific genetic sequence; rather, the observed malformations are due to insertional mutagenesis of a host gene. In this case, the construct that was microinjected into mouse eggs contained a cloned human mutant TTR gene, which codes for transthyretin containing a methionine at the 30th position instead of a valine residue.[180] The transgenic offspring were recognized by an abnormal phenotype consisting of a shortened snout and a twisted upper jaw that were secondary to malformations of the premaxillary and nasal bones. The jaw of the affected neonates was hypoplastic, and cleft lip was a consistent finding. The malformations were recognized in developmental studies as early as gestational day 15.5, at which time the bone formation did not seem delayed when compared with the severe hypoplasia found in the craniofacial tissues.[180] The authors thought that the primary cause of this malformation complex was a morphogenetic problem in the maxillary prominence of the first branchial arch.

The abnormal craniofacial phenotype was present in outbred progeny of transgenic animals, suggesting an autosomal dominant mode of transmission.[180] This dominant pattern indicates that the integration event of the construct does not involve a loss of function; rather, it only appears to change the pattern of expression in the final structure of the host gene product. Further work has indicated that the integration site is on mouse chromosome 13, on which another mutant gene *(dumpy),* resulting in growth retardation and limb malformations, has been mapped. This latter gene is inherited as a recessive disorder; therefore, it is unlikely that it is the same as the putative gene in this transgenic model of abnormal facial development. The original authors suggested that it could serve as a model for one of the many first branchial arch–related syndromes in humans, such as Crouzon syndrome or Treacher Collins syndrome, both of which are inherited as autosomal dominant disorders.[181]

Homeobox-induced malformations

Another group of transgenic mouse models provides a great deal of new information on normal developmental processes. These models all involve the insertion of *Hox* genes, which contain a homeobox within their sequence. The murine homeobox, like that of *Drosophila,* is a group of highly conserved sequences, 180 base pairs long, located near the 3′ end of the transcriptional unit. Homeobox genes in the mouse are designated by the name *Hox,* followed by two numerals indicating different subgroups. For example, *Hox-1.1* represents a murine homeobox gene that, under normal conditions, is found to have its peak transcriptional activity on gestational day 12; it has been localized in spinal ganglia, sclerotomes, and in the cells of the neural tube.[182] In the adult mouse, *Hox-1.1* transcripts are found in abundance in the testis, brain, and kidney, with minor amounts of transcripts recognized in the bone marrow, spleen, and ovary.[183]

Balling et al.[184] developed a transgenic mouse using the *Hox-1.1* gene under the control of the ubiquitous β-actin promoter. Mice carrying one to five copies of this construct in a single integration site have profound craniofacial defects and cannot survive the neonatal period. Affected animals are born with their eyes open, indicating incomplete eyelid fusion; they have clefts of the secondary palate, the pinnae of their ears are not fused, and they are growth retarded. It has been suggested that the observed defects are the result of an underlying connective tissue disorder, resulting in the hypoplastic palatal shelves and palpebral fissures, as well as the lack of fusion of the pinnae. Other organ systems appear to have developed normally in the transgenic animals, suggesting that the malformations observed are the result of specific, localized problems in development and not the result of an overall developmental delay.

This model shares a great deal of phenotypic homology with Treacher Collins syndrome in humans and with the retinoic acid embryopathy described in both humans and in mice.[154,170,181] Furthermore, this model produces many of the craniofacial abnormalities described in the murine mutant *far,* which has similarly been proposed as an animal model of human first arch syndrome defects, including mandibulofacial dysostosis and hemifacial microsomia.[185,186] The use of models such as this provides great insight into the molecular basis of important developmental processes and supports the prevailing hypothesis that homeobox genes are important regulators of normal morphogenesis. Furthermore, the fact that retinoic acid, a putative morphogen,[187] produces a similar phenotype as those observed in the ectopic expression of *Hox-1.1* suggests that the *Hox* genes may be induced by endogenous retinoic acid.

Another transgenic mouse model utilizing a *Hox* mutation was developed by Wolgemuth et al.[188] to take advantage of the overexpression of the homeobox-containing gene *Hox-1.4.* Using pronuclear injection, these investigators inserted a linear DNA construct that contained not only the whole *Hox-1.4* gene but also a 400 base pair sequence from the 3′ end untranslated region and a poly(A) addition site of the simian virus 40 T antigen as a tag to differentiate between the transgene and the endogenous sequence.[188] By developing such a construct, the transgenic animals should express the gene at the appropriate time and in the appropriate cells, only at an enhanced level. In fact, the levels of expression were determined to be elevated at least twofold in the central nervous system and lungs and even higher in the gut of the transgenic embryos.

Developmental studies of day 12.5 embryos revealed a high level of *Hox-1.4* expression in the presence of grossly distended colons, similar in phenotype to congenital megacolon. Those animals that survived to term had difficulty defecating, resulting in severely enlarged bowels with compacted feces, which was not compatible with long-term survival. Because of differences in the severities of the defects, some animals did survive and reproduce, in spite of carrying the transgene. Given that the offspring of several different lineages carrying the construct had the abnormal phenotype, it appears that the congenital defects are the result of overexpression of the *Hox-1.4* gene and not the result of dominant insertional mutagenesis.[188]

This model presents similarities with the mouse dominant megacolon mutant and with Hirschsprung disease in humans. The feature common to all three disorders is lack of ganglion cells in the colon, presumed to be due to failure of neural crest cells to migrate into the developing gut. It is possible that the *Hox-1.4* gene is involved in facilitating the migration of these cells so that the overexpression of this gene may disrupt an underlying mechanism or spatially disorient the cells from following proper cues and taking residence in the mesenchymal layer of the developing gut.

Osteogenesis imperfecta transgenic model

The final example of a transgenic mouse model of abnormal development to be discussed concerns a defective gene for collagen synthesis, resulting in mice with osteogenesis imperfecta. Stacey et al.[189] generated a cosmid carrying a mouse pro-α (I) collagen gene from a genomic clone in which two mutations were introduced, exchanging the glycine residue at position 859 with either a cysteine or an arginine. When cells in culture were transfected with the construct, they produced a normal as well as a slow-migrating form of collagen, as determined by polyacrylamide gel electrophoresis.[189] The latter was translated from the mutant collagen fiber, and its slow-migrating property was thought to be the result of an increased lysine hydroxylation and glycosylation.

To determine whether this abnormal collagen chain would produce the osteogenesis imperfecta phenotype, the cosmid was microinjected into fertilized mouse eggs that were then implanted into pseudopregnant dams. Some foster mothers delivered naturally and some by cesarean section, and the neonates were examined. While none of the liveborn pups carried the transgene, seven of nine stillborn pups, or those that died in the perinatal period, were determined by Southern analysis to be transgenic.[189] The affected pups were characterized by flabby, hypotonic limbs that could be flexed in any direction and by an unusually soft cranium. Radiographs of these animals revealed bones that were severely underdeveloped, with short wavy ribs and broad long bones that were poorly mineralized. These features are all observed in human osteogenesis imperfecta.[190]

Mechanistic models

By investigating abnormal development it is often possible to gain insight into normal development. Several animal models have helped us directly or indirectly to understand the mechanisms involved in the generation of congenital abnormalities.

Induction

Renal agenesis

In normal development the metanephros or permanent kidney originates from two mesodermal components. One of these is the epithelium of the metanephric diverticulum (a prominence that forms in the mesonephric duct, usually called the "ureteric bud"), which as it grows out comes in contact with the metanephrogenic mesenchyme. Both tissues interact with each other such that the ureteric bud elongates and branches, and the mesenchyme condenses at the tips of the branches (which are still blind at this point). The nephrogenic cells become arranged into vesicular masses that eventually change into the form of S-shaped tubes. A connection will develop between each of these tubes and the ureteric bud branches. Each S-shaped tube will become a nephron, and the ureteric bud will develop into the renal

ducts and the ureter. The idea that it is one tissue inducing the other one to differentiate (reciprocal induction) was first put forward and demonstrated in vitro in 1955 by Grobstein.[191]

The nature of the induction is through changes in the composition of the extracellular matrix; the mesenchymal cells are induced to synthesize collagen IV and laminin, which causes them to aggregate into an epithelium and to form a basement membrane.[192] These changes induce the epithelial cells to synthesize the transferrin receptor, which enables the cells to proliferate.[193]

Mechanical separation of both components (by malformations in the caudal end of the embryo) or lack of development of the ureteric bud will impede induction and lead to renal agenesis. In humans this defect results in oligohydramnios or lack of amniotic fluid that causes fetal compression and, subsequently, limb positioning defects, pulmonary hypoplasia, and growth deficiencies; the agenesis can be unilateral or bilateral, the latter being lethal.[194]

There are two mouse mutants whose phenotype include renal agenesis, each one exemplifying one of the two possible etiologies of the malformation:

Sd mutant. The *Sd* mutation was first described by Dunn et al. in 1940[195]; it segregates as a dominant allele that is lethal at the homozygous condition. The heterozygotes have short or absent tails and urogenital malformations, with one or both kidneys absent or reduced in size, which causes a high rate of perinatal mortality, 70% dying before weaning. The homozygotes are born with no tail and with a shortened spinal column; they present bilateral renal agenesis, a closed cloaca, and no urethral or anal openings. Their death occurs shortly after birth.[196]

Together with the described urogenital defects, these animals present malformations of the caudal region of the vertebral column. The number of thoracic vertebrae is usually normal; occasionally the number of lumbar vertebrae is reduced to five (the normal number is six), but the number of sacral vertebrae is commonly less than four, with the third and fourth being abnormal in shape or size if present at all. Often they are fused to each other or to the caudal vertebrae; these in turn are variable in number and are usually malformed and/or fused. These malformations are likely to be responsible for the renal agenesis, moving the nephrogenic parenchyma to a position relative to the ureteric bud such that the latter is unable to contact and induce the former.[194]

my mutant. The *my* mouse strain was created and described by Bagg and Little[198] in 1925. It was generated by x-ray irradiation, and the visceral defects were fixed by selection.

The major features of the strain are malformations of the genitourinary tract, eyes, and hindlimbs. The most ubiquitous defect is unilateral and bilateral renal agenesis, and the presence of polycystic and/or hydronephrotic kidneys is common as well. Many animals present with clubfeet accompanied by hypodactyly, syndactyly, or polydactyly. They also described liver and pancreatic hematomas, fetal hemorrhages in the region of the kidneys, and absent testis. In the cases in which kidney is absent, the ureter also fails to develop, and the single kidney can show hypertrophy to a variable extent.

In 1931 Alice Brown,[199] a graduate student, set out to find an explanation for the renal agenesis observed in Bagg and

Little's strain (at the time still unnamed). In a very meticulous study she concluded, among other things, that "during the maximum stress of the mechanical twisting of the posterior region of the early embryonic body, deficient kidney anlagen fail to come together and the excretory and drainage mechanisms remain ununited."[199] She goes on to explain that, to obtain a normal kidney, it is necessary for two "healthy anlagen" (the ureteric bud and the nephrogenic mesenchyme) to fuse. Because of retarded development of the former these two tissues do not come in contact, thereby failing to induce the formation of a definitive kidney.

Anophthalmia

The development of the eye, one of the miracles of the animal kingdom, consists of a more complex sequence of secondary inductions than that of the kidney. It is not surprising that anophthalmia, the lack of ocular structures, has been described for almost all vertebrate species, and it has been studied for over a century at the gross embryologic level.[200]

The cascade of events that lead to the formation of the normal eye in the mammalian embryo commences with the notochord inducing the neural tube to form a bulge: the optic vesicle. The vesicle in turn grows into the shape of a cup. When the optic cup makes contact with the head ectoderm, the latter is induced to form the lens. New ectoderm covers the developing lens, and this ectoderm is induced by the lens to form the cornea.

It is apparent that since this process occurs as a succession of required steps, any obstacle at one stage will inhibit the formation of all later structures. There is one mouse model that exemplifies this possibility. The anophthalmic mouse strain arose spontaneously in the Jackson Laboratory at Bar Harbor in Maine, and it was first described by Chase and Chase[201] in 1941. The genetic composition, although not yet well understood, seems to be that of a recessive gene or genes. Approximately 90% of the adult mice of this strain entirely lack all ocular structures. The orbit is occupied by a large lacrimal gland. The eyelids are normal, and, although not fused, they are not open. No remnants of eye structures, such as muscles, retina, or optic nerve, are present.

The remaining 10% of the adults show variable degrees of ocular development. The eyes tend to be small, in some cases with a ring of pigment. Occasionally there is a lens present, but it is smaller in diameter than in normal animals. Few or no muscles develop, which causes the eyes to have abnormal orientation, sometimes even facing the back of the orbit. The eyelids are only open if the eye is more than one-half the normal size.

Differences between normal and anophthalmic mice begin to be apparent as early as gestational day 9. Although all embryos have optic vesicles, anophthalmic embryos have smaller ones. The development rate of the optic vesicle is slower in the anophthalmic embryos. This growth inhibition was determined by Chase and Chase[201] in 1941 to last from gestational days 9 to 13. This causes the optic cup either not to be formed at all or, more often, not to come into contact with the surface ectoderm, thus failing to induce the formation of a lens and subsequently all other eye structures. In conclusion, anophthalmia is brought about by a specific inhibition of growth in the optic vesicle that persists for approximately 4 days during the embryonic development.

This study was not the first one to analyze anophthalmia in order to understand eye development; in fact, in 1905 Lewis[200] studied the formation of the cornea in the frog. By removing the rudimentary embryonic eye structures, he concluded that it is the presence of the eyeball that induces the formation of the cornea and the rearrangement of the mesenchyme superior to it. On the other hand, what is innovative about Chase and Chase's study is the fact that genetically determined anophthalmia is being analyzed, thus reinforcing the idea that genes are involved in specifically determining rates of growth and development during normal embryogenesis.

Cell death

The study of cell death under physiologic conditions as a significant process is relatively new. The very object of the study, the death of a cell, has only been considered to be relevant to the study of pathology for about 40 yr. Nevertheless, and in spite of the fact that it was recognized that cell death might play an important role during development,[202] embryologists displayed only limited curiosity until the early 1970s. In fact, the idea that cell death could be a programmed, active process rather than passive degeneration has been largely overlooked, probably because it is contrary to the instinct of self-conservation.

There are two different kinds of dying cells. First are those that die under circumstances that severely deviate from physiologic conditions, such as hypoxia, ischemia, disruption of the membranes, severe temperature changes, and so forth. These are said to undergo coagulative necrosis, which usually involves relatively large sections of tissue. The major features of this process are the swelling of the cytoplasm and the loss of organelle integrity. Second is the process known as *apoptosis,* which involves single, scattered cells, and usually occurs under normal conditions. The apoptotic cell is characterized by condensed chromatin and a contracting cytoplasm, which finally leads to the formation of separate bodies containing isolated organelles that will eventually be phagocytosed by neighboring cells.[203]

Apoptosis is involved in the programmed focal elimination of cells during embryonic and fetal development and metamorphosis, in regulating the size of organs and tissues in adult life, and in maintaining equilibrium in cell populations undergoing permanent turnover, such as lymphocytes. This form of cell death also plays a role in many types of atrophy and in the regression of hyperplasia. It also occurs spontaneously in neoplasms and is increased in both neoplastic and rapidly dividing cell populations by chemotherapeutic agents and ionizing radiation.

More extensive characterization of cell death is beyond the scope of this chapter. The reader is referred to the excellent reviews by Wyllie et al.[204] and Walker et al.[205]

Until recently, the predominant concept was that a developing cell population should follow a linear growth pattern in order to achieve its final fate, avoiding the potential loss or misuse of energy that generating "unuseful" intermediates would involve. It is now known that this is not the case, and growth, far from being linear, involves many different changes of function, shape, and relative size that are concomitant with drastic changes in the number of cells present in a given tissue at a given time. Thus it becomes obvious that a cell's death plays a main role in its progression. Following are some models that helped clarify the role that cell death plays in normal development.

Cell death in normal development

Digit formation in vertebrate development. Digit formation is probably one of the best studied models of the involvement of programmed cell death in normal development. In all amniote embryos, the digits initially develop from a hand or foot plate that consists of a core of mesenchymal cells covered by an ectodermal jacket. At one point, the mesenchymal cells that are part of the presumptive digital arrays start to chondrify, eventually originating in the anlagen of the phalanges, while the mesenchymal cells between the chondrifying digits degenerate.[206] Earlier studies of digit formation in avian species with webbed feet showed that cell death also occurs, but with less intensity, and that the degree of cell death observed correlates well with the general structure of the adult foot. Nevertheless, the correlation between digit shape and cell death is not precise enough to allow digit formation to be explained by cell death alone.

Induced and spontaneous soft tissue syndactyly has been observed in chickens with a mutation in the *Ta* locus *(Ta³)* that causes a deficiency in interdigital cell death. Janus green B dye or 5-bromodeoxyuridine, both of which inhibit interdigital cell death, also cause syndactyly in this model, but the results have been obscured by secondary anomalies, such as polydactyly and hypophalangy, indicating that digit formation is a more complex process than initially thought.[207,208] It should be noted that in amphibian embryos there is no interdigital cell death, and digits form by a differential growth mechanism, indicating that in phylogeny similar results can be obtained through different pathways.[209]

Palatal fusion. In mammals, palatal closure occurs by the fusion of two opposing palatal processes, each consisting of a mesenchymal core surrounded by epithelial tissue. After elevation of the palatal shelves from a vertical to a horizontal position over the tongue, palatal fusion takes place at the midline in a two step process: First, there is contact and adherence of the two edges with formation of an epithelial seam; second, there is epithelial breakdown followed by mesenchymal confluence.[210] The process has been experimentally reproduced in vitro by organ culture of murine palatal shelves. It has also been possible to demonstrate that cell death may occur independently of fusion by culture of a single palatal process, which undergoes epithelial breakdown in a time scale comparable to that observed in vivo and provides strong evidence to suggest that in this case cell death is preprogrammed and determined by the cell itself rather than by extracellular stimuli.[211] Moreover, this epithelial breakdown is mediated by the intracellular release of hydrolytic enzymes from lysosomes.[212]

Cell death in abnormal development

Cell death is a common feature of both induced and spontaneous abnormal development. Abnormal development can be caused by alterations in the spatial or temporal patterns of cell death or in its intensity. Cell death has been described in the abnormal development of virtually all organs. Some examples are described of both spontaneous and in-

duced malformations that involve cell death as a major mechanism of action.

Preaxial polydactyly. The mouse mutant strain *Pdn (polydactyly Nagoya)* is the model for this malformation. Animals carrying a mutation in this gene have an extra digit in both the forelimbs and hindlimbs.[213] The malformation is induced by excessive growth induction caused by the delay in ectodermal cell death in the preaxial segment of the apical ectodermal ridge (AER) of the affected limb.

In normal development the AER is responsible for the induction of the mesenchyme. Normally it degenerates, and this is followed by death of the underlying mesenchyme. If cell death in the AER is delayed—as is the case in *Pdn* mutants—the mesenchymal cells are rescued from cell death and induced to form the extra digit. A similar effect was induced in rats by treatment of pregnant dams with the antiproliferative agents cytosine arabinoside and 5-fluorodeoxyuridine, which inhibited mesenchymal cell death alone.[214]

Cell death and teratogenic agents. Many teratogenic insults result in cell death in different tissues. Why certain cells will die and others will not has not received much attention, and the assumption has been that the organ that is affected the most is that which was at the highest rate of growth or differentiation at the time of the teratogenic insult. Nevertheless, it has been shown that other variables, such as differential drug distribution and metabolism, state—rather than rate—of cellular differentiation, and other cellular characteristics,[215] do play a role.

Unfortunately, very little is known about the normal patterns of programmed cell death in the whole embryo. Therefore it is difficult to assess the changes in patterns of cell death that correlate with the teratogenic insult.

• *Ethanol.* In an effort to elucidate the relationship between cell death and teratogenesis, Sulik et al.[170] determined the normal patterns of cell death in murine embryos, as assessed by Nile Blue sulfate uptake, and compared them with those observed in treated animals. They noted that maternal treatment with ethanol between days 7 and 9 of gestation induced excessive cell death. Although the spatial patterns were respected, in some areas cell death was detected earlier in the treated embryos. It is possible that the mechanism generating the excess cell death is through lipid peroxide formation (which results from ethanol exposure), leading to the rupture of lysosomal membranes and consequently to the release of hydrolytic enzymes.[216] It is important to note that Nile Blue sulfate staining is not retained in tissues fixed for normal histologic analysis, which impedes precise morphologic description of the dying cells. It is not possible by this technique to distinguish clearly between necrosis and apoptosis.

• *Hypoxia.* It is possible to induce cleft lip in CL/Fr mice by regulating the amount of oxygen to which pregnant dams are exposed.[217] Bronsky et al.[218] observed an abnormally high amount of cellular debris in the invaginating nasal placodes of day 11 embryos from treated dams, which indicates that cell death, together with overall growth retardation, inhibited the fusion of the facial prominences, thus causing the clefting. It has been suggested that hypoxia acts through depletion of energy in those areas involved in the most active morphogenetic movements, such as invagination of the olfactory placodes, thus impeding fusion.

• *Glucocorticoid-induced cleft palate.* Programmed cell death is one of the primary morphogenetic processes involved in palate formation. During closure of the secondary palate, the palatal shelves first grow vertically and then horizontally where they meet in the midline. As the shelves meet, the covering epithelial cells undergo apoptosis, thereby allowing the underlying mesenchymal cores to meet and fuse.

It has been known for a long time that glucocorticoids delay the elevation of the palatal shelves in murine embryos.[219] It was thought that, due to this delay, by the time the shelves become horizontal, the maxillary growth was such that it was not possible for the shelves to contact each other in the middle, thus causing palatal clefts. In 1973, Greene and Kochhar[220] demonstrated that even if the shelves contacted each other they would not fuse because of the lack of epithelial cell death in the presence of corticoids. It is interesting to observe that glucocorticoid-induced cleft palate can be prevented by cotreatment with arachidonic acid, which somehow releases the inhibition of cell death; also cell death blockage can be removed by treatment with cycloheximide or with indomethacin (which competitively occupies the glucocorticoid receptor). Thus cell death inhibition requires ligand–receptor interaction and protein synthesis.[221,222]

Not all cell death observed during palate formation is of the apoptosis type. Various teratogens can directly disturb cells in the palatal shelves, resulting in cellular necrosis. Furthermore, it is also possible that environmental agents can disturb morphogenesis by altering cellular cues such that cells that were not normally programmed to die receive apoptotic signals. The end result would again be cell death although in this situation it would be misguided apoptosis rather than direct cellular necrosis.

Genetic control of cell death

Little is known about the control of cell death in higher vertebrates. It is logical to assume that mutations at the level of the effector mechanism would render the cell immune to cell killing by all those stimuli that act on that effector, although there probably is a much more complicated scheme of control acting on other variables as well. This is well exemplified in the nematode *Caenorhabditis elegans*. This organism, a free-living soil nematode, has long been used as a genetic developmental model mostly because all of its cell lineage has been mapped,[223,224] and found to be almost invariable between individuals.[225]

Five genes have been identified that are directly involved in the control of cell death: *ced-1, -2, -3,* and *-4* (for cell death deficient) and *nuc-1* (for nuclease deficient).[226,227] Mutants for the genes *ced-1, -2,* and *nuc-1* show abnormal cell death, while mutants at the *ced-3* or *ced-4* loci completely lack programmed cell death.[228] Interestingly, the gene product of each of these genes acts independently to cause the programmed death.[229]

The cells that are rescued from dying by mutations at these loci may take over the function of other cells but do not perform as well. Moreover, Avery and Horvitz[230] argue that since these cells are programmed to die they are not under selective pressure in the wild type; thus they play a similar role in development as that of pseudogenes in the evolution of the genomes such that new cellular functions may arise by drift of cellular fate.

This model has been of great importance, primarily by providing irrefutable proof of the existence of genetic control over programmed cell death. Although no cell death mutations have yet been found in higher organisms, little doubt is left that cell death is a necessary process during the normal development and morphogenesis of most, if not all, organisms.

Summary

This chapter reviews a small sampling of the many animal models for spontaneous and genetically determined congenital anomalies in humans.[98,231] These models provide the only means by which investigators can readily visualize morphologic changes as they occur developmentally, thereby generating hypotheses about the pathogenesis of the observed malformations that can later be tested experimentally. The models presented have certain attributes that make them more or less suitable as a model system to study a given genetic disorder or malformation complex. Craniofacial malformations such as the mouse mutant *first arch (far)* may be the model of choice if the particular interest concerns genetic epistatic interactions.[196] However, should the focus be on the underdevelopment of the mandible or the palate clefting, then the model of choice might be the *chondrodystrophic (cho)* mouse.[49] Finally, if one is focusing on the molecular basis of craniofacial defects, then one of the transgenic model systems with *Hox-1.1* or the transthyretin gene constructs would be appropriate.[179,183] It should be clear to the reader that no single model system is ideal for all purposes.

Based on our current understanding of genetics and of how genes interact in developing systems, it stands to reason that genetic differences between species influence the phenotypic expression of individual genes, even those with a great degree of homology. Therefore one must be cautious when claiming homology between an animal model and a human disorder, yet flexible enough to recognize the similarities that do exist and utilize them in creative ways to help broaden our knowledge of congenital anomalies.

Acknowledgments—This work was supported in part by U.S. Public Health Service grant ES-04326 and by grant 1-1170 from the March of Dimes Birth Defects Foundation.

References

1. Needham J: A History of Embryology. Abeland-Schuman, New York, 1959, p 18.
2. Landauer W: Hatchability of chicken eggs as influenced by environment and heredity. Storrs Agric Exp Station Bull 262:10, 1948.
3. Littré E: Oevres Complètes d'Hippocrate, Traduction Nouvelle Avec le Texte Grec, vol 7. Baillière, Paris, 1839–1861, p 531.
4. Aristotle: De Generatione Animalium, vol II. In: The Works of Aristotle Translated into English. WD Ross, ed. Oxford University Press, Oxford, 1908–1931.
5. Aristotle: Generatione Animalium, vol II, 4, 740a25–740b10; vol II, 7, 745b20–746a30. In: The Works of Aristotle Translated into English. WD Ross, ed. Oxford University Press, Oxford, 1908–1931.
6. Aristotle: Historia Animalium, vol VI, 10, 565b1–566a. Translated and edited by AW Thompson. Clarendon Press, Oxford, 1910.
7. Aristotle: Historia Animalium, vol VI, 2, 559b15. Translated and edited by AW Thompson. Clarendon Press, Oxford, 1910.
8. Aristotle: Historia Animalium, vol VI. Translated and edited by AW Thompson. Clarendon Press, Oxford, 1910.
9. Adelmann HB: The formation of the egg of the chick. In: The Embryological Treatises of Hieronymus Fabricius of Aquapendente, vol I. Cornell Univ Press, Ithaca, 1942, p 37.

10. Galen: De Foetum Formatione. In: Opera Omnia, vol 4. CG Kühn, ed. Cnoblock, Leipzig, 1828.

11. Leonardo da Vinci: Quaderni d'Anatomia, vol 3, plate 8. CL Vangesten, A Fonahn, H Hopstock, eds. Dybwad, Christiana, 1911.

12. Vesalius: De Humani Corporis Fabrica, vol V, Oportinum, Basileae, 1555.

13. Coiter V: Externarum et Internarum Principalium Humani Corporis Partium Tabulae et Exercitationes. T Gerlatzeni, Nürnberg, 1573.

14. Fabricius ab Aquapendente: De Formatione Ovi et Pulli tractatus acuratissimus. A Bencii, Patavii, 1621.

15. Harvey W: Exercitationes de Generatione Animalium. AJ Ravesteynium, Amsterdam, 1651.

16. Oppenheimer JM: Essays in the History of Embryology and Biology. MIT Press, Cambridge, 1967.

17. von Baer KE: Entwicklungsgeschichte der Thiere: Beobachtung und Reflexion. Bornträger, Konigsberg, 1828.

18. de Réaumur RAF: L'Art de Faire Éclore et Élevér en Toute Saison des Oiseaux Domestiques de Toutes Especies Soit par le Moyen de la Chaleur de Fumier Spit par le Moyen de Celle du Feu Ordinaire. Imp. Royale, Paris, 1749.

19. Warkany J: Teratology: Spectrum of a science. In: Issues and Reviews in Teratology, vol I. H Kalter, ed. Plenum, New York, 1983, p 19.

20. Wilson JG: Current status of teratology—General principles and mechanisms derived from animal studies. In: Handbook of Teratology, vol I. JG Wilson, FC Fraser, eds. Plenum, New York, 1977 p 47.

21. Ballantyne JW: Manual of Antenatal Pathology and Hygiene. The Embryo. William Green and Sons, Edinburgh, 1904.

22. Stockard CR: Developmental rate and structural expression: An experimental study of twins, "double monsters," and single deformities, and the interaction among embryonic organs during their origin and development. Am J Anat 28:115, 1921.

23. Warkany J, Nelson RC: Appearance of skeletal abnormalities in the offspring of rats reared on a deficient diet. Science 92:383, 1940.

24. Giroud A, Boisselot J: Repercussions de l'avitaminose B2 sur l'embryon du rat. Arch Fr Pediatr 4:317, 1947.

25. Gillman J, Gilbert C, Gillman T, et al.: A preliminary report on hydrocephalus, spina bifida, and other congenital anomalies in the rat produced by trypan blue. S Afr J Med Sci 13:47, 1948.

26. Fraser FC: Gene–environment interactions in the production of cleft palate. In: Methods for Teratological Studies in Experimental Animals and Man. H Nishimura, JR Miller, eds. Igaku Shoin, Tokyo, 1969, p 34.

27. Trasler DG: Pathogenesis of cleft lip and its relation to embryonic face shape in A/J and C57BL mice. Teratology 1:33, 1968.

28. Fraser FC, Pashayan H: Relation of face shape to susceptibility to congenital cleft lip: A preliminary report. J Med Genet 7:112, 1970.

29. Fraser FC: Relation of animal studies to the problems in man. In: Handbook of Teratology, vol I. JG Wilson, FC Fraser, eds. Plenum, New York, 1977, p 75.

30. Marin-Padilla M: Study of the skull in human cranioschisis. Acta Anat 62:1, 1965.

31. Langman J, Welch GW: Excess vitamin A and development of the central nervous system. J Comp Neurol 128:1, 1967.

32. Bannigan J, Cottell D: Ethanol teratogenicity in mice: An electron microscopic study. Teratology 30:281, 1984.

33. Stevenson RE, Kelly JC, Aylsworth AS, et al.: Vascular basis for neural tube defects. Proc Greenwood Genet Center 6:109, 1987.

34. Gardner WJ: The Dysraphic States. Excerpta Medica, Amsterdam, 1973, p 1.

35. Finnell RH, Moon SP, Abbott LC, et al.: Strain differences in heat-induced neural tube defects in mice. Teratology 33:247, 1986.

36. Morris GL, O'Shea KS: Anomalies of neuroepithelial cell associations in the splotch mutant embryo. Dev Brain Res 9:408, 1983.

37. Edwards MJ, Mulley R, Ring S, et al.: Mitotic cell death and delay of mitotic activity in guinea pig embryos following brief maternal hyperthermia. J Embryol Exp Morphol 32:593, 1974.

38. Edwards MJ, Gray CH, Beatson J: Retardation of brain growth of guinea pigs by hyperthermia: Effects of varying intervals between successive exposures. Teratology 29:305, 1984.

39. Watney M, Miller JR: Prevention of a genetically determined congenital eye anomaly in the mouse by the administration of cortisone during pregnancy. Nature 202:1029, 1964.

40. Juriloff DM, Harris MJ: A scanning electron microscope study of fetal eyelid closure accelerated by cortisone in SWV/Bc mice. Teratology 40:59, 1989.

41. Harris MJ: Cortisone cure of the eyelid closure defect in lidgap-Stein fetal mice: A dose–response and time–response study as a test of the Hypomorph Hypothesis for the lidgap alleles. Teratology 39:601, 1989.

42. Erway LC, Fraser AS, Hurley LC: Prevention of congenital otolith defect in pallid mutant mice by manganese supplementation. Genetics 67:97, 1971.

43. Rimoin DL, Hollister DW, Lachman RS, et al.: Histologic studies in the chondrodystrophies. BDOAS X(12):274, 1974.

44. Sillence DO, Horton WA, Rimoin DL: Morphologic studies in the skeletal dysplasias. Am J Pathol 96:813, 1979.

45. Rimoin DL, Lachman RS: The chondrodysplasias. In: Principles and Practice of Medical Genetics. AE Emery, DL Rimoin, eds. Churchill Livingstone, Edinburgh, 1983, p 703.

46. Johnson DR: The Genetics of the Skeleton. Clarendon Press, Oxford, 1986, p 40.

47. Rimoin DL: The chondrodystrophies. Adv Hum Genet 5:1, 1975.

48. Lalley PA, McKusick VA: Report of the committee on comparative mapping. HGM8, Cytogenet Cell Genet 40:536, 1985.

49. Rittenhouse E, Dunn LC, Cookingham J, et al.: Cartilage matrix deficiency (cmd): A new autosomal recessive lethal mutation in the mouse. J Embryol Exp Morphol 43:71, 1978.

50. Kimata K, Barrach HJ, Brown KS, et al.: Absence of proteoglycan core protein in cartilage from the cmd/cmd mouse. J Biol Chem 256:6961, 1981.

51. Seegmiller RE, Brown K, Chandrasekhar S: Histochemical, immunofluorescence, and ultrastructural differences in fetal cartilage among three genetically distinct chondrodystrophic mice. Teratology 38:579, 1988.

52. McKeown PJ, Goetinck PF: A comparison of the proteoglycans synthesized in Meckel's and sternal cartilage from normal and nanomelic chick embryos. Dev Biol 71:203, 1979.

53. Lane PW, Dickie MM: Three recessive mutations producing disproportionate dwarfing in mice. J Hered 59:300, 1968.

54. Orkin RW, Pratt RM, Martin GM: Undersulphated chondroitin sulphate in cartilage matrix of brachymorphic mice. Dev Biol 50:82, 1976.

55. Miller WA, Flynn-Miller KL: Achondroplastic, brachymorphic and stubby chondrodystrophies in mice. J Comp Pathol 86:349, 1976.

56. Bonucci E, Del Marco A, Nicoletti B, et al.: Histological and histochemical investigations of achondroplastic mice: A possible model of human achondroplasia. Growth 40:241, 1976.

57. Silberberg R, Lesker P: Skeletal growth and development of achondroplastic mice. Growth 39:17, 1975.

58. Silberberg R, Hasler M, Lesker P: Ultrastructure of articular cartilage of achondroplastic mice. Acta Anat 96:162, 1976.

59. Thurston MN, Johnson DR, Kember NF: Cell kinetics of growth cartilage of achondroplastic (cn) mice. J Anat 140:425, 1985.

60. Konyukhov BV, Paschin YV: Abnormal growth of the body, internal organs and skeleton in the achondroplastic mouse. Acta Biol Acad Sci Hung 21:347, 1970.

61. Seegmiller RE, Fraser FC, Sheldon H: A new chondrodystrophic mutant in mice: Electron microscopy of normal and abnormal chondrogenesis. J Cell Biol 48:580, 1971.

62. Seegmiller RE, Cooper CA, Houghton MJ, et al.: Pulmonary hypoplasia in chondrodystrohic mice. Teratology 33:339, 1986.

63. Seegmiller RE, Fraser FC: Mandibular growth retardation as a cause of cleft palate in mice homozygous for the chondrodysplasia gene. J Embryol Exp Morphol 38:227, 1977.

64. Monson CB, Seegmiller RE: Ultrastructural studies of cartilage matrix in mice homozygous for chondrodysplasia. J Bone Joint Surg 63-A:637, 1981.

65. Seegmiller RE, Myers RA, Dorfman A, et al.: Structural and associative properties of cartilage matrix constituents in mice with hereditary chondrodysplasia. Connect Tissue Res 9:69, 1981.

66. Ferguson JM, Wallace ME, Johnson DR: A new type of chondrodystrophic mutation in the mouse. J Med Genet 15:128, 1978.

67. Johnson DR: The growth of the femur and tibia in three genetically distinct chrondrodystrophic mutants of the house mouse. J Anat 125:267, 1978.

68. Johnson DR: Abnormal cartilage from the mandibular condyle of stumpy (stm) mutant mice. J Anat 137:715, 1983.

69. Brown KS, Cranley RE, Greene R, et al.: Disproportionate micro-

melia *(Dmm)* an incomplete dominant mouse dwarfism with abnormal cartilage matrix. J Embryol Exp Morphol 62:165, 1981.

70. Mackenson JA, Stevens LC: Rib-fusions, a new mutation in the mouse. J Hered 51:264, 1960.

71. Theiler K, Stevens LC: The development of rib-fusions, a mutation in the house mouse. Am J Anat 106:171, 1960.

72. Dunn LC, Gluecksohn-Schoenheimer S: Stub, a new mutation in the mouse, J Hered 33:235, 1942.

73. Gruneberg H: Genetical studies on the skeleton of the mouse. XXIX. Pudgy. Genet Res 2:384, 1961.

74. Theiler K, Varnum DS, Southard JL, et al.: Malformed vertebrae: A new mutant with the "Wirbel-Rippen" syndrome in the mouse. Anat Embryol 147:161, 1975.

75. Morgan WC: A new crooked tail mutation involving distinctive pleiotropism. J Genet 52:354, 1954.

76. Theiler K, Varnum DS, Stevens LC: Development of rachiterata, a mutation in the house mouse with 6 sacral vertebrae. Z Anat Entwickl 145:75, 1974.

77. Campbell LR, Dayton DH, Sohal GS: Neural tube defects: A review of human and animal studies on the etiology of neural tube defects. Teratology 34:171, 1986.

78. Holmes LB, Driscoll SG, Atkins L: Etiologic heterogeneity of neural tube defects. N Engl J Med 294:365, 1976.

79. Carter CO: Clues to the aetiology of neural tube malformations. Dev Med Child Neurol [Suppl] 32:3, 1974.

80. Baird PA: Neural tube defects in Sikhs. Am J Med Genet 16:49, 1983.

81. Jorde LB, Fineman RM, Martin RA: Epidemiology of neural tube defects in Utah, 1940–1979. Am J Epidemiol 119:487, 1984.

82. Windham GC, Sever LE: Neural tube defects among twin births. Am J Hum Genet 34:988, 1982.

83. Khoury MJ, Erickson JD, James LM: Etiologic heterogeneity of neural tube defects. II. Clues from family studies. Am J Hum Genet 32:980, 1982.

84. Baraitser M, Burns J: Brief clinical report: Neural tube defects as an X-linked condition. Am J Med Genet 17:383, 1984.

85. Kousseff BG: Sacral meningocele with conotruncal heart defects: A possible autosomal recessive trait. Pediatrics 74:395, 1984.

86. Robertson RD, Sarti DA, Brown WJ, et al.: Congenital hydrocephalus in two pregnancies following the birth of a child with a neural tube defect: Aetiology and management. J Med Genet 18:105, 1981.

87. Sever LE: Spinal anomalies and neural tube defects. Am J Med Genet 15:343, 1983.

88. Jones MC, Jones KL, Chernoff GF: Possible mesodermal origin for axial dysraphic disorders. J Pediatr 101:845, 1982.

89. Ferguson JW, Rouse BM, Lockhart L: Mesodermal origin of axial dysraphism. J Pediatr 103:498, 1983.

90. Opitz JM, Gilbert EF: Editorial comment: CNS anomalies and the midline as a "developmental field." Am J Med Genet 12:443, 1982.

91. Bennett D: The T-locus of the mouse. Cell 6:441, 1975.

92. Fellous M, Boue J, Malbrunot C, et al.: A five-generation family with sacral agenesis and spina bifida: Possible similarities with the mouse T-locus. Am J Med Genet 12:465, 1982.

93. Erickson JD: Racial variation in the incidence of congenital malformations. Ann Hum Genet 39:315, 1976.

94. Carter CO, Evans K: Spina bifida and anencephalus in Greater London. J Med Genet 10:209, 1973.

95. Lemire RJ, Beckwith JB, Warkany J: Anencephaly. Raven, New York, 1978, p 11.

96. Vogel FS: The anatomic character of the vascular anomalies associated with anencephaly: With consideration of the role of abnormal angiogenesis in the pathogenesis of the cerebral malformation. Am J Pathol 39:163, 1961.

97. Abd-El-Malek S: The anencephalic skull and a vascular theory of causation. J Egypt Med Assoc 40:216, 1957.

98. Winter RM: Malformation syndromes: A review of mouse/human homology. J Med Genet 25:480, 1988.

99. Seller MJ, Embury S, Polani PE, et al.: Neural tube defects in curly tail mice. II. Effect of maternal administration of vitamin A. Proc R Soc Lond [Biol] B206:95, 1979.

100. Auerbach R: Analysis of the developmental effects of a lethal mutation in the house mouse. J Exp Zool 127:305, 1954.

101. Wilson DB: Proliferation in the neural tube of the splotch *(Sp)* mutant mouse. J Comp Neurol 154: 249, 1974.

102. Kapron-Bras CM, Trasler DG: Interaction between the splotch mutation and retinoic acid in mouse neural tube defects in vitro. Teratology 38:165, 1988.

103. Kapron-Bras CM, Trasler DG: Histological comparison of the effects of the splotch gene and retinoic acid on the closure of the mouse neural tube. Teratology 37:389, 1988.

104. Gruneberg H: Genetical studies on the skeleton of the mouse. VIII. Curly tail. J Genet 52:52, 1954.

105. Embury S, Seller MJ, Adionolfi M, Polani PE: Neural tube defects in curly tail mice. I. Incidence, expression, and similarity to the human condition. Proc R Soc Lond [Biol] B206:85, 1979.

106. Copp AJ, Seller MJ, Polani PE: Neural tube development in mutant (curly tail) and normal mouse embryos: The timing of posterior neuropore closure. J Embryol Exp Morphol 69:151, 1982.

107. Seller MJ, Adinolfi M: Minireview: The curly tail mouse: An experimental model for human neural tube defects. Life Sci 29:1607, 1981.

108. Seller MJ, Perkins KJ: Prevention of neural tube defects in curly tail mice by maternal administration of vitamin A. Prenat Diagn 2:297, 1983.

109. Adinolfi M, Beck S, Embury S, et al.: Levels of alpha-fetoprotein in amniotic fluids by mice (curly tail) with neural tube defects. J Med Genet 13:511, 1976.

110. Searle AG: Curtailed, a new dominant t-allele in the house mouse. Genet Res 7:86, 1966.

111. Chesley P: Development of the short-tailed mutant in the house mouse. J Exp Zool 70:429, 1935.

112. Park C-HT, Pruitt JH, Bennett D: A mouse model for neural tube defects: *The Curtailed (T^C)* mutation produces spina bifida occulta in $T^C/+$ animals and spina bifida with meningomyelocele in T^C/t. Teratology 39:303, 1989.

113. Macdonald KB, Juriloff DM, Harris MJ: Developmental study of neural tube closure in a mouse stock with a high incidence of exencephaly, Teratology 39:195, 1989.

114. Fraser FC: The multifactorial/threshold concept—Uses and misuses. Teratology 14:247, 1976.

115. Kurnit DM, Layton WM, Matthysse S: Genetics, chance, and morphogenesis. Am J Hum Genet 41:979, 1987.

116. Juriloff DM, Macdonald KB, Harris MJ: Genetic analysis of the cause of exencephaly in the SELH/Bc mouse stock. Teratology 40:395, 1989.

117. Seller MJ, Perkins-Cold KJ: Sex differences in mouse embryonic development at neurulation. J Reprod Fertil 79:159, 1987.

118. Kaufmann MH: Cephalic neurulation and optic vesicle formation in the early mouse embryo. Am J Anat 155:425, 1979.

119. Jacobson AG, Tam PPL: Cephalic neurulation in the mouse embryo analyzed by SEM and morphometry. Anat Rec 203:375, 1982.

120. Golden JA, Chernoff GF: Anterior neural tube closure in the mouse: Fuel for disagreement with the classical theory. Clin Res 31:127A, 1983.

121. Finnell RH, Buehler BA, Kerr BM, et al.: Clinical and experimental studies linking oxidative metabolism to phenytoin-induced teratogenesis. Neurol, 1992 (in press).

122. Putz B, Morriss-Kay G: Abnormal neural fold development in trisomy 12 and trisomy 14 mouse embryos. I. Scanning electron microscopy. J Embryol Exp Morphol 66:141, 1981.

123. Cox DR, Epstein LB, Epstein CJ: Genes coding for sensitivity to interferon *(IfRec)* and soluble superoxide dismutase *(SOD-1)* are linked in mouse and man and map to mouse chromosome 16. Proc Natl Acad Sci USA 77:2168, 1980.

124. Cox DR, Smith SA, Epstein LB, et al.: Mouse trisomy 16 as an animal model of human trisomy 21 (Down syndrome): Production of viable 16-diploid mouse chimeras. Dev Biol 101:416, 1984.

125. Epstein CJ, Cox DR, Epstein LB: Mouse trisomy 16: An animal model of human trisomy 21 (Down syndrome). Ann NY Acad Sci 450:157, 1985.

126. Buselmaier W, Bacchus C, Grohe G, et al.: Behavioral and developmental abnormalities in mouse trisomy 19: An animal model of mental retardation induced by chromosomal imbalance. Teratology 37:167, 1988.

127. White BJ, Tijo JH, Van de Water LC, et al.: Trisomy for the smallest autosome of the mouse and identification of the T1Wh translocation chromosome. Cytogenet Cell Genet 11:363, 1972.

128. Gropp A, Giers D, Kolbus U: Trisomy in the fetal backcross prog-

eny of male and female metacentric heterozygotes of the mouse. I. Crytogenet Cell Genet 13:511, 1974.

129. Gropp A, Kolbus U, Giers D: Systematic approach to the study of trisomy in the mouse. II. Cytogenet Cell Genet 14:42, 1975.

130. Gropp A, Winking H, Herbst EW, et al.: Murine trisomy: Developmental profiles of the embryo and isolation of trisomic cellular systems. J Exp Zool 228:253, 1983.

131. Epstein CJ: Mouse monosomies and trisomies as experimental systems for studying mammalian aneuploidy. Trends Genet 1:129, 1985.

132. Epstein CJ: The Consequences of Chromosome Imbalance. Cambridge University Press, Cambridge, 1986.

133. Dyban AP, Baranov VS: Cytogenetics of Mammalian Embryonic Development. Clarendon Press, Oxford, 1987.

134. Kochhar DM: Teratogenic activity of retinoic acid. Acta Pathol Microbiol Scand 70:398, 1967.

135. Cohlan SQ: Congenital anomalies in the rat produced by excessive intake of vitamin A during pregnancy. Pediatrics 13:556, 1954.

136. Chernoff GF: The fetal alcohol syndrome in mice: An animal model. Teratology 15:223, 1977.

137. Chernoff GF: The fetal alcohol syndrome in mice: Maternal variables. Teratology 22:71, 1980.

138. Finnell RH: Phenytoin-induced teratogenesis: A mouse model. Science 211:483, 1981.

139. Finnell RH, Chernoff GF: Variable patterns of malformation in the mouse fetal hydantoin syndrome. Am J Med Genet 19:463, 1984.

140. Jones KL, Smith DW: Recognition of the fetal alcohol syndrome in early infancy. Lancet 2:999, 1973.

141. Jones KL, Smith DW, Ulleland CW, et al.: Pattern of malformation in offspring of chronic alcoholic women. Lancet 1:1267, 1973.

142. Ferrier PE, Nicod I, Ferrier S: Fetal alcohol syndrome. Lancet 2:218, 1973.

143. Sandor S, Elias S: The influence of aethyl-alcohol on the development of the chick embryo. Rev Roum Embryol Cytol Ser Embryol 5:51, 1968.

144. Sandor S, Amels D: The action of aethanol on the prenatal development of albino rats. Rev Roum Embryol Cytol Ser Embryol 8:105, 1971.

145. Sulik KK, Johnston MC: Sequence of developmental alterations following acute ethanol exposure in mice. Craniofacial features of the fetal alcohol syndrome. Am J Anat 116:257, 1983.

146. Sulik KK, Johnston MC, Webb MA: Fetal alcohol syndrome: Embryogenesis in a mouse model. Science 214:936, 1981.

147. Finnell RH, Chernoff GF: The mouse fetal hydantoin syndrome: Effects of maternal seizures. Epilepsia 23:423, 1982.

148. Finnell RH, Abbott LC, Taylor SM: The fetal hydantoin syndrome: Answers from a mouse model. Reprod Toxicol 3:127, 1989.

149. Buehler BA: Epoxide hydrolase activity and fetal hydantoin syndrome. Proc Greenwood Genet Center 3:109, 1984.

150. Finnell RH, Bennett GD, Karras SB, et al.: Common hierarchies of susceptibility to the induction of neural tube defects in mouse embryos by valproic acid and its 4-propyl-4-pentenoic acid metabolite. Teratology 38:313, 1988.

151. Naruse I, Collins MD, Scott WJ, Jr: Strain differences in the teratogenicity induced by sodium valproate in cultured mouse embryos. Teratology 38:87, 1988.

152. Bennett GD, Mohl VK, Finnell RH: Embryonic and maternal heat shock responses to known teratogenic insults. Reprod Toxicol 4:113, 1990.

153. Finnell RH: Genetic differences in susceptibility to anticonvulsant drug-induced developmental delay. Pharmacol Toxicol 69:223, 1991.

154. Lammer EJ, Chen DT, Hoar RM, et al.: Retinoic acid embryopathy. N Engl J Med 313:837, 1985.

155. Cohlan SQ: Excessive intake of vitamin A as a cause of congenital anomalies in the rat. Science 117:535, 1953.

156. Giroud A, Martinet M: Malformations embryonnaires par hypervitaminose A. Arch Fr Pediatr 12:292, 1955.

157. Kalter H, Warkany J: Experimental production of congenital malformations in strains of inbred mice by maternal treatment with hypervitaminosis A. Am J Pathol 38:1, 1961.

158. Fantel AG, Shepard TG, Newell-Morris LL, et al.: Teratogenic effects of retinoic acid in pigtail monkeys *(Macaca nemestrina).* 1. General features. Teratology 15:65, 1977.

159. Wiley MJ, Cauwenbergs P, Taylor IM: Effects of retinoic acid on the development of the facial skeleton in hamsters: Early changes involving cranial neural crest cells. Acta Anat 116:180, 1983.

160. Newell-Morris LL, Sirianni JE, Shepard TH, et al.: Teratogenic effects of retinoic acid in pigtail monkeys *(Macaca nemestrina).* II. Craniofacial features. Teratology 22:87, 1980.

161. Kraft JC, Kochhar DM, Scott WJ, et al.: Low teratogenicity of 13-*cis*-retinoic acid (isotretinoin) in the mouse corresponds to low embryo concentrations during organogenesis: Comparison to the all-*trans* isomer. Toxicol Appl Pharmacol 87:474, 1987.

162. Slough CL, Yonker J: Dose-related teratogenic effects of vitamin A palmitate and *trans*-retinoic acid in the rat. Teratology 33:73C, 1986.

163. Nolen GA: Effect of a high systemic background level of vitamin A on the teratogenicity of all-*trans* retinoic acid given either acutely or subacutely. Teratology 39:333, 1989.

164. Alles AJ, Sulik KK: Retinoic acid–induced limb reduction defects: Perturbations of zones of programmed cell death as a pathogenetic mechanism. Teratology 40:163, 1989.

165. Satre MA, Penner JD, Kochhar DM: Pharmacokinetic assessment of teratologically effective concentrations of an endogenous retinoic acid metabolite. Teratology 39:341, 1989.

166. Morriss GM: The ultrastructural effects of excess maternal vitamin A on the primitive streak stage rat embryo. J Embryol Exp Morphol 30:219, 1973.

167. Marin-Padilla M: Mesodermal alterations induced by hypervitaminosis A. J Embryol Exp Morphol 15:261, 1966.

168. Geelen JAG: Skullbase malformations in rat fetuses with hypervitaminosis A–induced exencephaly. Teratology 7:49, 1973.

169. Theodosis D, Fraser FC: Pathogenesis of vitamin A–induced exencephaly in the mouse. Teratology 7:29a, 1973.

170. Sulik KK, Cook CS, Webster WS: Teratogens and craniofacial malformation: Relationships to cell death. Development 103(Suppl):213, 1988.

171. Sulik KK, Dehart DB: Retinoic acid–induced limb malformations resulting from apical ectodermal ridge cell death. Teratology 37:527, 1988.

172. Gordon JW, Scangos GA, Plotkin DJ, et al.: Genetic transformation of mouse embryos by microinjection of purified DNA. Proc Natl Acad Sci USA 77:7380, 1980.

173. van Lohuizen M, Verbeek S, Krimpenfort P, et al.: Predisposition to lymphomagenesis in *pim-1* transgenic mice: Cooperation with *c-myc* and *N-myc* in murine leukemia virus-induced tumors. Cell 56:673, 1989.

174. Lucy MC, Petters RM: Production of chimeric mice by reciprocal exchange of split embryo halves. Theriogenology 28:899, 1987.

175. Palmiter RD, Brinster RL: Germ-line transformation of mice. Annu Rev Genet 20:465, 1986.

176. Brinster RL, Chen HY, Trumbauer ME, et al.: Factors affecting the efficiency of introducing foreign DNA into mice by microinjecting eggs. Proc Natl Acad Sci USA 82:4438, 1985.

177. Jahner D, Haase K, Mulligan R, et al.: Insertion of the bacterial *gpt* gene into the germ line of mice by retroviral infection. Proc Natl Acad Sci USA 82:6927, 1985.

178. Epstein CJ, Avraham KB, Lovett M, et al.: Transgenic mice with increased Cu/Zn–superoxide dismutase activity: An animal model of dosage effect in Down syndrome. Proc Natl Acad Sci USA 84:8044, 1987.

179. McNeish JD, Scott WJ, Potter SS: Legless, a novel mutation found in PHT1-1 transgenic mice. Science 241:837, 1988.

180. Wakasugi S, Iwanaga T, Inomoto T, et al.: An autosomal dominant mutation of facial development in a transgenic mouse. Dev Genet 9:203, 1988.

181. Jones KL: Smith's Recognizable Patterns of Human Malformation, ed 4. WB Saunders, Philadelphia, 1988, p 210.

182. Mahon KA, Westphal H, Gruss P: Expression of homeobox gene *Hox-1.1* during mouse embryogenesis. Development 104(Suppl):187, 1988.

183. Fienberg AA, Utset MF, Bogarad LD, et al.: Homeobox genes in murine development. Curr Top Dev Biol 23:233, 1987.

184. Balling R, Mutter G, Gruss P, et al.: Craniofacial abnormalities induced by ectopic expression of the homeobox gene *Hox-1.1* in transgenic mice. Cell 58:337, 1989.

185. Juriloff DM, Harris MJ: Abnormal facial development in the mouse mutant first arch. J Craniofac Genet Dev Biol 3:317, 1983.

186. Juriloff DM, Harris MJ, Froster-Iskenius U: Hemifacial deficiency

induced by a shift in dominance of the mouse mutation far: A possible genetic model for hemifacial microsomia. J Craniofacial Genet Dev Biol 7:27, 1987.

187. Thaller C, Eichelle G: Identification and spatial distribution of retinoids in the developing chick limb bud. Nature 327:625, 1987.

188. Wolgemuth DJ, Behringer RR, Mostoller MP, et al.: Transgenic mice overexpressing the mouse homeobox containing gene *Hox-1.4* exhibit abnormal gut development. Nature 337:464, 1989.

189. Stacey A, Bateman J, Choi T, et al.: Perinatal lethal osteogenesis imperfecta in transgenic mice bearing an engineered mutant pro-alpha (I) collagen gene. Nature 332:131, 1988.

190. Wynne-Davies R: Heritable Disorders in Orthopaedic Practice. Blackwell, London, 1973, p 80.

191. Grobstein C: Induction interaction in the development of the mouse metanephros. J Exp Zool 130:319, 1955.

192. Ekblom P, Thesleff I, Saxén L, et al.: Transferrin as a fetal growth factor: Acquisition of responsiveness related to embryonic induction. Proc Natl Acad Sci USA 80:2651, 1983.

193. Thesleff I, Partanen AM, Landschulz W, et al.: The role of transferrin receptors and iron delivery in mouse embryonic morphogenesis. Differentiation 30:152, 1985.

194. Potter EL: Bilateral renal agenesis. J Pediatr 29:68, 1946.

195. Dunn LC, Gluecksohn-Schoenheimer S, Bryson V: A new mutation in the mouse affecting spinal column and urogenital system. J Hered 31:343, 1940.

196. Gluecksohn-Schoenheimer S: The morphological manifestations of a dominant mutation in mice affecting tail and urogenital system. Genetics 28:341, 1943.

197. Gluecksohn-Waelsch S, Rota TR: Development in organ tissue culture of kidney rudiments from mutant mouse embryos. Dev Biol 7:432, 1963.

198. Bagg HJ, Little CC: Hereditary abnormalities of the viscera: A morphological study with special reference to abnormalities of the kidneys in the descendants of x-rayed mice. Am J Anat 36:275, 1925.

199. Brown AL: An analysis of the developing metanephros in mouse embryos with abnormal kidneys. Am J Anat 47:117, 1931.

200. Lewis WH: Experimental studies on the development of the eye in Amphibia. II. On the cornea. J Exp Zool 2:431, 1905.

201. Chase HB, Chase E: Studies on an anophthalmic strain of mice. I. Embryology of the eye region. J Morphol 68:279, 1941.

202. Glücksman A: Cell death in normal vertebrate ontogeny. Biol Rev 26:59, 1951.

203. Kerr JFR, Wyllie AH, Currie AR: Apoptosis: A basic biological phenomenon with wide-ranging implications in tissue kinetics. Br J Cancer 26:239, 1972.

204. Wyllie AH, Kerr JFR, Currie AR: Cell death: The significance of apoptosis. Int Rev Cytol 68:251, 1980.

205. Walker NI, Harmon BV, Gobé GC, et al.: Patterns of cell death. Methods Achiev Exp Pathol 13:18, 1988.

206. Hinchliffe JR: Cell death in vertebrate limb morphogenesis. In: Progress in Anatomy, vol 2. RJ Harrison, V Navaratnam, eds. Cambridge University Press, Cambridge, 1982, p 1.

207. Hinchliffe JR, Thorogood PV: Genetic inhibition of mesenchymal cell death and the development of form and skeletal pattern in the limbs of talpid³ *(Ta³)* mutant chick embryos. J Embryol Exp Morphol 31:747, 1974.

208. Hurle JM: Cell death in developing systems. Methods Achiev Exp Pathol 13:55, 1988.

209. Cameron JA, Fallon JF: The absence of cell death during development of free digits in amphibians. Dev Biol 55:331, 1977.

210. Greene RM, Pratt RM: Developmental aspects of secondary palate formation. J Embryol Exp Morphol 36:225, 1976.

211. Tyler MS, Koch WE: In vitro development of palatal tissues from embryonic mice. J Embryol Exp Morphol 38:19, 1977.

212. Greene RM, Pratt RM: Inhibition of epithelial cell death in the secondary palate in vitro by alteration of lysosome function. J Histochem Cytochem 26:1109, 1978.

213. Hayasaka L, Nakatsuka T, Fujii T, et al.: Polydactyly Nagoya, *Pdn:* A new mutant gene in the mouse. Exp Anim 29:391, 1980.

214. Scott WJ, Ritter EJ, Wilson JG: Delayed appearance of ectodermal cell death as a mechanism of polydactyly induction. J Embryol Exp Morphol 42:93, 1977.

215. Scott WJ: Cell death and reduced proliferative rate. In: Handbook of Teratology, vol 2. JG Wilson, FC Fraser, eds. Plenum, New York, 1977, p 81.

216. Wills ED, Wilkinson AE: Release of enzymes from lysosomes by irradiation and the relation of lipid peroxide formation to enzyme release. Biochem J 99:657, 1966.

217. Millicovsky G, Johnston MC: Hyperoxia and hypoxia in pregnancy: Simple experimental manipulation alters the incidence of cleft lip and palate in CL/Fr mice. Proc Natl Acad Sci USA 9:4723, 1981.

218. Bronsky PT, Johnston MC, Sulik KK: Morphogenesis of hypoxia-induced cleft lip in CL/Fr mice. J Craniofac Gen Dev Biol 2(Suppl):113, 1986.

219. Walker BE, Fraser FC: The embryology of cortisone-induced cleft palate, J Embryol Exp Morphol 5:201, 1957.

220. Greene RM, Kochhar DM: Spatial relations in the oral cavity of cortisone-treated mouse fetuses during the time of secondary palate closure. Teratology 8:153, 1973.

221. Goldman AS, Baker MY, Piddington R, et al.: Inhibition of programmed cell death in mouse embryonic palate in vitro by cortisol and phenytoin: Receptor involvement and requirement of protein synthesis. Proc Soc Exp Biol Med 174:239, 1983.

222. Goldman AS: Biochemical mechanism of glucocorticoid- and phenytoin-induced cleft palate. Curr Top Dev Biol 19:217, 1984.

223. Sulston JE, Horvitz HR: Postembryonic cell lineages of the nematode *Caenorhabditis elegans.* Dev Biol 56:110, 1977.

224. Kimble J, Hirsch D: The postembryonic cell lineages of the hermaphrodite and male gonads in *Caenorhabditis elegans.* Dev Biol 70:396, 1979.

225. Sulston JE, Schierenberg J, White J, et al.: The embryonic cell lineage of the nematode *Caenorhabditis elegans.* Dev Biol 100:64, 1983.

226. Sulston JE: Post-embryonic development in the ventral cord of *Caenorhabditis elegans.* Philos Trans R Soc Lond [Biol] 275:287, 1976.

227. Hedgecock E, Sulston JE, Thomson N: Mutations affecting programmed cell deaths in the nematode *Caenorhabditis elegans.* Science 220:1277, 1983.

228. Ellis HM, Horvitz HR: Genetic control of programmed cell death in the nematode *C. elegans.* Cell 44:817, 1986.

229. Yuan JY, Horvitz HR: The *Caenorhabditis elegans* genes *ced-3* and *ced-4* act cell autonomously to cause programmed cell death. Dev Biol 138:33, 1990.

230. Avery L, Horvitz HR: A cell that dies during wild-type *C. elegans* development can function as a neuron in a *ced-3* mutant. Cell 51:1071, 1987.

231. Searle AG, Peters J, Lyon MF, et al.: Chromosome maps of man and mouse IV. Ann Hum Genet 53:89, 1989.

6

The Genetic Basis of Human Anomalies

ROGER E. STEVENSON

The genetic content of egg and sperm brings to the conceptus all instructions necessary for the formation and function of a new life. Disturbances in the amount of genetic material (aberrations in chromosome number or structure) or in the nature of this material (gene mutations) may preclude normal formation, causing a wide range of anomalies or other morphologic changes and an equally broad range of functional impairments.

Normal human formation, however, is not assured by normal chromosomes and genes; environmental insults during pregnancy can exert an equally potent influence on human morphology. Current clinical and technological methods can determine the cause of approximately one-half of the anomalies found in newborn infants (Table 6–1). One-half of the identifiable causes are either wholly or partially genetic.

The chromosomal basis for human anomalies

Over 75 years passed between Flemming's observations[1] of chromosomes in the epithelium of the human cornea (1882) and the first demonstration (by Lejeune[2] in 1959) of the chromosomal basis for a human malformation syndrome, although the link between chromosomes and malformations had been suggested in the interim. As early as the 1930s, Waardenburg[3] and Bleyer[4] independently predicted that nondisjunction of chromosomes during meiosis, resulting in abnormal chromosome number, might be the cause of Down syndrome.

Determination of the correct number of human chromosomes took an equivalent period of time. Flemming[1] gave the name *chromatin* to the stained material of the nucleus that he identified and followed through several stages of cell division, termed *mitosen* (Fig. 6–1). He considered chromatin to be a single strand of material that resolved itself into individual stained bodies at certain times in the cell cycle. Early attempts to count the number of chromosomes depended on finding naturally occurring mitoses in tissue sections.[5–7] The sections proved unsatisfactory for this purpose because the chromosomes appeared indistinct and poorly separated from each other. Hansemann[5] analyzed three such human cells in 1891, finding in them counts of 18, 24, and "more than 40" chromosomes. For several decades thereafter the diploid chromosome number in man was thought possibly to be 24.

On the basis of counts made on testicular sections, von Winiwarter[7] concluded in 1912 that the human chromosome number differed in the two sexes, females having a 48 count with two X chromosomes and males a 47 count with one X chromosome. In 1924, Painter[8] demonstrated an X and a Y chromosome in males, but his findings were not universally accepted.

In the 1940s and 1950s, bone marrow preparations were investigated as a source of mitoses for chromosome analyses, but were found to be nearly as unsatisfactory as tissue sections had been.[9] The belief that 48 was the correct number of chromosomes in humans was maintained into the mid-1950s. Analysis and correct counting had to await the development of more satisfactory cytologic techniques.

Tjio and Levan[10] surprised the scientific community in 1956 with their report of 46 chromosomes found in the culture of fibroblasts from fetal lung (Fig. 6–2). Rapid refinement in tissue culture and metaphase preparation and agreement on nomenclature followed so that within three years chromosome analysis became commonplace in laboratories throughout the world. The discovery of numerical chromosome aberrations followed (Table 6–2), opening an era when an answer to nearly all human maladies was sought in the chromosomes. Cancer, malformations, mental retardation, abortion, sexual aberrations, and other disorders were investigated.

A rich yield rewarded investigators who sought the explanation of spontaneous abortion in chromosome analysis.[11–14] In 1961, Penrose and Delhanty[12] demonstrated triploidy in a macerated fetus. In the reports that followed chromosome aberrations were found in approximately one-half of early spontaneous abortions.[11,13–16] The 45,X karyotype was found most frequently, but tetraploidy, triploidy, and numerous other trisomies not seen in liveborn infants constituted a major portion of chromosomally abnormal abortuses (Table 6–3).

Prenatal diagnosis of chromosome aberrations became possible in 1966, when Steele and Breg[17] combined the technique of amniocentesis with culture of amniotic fluid cells. The reliability and safety of the combined procedures contributed to rapid acceptance of the techniques for pregnancies determined to be at increased risk of chromosome abnormalities and certain biochemical defects.

The utility of chromosomes in expanding and understand-

Table 6–1. Causes of anomalies among liveborn infants

Cause	Percent incidence
Genetic	15–25
Chromosome	10–15
Single gene	2–10
Multifactorial	20–25
Environmental	8–12
Maternal diseases	6–8
Uterine/placental	2–3
Drugs/chemicals	0.5–1
Twinning	0.5–1
Unknown	40–60

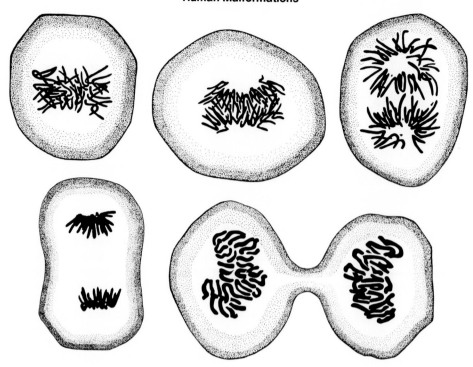

Fig. 6–1. Chromosomes were first visualized by Walther Flemming prior to 1880 in several different stages of cell division he called *mitosen.* He gave the term *chromatin* to the colored material that he found in the nucleus of cells from numerous organisms, including human. Redrawn from Flemming.[122]

ing of human disease reached a plateau in the late 1960s. Excitement was returned to the field of cytogenetics with the introduction of banding techniques by Caspersson et al.[18] in 1971, demonstration of fragile sites by Sutherland[19] in 1977, and analysis of prophase and prometaphase (high resolution)[20] chromosomes in the early 1980s (Figs. 6–3, 6–4). A greater understanding of the chromosomal basis for malformations, mental retardation, cancer, and other human disorders accompanied these advances. The search for structural chromosome abnormalities now includes molecular

technology that permits the detection of deletions and duplications that are beyond the resolution of the light microscope.[21–24]

Chromosome watching provides only a crude view of genetic events. Best regarded as carrier structures, the chromosomes keep the genes together in a limited number of packets, perhaps maintain the genes in some necessary sequence, and provide for the orderly transmission of the genes they contain to daughter cells through mitotic division and to new offspring through meiotic division.

Through mitosis, all chromosomes can be replicated and a full diploid complement of chromosomes distributed to daughter cells (Fig. 6–5). This process is fundamental to growth, allowing multiplication of cell numbers, with each cell retaining the genetic capacity of the initiating cell.

Chromosomes transfer representative genes to a new generation through gametogenesis and allow the admixing of genes from the parental generation through the phenomenon of crossing-over (Fig. 6–6). An offspring does not receive any single chromosome in sperm or egg that is identical to that in either parent's somatic cells. Rather, as chromosomes pass

Fig. 6–2. Metaphase chromosome preparation from fibroblasts of fetal lung that accompanied Tjio and Levan's 1956 report[10] establishing 46 as the number of chromosomes in human cells.

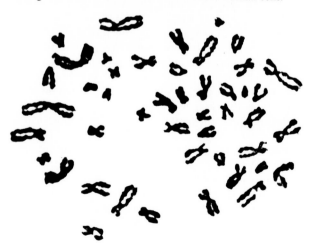

Table 6–2. Sequence of discovery of chromosome aberrations

1959	Trisomy 21; 45,X; 47,XXY
1960	Trisomy 18; trisomy 13
1961	47,XYY
1963	Del 5p
1965	Del 4p
1969	Fragile X
1971	Trisomy 8
1973	Trisomy 9

Table 6-3. Prevalence of chromosomal aberrations among spontaneous abortions

Type aberration	Percent
All chromosome aberrations	40
Trisomies	20
T-16	8
T-13,15,21,22	2[a]
T-2,7,8,14,18	1[a]
T-4,9,10,20	0.5[a]
T-3,5,6,12,17	0.1[a]
T-1,11,19	<0.1[a]
Sex chromosome	<0.5
Monosomy X	8
Autosomal monosomy	<0.1
Polyploidies	9
Triploidy	7
Tetraploidy	2
Other rearrangements	3
Mosaicism	2
Unbalanced rearrangement	1
Balanced rearrangement	<0.5

[a]Approximate rate for each of the trisomies named

through meiosis I of gametogenesis, there occurs an interchange of the genes along homologs through the process of crossing-over. This phenomenon results in the construction of chromosomes with new combinations of parental genes, each a mosaic structure of the two somatic homologs of the parent. Because of the unpaired sex chromosomes in males, the possibility for crossover between the X and Y chromosomes is limited to a small region of homologous sequences on these chromosomes, the so-called pseudoautosomal regions. The chromosomal repertoire thus is limited to replication through mitotic division to form identical daughter cells, reduction division (meiosis) for sexual reproduction, and crossing-over, which provides an almost infinite variety of gene combinations for each generation.

Errors can occur and in fact are commonplace in each of these processes. Nondisjunction or anaphase lag can occur in mitosis or meiosis, resulting in an abnormal chromosome number in daughter cells or gametes.[25,26] Translocation, inversion, deletion, and duplication may occur because of faulty crossing-over and result in imbalanced chromosome complement of gametes.

In at least four circumstances, regions of chromosomes can become altered, rendering the involved region functionally inert. The phenomenon is called "inactivation," involves no change in DNA structure, and is reversed in oogonia prior to meiosis. Inactivation involving most of the X chromosome is a well-documented phenomenon. One X chromosome in normal females and all but one X chromosome in individuals with multiple X chromosomes become inactivated during the 1000–2000 cell stage of embryogenesis. Inactivation appears random; that is, either the maternal or the paternal chromosome can be inactivated, but once this is established it remains fixed for all descendants of all the initially inactivated cell. With the exception of certain small segments of short arm (p) and proximal long arm (q), all of the X chromosome participates in the inactivation

Fig. 6-3. Human female metaphase (left) and karyotype (right). In each, trypsin Giemsa banding is used, and the resolution is 400–500 bands.

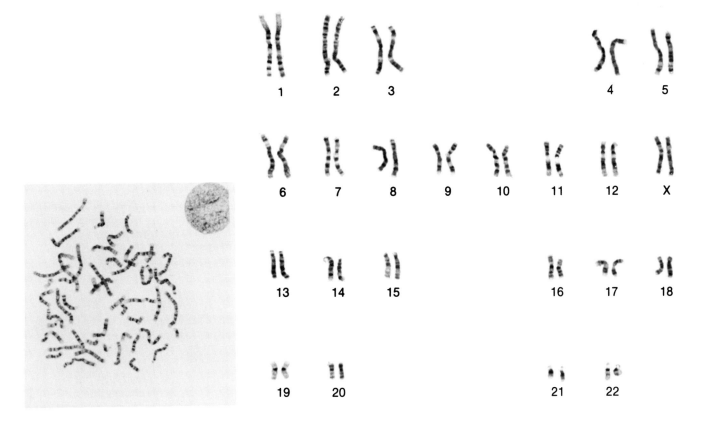

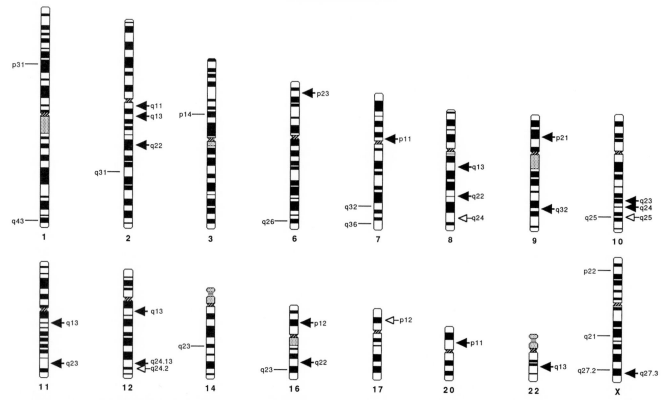

Fig. 6–4. Schematic of human chromosomes showing locations of major heritable fragile sites. Closed arrows indicate folate-sensitive sites, including the fragile X site Xq27.3. Open arrows indicate sites that are induced by bromodeoxyuridine (BrdU) and distamycin A. Bars indicate common constitutive fragile sites that are folate sensitive and induced by aphidicolin. After Jacky.[123]

(Fig. 6–7). Because of this phenomenon, normal females are genetically mosaic, a portion of their cells having one "active" X chromosome and the remaining cells having the alternative X chromosome active. At the molecular level, X chromosome inactivation is thought to be achieved by methylation of DNA. Inactivation of segments of other chromosomes is presumed to be responsible for partitioning of gene activity temporally (genes that are active during embryogenesis may become inactive thereafter) and by cell type (genes that are transcribed in hepatic cells may not be transcribed in muscle cells and vice versa).

Considerable attention has recently been given to the potential of certain genes to be expressed differently depending on whether they were inherited from the mother or the father. This special type of altered gene activity has been called *imprinting*. As with other types of nonpermanent DNA modification, imprinting may involve methylation of DNA, generally persists for life, and may be reversible during gametogenesis.[27–29]

In the end analysis, chromosome changes of consequence cause an imbalance in a number of genes. Assuming equal size of genes and even distribution along the chromosome, the smallest resolvable chromosome change, one band of a 1000 band microscopic preparation, would affect 50–100 genes. Of course genes are not of equal size, and they are not evenly distributed along the chromosomes. Genes appear to be more concentrated in the guanine–cytosine-rich regions of the chromosome, i.e., regions that appear as light bands in giemsa–trypsin preparations.[26] Certain large genes, such as the dystrophin gene, which contains 2300 kb of DNA and spans 2.3 cM of the genome, would occupy most of an av-

erage band.[30] More than 500 small genes the size of β-globin could crowd into a single average band.

Deletion of a representative band would leave the individual with only a single copy (hemizygosity) for 50–100 genes rather than the normal two copies of each (Fig. 6–8). Deleterious recessive characteristics, if present on the normal homolog, could be uncovered and expressed by such a deletion. Phenotype alterations different from those found in the heterozygous state might also accompany the hemizygous state for genes coding for dominant characteristics.

Duplication of a "typical" band would, in effect, cause partial trisomy for 50–100 genes, allowing for a triple dose of each gene within the duplicated band (Fig. 6–9). Three genes for each locus over even such a small region appear to be accommodated no more harmoniously than would three partners in a marriage.

It is possible for all genes on a duplicated chromosome or a duplicated chromosome band to be "normal" and yet cause structural and functional abnormalities. This suggests that quantitative expression of genes may be an important determinant of structure and function. In fact, all of human variability may owe more to variation in quantitative expression at each gene locus than to the quality of the gene expression controlled by its nucleotide sequence. Further augmentation or reduction of gene expression may be produced by inactivation or imprinting of genes, chromosome regions, or entire chromosomes.[27–29]

Chromosome abnormalities of all types exert their influence from conception onward. The possibility that they also influence function and survival of the gametes cannot be dismissed. Chromosome abnormalities of a great variety can

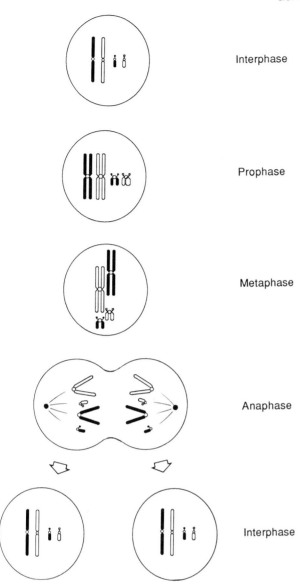

Fig. 6-5. Schematic of mitosis using only 2 of the 23 chromosome pairs. The single chromatin strands replicate in prophase and align along the equatorial plate in metaphase. During anaphase the chromatids of each chromosome migrate to opposite poles (centrosomes). The cell completes its division in telophase, and two daughter chromosomes (interphase) have identical chromosome (DNA) content as the parent cell.

cause substantial disorganization of the conceptus, embryodysgenesis, and fetal pathology. Postnatally, chromosomally abnormal babies that survive such pregnancies have abnormal morphology and mentation, and poor general health.[31,32] Malformations, disturbances in growth, mental impairment, and other features accompany even the most minute change in the chromosomes.

No human population has diverged from the chromosome number of 46 or in the appearance of the 46 chromosomes. There are certain polymorphisms comprising nongenomic repeat sequences that appear in heterochromatic regions of the chromosomes (notably in chromosomes 1, 9, 16, and Y) and the satellites of the acrocentric chromosomes (13–15, 21, and 22). The failure to find any chromosomal difference among the various populations of humans suggests ascent

from common ancestors and along a single evolutionary line. Presumably those who diverted in chromosome number or content from the main line failed to reproduce, bringing that divergence to an end.

Numerical abnormalities

Reproduction in man depends on the production of gametes through the process of reduction division, or meiosis. The number of chromosomes in the primordial cell must be reduced by one-half during maturation of the gametes in the ovary and testis. It is during this process of meiosis that most numerical chromosome abnormalities arise, due mostly to failure of normal disjunction of homologous chromosomes (nondisjunction). When a gamete with other than 23 chromosomes participates in fertilization, the resulting zygote has an abnormal number of chromosomes. The consequence of this is that the pregnancy is usually lost, the conceptus either failing to implant or aborting during the early weeks of formation.[15,16,31–39] With few exceptions, those conceptuses that are maintained are destined to be born with malformations and disturbances of growth and mental function.[31,32]

Nondisjunction can occur in production of either egg or sperm. Meiosis appears to be most susceptible to nondisjunction, but nondisjunction in the numerous mitoses of oogonia and spermatogonia leading to meiosis could result in gametic aneusomy. Furthermore, nondisjunction leading to mosaicism (an individual having cells with both normal and abnormal chromosome numbers) can occur in mitotic cell divisions subsequent to conception.

Through a series of mitoses, the female accumulates a large number of oogonia (6.8 × 10⁶) by the fifth month of fetal life.[40] Prior to birth most oogonia degenerate, but about 2 million progress to the oocyte stage, entering prophase of meiosis I. These oocytes remain suspended in prophase of meiosis I for a variable number of years. Following puberty, the oocytes mature, usually at the rate of one per month, by completing the first meiotic division and entering meiosis II. Completion of meiosis II occurs only after fertilization by a sperm. Nondisjunction can occur at either meiotic division, although the vast majority of nondisjunctions occur in meiosis I of oogenesis.

With the advent of in vitro fertilization programs, small numbers of oocytes have become available for cytogenetic analysis. From these studies, aneuploidy (hypo- or hyperhaploidy) has been found in 4%–30% of oocytes.[41,42]

Spermatogenesis begins in the male at about the same time as oogenesis in the female, that is, during the second month of embryonic life.[40] During fetal life, infancy, and childhood spermatogonia increase in numbers through repeated mitoses. After puberty, a spermatogonial division produces a dark (Ad) spermatogonium that is retained as the parent cell for future mitotic divisions and a pale (Ap) spermatogonium. The pale spermatogonium undergoes two mitoses, forming four spermatocytes, each of which enters meiosis, producing four spermatozoa. The number of mitoses preceding spermatocyte production thus increases with age and ultimately becomes many times greater than the fixed number of mitoses that precedes oocyte formation.

The technique of sperm penetration of hamster eggs has permitted the cytogenetic analysis of human spermatozoa. Numerical chromosome abnormalities have been found in 1%–5% of sperm from normal males.[43–45]

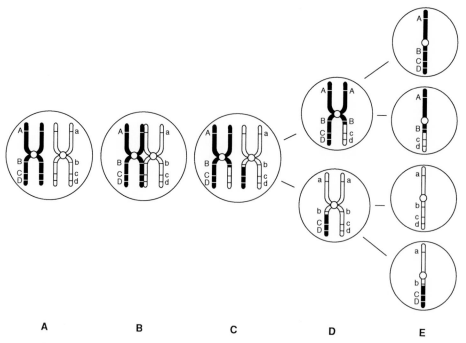

Fig. 6–6. Crossover. A paternal chromosome is shown in black and its maternal homolog in white (A). In preparation for the first cell division in meiosis, pairs of chromosomes come to lie adjacent to each other (B), during which time adjacent chromatids may exchange genetic material (crossover). The chromosomes distributed to daughter cells following the meiosis I division (D) are therefore mosaic chromosomes of the maternal and paternal homologs. These mosaic chromosomes are distributed to gametes (E) at the second meiotic division.

Trisomies

Aneuploidies are tolerated poorly in humans. Most produce such disorganization of the conceptus that implantation cannot be accomplished and maintained. Trisomy for each autosome, except chromosome 1, has been detected in conceptuses (Table 6–3). Trisomy 16 is the most common autosomal trisomy and one with near total loss during pregnancy.[16,46] Certain trisomies (i.e., trisomies 13, 18, and 21) are met with limited tolerance. Although these defects, too, regularly cause abortion, they constitute the most common autosomal trisomies among liveborn infants. Full trisomies for most other autosomes uniformly cause abortions.[16,31,32]

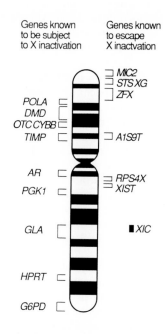

Fig. 6–7. X inactivation. Idiogram showing areas of the X chromosome subject to inactivation (left) and areas that escape inactivation (right). From Hall.[124]

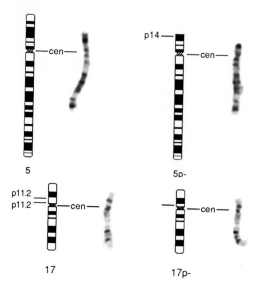

Fig. 6–8. Deletion. Top: idiograms and photomicrographs of a normal chromosome 5 (left) and of a terminal deletion of the short arm of chromosome 5 (right) in a patient with the cri du chat syndrome. Bottom: idiograms and photomicrographs of a normal chromosome 17 (left) and an interstitial deletion of a portion of band p11.2 from the short arm of chromosome 17 (right)

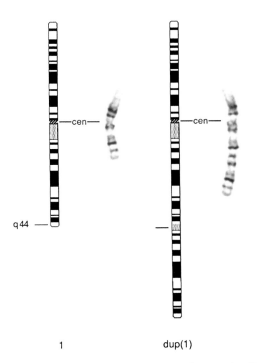

1   dup(1)

Fig. 6–9. Duplication. Idiograms and photomicrographs of normal chromosome 1 (left) and duplication of most of the long arm of chromosome 1 (right). The duplicated region extends from the heterochromatic region (stippled) to the terminal band (q44).

Table 6–4. Prevalence of chromosomal aberrations among liveborn infants

Trisomy 21	1/700
Trisomy 13	1/7000
Trisomy 18	1/8000
Trisomy 8[a]	<1/100,000
Trisomy 9	<1/100,000
Monosomy X	1/2500 (females)
47,XXX	1/1200 (females)
47,XXY	1/1000 (males)
47,XYY	1/1000 (males)
Fragile Xq27.3	1/1200 (males)
48,XXYY	1/25,000 (males)
48,XXXX	<1/100,000 (females)
48,XXXY	<1/100,000 (males)
49,XXXXX	<1/100,000 (females)
49,XXXXY	<1/100,000 (males)

[a]Usually mosaic.

Each autosomal trisomy produces a more or less characteristic pattern of malformations.[31,32]

Extra sex chromosomes are among the most common chromosome abnormalities in liveborn infants (Table 6–4). In general, malformations do not accompany the presence of one or more additional X or Y chromosomes. This is due in part to routine inactivation of all except one X chromosome in each cell and the paucity of active genes located on the Y chromosome. Extra sex chromosomes can produce alterations of growth (XXY, XYY, XXX), habitus (XXY), sexual maturation (XXY), and behavior (XXY, XYY).

Monosomies

Full monosomies for other than the X chromosome do not exist in liveborn infants.[47,48] Autosomal monosomies leave the organism at such risk for hemizygous expression of deleterious genes that they cannot survive the formative and fetal months. Likewise, Y monosomy is lethal in humans since numerous genes on the X chromosome are required for even the rudiments of embryonic development.

In contrast, X monosomy is one of the most common aneuploidies. While highly lethal prenatally (95% of affected conceptuses spontaneously abort), X monosomy has an incidence of 1 in 2500 liveborn females. Affected girls show growth impairment, ovarian dysgenesis with failure of sexual maturation, and anomalies of the skeleton, heart, kidneys, and craniofacies.[31,32,49]

Mosaicism

Numerical chromosome abnormalities can also occur by nondisjunction or anaphase lag subsequent to fertilization, leading to mosaicism.[50] The affected individual has two or more chromosomally different cell lines, all derived from a single zygote. One cell line is usually normal. The timing of the misdivision after fertilization, the lineage of the initiating cell, and the viability of the aberrant cell line(s) determine the proportion and type of tissue(s) affected and the impact. Nondisjunction or anaphase lag occurring during the preimplantation and embryonic period can lead to malformations. Misdivision at a later time would not cause malformations, but could cause a mosaic pattern of skin or hair pigmentation, segmental dyssymmetry, and other growth disturbances.[51] Mosaicism can be demonstrated in a single cell type (e.g., lymphocytes) or may require examination of different tissues. Cultured lymphocytes and skin fibroblasts are generally used for this purpose.[52–55] Mosaicism confined to other tissues cannot be excluded with this approach.

In most cases, mosaicism for numerical chromosome aberrations occurs sporadically and transmission to the next generation is not to be anticipated. Only if the germinal cells (oogonia or spermatogonia) are affected with the aneuploidy would there be risk of full aneuploidy in the offspring. Juberg et al.[55] have suggested that a predisposition to anaphase lag may explain the recurrence of chromosomal mosaicism within a family.

Mosaicism arising during the first few days after fertilization may affect the embryo, the extraembryonic tissues, or both. This phenomenon complicates the use of extraembryonic tissues such as chorionic villi for prenatal diagnosis and may explain survival of fetuses with certain severe trisomies. Kalousek et al.[56] have demonstrated that trisomy 13 and trisomy 18 fetuses who survive pregnancy have placentas that are euploid, at least in part. Alternatively, aneuploidy confined to the placenta may explain growth retardation or spontaneous abortion of chromosomally normal fetuses.[57,58]

Structural abnormalities

Structural abnormalities presumably arise during meiosis through abnormal pairing of homologous sequences and interchange of genetic material between chromosomes or between parts of the same chromosome. The same mechanism may underlie all types of structural rearrangements: translocations, deletions, duplications, inversions, and insertions. Certain structural rearrangements may remain balanced and nondisruptive, that is, resulting in no total loss or gain of genetic material, occurring between genes, and failing to interrupt the regulatory sequences of adjacent genes. In this circumstance no phenotypic consequence results from the rearrangement. Carriers of balanced rearrangements, however, have a 50% probability of producing unbalanced gametes.

Other chromosome rearrangements are balanced but disruptive. A rearrangement of this type bisects a gene, preventing transcription, or disturbs the gene's regulatory sequence and may be accompanied by phenotypic consequences.

Unbalanced rearrangements result in a loss or a gain of chromosome material, or both. They can occur de novo or can result from unbalanced segregation of a balanced rearrangement in one of the parents.

Deletion

A deletion is the loss of a portion of a chromosome (Fig. 6–8). Deletions can affect a single gene, being submicroscopic and requiring molecular techniques for detection, or may be large enough to be seen under the microscope.[21–24,59,60] Deletion of a region of a chromosome has the same effect as monosomy. It leaves the involved region of the chromosome unpaired, a situation permitting deleterious genes to be expressed with no possibility of compensation by the missing allele.

A ring chromosome is formed by fusion of the two ends of a chromosome after deletion of the two telomeres and variable segments of juxtatelomeric genes (Fig. 6–10). Ring chromosomes are unstable, can vary considerably in size in different cells, and tend to be lost during cell division, leading to mosaicism.[61] Phenotypic consequences are quite variable, depending on the genetic material deleted. It is unusual for ring chromosomes to persist for more than one generation.

Duplication

A portion of a chromosome can become duplicated by unequal crossover involving a normal chromosome, by a crossover between the breakpoints of a pericentric inversion, or by unbalanced segregation of a translocation (Fig. 6–9).[62,63] Trisomy for the duplicated region of the chromosome results in phenotypic changes.

Translocation

Several types of translocations occur in which chromosome material is interchanged between two chromosomes or transferred from one chromosome to another.[64–67] Robertsonian translocations, the most common type, involve only the acrocentric chromosomes (13–15, 21, and 22) and arise by fu-

Fig. 6–10. Ring chromosome. Idiograms and photomicrographs of normal chromosome 22 (left) and a ring chromosome 22 (right). The satellites and the telomere of 22q have been lost.

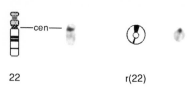

22   r(22)

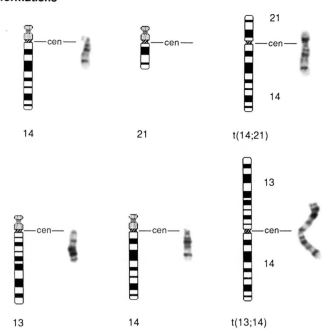

Fig. 6–11. Robertsonian translocation. Top: idiograms and photomicrographs of normal chromosomes 14 and 21 (left and middle) and a Robertsonian (centromeric) translocation involving chromosomes 14 and 21 (right). The combined chromosome retains all the active genes on chromosomes 14 and 21. The short arms are genetically inactive and presumed to be lost from most cells. Balanced translocation carriers have the combined chromosome in addition to one normal 14 chromosome and one normal 21 chromosome. A small percentage of patients with Down syndrome have the combined chromosome in addition to one normal 14 and two normal 21 chromosomes. Bottom: idiograms and photomicrographs of normal chromosomes 13 and 14 (left and middle) and a Robertsonian translocation involving these two chromosomes. This is the most common translocation in humans.

sion of two chromosomes at the centromere, forming a single composite (compound) chromosome (Fig. 6–11).[64] Residual fragments of the short arms of the two chromosomes are lost in subsequent divisions. Loss of the short arms, known to contain redundant ribosomal RNA genes, does not appear to influence health. Carriers of Robertsonian translocations between homologous acrocentric chromosomes produce only abnormal gametes, either containing the compound chromosome or missing one acrocentric altogether. Resulting pregnancies are trisomic or monosomic. Carriers of Robertsonian translocations between different acrocentric chromosomes produce normal gametes (25%), gametes lacking the homolog of one of the acrocentrics involved in the translocation (25%), gametes having the translocation (25%), or gametes that have the translocation plus the homolog of one of the acrocentrics involved (25%). Theoretically, an offspring has an equal chance of being a normal, balanced carrier, trisomic, or monosomic. Empirical observations document the risk for trisomy in offspring to be less than 25% and to differ depending on whether the mother or father is the translocation carrier.[68] The risk for Down syndrome among offspring of mothers with balanced 14;21 translocations is 15%. When the father has a balanced 14;21 translocation, the risk decreases to 2%–3%. Monosomy 14 and monosomy 21 fetuses are uniformly lost to spontaneous abortion.

Reciprocal translocations involve exchange of material be-

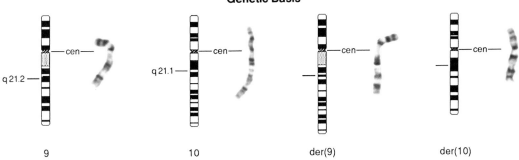

9   10   der(9)   der(10)

Fig. 6–12. Reciprocal translocation. Idiograms and photomicrographs of normal 9 and 10 chromosomes (left and left center) and the derivative 9 and 10 chromosomes formed by reciprocal trans-location between the two chromosomes at breakpoints 9q21.2 and 10q21.1 (right center and right).

tween two chromosomes, resulting in the formation of two abnormal composite (compound) chromosomes (Fig. 6–12).[65] Balanced and nondisruptive translocations cause no phenotypic effects. One-half of the gametes produced by carriers of a balanced reciprocal translocation will be unbalanced.

An insertion is a rare type of nonreciprocal translocation in which a segment of a donor chromosome is inserted into a nonhomologous chromosome.[66] In the process, the donor chromosome becomes deleted. The phenomenon requires three breakpoints, one in the recipient chromosome and two in the donor. As with other translocations involving nonhomologous chromosomes, this rearrangement can lead to abnormal gametes depending on the segregation of the two chromosomes involved and their homologs.

Inversion

In pericentric inversions, a chromosome has breakpoints on both arms, with reversal of the intervening centromeric segment (Fig. 6–13). When balanced and nondisruptive, the rearrangement is benign.[69,70] During meiosis I the inverted chromosome is required to form a loop in order to pair with its noninverted homolog. If an uneven number of crossovers occurs within the loop, the gamete will be unbalanced, hav-

ing one part of the chromosome duplicated and another part deleted. Gametes formed with the duplication–deletion chromosomes are unbalanced. Theoretically, one-half of gametes formed by a parent with a pericentric inversion will be unbalanced if crossing-over occurs in the inverted segment.

In paracentric inversions, a segment of genes on one arm of a chromosome is reversed.[71,72] In the absence of a bisected gene or disrupted regulation of adjacent genes, this rearrangement is benign. As with pericentric inversions, paracentric inversions must form a loop in order for pairing of sequences along the inverted segment during meiosis. An unequal number of crossovers during this pairing can produce two different types of duplication–deletion chromosomes, one of which is acentric and one dicentric. Theoretically, one-half of the gametes produced by a carrier of a balanced paracentric inversion would be unbalanced, having one of these two duplication–deletion chromosomes if crossing-over occurred in the inverted segment.

Isochromosomes

Cleavage of the centromere perpendicular to the plane of usual cleavage results in isochromosome formation (Fig. 6–14). This misdivision occurs at metaphase (meiosis or mitosis), leaving the anaphase chromosome with two long arm (q) chromatids or two short arm (p) chromatids rather than one of each. The resulting isochromosome has two identical arms

Fig. 6–13. Pericentric inversion. Idiograms and photomicrographs of normal chromosome 2 (left) and pericentric inversion involving the segment p11 to q13 of chromosome 2 (right). The resulting inversion chromosome 2 has reduced short arm length and increased long arm length.

Fig. 6–14. Isochromosome. Idiograms and photomicrographs of normal X chromosome (left) and an isochromosome for the long arms of the X chromosome (right). The original chromosome is presumed to have divided horizontally rather than longitudinally, resulting in a long arm isochromosome shown here and a short arm isochromosome lost from this cell line.

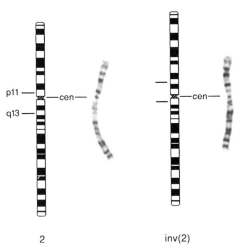

2   inv(2)

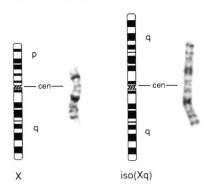

X   iso(Xq)

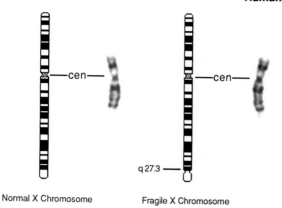

Normal X Chromosome   Fragile X Chromosome

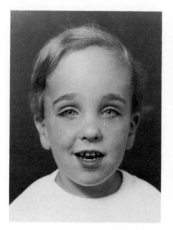 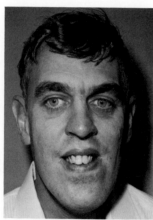

Fig. 6–15. Fragile X chromosome. Idiograms and photomicrographs of normal X chromosome (top left) and fragile site at q27.3 of the X chromosome (top right). Photographs show facial features of males with the fragile X syndrome. Child at age 3 years (bottom left) shows prominent forehead but little other distinctive facial changes. In adulthood (age 37 years; bottom right) the typical facies with long face, prominent forehead, large ears, and large lower jaw is apparent.

and functionally represents duplication of one arm of the chromosome and deletion of the other. Autosomal isochromosomes are unusual, but Xq isochromosomes occur not infrequently.[73,74]

Fragile sites

Heritable regions of chromosomes that show a tendency to separation, breakage, or attenuation under certain cell conditions have been termed "fragile sites."[75] Numerous fragile sites have been identified (see Fig. 6–4). Fragile sites give variable appearance under the microscope and are enhanced by folate or thymidine depletion of the culture media or by the addition of 5-fluoro-2′-deoxy-β-uridine or folate antagonists. Only the fragile site located at q27.3 of the X chromosome has been associated with human dysmorphism and mental retardation, the so-called fragile X syndrome (Fig. 6–15).

Other chromosome aberrations

Breakage and rearrangement of chromosomes occur in a small group of autosomal recessive disorders. The number of breaks can be increased over the spontaneous number found in cell cultures by exposure to radiation, mitomycin-C, or diepoxybutane.[76,77] Chromatid breaks are typically found in Fanconi anemia; breaks, triradial and quadriradial associations between chromosomes, and sister chromatid exchanges in Bloom syndrome; breaks and nonrandom rearrangements of chromosomes 7 and 14 in ataxia-telangiectasia; and breaks in progeria and Werner syndrome. Whether the growth impairment, malformations, and other dysmorphic features in these conditions can be attributed to the influence of these chromosomal changes during development or represent pleiotropic effects of the underlying mutation is not known.

Centromere separations (chromosome puffs), primarily involving the acrocentric chromosomes and chromosomes 1, 9, and 16, have been found in numerous patients with the Roberts syndrome (SC phocomelia).[78] The centromeric constriction of these chromosomes is lost, and two distinct centromeres in alignment with the two chromatids can be demonstrated with C-banding (Fig. 6–16). Although centromere separation has been noted in normal individuals, those with a variety of hematologic disorders, and in aging women, it is a useful marker to distinguish Roberts syndrome from other limb reduction syndromes.

Uniparental disomy

Normally one of each pair of chromosomes derives from each parent. When both chromosomes derive from one parent (uniparental disomy), the offspring can be affected with dysmorphic features, growth disturbance, and mental impairment. The mechanism underlying these phenotypic changes is not known, but it appears possible that the maternal and paternal chromosomes are modified (imprinted) differently during gametogenesis and that each is necessary for normal growth and development.[27]

Heterodisomy exists when the homologous chromosomes are different but both inherited from one parent. In isodisomy, both members of a chromosome pair are identical and the individual is homozygous for all genes on the chromosome involved. Both types of uniparental disomy have been identified in humans. Maternal disomy has been found in 10%–25% of individuals with Prader-Willi syndrome and paternal disomy in 3%–4% of individuals with Angelman syndrome.[29,79] Uniparental disomy has also been documented in Beckwith-Wiedemann syndrome and in individuals with short stature, mental retardation, and multiple anomalies.[80,81] It is anticipated that other sporadically occurring syndromes (e.g. Williams, Russell-Silver, Sotos, Rubinstein-Taybi, de Lange) may be caused by uniparental disomy.

Role of genes in human anomalies

Genes are the physical units of heredity by which characteristics are transmitted from generation to generation in all living organisms. They are the functional units under whose instructions all metabolism is activated and structure formed. Genes constitute the primary elements of the chromosomes along the length of which they are irregularly distributed.

An understanding of the function of genes preceded knowledge of the physical nature of genes. To Gregor Men-

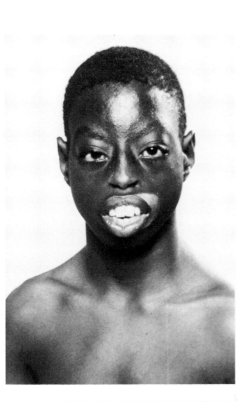
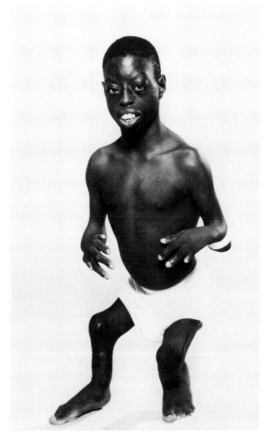
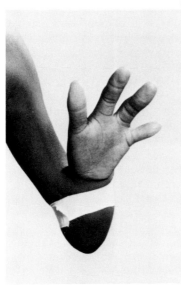
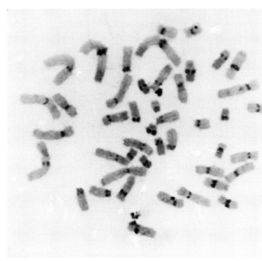

Fig. 6–16. Roberts syndrome patient showing limb reduction defects and premature separation of the centromere in metaphase chromosome preparation. Courtesy Dr. G. S. Pai, Medical University of South Carolina, Charleston.

del, an Augustinian monk from Moravia (present-day Czechoslovakia), must go credit for discovery of the principles of heredity.[82] Working with *Pisum* hybrids, Mendel found that hereditary characters were transmitted as units that retained their integrity generation to generation, even when their expression was masked by another character. Those characters expressed in the hybrid (heterozygote) he called *dominant* and those whose expression could be masked in the hybrid *recessive.*

Those characters which are transmitted entire, or almost unchanged in the hybridization, and therefore in themselves constitute the characters of the hybrid, are termed *dominant,* and those which become latent in the process, *recessive.* The expression "recessive" has been chosen because the characteristics thereby designated withdraw or entirely disappear in the hybrids, but nevertheless reappear in their progeny.

On this basis Mendel could predict the behavior of selected characteristics generation to generation and express the pre-

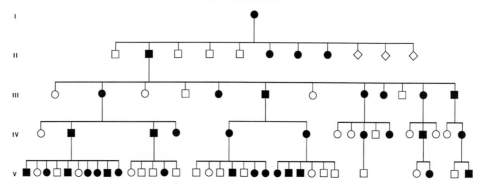

Fig. 6-17. Pedigree of brachydactyly transmitted as an autosomal dominant trait published by Farabee in 1905. This trait was the first recognized to demonstrate that the laws of Mendel applied to humans as well as to plants and the lower animals.

dictions in mathematical terms. His findings were contrary to the prevailing view that hereditary characteristics were blended in each new generation, and his work went unnoticed by the scientific community for 30 years.[83-85]

Shortly after 1900, examples of Mendel's dominant and recessive inheritance were suggested as the basis for human disorders. Farabee[86] attributed the malformation brachydactyly, found in five generations of a Pennsylvania family, to a dominant hereditary factor (Fig. 6-17). At the same time, Garrod[87,88] described three inborn errors of metabolism, alkaptonuria, cystinuria, and albinism, and on the advice of Bateson indicated that they could be caused by rare recessive factors. He further believed that these conditions and a fourth, pentosuria, which he added later, resulted from blocks in normal enzyme activities, anticipating the relationship between genes and enzymes that would be elucidated some 40 years later.

In 1911, Johannsen[89] suggested the term *gene* be used for a hypothetical unit of heredity, acknowledging that no structure or specific mechanism of action for the unit could at the time be assigned. He also used the terms *phenotype* to indicate the features caused by a gene and *genotype* for the gene basis for a given phenotype.

That genes controlled cell biology by acting as enzymes or regulating enzymes was concluded by Beadle and Tatum[90] on the basis of studies on the nutritional requirements of *Drosophila* and *Neurospora*. Their one gene–one enzyme concept forms the crux of current understanding of gene function. Some revision of the concept has occurred: initially to one gene–one protein to include gene control over production of enzymatic and nonenzymatic proteins, then to one gene–one polypeptide to accommodate the fact that complex proteins can be assembled from gene products of more than one gene, and finally to one cistron–one polypeptide to indicate the DNA actually transcribed into a polypeptide sequence.

Specialists in metabolism, endocrinologists, clinical geneticists, and dysmorphologists generally focus their studies on the functional and structural consequences of mutant genes. Such genes underly no small portion of human dysmorphology and impaired function. They constitute all entries in McKusick's *Mendelian Inheritance in Man*[91] and 63% of the entries in Jones' *Smith's Recognizable Patterns of Human Malformations.*[92]

Defining the structure of the gene involved the efforts of numerous investigators using a variety of experimental organisms, work that has pervaded the twentieth century. The first insights into the physical nature of the gene came early in the century from observations on meiosis in the great "Lubber" grasshopper, *Brachystola*, by Sutton[93] and on mutants of *Drosophila* by Morgan and associates[94,95] of Columbia University's famed "fly room." They placed the units responsible for individual hereditary characteristics on the chromosomes and determined that such units were numerous, were distributed in linear fashion along the chromosomes, and could be exchanged between homologous chromosomes by the process of crossing-over during meiosis. Contrary to the long-held suspicion that genes were proteins, the chemical composition of genes turned out to be deoxyribonucleic acid (DNA) as determined by Avery et al.[96] Watson and Crick[97] demonstrated that the configuration of DNA was a double-helical structure in which nucleotide pairs were linked together by an external sugar–phosphate backbone (Fig. 6-18).

Yet to be explained was how the structure of the gene correlated with its function. How was DNA coded for protein structure, and how was this information conveyed to the synthetic processes of the cell? At midcentury, Dounce[98] set forth the idea that a second nucleic acid, ribonucleic acid (RNA), could serve as a template for protein synthesis and that the amino acid sequence of the protein could be determined by the nucleotide sequence of the RNA. This intermediary role for RNA was later confirmed. The code problem was resolved by Nirenberg and Matthaei[99] who determined that the amino acid sequence of protein was indeed dictated by the nucleotide sequence of DNA, a sequence of three particular nucleotides specifying one amino acid.

Molecular techniques developed during the past two decades continue to provide a rich yield of information about gene structure.[100-102] Individual genes have been isolated, cloned, and sequenced. Genes have been shown to vary remarkably in size, to be configured of variable numbers of translated sequences (exons) separated by noncoding intervening sequences (introns), and to be closely flanked by regulatory sequences at the upstream (5') and downstream (3') ends (Fig. 6-19). Messenger RNA, formed of exons spliced together after the introns have been removed from precursor nuclear RNA (Hn RNA), provides the template for polypeptide assembly.

It has been estimated that humans may have as many as 50,000–100,000 gene pairs distributed along the 46 chromosomes.[91] For the most part, genes have come to light only

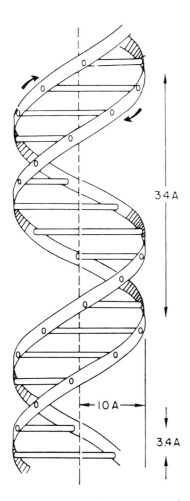

Fig. 6–18. Double-stranded helical structure of DNA as determined by Watson and Crick. Nucleotide pairs (horizontal bars) are spaced along the helix every 3.4 Å and each turn of the helix (34 Å) contains 10 nucleotide pairs.

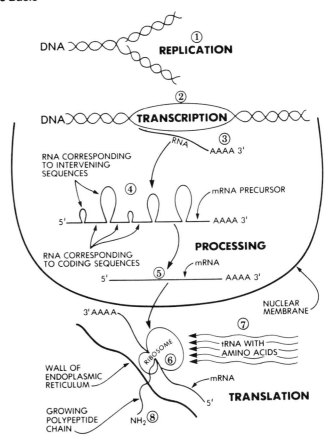

Fig. 6–19. The repertoire of DNA in somatic cells is shown in this schematic. Through the process of replication (1), DNA duplicates itself prior to cell division so that identical genetic information can be transmitted to daughter cells. Through the processes of transcription, RNA processing, and translation (2–8) the genetic information is utilized within the cell to synthesize polypeptides or proteins. Reprinted with permission from Miller WL: J Pediatr 99:1, 1981.[125]

if they produce some distinctive change—morphologic or functional—within an individual. Other than acknowledging the existence of the gene that causes such a distinctive phenotype, little more can be said about most genes. The exact functions of relatively few genes have been determined, and even fewer genes have been sequenced. With the advent of large-scale mapping and sequencing projects, this situation will rapidly change.[103,104] Extensive characterization of a gene and its chromosomal location, sequence, and gene product may be accomplished before a link between the gene and the human phenotype is recognized.

McKusick lists 4397 gene loci in the ninth edition of *Mendelian Inheritance in Man,* representing only 4%–8% of the human genome.[91] Virtually all of these loci were ascertained through the recurrence of phenotypic alterations within families. 2325 genes have been mapped to a regional or specific position on one of the chromosomes (Human Gene Mapping 11).[105] The X chromosome is most heavily mapped, containing 221 loci as of this writing. The list of genes and gene localizations grows weekly. Complete mapping and sequencing of the human genome by the year 2005 is the goal of the human genome project.[103,104]

1616 gene loci, 33% of the total loci identified in *Mende-*

lian Inheritance in Man, are linked to malformations or morphologic features.[91] Since gene ascertainment has depended predominantly on phenotype, it might be anticipated that a significant portion of genes associated with human dysmorphism have already been identified. Regarding these genes, the tasks ahead include localizing the genes on the chromosomes, determining their structure, identifying the gene products, and determining how they cause phenotypic alteration. As yet, no gene that produces malformations in man has been thus characterized.

Chromosome rearrangements and linkage analyses have allowed a number of genes that cause human anomalies to be localized on various chromosomes.[106–108] Table 14–6 lists the localizations that are currently known and gives the chromosome locations of other genes that are related to human morphology.

Mutations are alterations in the structure or regulatory apparatus of a normal gene. They result in altered amino acid sequences in the polypeptide gene product or in the amount of polypeptide produced. For each gene, the number of possible mutations is great. Many, perhaps most, do not cause phenotypic effects and exist as innocuous molecular polymorphisms in the population. Other mutations interfere

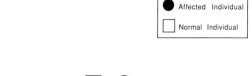

with normal biologic processes sufficiently to prevent survival of the organism. Intermediate between these extremes are mutations that produce nonlethal changes in the phenotype. These constitute the single gene disorders that provide diagnostic and research challenges for the dysmorphologists and clinical geneticists.

Most genes exist in pairs, or alleles, one located on each member of a pair of homologous chromosomes. The exceptions occur in males in whom most genes on the X and Y chromosomes are unpaired, or hemizygous. Unless inactivated by one of the mechanisms described above, all genes are expressed within the metabolic machinery of the cell. This metabolic expression, however, may not be reflected in discernible features (phenotype) of the individual. For this reason, the terms *recessive* and *dominant* are useful in the clinical setting to describe the phenotypic consequences of gene mutations. In the strict sense, use of these terms in reference to genes may be considered inappropriate, since expression can be equally evident at the cellular level for genes that produce no phenotypic changes as for those that produce dramatic change. However technically incorrect, common usage permits one to speak of recessive or dominant genes and gene mutations.

Dominant phenotypes

Phenotypic changes produced by a single dose of a given gene are termed *dominant,* or, as noted above, the terms *dominant genes* and *dominant mutations* are commonly used to characterize genes that can produce phenotypic manifestations when present in a single dose. To date, dominant phenotypes outnumber recessive phenotypes, a finding likely related to easier ascertainment of the former.[88] There is no a priori reason to suspect that the mutations leading to dominant phenotypes occur more frequently than those leading to recessive phenotypes, and work with experimental animals and plants indicates that most mutations are recessive (require a double dose for manifestation).

It is anticipated that mutations leading to dominant phenotypes will in most cases affect genes coded for structural proteins. Examples include mutations of collagen genes resulting in Stickler syndrome and osteogenesis imperfecta.[108,109] Mutation of a single gene controls the amount or structure of 50% of the gene product produced, which in the case of structural protein can be sufficient to cause phenotypic changes. For this reason, these mutations are good candidates to cause structural abnormalities during embryogenesis.

The study of rare pathologic phenotypes in the population allows certain generalizations about the mode of inheritance to be made. The implications of dominant phenotypes differ depending on whether the responsible gene is located on an autosome or on the X chromosome (Figs. 6–20, 6–21). Characteristics common in autosomal dominant phenotypes include the following.

1. Males and females are affected in equal proportions.
2. Male to male inheritance does occur.
3. Only one parent is usually affected.
4. Each offspring of an affected parent has a 50% risk of being affected.
5. Normal children of an affected parent will not transmit the condition to their children.

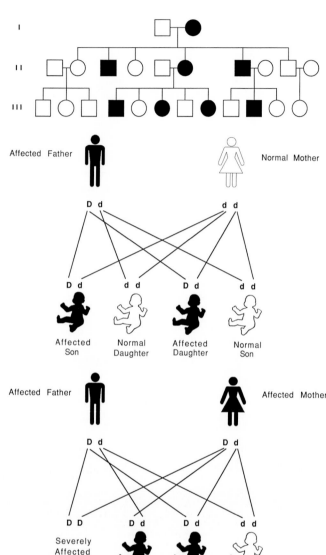

Fig. 6–20. Autosomal dominant inheritance. Top: pedigree showing autosomal dominant inheritance. Note that males and females are affected and that male to male transmission occurs. Middle: segregation of an autosomal dominant trait when one parent is affected. Each child, male or female, has a 50% chance of being affected. Bottom: segregation of an autosomal dominant trait when both parents are affected. Each child has a 50% chance of being affected (receiving the trait from one or the other parent), a 25% chance of being normal, and a 25% chance of being severely affected (receiving trait from both parents).

Characteristics common in X-linked dominant phenotypes include the following.

1. Males and females are affected in a 1:2 ratio.
2. Male to male inheritance does not occur.

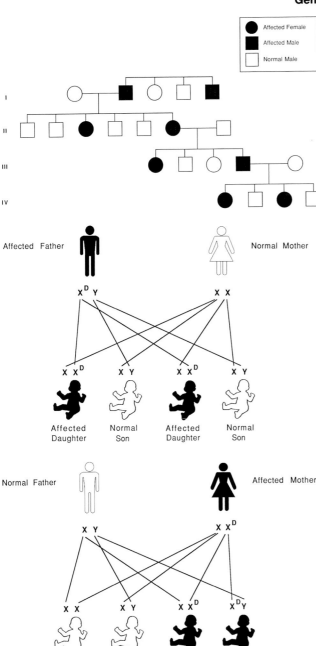

Pleiotropy

The mutation of a single gene can produce multiple effects (pleiotropism) in the phenotype. These effects may appear unrelated, but in some cases the underlying metabolism or the developmental process by which the features arise during embryogenesis provides an explanation for the pleiotropism. In other cases the explanations remain obscure.

Genetic heterogeneity

Identical or similar phenotypic disturbances can be caused by different gene mutations or chromosome imbalances. When genetically determined phenotypes mimic each other they are termed *genocopies* (e.g., Marfan syndrome and homocystinuria). Environmentally caused mimics of a genetically determined phenotype can occur as well and are termed *phenocopies* (e.g., the limb malformation condition produced by thalidomide exposure during pregnancy is a phenocopy of the genetic entity SC phocomelia). For this reason, precise ascertainment of the cause of a given phenotypic change is fundamental to accurate counseling and rational preventive efforts.

Penetrance

The frequency with which evidence of a mutant gene can be found in the phenotype is called *penetrance*. Usually used in reference to dominant phenotypes, *full* or *complete* penetrance describes phenotypic effects found in every individual possessing a given gene mutation. *Incomplete* or *reduced* penetrance occurs when some proportion of persons possessing a gene mutation show no phenotypic effect.

Expressivity

Expressivity indicates the degree to which a mutant gene is manifest in the phenotype. Some degree of variable expressivity can be expected in most phenotypes depending in part on the influence of other genes, various types of inactivation, and environmental forces.

Recessive phenotypes

Phenotypes that require a double dose of a given gene are termed *recessive*. The abnormal gene product is usually an enzyme or transport protein. In the individual homozygous for these mutations, the structure of all of the gene product or the quantity produced is affected by the mutation. Individuals having only one mutant gene are called *carriers* or *heterozygotes,* have 50% of their gene product affected by the mutation, and generally exhibit no phenotypic consequences. Because of the nature of the gene product affected by these mutations, the recessive phenotypes are often metabolic disturbances that impair function rather than morphology. Morphologic changes, if they occur, usually develop after embryogenesis or even postnatally. Exceptions to this generalization, e.g., extra digits in Carpenter syndrome, radial aplasia in Fanconi pancytopenia syndrome, and marked prenatal growth impairment in achondrogenesis, are readily called to mind.

Fig. 6-21. X-linked dominant inheritance. Top: pedigree showing X-linked dominant inheritance. Note males and females are affected, but male to male transmission does not occur. Middle: segregation of X-linked dominant trait when the father is affected. All daughters are affected, and all sons are normal. Right: segregation of X-linked dominant trait when the mother is affected. Each son or daughter has a 50% risk of being normal and a 50% risk of being affected.

3. Affected males transmit the phenotype to all of their daughters.
4. Offspring of affected females have a 50% risk of being affected whether male or female.
5. Only one parent is usually affected.
6. Heterozygous females are affected less severely than are hemizygous males.

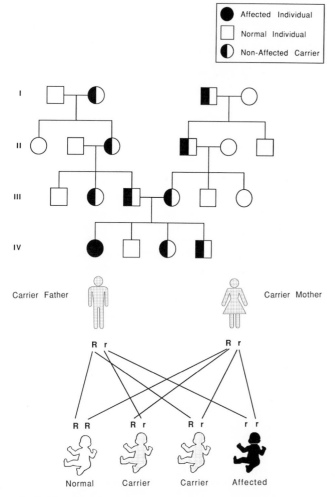

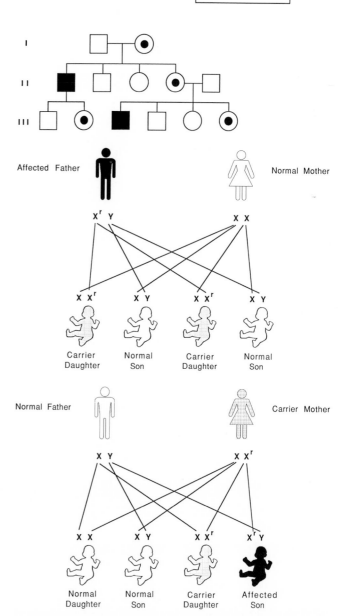

Fig. 6–22. Autosomal recessive inheritance. Top: pedigree showing autosomal recessive inheritance. Note that both parents must be carriers, and the affected offspring may be male or female. Bottom: segregation of autosomal recessive trait in offspring when both parents are carriers. Each offspring has a 25% risk of being normal noncarrier, a 50% risk of being a carrier, and a 25% risk of being affected (inheriting the trait from both parents).

Implications of recessive phenotypes also depend on whether the responsible gene is located on an autosomal or a sex chromosome (Figs. 6–22, 6–23). Characteristics of autosomal recessive phenotypes include the following.

1. Males and females are affected in equal proportions.
2. Both parents must be carriers of a single copy of the responsible gene in order for a child to be affected.
3. Parents (heterozygous carriers) are usually normal.
4. Each child of carrier parents has
   a. A 25% risk of being affected.
   b. A 50% risk of being a carrier.
   c. A 25% risk of being a nonaffected noncarrier.
5. The rarer the mutant gene is in the population, the greater the likelihood that parents of affected children will be consanguineous.

A single gene spans a long segment of DNA, and alterations (mutations) can occur virtually anywhere along its length. Many different mutations exist in the population for most genes. This being the case, it is to be expected that some

Fig. 6–23. X-linked recessive inheritance: Top: pedigree of X-linked recessive inheritance. Note that males can be affected in multiple generations and that they inherit the X-linked trait from their mothers. Middle: segregation of X-linked recessive trait when the father is affected. All daughters are carriers, and all sons are normal noncarriers. Bottom: segregation of X-linked trait when the mother is a carrier. Each son has a 50% risk of being affected and each daughter a 50% risk of being a carrier.

recessive phenotypes result from two different mutations of the same gene rather than homozygosity for a single mutation. Hemoglobin SC disease is a well-recognized example. This phenomenon, termed *compound heterozygosity*, may be responsible for much of the variability present in recessive phenotypes. Only in cases of parental consanguinity can one be reasonably certain of homozygosity at the gene level.

Conditions caused by genes on the X chromosome exhibit distinctly different pedigrees from conditions caused by autosomal genes. The differences are determined primarily by the presence of a single X chromosome in males and two X chromosomes in females and by the obligatory transfer of the male's single X chromosome to all daughters but not to sons. Characteristics of X-linked recessive phenotypes include the following.

1. Only males are affected.
2. Sons of carrier females have a 50% risk of being affected.
3. Daughters of carrier females have a 50% risk of being carriers.
4. Male to male transmission does not occur.
5. All daughters of affected males will be carriers.
6. Unaffected males cannot transmit the phenotype.

Carrier detection using metabolic parameters or molecular techniques (linkage or gene analysis) has become possible for many autosomal and X-linked recessive phenotypes. Such testing will become increasingly important in the prevention of birth defects and functional impairments.

Mosaicism

When mutations occur after fertilization of an egg, a mosaic condition results in which the lineage of one cell harbors the mutation and one cell line remains normal.[110] Depending on the type of gene affected, on the timing of the mutation, and on the lineage and viability of the cells bearing the mutation, phenotypic disturbances of various magnitudes can result. Certain conditions of unknown causation have been identified as candidates for single gene mosaicism, primarily because of the clonal or segmental nature of their phenotypic changes. Among these are Proteus syndrome, various pigmentary disturbances, McCune-Albright syndrome, Klippel-Trenaunay-Weber syndrome, and tumors.

Germinal mosaicism describes the presence of a mutant germ line that is not found in the individual's somatic cells. Although rarely documented, this phenomenon may explain the occurrence of several offspring affected with a dominant phenotype born of normal parents. Such has been suspected in some cases of achondroplasia and has been demonstrated by molecular techniques in the case of osteogenesis imperfecta.[111]

Alteration of a single gene can have a profound phenotypic effect, indeed as great as adding or deleting an entire chromosome. The effect of a mutation, while limited to a single metabolic reaction (at the cellular level), can shape the entire individual. The power of such mutations to malform if expressed during embryogenesis or to otherwise disturb morphology if expressed later is not ordinarily offset by other genes or by the environment; i.e., the penetrance of such abnormal genes is often very high.

Polygenic phenotypes

Although no example of a polygenic phenotype related to human anomalies can be given, it must be surmised that in some cases mutations of more than one gene may collaborate to produce phenotypic changes. Fingerprint patterns appear to be determined polygenically.[112,113] It is most appropriate to consider polygenic inheritance in its role as the genetic component of multifactorial causation (see Multifactorial causation of human anomalies, below).

Contiguous gene phenotypes

Local groupings of separate genes that can be simultaneously affected by microdeletions and possibly by mutations have been termed *contiguous gene complexes.*[21-24] The phenomenon, also termed *segmental aneusomy,* has been helpful in localizing genes to a specific chromosomal region and in determining their order. It provides a basis for phenotypic variability that might otherwise be attributed to variable expressivity or pleiotropism of a single gene. The phenotypes produced may have diverse components, each of which may be caused by alteration of a separate gene. Alternatively, mutations can occur independently in any single gene in a contiguous gene complex without disturbing adjacent genes.

Multifactorial (bifactorial) causation of human anomalies

At the interface of genetic etiology and environmental etiology is multifactorial (bifactorial) causation, which requires the combined influences of both. Hereditary and environmental factors collaborate to cause certain malformations, other morphologic characteristics, and functional disabilities. Implicit in the multifactorial concept is the notion that the individual genetic or environmental factors involved lack the power to produce an abnormal phenotype but that multiple factors, heritable and environmental, can do so through their additive influence.[114-116] By definition, if genes from two or more loci participate, the genetic component is polygenic.

Multifactorial causation is broadly accepted, the evidence for it based on the recurrence risks for certain phenotypes within a family being greater than that for the general population but significantly lower than Mendelian expectation, the high but incomplete concordance in monozygotic twins, and the significantly lower but not negligible concordance in dizygotic twins. No example can be given, however, in which the genetic components and the environmental components have been elucidated. Multifactorial causation is considered responsible for phenotypes found in the extremes of continuous morphologic variation and for phenotypes found only beyond a developmental threshold.

Continuous traits

Human characteristics that vary by measurable increments across a broad spectrum are called *continuous traits.* Morphologic features included among the continuous traits are head circumference, height, and interpupillary measurement. No abrupt change separates normal from abnormal (Fig. 6-24). Abnormalities of these characteristics are arbitrarily defined as those variations that fall beyond 2 SD in ei-

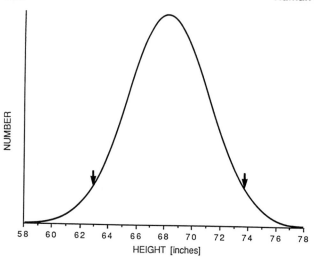

Fig. 6–24. Distribution curve for height, a trait with continuous variation; 95% of individuals will have measurements between the two arrows (mean ± 2 SD).

ther direction from the mean for a given population. Hence macrocephaly can be defined as head circumference or volume greater than 2 SD above the mean, microcephaly as head circumference or volume less than 2 SD below the mean, short stature as height less than 2 SD below the mean, and so forth. It should be cautioned that phenotypes defined as abnormal in this system should not be considered absolute, fixed for all time and all populations.[117] Rather, they should be considered abnormal only for a given subpopulation and at a given point in time.

Threshold traits

Traits that do not vary continuously but appear only above a given threshold are called *discontinuous* or *threshold* traits. Several of the more common human malformations, notably neural tube defects and cleft lip and palate, are included among these traits (Table 6–5).

Characteristics that can be expected in multifactorial causation are as follows.

1. Males and females are affected but often with unequal frequencies.

Table 6–5. Incidence of selected malformations which often have multifactorial causation

Malformation	Incidence per 10,000 births
Neural tube defects	
Anencephaly	5
Spina bifida	5
Encephalocele	1
Cleft lip/palate	10
Congenital dislocation of the hip	10
Club foot	12
Pyloric stenosis	30
Cardiac defects	70

2. There is an increased risk for recurrence in first-, second-, and third-degree relatives of an index case: 2%–5% for first-degree relatives, about one-fourth as high for second-degree relatives and one-tenth as high for third-degree relatives. (Edward's approximation[118] states that the recurrence risk for first-degree relatives is $\sqrt{p}$, where the incidence in the population is p.)
3. The recurrence risk doubles after a second first-degree relative is affected.
4. The recurrence risk increases with severity of the phenotype in the index case.
5. The recurrence risk increases if the index case is of the sex less frequently affected.

The nature and number of genes and environmental factors involved in the production of any multifactorial malformation cannot be given. The concept that a vast number of genes and environmental factors must be operative is probably incorrect. Assuming equal environmental and genetic contributions to a hypothetical malformation with a recurrence risk of 2%–5%, the number of genes involved in producing the malformation can be as few as three. The only requirement of the environmental factor is that it be operative during the period of embryogenesis. One might suspect nutritional variations to be a strong environmental contributor prenatally, as they are in many multifactorial phenotypes postnatally.

Human anomalies with unknown causes

Clinicians attempt to assign causation in all human anomalies to gain a foundation for counseling and preventive efforts. As desirable as that goal may be, it is not attainable in every case. The causes of many malformations and recognized syndromes simply are not known. This is the case for approximately 43% of malformations.[119] In Jones' *Smith's Recognizable Patterns of Human Malformations,* 44 (16%) of the 278 entities have unknown etiology.[92] Assignment of causation of a malformation in one individual may not be possible although the cause of the same malformation is readily determined in other cases.

Lethality can pose a barrier to determining causation of certain malformations and patterns of malformations; sirenomelia and Rubinstein-Taybi syndrome might be examples (Fig. 6–25).[120,121] These conditions always occur as isolated cases (except for monozygous twins) within a family. All affected individuals die early (sirenomelia) or fail to reproduce (Rubinstein-Taybi syndrome). The possibilities that either represents a dominant phenotype caused by a new mutation, a multifactorial phenotype with a low recurrence rate, or a chromosomal disorder caused by submicroscopic deletion cannot be determined with current technology. Hence the causes of these conditions will remain unknown until one of the possibilities or another alternative is confirmed.

If heritable factors, environmental factors, or some combination of the two is accepted as the only etiologic possibility for human anomalies, then one assumes that entities of unknown etiology will eventually be explained in terms of one of these three cases. Should factors other than hereditary and environmental be identified, the new influence must be woven into the causation schema.

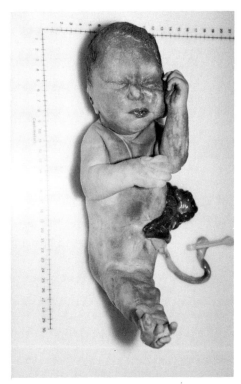
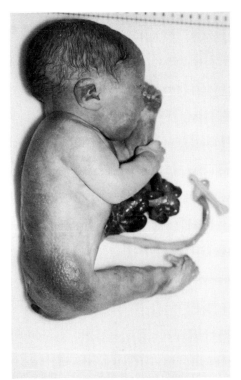
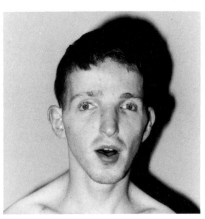
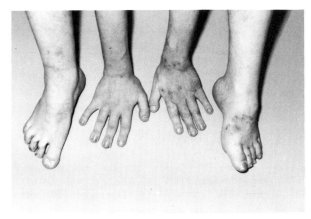

Fig. 6–25. Top: sirenomelia and gastroschisis in newborn infant. Virtually all affected infants have renal agenesis in addition to the skeletal, genital, and anal anomalies and die soon after birth. Bottom: facial features and hands and feet of a 23-yr-old male with Rubinstein-Taybi syndrome. Affected individuals do not have lethal anomalies but do not reproduce.

References

1. Flemming W: Beitrage zur Kenntniss der Zelle und ihrer Lebenserscheinungen. Arch Mikrosk Anat Entwickl 20:1, 1882.
2. Lejeune J: Le mongolisme. Premier example d'aberration autosomique humaine. Ann Genet Semaine Hop 1:41, 1959.
3. Waardenburg PJ: Das menschliche Auge und seine Erbanlagen. Martinus Nijhoff, Haag, 1932.
4. Bleyer A: Indications that mongoloid imbecility is a gametic mutation of degressive type. Am J Dis Child 47:342, 1934.
5. Hansemann D: Ueber pathologische mitosen. Arch Pathol Anat Physiol 123:356, 1891.
6. Wieman HL: Chromosomes in man. Am J Anat 14:461, 1912.
7. von Winiwarter H: Estudes sur la spermatogenese humaine. Arch Biol 27:97, 1912.
8. Painter TS: The sex chromosomes of man. Am Nat 58:506, 1924.
9. Slizynski BM: Human chromosomes. Nature 155:427, 1945.
10. Tjio JH, Levan A: The chromosome number of man. Hereditas 42:1, 1956.
11. Carr DH: Chromosome studies in abortuses and stillborn infants. Lancet 2:603, 1963.
12. Penrose LS, Delhanty JDA: Triploid cell cultures from a macerated fetus. Lancet 1:1261, 1961.
13. Hall B, Kallen B: Chromosome studies in abortuses and stillborn infants. Lancet 1:110, 1964.
14. Aula P, Hjeh L: A structural chromosome anomaly in a human fetus. Ann Paediatr Fenn 8:297, 1962.
15. Boue J, Boue A, Lazar P: The epidemiology of human spontaneous abortions with chromosomal anomalies. In: Aging Gametes. RJ Blandau, ed. Karger, Basel, 1975, p 330.
16. Warburton D, Stein Z, Kline J, et al.: Chromosome abnormalities in spontaneous abortion: data from the New York City study. In: Human Embryonic and Fetal Death. IH Porter, EB Hook, eds. Academic Press, New York, 1980, p 261.
17. Steele MW, Breg WR: Chromosome analysis of human amniotic fluid cells. Lancet 1:383, 1966.
18. Caspersson T, Lomakka G, Zech L: The 24 fluorescence patterns

of human metaphase chromosomes—distinguishing characters and variability. Hereditas 67:89, 1971.

19. Sutherland GR: Heritable fragile sites on human chromosomes. I. Factors affecting expression in lymphocyte culture. Am J Hum Genet 31:125, 1979.

20. Yunis JJ: High resolution of human chromosomes. Science 191:1268, 1976.

21. Murachi S, Nogami H, Oki T, et al.: The tricho-rhino-phalangeal syndrome with exostoses: four additional patients without mental retardation, and review of the literature. Am J Med Genet 19:111, 1984.

22. Schmickel RD: Contiguous gene syndromes: a component of recognizable syndromes. J Pediatr 109:231, 1986.

23. Narahara K, Nikkawa K, Kimira S, et al.: Regional mapping of catalase and Wilms tumor—aniridia, genitourinary abnormalities, and mental retardation triad loci to the chromosome segment 11p1305 → p1306. Hum Genet 66:181, 1984.

24. Ledbetter DH, Ledbetter SA, van Tuinen P, et al.: Molecular dissection of a contiguous gene syndrome: frequent submicroscopic deletions, evolutionarily conserved sequences, and a hypomethylated "island" in the Miller-Dieker chromosome region. Proc Natl Acad Sci USA 86:5136, 1989.

25. Hassold TJ: The origin of aneuploidy in humans. In: Aneuploidy, Etiology and Mechanisms. VL Dellarco, PE Voytek, A Hollaender, eds. Plenum Press, New York, 1985, p 103.

26. Therman E: Human Chromosomes, Structure, Behavior, Effects, ed 2. Springer-Verlag, New York, 1986.

27. Hall JG: Genomic imprinting: review and relevance to human diseases. Am J Hum Genet 46:857, 1990.

28. Lyon MF: Mechanisms and evolutionary origins of varible X-chromosome activity in mammals. Proc R Soc Lond [Biol] 187:243, 1974.

29. Nicholls RD, Knoll JHM, Butler MG, et al.: Genetic imprinting suggested by maternal heterodisomy in non-deletion Prader-Willi syndrome. Nature 342:281, 1989.

30. Burmeister M, Monaco AP, Gillard EF, et al.: A 10-megabase physical map of human Xp21, including the Duchenne muscular dystrophy gene. Genomics 2:189, 1988.

31. de Grouchy J, Turleau C: Clinical Atlas of Human Chromosomes, ed 2. John Wiley & Sons, New York, 1984.

32. Schinzel A: Catalogue of Unbalanced Chromosome Aberrations. Walter de Gruyter, Berlin, 1984.

33. Warburton D: Chromosomal causes of fetal death. Clin Obstet Gynecol 30:268, 1987.

34. Porter IH, Hook EB: Human Embryonic and Fetal Death. Academic Press, New York, 1980.

35. Milunsky A: Genetic Disorders and the Fetus: Diagnosis, Prevention, and Treatment, ed 2. Plenum Press, New York, 1986, p 120.

36. Shiota K, Uwabe C, Nishimura H: High prevalence of defective human embryos at the early postimplantation period. Teratology 35:309, 1987.

37. Shepard TH, Fantel AG, Fitzsimmons J: Congenital defect rates among spontaneous abortuses: Twenty years of monitoring. Teratology 39:325, 1989.

38. Hassold T, Chen N, Funkhouser J, et al.: A cytogenetic study of 1000 spontaneous abortions. Ann Hum Genet 44:151, 1980.

39. Kajii T, Ferrier A, Niikawa N, et al.: Anatomic and chromosomal anomalies in 639 spontaneous abortuses. Hum Genet 55:87, 1980.

40. Vogel F, Rathenberg R: Spontaneous mutation in man. Adv Hum Genet 5:223, 1975.

41. Martin RH, Mahadevan MM, Taylor PJ, et al.: Chromosomal analysis of unfertilized human oocytes. J Reprod Fertil 78:673, 1986.

42. Pellestor F, Sele B, Raymond L: Human oocyte chromosome analysis. Am J Hum Genet 45:A104, 1989.

43. Brandiff B, Gordon L, Ashworth L, et al.: Chromosomes of human sperm: variability among normal individuals. Hum Genet 70:18, 1985.

44. Kamiguchi Y, Mikamo K: An improved, efficient method for analysing human sperm chromosomes using zona-free hamster ova. Am J Hum Genet 38:724, 1986.

45. Martin RH, Rademaker AW, Hildebrand K, et al.: Variation in the frequency and type of sperm chromosomal abnormalities among normal men. Hum Genet 77:108, 1987.

46. Creasy MR, Crolla JA, Alberman ED: A cytogenetic study of human spontaneous abortions using banding techniques. Hum Genet 31:177, 1976.

47. Jacobson CB, Barter RA: Some cytogenetic aspects of habitual abortion. Am J Obstet Gynecol 97:666, 1967.

48. Czulman AE: Chromosomal aberrations in spontaneous human abortions. N Engl J Med 272:811, 1965.

49. Rosenfeld RG, Grumbach MM: Turner Syndrome. Marcel Dekker, New York, 1990.

50. Stern C: Genetic mosaics in animals and man. In: Genetic Mosaics and Other Essays. C Stern, ed. Harvard University Press, Cambridge, 1968.

51. Happle R: Lyonization and the lines of Blaschko. Hum Genet 70:200, 1985.

52. Pagon RA, Hall JG, Davenport SLH, et al.: Abnormal skin fibroblast cytogenetics in four dysmorphic patients with normal lymphocyte chromosomes. Am J Hum Genet 31:54, 1979.

53. Donnai D, McKeown C, Andrews T, et al.: Diploid/triploid mixoploidy and hypomelanosis of Ito. Lancet 1:1443, 1986.

54. Thomas IT, Frias JL, Cantu ES, et al.: Association of pigmentary anomalies with chromosomal and genetic mosaicism and chimerism. Am J Hum Genet 45:193, 1989.

55. Juberg RC, Holliday DJ, Hennesy VS: Familial sex chromosomal mosaicism. Pediatr Res 23:330A, 1988.

56. Kalousek DK, Barrett IJ, McGillivray BC: Placental mosaicism and intrauterine survival of trisomies 13 and 18. Am J Hum Genet 44:338, 1989.

57. Gartner AB, Barrett IJ, Kalousek DK: Confined placental mosaicism in spontaneous abortions. Am J Hum Genet 43:A130, 1988.

58. Kalousek DH, Dill FJ: Chromosomal mosaicism confined to the placenta in human conceptions. Science 221:665, 1983.

59. Epstein CJ: The Consequences of Chromosome Imbalance. Cambridge University Press, Cambridge, 1986.

60. Schinzel A: Microdeletion syndromes, balanced translocations, and gene mapping. J Med Genet 25:454, 1988.

61. Wyandt HE: Ring autosomes: identification, familial transmission, causes of phenotypic effects and in vitro mosaicism. In: The Cytogenetics of Mammalian Autosomal Rearrangements. A Daniel, ed. AR Liss, New York, 1988, p 667.

62. van Dyke DL: Isochromosomes and interstitial tandem direct and inverted duplications. In: The Cytogenetics of Mammalian Autosomal Rearrangements. A Daniel, ed. AR Liss, New York, 1988, p 635.

63. Mattei MG, Souiah N, Mattei JF: Chromosome 15 anomalies and the Prader-Willi syndrome: cytogenetic analysis. Hum Genet 66:313, 1984.

64. Schwartz S, Palmer CG, Yu P-L, et al.: Analysis of translocations observed in three different populations. II. Robertsonian translocations. Cytogenet Cell Genet 42:53, 1986.

65. Schwartz S, Palmer CG, Yu P-L, et al.: Analysis of translocations observed in three different populations. I. Reciprocal translocations. Cytogenet Cell Genet 42:42, 1986.

66. Abuelo DN, Barsel-Bowers G, Richardson A: Insertional translocations: report of two new families and review of the literature. Am J Med Genet 31:319, 1988.

67. Davis JR, Rogers BB, Hagaman RM, et al.: Balanced reciprocal translocations: risk factors for aneuploid segregant viability. Clin Genet 27:1, 1985.

68. Stene J, Stengel-Rutkowski S: Genetic risks of familial reciprocal and robertsonian translocation carriers. In: The Cytogenetics of Mammalian Autosomal Rearrangements. A Daniel, ed. AR Liss, New York, 1988, p 3.

69. Groupe de Cytogénéticiens Français: Pericentric inversions in man: a French collaborative study. Am Genet 29:129, 1986.

70. Kleczkowska A, Fryns JP, Van den Berghe H: Pericentric inversions in man: personal experience and review of the literature. Hum Genet 75:333, 1987.

71. Groupe de Cytogénéticiens Français: Paracentric inversions in man: a French collaborative study. Ann Genet 29:169, 1986.

72. Madan K, Seabright M, Lindenbaum RH, et al.: Paracentric inversions in man. J Med Genet 21:407, 1984.

73. Harbison M, Hassold T, Kobryn C, et al.: Molecular studies of the parental origin and nature of human X isochromosomes. Cytogenet Cell Genet 47:217, 1988.

74. Schmutz SM, Pinno E: Morphology alone does not make an isochromosome. Hum Genet 72:253, 1986.

75. Tedeschi B, Porfirio B, Vernole P, et al.: Common fragile sites: their prevalence in subjects with constitutional and acquired chromosomal instability. Am J Med Genet 27:471, 1987.

76. German J: Chromosome Mutations and Neoplasia. AR Liss, New York, 1983.

77. Auerbach AD, Alder B, Chaganti RSK: Prenatal and postnatal diagnosis and carrier detection of Fanconi anemia by a cytogenetic method. Pediatrics 67:128, 1981.

78. Parry DM, Mulvihill JJ, Tsai S, et al.: SC phocomelia syndrome, premature centromere separation, and congenital cranial nerve paralysis in two sisters, one with malignant melanoma. Am J Med Genet 24:653, 1986.

79. Nicholls RD, Rinchik EM, Driscoll DJ: Genomic imprinting in mammalian development: Prader-Willi and Angelman syndromes as disease models. Semin Dev Biol (in press, 1992).

80. Frézal J, Schinzel A: Report of the committee on clinical disorders, chromosome aberrations and uniparental disomy. Cytogenet Cell Genet 58:986, 1991.

81. Henry I, Bonaiti-Pellié C, Chehensse V et al.: Uniparental paternal disomy in a cancer-predisposing syndrome. Nature 351:665, 1991.

82. Mendel G: Experiments in Plant Hybridisation. Translated by The Royal Horticultural Society of London. Harvard University Press, Cambridge, 1965.

83. Corcos AF, Monaghan FV: Role of DeVries in the recovery of Mendel's work. J Hered 76:187, 1985; 78:275, 1987.

84. Corcos AF, Monaghan FV: Tschermak, a non-discoverer of mendelism. J Hered 77:468, 1986; 78:208, 1987.

85. Corcos AF, Monaghan FV: Correns, an independent discoverer of Mendelism? J Hered 78:330, 1987; 78:404, 1987.

86. Farabee WC: Inheritance of digital malformations in man. In: Papers of the Peabody Museum of American Archaeology and Ethnology, vol 3. Harvard University Press, Cambridge, 1905, p 69.

87. Garrod AE: Inborn errors of metabolism. Lancet 2:1, 73, 142, 214, 1908.

88. Garrod AE: The incidence of alkaptonuria: a study in chemical individuality. Lancet 2:1616, 1902.

89. Johannsen W: The genotype conception of heredity. Am Nat 45:129, 1911.

90. Beadle GW, Tatum EL: Genetic control of biochemical reactions in *Neurospora*. Proc Natl Acad Sci USA 27:499, 1941.

91. McKusick VM: Mendelian Inheritance in Man, ed 8. Johns Hopkins University Press, Baltimore, 1988.

92. Jones KL: Smith's Recognizable Patterns of Human Malformations, ed 4. WB Saunders, Philadelphia, 1988.

93. Sutton WS: On the morphology of the chromosome group in *Brachystola magna*. Biol Bull 4:24, 1902.

94. Morgan TH: Random segregation versus coupling in Mendelian inheritance. Science 34:384, 1911.

95. Morgan TH: On the mechanism of heredity. Proc R Soc Biol 94:162, 1922.

96. Avery OT, MacLeod CM, McCarty M: Studies on the chemical nature of the substance inducing transformation of pneumococcal types. I. Induction of transformation by a desoxyribonucleic acid fraction isolated from pneumococcus type III. J Exp Med 79:137, 1944.

97. Watson JD, Crick FHC: A structure of deoxyribose nucleic acid. Nature 171:737, 1953.

98. Dounce A: Duplicating mechanisms for peptide chains and nucleic acid synthesis. Enzymologia 15:251, 1952.

99. Nirenberg MW, Matthaei HJ: The dependence of cell-free protein synthesis in *E. coli* upon naturally occurring or synthetic polyribonucleotides. Proc Natl Acad Sci USA 47:1589, 1961.

100. Watson JD, Hopkins NH, Roberts JW, et al.: Molecular Biology of the Gene, vols I and II. Benjamin/Cummings, Menlo Park, CA, 1987.

101. Padgett RA, Grabowski PJ, Konarska MM, et al.: Splicing of messenger RNA precursors. Annu Rev Biochem 55:1119, 1986.

102. Gilbert W: Genes-in-pieces revisited. Science 228:823, 1985.

103. Watson JD, Jordan E: The human genome program at the National Institutes of Health. Genomics 5:654, 1989.

104. Barnhardt BJ: The Department of Energy (DOE) human genome initiative. Genomics 5:657, 1989.

105. Human Gene Mapping 11. Eleventh International Workshop on Human Gene Mapping. Cytogenet Cell Genet 58:1, 1991.

106. McKusick VA: The morbid anatomy of the human genome. In: Mendelian Inheritance in Man. VA McKusick, ed. Johns Hopkins University Press, Baltimore, 1990, p cliv.

107. McKusick VA: Mapping the genes for hormones and growth factors and the mutations causing disorders of growth. Growth Genet Hormones 5:1, 1989.

108. Tsipouras P, Ramirez F: Genetic disorders of collagen. J Med Genet 24:2, 1987.

109. Knowlton RG, Weaver EJ, Struyk AF, et al.: Genetic linkage analysis of hereditary arthro-ophthalmopathy (Stickler syndrome) and the type II procollagen gene. Am J Hum Genet 45:681, 1989.

110. Hall JG: Review and hypothesis: somatic mosaicism: observations related to clinical genetics. Am J Hum Genet 43:355, 1988.

111. Cohn DH, Starman BJ, Blumberg B, et al.: Recurrence of lethal osteogenesis imperfecta due to parental mosaicism in a human type I collagen gene (Col 1A1). Am J Hum Genet 46:591, 1990.

112. Carter CO: Principles of polygenic inheritance. BDOAS XIII(3A):69, 1977.

113. Holt SB: Quantitative genetics of fingerprint patterns. Br Med Bull 17:247, 1961.

114. Carter CO: Genetics of common disorders. Br Med Bull 25:52, 1969.

115. Roberts JAF: Multifactorial inheritance in relation to normal and abnormal human traits. Br Med Bull 17:241, 1961.

116. Fraser FC: Interactions and multiple causes. In: Handbook of Teratology, vol 1. JG Wilson, FC Fraser, eds. Plenum, New York, 1977, p 445.

117. Chinn S, Price CE, Rona RJ: Need for new reference curves for height. Arch Dis Child 64:1545, 1989.

118. Edwards JG: The simulation of mendelism. Acta Genet (Basel) 10:63, 1960.

119. Nelson K, Holmes LB: Malformations due to presumed spontaneous mutations in newborn infants. N Engl J Med 320:19, 1989.

120. Stevenson RE: Jones KL, Phelan MC, et al.: Vascular steal: the pathogenetic mechanism producing sirenomelia and associated defects of the viscera and soft tissues. Pediatrics 78:451, 1986.

121. Rubinstein JH, Taybi H: Broad thumbs and toes and facial abnormalities. Am J Dis Child 105:588, 1963.

122. Flemming W: Zellsubstanz, Kern, und Zelltheilung. Vogel, Leipzig, 1882.

123. Jacky P: Fragile X and other heritable fragile sites on human chromosomes. In: The ACT Cytogenetics Laboratory Manual, ed 2. MJ Barch, ed. Raven Press, New York, 1991, p 489.

124. Hall JG: Review and editor's comment: X inactivation of the X chromosome is not complete. Growth Genet Horm 7(3):9, 1991.

125. Miller WL: Recombinant DNA and the pediatrician. J Pediatr 99:1, 1981.

7

The Environmental Basis of Human Anomalies

ROGER E. STEVENSON

The uterus serves to shelter, nourish, and protect the conceptus until maturity sufficient for extrauterine viability is reached. When any of these basic functions fails, the organism can suffer pathologic consequences. The available safeguards are simply insufficient to protect against every environmental exigency that may be imposed through the maternal host.[1-4] Noxious insults from the environment usually reach the developing organism by way of the vascular system and placenta, less commonly by direct penetration through the uterine wall, and rarely by ascent through the os cervix.

Environmental insults after fertilization that produce structural defects are termed *teratogens,* from the Greek word *teratos* (monster) and *gen* (producing). Because of this derivation, it seems inappropriate to classify influences as teratogenic unless they can cause structural defects. Agents that cause visual impairments, hearing impairments, or mental retardation are not teratogens unless (in the process) they malform the eyes, ears, or brain. Nor should chromosome aberrations or mutations be considered teratogenic. The term is reserved for environmental insults. Teratogenic potential is largely limited to the period of organogenesis, although certain insults, primarily ones mechanical in nature, can produce deformation or destruction of tissues after the embryonic period.

After the period of organ formation, fetal energies are devoted to maturation and growth of tissues. Detrimental insults during this period exert their influence chiefly by inhibiting growth, disrupting the normal pattern of maturation, and interfering with the function of cellular components of various tissues. The term *hadegen*, after *Hades*, the mythological Greek god of the underworld and possessor of the helmet of invisibility, is used to identify those environmental influences that interfere with maturation, resulting in functional impairments. *Trophogen* is used to identify prenatal influences that alter growth. Hadegens and trophogens can exert their influences at any time during gestation; with few exceptions teratogens affect development only during the period of organogenesis.

Whereas chromosome and single gene aberrations are innate to the conceptus, teratogens, hadegens, and trophogens arise externally and are imposed on the conceptus. They exert their primary influence only during the time of actual exposure. In many cases, e.g., radiation and certain chemical insults, damage can result from a brief exposure. In other cases, the insult may be present for an extended period of time, sometimes persisting throughout pregnancy, as in chronic chemical or metabolic exposures and certain infectious processes.

By and large, environmental exposures are sporadic events with a low liklihood of recurrence. Teratogenic, hadegenic, and trophogenic effects recur in successive pregnancies only if the environmental exposure recurs.

Environmental insults can indirectly affect the conceptus by causing ill health in the mother. General systemic toxicity may accompany radiation exposure or certain infections, leading to abortion although no specific damage has been caused to the tissues of the conceptus. Alternatively, environmental insults can produce chromosome damage or mutation in the developing conceptus that in turn leads to abortion, malformation, or other injury. Radiation and certain chemicals have this potential. Occurring after fertilization, such induced genetic damage will affect only a portion of the cells, will become heritable only if germ cells are involved, and should not be considered teratogenic or hadegenic.

Teratogens, hadegens, and trophogens directly influence development by interfering with cellular metabolism, placing pressure on developing parts, disturbing regional vascular supply, and killing cells. Metabolism may be disturbed by altering the availability of essential nutrients, inhibiting enzyme activities, blocking mitosis, interfering nonmutationally with nucleic acid function, and impairing membrane function, osmolar balance, and energy production.[5]

A certain degree of protection against prenatal environmental insults may be afforded by the genetic constitution of a conceptus. This can be surmised from the variable rates at which identical insults induce malformations in different strains of experimental animals.[6] It explains in part the variable rates of specific malformations among the different human races.[7] However, some teratogens and hadegens have sufficient potency that they cannot be neutralized by genomic protection. Thalidomide apparently represents such a teratogen; hypoxia represents such a hadegen. It must be suspected that the genotype of the mother can diminish or enhance the susceptibility to teratogenic or hadegenic influences as well.

The time during pregnancy when the environmental exposure occurs greatly influences the effects. An insult that produces teratogenic effects during organogenesis may produce hadegenic effects, trophogenic effects, or no effects later in fetal life. For example, prenatal rubella infection during the first 2 months produces cardiac defects, infection after the fourth month produces deafness, and infection at any time causes growth impairment.

For teratogenic, hadegenic, or trophogenic effects to occur, the environmental agent must gain access to the conceptus or induce disturbances in the mother that are then reflected in the conceptus. Certain chemical agents, because of their size, transport, or binding properties, do not reach the conceptus even though they may be present in the maternal circulation. Many hormones are typical. They exert their influence via metabolic changes in the mother that can then be imposed transplacentally.

Most teratogenic, hadegenic, and trophogenic influences are dose dependent: the greater the exposure, the greater the likelihood of adverse effects and the greater the severity of the effects produced. During early embryogenesis, the same agent may in high doses be lethal, in moderate doses teratogenic or trophogenic, and in lower doses hadegenic.

Radiation

Radiation, a ubiquitous environmental influence, has the potential to produce fetal death, growth impairment, somatic abnormalities, mutation, chromosome fragmentation, and malignancy. Ionizing radiation from any source—natural, conventional x-ray machines, isotopes, or nuclear explosions—carries this potential. Radiation-induced pathology in the conceptus presumably arises because of impairment of cell division, cell death, mutation, and chromosome damage.[8]

All persons are inescapably exposed to low doses of naturally occurring radiation. At the surface of the earth the magnitude of this exposure is about 125 mrad per person per year, but can vary severalfold in different locations around the world (a rad is the unit of absorbed energy equivalent to 100 ergs per gram of tissue. From a chest x-ray, an individual receives one-thirtieth of a rad of radiation to the chest wall). Nearly one-half of naturally occurring radiation derives from the land, the structures thereon, and the air, 30% from cosmic sources, and 20% from ingested radionuclides. Less than 5% of radiation in the general environment derives from nuclear-powered reactors or residual fall-out from nuclear explosions.

The discovery of x-rays in 1895 and subsequent efforts to exploit the properties of ionizing radiation for diagnostic and treatment purposes have increased the average exposure 50%–100% over the natural background radiation. An approximation of the radiation dosage to the fetus or embryo from diagnostic radiographic examinations of the mother can be deduced from the ovarian dosages given in Table 7–1.[9]

Although the total human exposure to intrauterine radiation fortunately is limited, sufficient data have been gained from medical radiation and from the nuclear explosions at Hiroshima and Nagasaki to delineate the major effects on the conceptus. By the time of birth, the usual infant will have received about 90 mrad of radiation from the natural environment and possibly an equal amount from medical procedures. The effects from this low level of radiation exposure are not measurable. Although the low level of radiation exposure may contribute in some minor way to mutation rate, it does not make a discernible contribution to the abortion, congenital malformation, and growth impairment rates or to any other measure of ill health in the embryo or fetus. Much higher exposures are required to reach the threshold of overt effects.

Impairment of growth is the most sensitive measure of radiation effect on the embryo and fetus.[8] During embryogenesis, 25 rads or more are required to impair growth. Some degree of recovery from growth impairments caused during embryogenesis may be anticipated postnatally. Fifty or more

Table 7–1. Estimated ovarian radiation dose from various diagnostic radiographic procedures[a]

Examination	Estimated ovarian radiation dose (millirads)
Barium enema	
Total	805
Radiography	439
Fluoroscopy	366
Upper gastrointestinal series	
Total	558
Radiography	360
Fluoroscopy	198
Intravenous or retrograde pyelography	407
Hip	309
Abdomen	289
Lumbar spine	275
Cholecystography	193
Pelvis	41
Thoracic spine	9
Chest	
Radiography	8
Photofluorography	8
Fluoroscopy	71
Skull	4
Cervical spine	2
Upper extremity (excluding shoulder)	1
Shoulder	<1
Lower extremity (excluding hip)	<1

[a]From Penfil and Brown.[9]

rads are required to impair fetal growth. Growth impairment during this period is less likely to improve during the postnatal period.

The brain and eyes sustain the brunt of radiation injury during embryogenesis.[10–12] Dosages in excess of 25 rads are required for discernible damage. Microcephaly, hydrocephaly, microphthalmia, optic atrophy, retinal dysplasia, and cataracts have all been reported, usually following exposures to 100 rads or more.[10–12] Skeletal, visceral, and genital abnormalities have been noted less commonly. Growth impairments always accompany these more specific abnormalities.

Progressively greater resistance to the lethal effect of radiation is gained as the conceptus passes through the preimplantation, embryonic, and fetal periods. Exposure during the preimplantation period either kills the conceptus or leaves no overt trace of injury, suggesting that the teratogenic, hadegenic, and lethal doses do not differ significantly during this time. Radiation doses in excess of 10 rads may be lethal during the first week postfertilization. The minimum lethal dosage steadily increases from 25 to over 100 rads between the first and last weeks of embryogenesis. In the early decades of this century x-rays were used to induce abortion. In the majority of cases (96%) a single dose of 360 rads to the uterus prior to 14 weeks gestation resulted in abortion.[13]

Each year approximately 15%–20% of women between ages 15 and 35 yr will have abdominal or pelvic x-rays. The

Table 7–2. Average absorbed dose of radiation to the fetus and to the fetal thyroid gland from maternal radioisotopic procedures[a]

Radionuclide	Purpose	Dose to fetus (millirems)	Dose to fetal thyroid (millirems)
Na [131]I	Thyroid scan	15	5000
R [131]ISA	Plasma volume	10	5000
Oleic acid [131]I	Lipid absorption	17	5000
Rose Bengal sodium [131]I	Liver function scan	19	5000
R [131]ISA	Placentography	7	4900
Hippuran [131]I	Kidney function scan	0.3	100
[99m]Tc	Placentography	2	10
[51]Cr	Placentography	3–4	3–4
[99m]Tc pertechnetate	Brain scan	—	—
[99m]Tc sulfur colloid	Liver scan	—	—

[a]From Brent[19] and Tabuchi.[17]

radiation dosage from such exposures is usually low, but always causes alarm if the woman is subsequently found to be pregnant. The radiation doses received by the uterus during various medical procedures are listed in Table 7–1.[9] The most commonly encountered exposure is a dose of 0.5–2 rads from intravenous pyelography, barium enema, or pelvic computerized tomography. With these levels of exposure no gross defect or growth impairment is to be expected in the offspring regardless of the time of the exposure. The possibility of mutational injury must be considered, but no means of detecting such injury exists.[14]

Isotopes

Radiation from radionuclide use during pregnancy occurs much less commonly than radiation from x-rays. Various ^{131}I preparations commonly used prior to the 1970s for isotopic scanning have the disadvantage of concentration in the thyroid gland. If administered to a pregnant woman after 10 weeks gestation in sufficiently high doses, ^{131}I can ablate the fetal thyroid gland, resulting in hypothyroidism.[15,16] [131]I has been largely replaced by technetium pertechnetate, which causes less total radiation dosage and less concentration in the thyroid gland. Fetal radiation doses received from various diagnostic isotopic procedures are listed in Table 7–2.[17] Diagnostic procedures with isotopes other than ^{131}I are unlikely to expose the fetus to hazardous levels of radiation.

Microwaves, shortwaves, and radiowaves

Radiation from exposure to radiowaves, shortwaves, and microwaves can produce tissue heating, and hence the possibility of disturbing embryonic development exists. Shortwave radiation can penetrate deeply enough into solid tissues to reach the human fetus and thus has a greater potential hazard than microwaves.[18,19] Microwaves have limited penetration power, reaching 3–4 cm below the skin surface, and thus have limited access to the human embryo and fetus. Microwave ovens and diathermy machines produce radiation in this wave length (2450 mHz). There is no evidence at present to indicate that radiowaves, shortwaves, or microwaves can cause nonthermal injury to the developing embryo.

Magnetic fields

Human exposures to magnetic fields result primarily from video display terminals and magnetic resonance imaging (MRI) machines. Neither type of exposure has caused malformations, but the risk for pregnancy loss may be increased.[20]

Ultrasound

Diagnostic ultrasound is utilized in the majority of pregnancies during the first and second trimesters. Although usually performed to determine fetal age, ultrasound is also used to document fetal movement, placental location, number of fetuses, growth increments, and certain malformations. Such examinations use ultrasound in microsecond pulses separated by 1–2 sec pauses, and have not been associated with any adverse effect on the fetus.[21] Continuous wave ultrasound can, of course, disrupt cellular structure and can generate tissue destruction through thermal effects. McLeod and Fowlow[22] described growth impairment, microcephaly, sacral dysgenesis, and developmental impairment in an infant born following therapeutic ultrasound to the psoas bursa of the mother at days 6–29 postovulation.

Hyperthermia and hypothermia

Elevation of maternal temperature, primarily from sauna or hot tub bathing and from infection, has been implicated as a hazard to the human embryo.[23–25] While much of the information on this subject has been retrospectively collected, its consistency with results from animal experiments makes hyperthermia a plausible teratogen. Abnormalities have been experimentally induced in a variety of species by raising the core temperature of pregnant dams with pyrogens, external heat sources, microwaves, and shortwaves. Abortion can result from heating prior to implantation, and abortion, resorption, malformation, growth impairment, perinatal death, and functional impairments can result from heating after implantation. Early in embryogenesis, the central nervous system appears most vulnerable, presumably because of its rapid rate of mitosis. Heat injury to this target tissue is manifested by temporary interruption of mitosis and cell death of periventricular cells and, to a lesser extent, of deeper mesenchymal cells.[26] Depending on the timing, duration, and degree of hyperthermia, growth impairment and various structural changes can be produced.

Smith and associates provided suggestive evidence that in humans 11% of pregnancies resulting in anencephaly and 7% of those resulting in spina bifida had a history of temperature elevation during the first few weeks of gestation.[23-25] They subsequently found that a maternal temperature elevation of 1.5°C or more, prolonged for 1 day or longer between weeks 4 and 14, could result in more subtle damage to the conceptus. All infants born after such exposures were mentally retarded, usually showing other evidence of neurologic insult, including hypotonicity, hypertonicity, contractures, or seizures. Microcephaly was found in two patients, and neuronal heterotopias were present in the two cases at autopsy. Facial changes, predominantly seen in those exposed prior to 7 weeks, included microphthalmia, micrognathia, midface hypoplasia, abnormal pinnae, and cleft lip and/or palate. Maternal hyperthermia has also been noted in the pregnancy history of infants born with Möbius syndrome (oromandibulo-limb hypogenesis syndrome).[27,28]

Prolonged and limited periods of hypothermia have been associated with fetal death and malformations in experimental animals as well. Damage from gestational hypothermia has not been reported in humans.

Infection

A substantial dichotomy often exists between the severities of infections in the maternal and prenatal organisms. Covert maternal infection is the rule. In contrast, the embryo or fetus may sustain devastating injury to all organ systems. Not uncommonly, the first evidence that the mother has harbored an infection comes with the birth of the affected infant.

A wide spectrum of microbial organisms can adversely affect the embryo or fetus.[1,29-31] It must be suspected, in fact, that any organism that can gain access to the conceptus can act as a pathogen. Women acquire certain important infections, including syphilis, gonorrhea, herpesvirus, cytomegalovirus, immunodeficiency virus, and chlamydia, through venereal transmission. Other infections can be acquired through respiratory spread (rubella, varicella, coxsackievirus, parvovirus), through contact with infected blood products (immunodeficiency virus, hepatitis virus, malaria), through cat litter exposure (toxoplasma), or through uncooked meat (toxoplasma).[1,29-31] In virtually all circumstances the conceptus becomes infected through hematogenous spread. Organisms causing maternal septicemia cross the placenta and reach fetal tissues through the fetal circulation. In some cases a placentitis may become established as an intermediate state that seeds the umbilical vessels. Less commonly, organisms from the genital tract may reach the placenta and fetal membranes by retrograde migration. Early postnatal infections can be established through direct contact with microorganisms in the lower genital tract during birth; this mode is responsible for many newborn herpes simplex virus, chlamydial, monilial, streptococcal, and other bacterial infections.

Twenty-five percent of women between ages 15 and 35 yr lack immunity for viral organisms known to be embry-

opathic or fetopathic. A primary infection by these organisms can result in maternal septicemia and the accompanying risk for transplacental spread. Recurrence in subsequent pregnancies should not be anticipated. Since prior infection with certain organisms, including *Treponema pallidum*, gonococcus, *streptococcus,* and herpesvirus does not confer immunity, all women are susceptible to infection or reinfection during pregnancy. All woman as well are susceptible to human immunodeficiency virus infection. Recurrence or persistence of infection through several pregnancies is possible for organisms of this type.

Infectious processes influence the developing organism through a number of well-defined and theoretical mechanisms.[32] Cell death and depletion result in tissue or organ hypoplasia and generalized growth impairment. Continuing nonlethal infection of cells can impair mitosis, which again inhibits local and overall growth. Vasculitis can lead to microinfarcts, calcium deposition, and cavitation of tissues. Suppressed hematopoiesis and hemolysis can cause anemia and increased cardiac burden.

With the exception of *T. pallidum,* organisms that cause septicemia can cross the placenta at any stage during pregnancy. The time of infection to some degree influences the effects on the fetus, as does the fetus' immunologic response to the infection. Infectious processes can further influence pregnancy maintenance and development of the conceptus by causing hyperthermia, general toxicity in the mother, or mutation or chromosomal damage in the conceptus.[32]

Viruses

Cytomegalovirus

Once considered a uniformly fatal process, prenatal cytomegalovirus infection is now known to cause remarkably diverse pathology.[33-35] In its most severe form, cytomegalovirus causes intrauterine growth retardation, hepatitis, meningoencephalitis, and pneumonitis. Growth impairment continues postnatally. The necrotizing meningoencephalitis results in microcephaly, periventricular calcification, mental retardation, seizures, deafness, and motor deficits (Fig. 7–1). Uncommonly, obstructive hydrocephalus occurs. Optic atrophy and chorioretinitis can leave residual visual impairment. Other findings include hepatosplenomegaly, thrombocytopenia, and hemolytic anemia. Morphologic features, inguinal hernias, microcephaly, hydrocephaly, and microphthalmia result from the continuing infectious damage rather than from developmental disturbance during the period of organogenesis.

Milder infections can cause functional deficits without morphologic changes. Subclinical cases with neither morphologic nor functional changes have been documented with serologic testing.

Herpesvirus

Type I herpes simplex virus generally infects the cornea, the skin of the face and upper trunk, and the oral mucosa; type II usually infects the genitalia. The type can be determined by serologic and virologic methods. Type II herpesvirus (genital type) appears to be the more important in prenatal infections. Antibodies against the two types cross react, but the antibody of one type does not prevent infection by the other

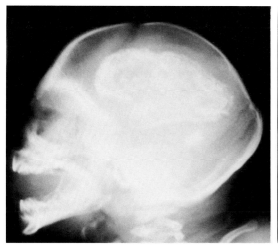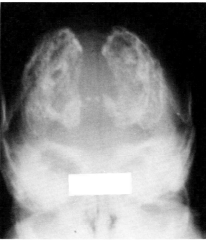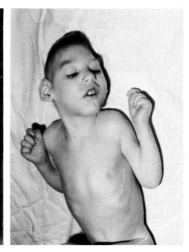

Fig. 7-1. Prenatal cytomegalovirus infection. Left and middle: dense periventricular calcification in severely microcephalic infant. Right: marked microcephaly, spasticity, and mental retardation in a 30-mo-old male with prenatal cytomegalovirus infection. Courtesy Dr. Charles I. Scott, Jr, A.I. duPont Institute, Wilmington, DE.

type, although spread of the virus may be limited. It has been suggested that transplacental infection might occur only in the absence of prior maternal infection by either type.

Of the few case reports of herpes simplex virus infection during early gestation, only the cases of Schaffer[36] and South et al.[37] can be accepted without reservation. In both infants the virus significantly involved the central nervous system with residual microcephaly, cerebral calcifications, microphthalmia, retinal dysplasia, tone disturbance, and seizures. Vesicles containing the virus were present on the extremities of both infants at birth.

Late infection is usually contracted at birth rather than prenatally. Severe infection occurs, nonetheless, with most cases being fatal during the first year of life. The cutaneous vesicle is a hallmark of infection and may be present at birth if infection occurred transplacentally or may develop during the first 2 weeks of life if infection was contracted during birth. Widespread infection with tissue necrosis involves most organs, particularly the brain and liver.

Varicella-zoster virus

Varicella can be transmitted transplacentally at any time during pregnancy. First-trimester varicella can cause meningoencephalitis, cutaneous lesions, and diffuse visceral involvement (Fig. 7-2).[38,39] Such infections are usually fatal; those who survive may have residual optic atrophy, microphthalmia, chorioretinitis, cortical atrophy, seizures, or motor disabilities. Similar features have been observed following herpes-zoster infection during the first trimester. Infection with varicella late in pregnancy may cause fetal infection, which is manifest by cutaneous vesicles at birth or during the initial weeks of life.[40]

Rubeola

While there is no doubt that rubeola virus can reach the conceptus during the phase of maternal viremia, malforming and destructive effects on the fetus have not been recognized. Abortion and stillbirth rates following maternal rubeola are not excessive. Scattered reports of congenital defects have documented no consistent pattern, and the defects should not be considered rubeola defects.

Influenza

Following the 1957 influenza pandemic, Coffey and Jessop[41] reported an increased incidence of central nervous system malformations among infants born of Irish mothers who had

Fig. 7-2. Prenatal varicella. Irregular scars along leg of infant whose mother had varicella during the fourth month of pregnancy. Infant also had chorioretinitis, cortical atrophy, seizures, and atrophy of the affected limb. Courtesy Dr. Roald Rinvik, Ullevaal Hospital, Oslo, Norway.

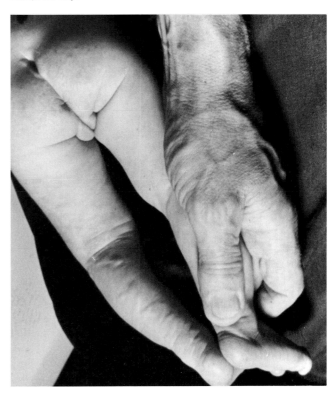

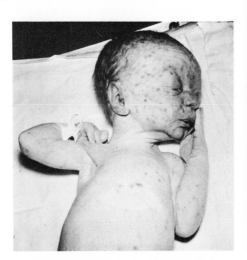

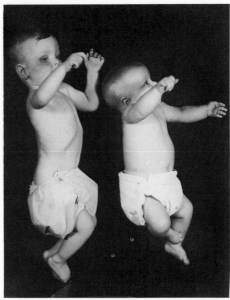

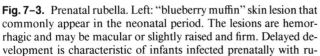

Fig. 7–3. Prenatal rubella. Left: "blueberry muffin" skin lesion that commonly appear in the neonatal period. The lesions are hemorrhagic and may be macular or slightly raised and firm. Delayed development is characteristic of infants infected prenatally with ru-

bella virus. Right: an 18-mo-old infant is shown with his 5-mo-old sibling on the right. Their development is comparable. Courtesy Dr. Janet B. Hardy, Johns Hopkins Hospital, Baltimore, MD.

influenza during pregnancy. An increased incidence of malformations was not found in other studies that utilized serologic evidence to confirm influenza virus infection. There is no compelling evidence to incriminate influenza virus infection as a cause of malformations. Maternal fever and increased drug use often accompany influenza and must be taken into account in cases of malformations following infection during pregnancy.

Mumps virus

Infection with mumps during pregnancy does not cause malformations but may result in abortion or stillbirth. Patients with endocardial fibroelastosis have been noted to have a positive mumps antigen skin test, but the relationship of mumps virus infection to this cardiomyopathy is obscure.[42]

Rubella

In the decades since Gregg's report of cataracts in infants born of mothers who had a rubella infection during the first trimester, a vast body of information on the embryopathy caused by this virus has accumulated.[43–47] The risk of fetal involvement resulting from maternal infection during the first month is 50% or greater and decreases with each successive month. Infection following the 8 weeks of organogenesis can cause deafness, microcephaly, or mental retardation. Rubella infection during the first trimester is accompanied by abortion (10%) and stillbirth (4%), with higher rates of fetal death during the first 2 mo.

Characteristically, rubella virus infection during the first trimester affects the developing eye, ear, and heart. Over one-half of infants have unilateral or bilateral hearing loss, primarily of the sensorineural type. Likewise, retinopathy, nuclear cataract, glaucoma, microphthalmia, and myopia affect

over one-half of infected infants (Fig. 7–3). Defects of the major arteries far outnumber the intracardiac lesions caused by rubella. Patent ductus arteriosus and pulmonary artery stenosis are the two most common cardiovascular defects. Intracardiac lesions, although less frequent, may be more significant in terms of hemodynamic disturbance. Pulmonary valvular stenosis, aortic valvular stenosis, and ventricular septal defects are the most common intracardiac lesions.

Continuing infection impairs growth, interrupts bone growth and maturation, causes pancytopenia, and produces widespread visceral involvement. Surviving infants have residual growth and neurologic impairments. The degree of postnatal growth impairment parallels the degree of mental deficit, presumably reflecting the duration and severity of infection.[46]

Parvovirus

Human parvovirus B19 causes erythema infectiosum in children and a nonspecific arthropathy in children and adults. The virus can also cause erythrocyte aplasia in patients with chronic hemolytic anemias or immunological impairments. As many as one-third of the fetuses born to women who have a primary B19 infection during pregnancy become infected.[48] Fetal infection generally results in nonimmune hydrops fetalis and in death. The pathogenesis has not been clarified, but presumably involves impairment of erythrocyte production, hemolysis, or direct infection of cardiac muscle alone or in some combination. Malformations do not result from human parvovirus B19 infection.

Human immunodeficiency virus

In the decade since its introduction into the United States, human immunodeficiency virus (HIV) infection has become the most common serious infection during pregnancy and the most common prenatal infection. From 30% to 50% of infants born of HIV seropositive women will develop AIDS or HIV-mediated disease.[49–53] It is thought that prenatal infection usually occurs transplacentally, although intrapartum infection may account for some cases. During the first year of life, infected infants exhibit growth retardation, microcephaly, seborrheic dermatitis, adenopathy, and recurrent infections.[49–51] Anemia, reversal of the T4:T8 lymphocyte ratio (<1), and hypergammaglobulinemia usually accompany the clinical findings. Mortality is high, with the majority of deaths occurring during the first 2 years of life.

Malformations as a part of prenatal HIV infection have not been reported. Facial features consisting of a box-like cranial configuration with frontal bossing, prominent eyes, oblique palpebral fissures, hypertelorism, depressed nasal root, triangular philtrum, and patulous lips have been described in two cohorts of infants and children with prenatally acquired AIDS.[52,53] Prudence requires further observation before these morphologic features can be attributed to HIV infection rather than to other environmental or ethnic influences.

Other viruses

Prenatal infections from a number of other viruses have also been documented. They have not resulted in malformations, but they have resulted in significant fetal pathology. Coxsackievirus infections have been associated with fetal pancarditis and meningoencephalitis; poliovirus with abortion, stillbirth, and meningomyelitis; echovirus with disseminated viremia; variola and vaccinia with necrotizing cutaneous and visceral infection; and hepatitis viruses with neonatal hepatitis.[1,54–61]

Chlamydia

Infection with *Chlamydia trachomatis* is considered to be the most prevalent venereally transmitted disease among pregnant women. While some studies have found infection to be associated with premature rupture of fetal membranes, premature delivery, and perinatal mortality, no association with malformations has been documented.[62]

Mycoplasma

Placental colonization with *Mycoplasma* is commonly found at delivery.[63] Prematurity and low birth weight may be associated with genital mycoplasmic colonization.[64] Malformations are not known to be caused by *Mycoplasma.*

Bacteria

Sepsis from a number of bacterial organisms can cause abortion or stillbirth, but does not cause malformations.[1,65] Bacterial infections are of greater concern as a cause of perinatal or newborn infections. Sepsis, pneumonitis, and meningitis can be caused by *Listeria monocytogenes, vibrio fetus,* nongroup A β-hemolytic *streptococcus, Staphylococcus, Escherichia coli,* and other coliform organisms. *Neisseria gonorrhea* is an important cause of generalized ophthalmitis in the newborn. Tuberculosis can be transmitted transplacentally or postnatally.

Spirochetes

T. pallidum

Syphilis is the major spirochetal infection of significance to the fetus. Always one of the most prevalent and devastating fetal infections, it has not disappeared with the advent of affective therapy.[66,67] For unknown reasons, the syphilis spirochete usually does not reach the conceptus during the first trimester; hence it is not an important cause of abortion or malformation.[68] Malformations of the permanent teeth may occur and include abnormal tapering of the incisors, enamel-covered notching of the central incisors, and crowding of the cusps of the first molars (Fig. 7–4).[69] These malformations are caused by infection after the period of organogenesis.

T. pallidum is disseminated through hematogenous spread to every organ system, but with predilection for skin, mucous membranes, liver, central nervous system, and bones (Fig. 7–5). Most severely involved fetuses die from widespread tissue damage. Hydrops fetalis is a well recognized but uncommon presentation.[70] Less severe infection can produce intrauterine growth retardation with or without active signs of syphilitic involvement at birth.[1]

Scarring or destruction of tissues and incomplete resolu-

Fig. 7–4. Prenatal rubella. Cataracts (top; left removed) and glaucoma (bottom) in prenatally infected children.

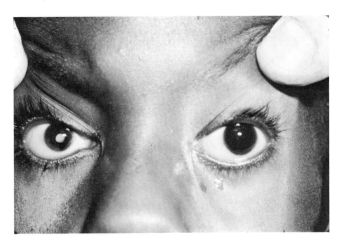

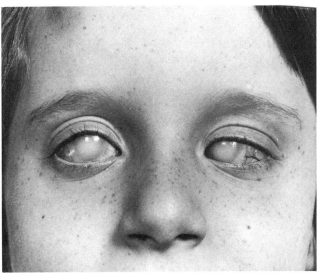

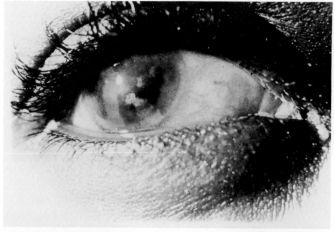
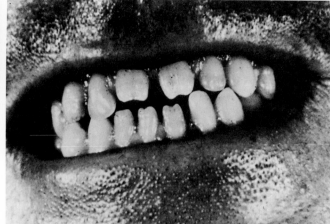
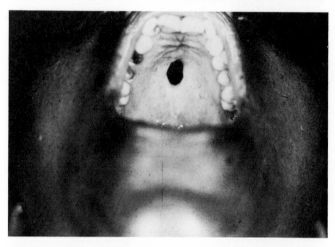
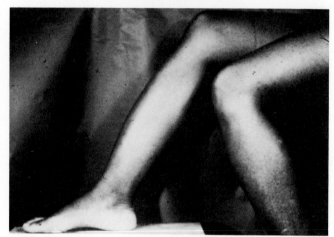

Fig. 7–5. Prenatal syphilis. Four stigmas of prenatal infection with syphilis: Top left: corneal scarring from interstitial keratitis. Top right: enamel-covered notching of permanent central incisors. Bottom left: perforation of the palate from gummatous involvement.

Bottom right: saber shins from incomplete resorption of periosteal bone formation. Courtesy Dr. James Millar, Centers for Disease Control, Atlanta, GA.

tion of proliferative processes produce certain morphologic changes after the active infectious stage of prenatal syphilis.[71] These predominantly facial changes include frontal or frontoparietal bossing, saddle nose, rhagades, and mandibular overgrowth. Chorioretinal lesions can also occur. Perforation of the palate or nasal septum can result from gummatous tissue reaction and destruction. Saber chins and hydrarthrosis can result from skeletal involvement. Most of these morphologic changes can be prevented or made less severe by early detection and treatment.

Leptospirosis and Lyme disease

Fatal leptospirosis, presumably acquired in utero, has been described in a newly born infant, but was not associated with congenital anomalies.[72] Transplacental passage of the Lyme spirochete has been documented, and it has been associated with a variety of adverse pregnancy outcomes.[73] A causal relationship between infection during pregnancy and fetal anomalies has not been established.

Fungi

One-third or more of pregnant woman harbor *Candida* species in the genital tract. In most instances these organisms are

nonpathogenic, existing in a saprophytic relationship with the host. By virtue of their location in the birth canal, they can contaminate the infant during birth and, in rare instances, have reached the fetus during intrauterine life. *Candida* species have not been implicated as a cause of malformations. Chorioamnionitis uncommonly occurs, often related to a retained contraceptive device or to cerclage.[74] Extension to the fetus can cause death or early delivery of an infant with disseminated infection.

Protozoa

Toxoplasma gondii

Primary maternal infection with *T. gondi* occurs in 1 per 1000 pregnancies in the United States.[1,75] Higher incidences can be found in other countries, notably Mexico and France. Infection is disseminated to the fetus in 40% of the cases. The organisms gain access to the fetal circulation from foci in the placenta and become widely distributed to all tissues. The clinical signs of toxoplasmosis result from chronic destructive infection of the tissues. The height of the tissue reaction occurs during the first few months of life. Thereafter the signs of active infection may not be discernible, even on pathologic

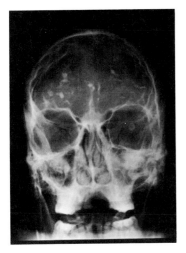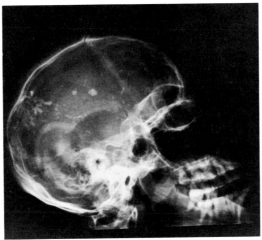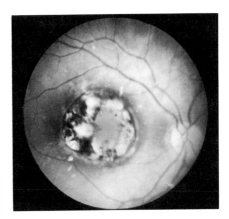

Fig. 7-6. Prenatal toxoplasmosis. Left and middle: microcephaly and diffuse cerebral calcifications in a mentally retarded adult with prenatal toxoplasma infection. Right: punched out chorioretinal lesion in macular region. Courtesy Dr. David Knox, Johns Hopkins Hospital, Baltimore, MD.

examination. However, the consequences, generally cerebral and ocular, may continue to appear over a number of years. Organisms have been recovered from the brain of a congenitally infected infant at age 5 yr.

Malformations are not a part of the pathology of prenatal toxoplasmosis. Hydrocephaly and microcephaly result from chronic destructive meningoencephalitis and should not be considered teratologic effects of the parasite. Little evidence has been accumulated to demonstrate fetal involvement during the period of organogenesis. The classic triad of congenital toxoplasmosis—chorioretinitis, hydrocephaly, and cerebral calcifications—has become accepted as the most common presentation of infants infected prenatally. This is unfortunate in that it encourages the observer to dismiss the diagnosis if cerebroocular signs are lacking. Signs and symptoms vary considerably in different infants and can change over time in the same infant.[75-77] Regardless of the predominant signs in a particular infant, significant residual damage to the central nervous system may become apparent after a period of years. This can occur even in children who show no signs of infection during infancy. The most common residual findings are chorioretinitis, blindness, and impaired intellect (Fig. 7–6).

Malaria

Although placental infection with malaria is a common event, prenatal infection of the fetus is decidedly rare. Infected fetuses can be growth impaired, and the infection usually results in stillbirth or in continuing infection in the neonatal period that is usually fatal.[78]

Prenatal chemical influences

The intimate intraplacental relationship between maternal and fetal circulations that permits the exchange of essential chemical substances also allows chemical disturbances to be reflected transplacentally. Most soluble constituents of maternal serum cross the placenta by simple or facilitated diffusion. Substances that diffuse poorly because of molecular size, degree of ionization, lipid insolubility, or adverse concentration gradient may be delivered to the fetus by active transport or by pinocytosis. Small leaks in the villous membrane would allow gross cross contamination of maternal and fetal circulations, but this leakage is probably not an important mechanism in the transfer of physiologically active substances. In any given case, the transport of a substance across the placenta may be altered by pathologic changes in the placenta, disturbances in maternal or fetal blood flow, or aberrant metabolism by the mother, fetus, or placenta. Transport is facilitated late in pregnancy by a thinning of the villous membrane.

Disorders of fetal metabolism are in most cases compensated for by the mother. Hence the fetus with phenylketonuria or hypothyroidism is protected, at least in part, during intrauterine life. Conversely, the limited metabolic capabilities of the fetus may not be sufficient to sustain homeostasis in the face of chemical disturbances imposed by the mother. Both exogenous substances, usually in the form of drugs, and metabolic deficiencies and excesses reflecting maternal disease states are important in this regard.

Deficiencies of essential metabolites

Hormone deficiencies

Diabetes mellitus

Distinguished as being the most common hormone deficiency during pregnancy, diabetes mellitus is the prototypic maternal metabolic disease that influences the health of the embryo and fetus. The maternal disease varies considerably in its severity and in its impact on the conceptus. The chemical imbalance inherent in diabetes is readily reflected transplacentally, placing stress on fetal homeostatic mechanisms. Diabetic pregnancies are subject to secondary complications that can further jeopardize the fetus. Since diabetes mellitus can exist throughout pregnancy, prenatal consequences include malformations, growth disturbances, stillbirth, and homeostatic derangements that can persist into the newborn period.

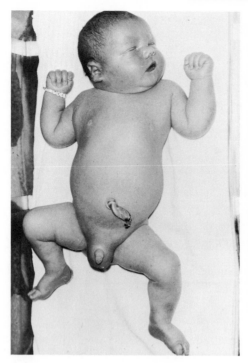

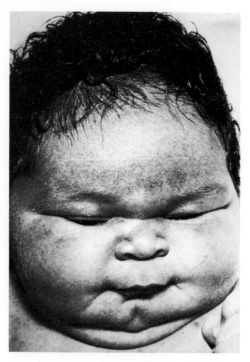

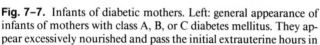

Fig. 7–7. Infants of diabetic mothers. Left: general appearance of infants of mothers with class A, B, or C diabetes mellitus. They appear excessively nourished and pass the initial extrauterine hours in a limp and quiet manner unless disturbed by stimuli from the environment or by their own respiratory distress, hypoglycemia, or hypocalcemia. Right: plethoric and cushingoid facies.

Infants born of mothers with diabetes mellitus types A, B, or C grow excessively before birth, presumably because of excessive glucose availability and fetal hyperinsulinism.[79–81] The macrosomia is generalized, affecting linear growth and weight, and with the notable exception of the brain it is shared by most internal organs (Fig. 7–7). In contrast, infants born of diabetic mothers with vascular complications can be growth impaired during fetal life. In neither case does the altered growth rate continue postnatally.

An overall threefold increase in malformations occurs among infants of diabetic mothers, the incidence bearing direct correlation with the severity and the degree of control of maternal diabetes.[82–87] Defects of the heart, central nervous system, kidneys, and skeleton predominate. Abnormalities of the major arteries, particularly transposition of the great vessels and conus arteriosus, ventricular septal defects, and dextrocardia occur with greatest frequency, but a variety of cardiovascular defects have been reported. Anencephaly, spina bifida, hydrocephaly, and holoprosencephaly are the major central nervous system malformations that occur in infants of diabetic mothers.

A spectrum of malformations involving the lower spine has been associated with diabetes mellitus. Collectively termed "caudal regression syndrome," the spine may have faulty segmentation or may terminate altogether in the lumbar or sacral region with disturbance in neurologic function below the level of spine disruption (Fig. 7–8). Anal and urethral spincters may be incompetent and motor function of the lower extremity impaired. Defective development of the long bones, joint dislocations, and malpositions can result as well. Sirenomelia occurs as a part of this spectrum of defects, and malformations of the lower and upper extremities can occur independently of the caudal regression syndrome.

While an overall increase in many types of malformations occurs among infants of diabetic mothers, holoprosencephaly and caudal regression syndrome in particular might be considered "diabetic malformations" because they occur with several hundredfold increase in these infants. Yet it is appropriate to remember that most cases of these uncommon malformations occur in nondiabetic pregnancies.[1,82] Other significant difficulties encountered by the infants of diabetic mothers include hyperbilirubinemia, hypocalcemia, hypoglycemia, vascular thromboses, respiratory distress syndrome, and birth injury.

Hypothyroidism

Since thyroxin fails to cross the placenta in early pregnancy and fetal synthesis of thyroxin begins after the first trimester, it may be surmised that organogenesis and early fetal growth proceed independently of thyroid hormone. Further evidence that thyroid hormone is not necessary for early development is the birth of normally formed infants to untreated cretinous and myxedematous women.[88] Later in pregnancy thyroid hormone does become important to fetal growth, osseous development, and neuronal maturation. However, the fetus should be capable of supplying its own hormone by the time the hormone is needed. Thyroid hormone may have some function in the maintenance of the placenta as demonstrated by an increased risk of abortion in pregnant women who have low thyroxin levels.[89] The exact relationship between hypothyroxemia and abortion in these pregnancies has not been clearly delineated. Pregnancies in women with frank and untreated hypothyroidism certainly do not consistently terminate in abortion. Only in cases in which the fetal thyroid gland has been impaired by antithy-

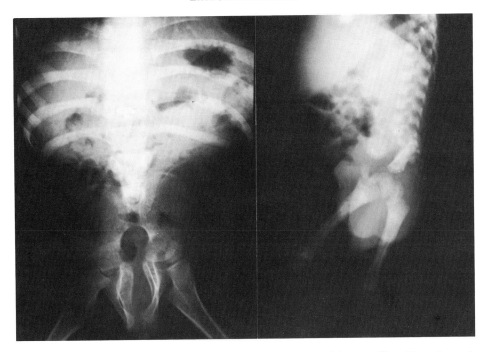

Fig. 7–8. Caudal deficiency in a 3-yr-old child whose mother had diabetes mellitus. The spine ends at L2, and the ilia are fused in the midline.

roid drugs (propylthiouracil, carbamizole, iodides), radioactive iodine (^{131}I), or possibly maternal antibodies does one expect effects on the fetus.[90,91]

Hypoparathyroidism

Infants of mothers with untreated hypoparathyroidism may have transient hyperparathyroidism during the fetal and neonatal periods.[92] The fetal parathyroid hyperplasia occurs in response to low maternal and fetal serum calcium concentrations mediated by the maternal parathyroid dysfunction. Excessive fetal parathyroid hormone predominantly affects the skeletal system, but other systemic effects of fetal hypercalcemia may result as well. All bones show demineralization, and subperiosteal reabsorption occurs in the long bones. Long bones may also show considerable bowing, and fractures may be present. Intrauterine growth retardation, pulmonary artery stenosis, ventricular septal defects, and muscle hypotonia have been described in individual cases.

Vitamin and mineral deficiencies

Folic acid

Minor deficiencies of folic acid and/or other vitamins have been suggested as a cause of defects in neural tube closure.[93–95] On the basis of this suggestion, supplementation of high-risk pregnancies in the periconceptional period (4 weeks before conception and 8 weeks after) has been carried out in Great Britain. Smithells et al.[94,95] used a multivitamin supplement (Pregnavite), and Laurence et al.[96] used a supplement of folic acid alone. In both studies, supplementation was found to protect against recurrence of neural tube defects in infants of mothers who had previously had an infant with a neural tube defect, reducing the recurrence rate to less that 0.5%. Two retrospective studies in the United States have

supported the British findings.[97,98] A third retrospective study in the United States failed to find any protection against neural tube defects from preconceptional vitamin usage.[99]

Infants born of women frankly folate deficient during pregnancy have not been found to show any measure of ill health, including intrauterine growth retardation, neural tube defects, or hematologic abnormalities.[100] Several infants born after exposure to the folic acid antagonist aminopterin have, however, had neural tube defects.[1]

Although the relationship between periconceptional folate deficiency and neural tube defects is unclear, a multinational study has confirmed that folic acid supplementation before and after conception protects against recurrence of neural tube defects.[101] Based on this evidence, folic acid supplementation is now recommended for women with a previously affected infant.

Vitamin D

Rickets has been present in newborn infants of mothers with osteomalacia and of women not overtly vitamin D deficient.[102] Clinical signs of rickets, rachitic rosary, Harrison groove, delayed maturation of skull bones with large fontanels, and expansion of the osteochondral junctions may be obvious at birth. Alternatively, radiographic histologic evidence may be found in the absence of physical findings. Dental enamel deposited during the period of intrauterine deficiency will be hypoplastic, dentin will be unevenly calcified, and the predentin will be excessively wide. The fetus may be endangered by hypocalcemic tetany in utero or by uterine tetany or dystocia secondary to pelvic contracture.

Calcium

Maternal hypocalcemia can result from hypoparathyroidism, inadequate dietary calcium or vitamin D, and heritable

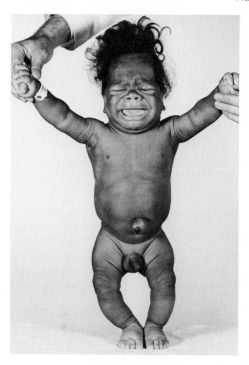

Fig. 7–9. Coarse facies, anteverted nostrils, large tongue, umbilical hernia, and muscular appearance of male infant with hypothyroidism. Courtesy Dr. Charles I. Scott, Jr, A. I. duPont Institute, Wilmington, DE.

vitamin D deficiencies. Although there is a calcium gradient favoring the fetus, fetal hypocalcemia can occur and result in osteopenia, rickets, or osteitis fibrosa, depending on the degree of calcium deficiency and other compensatory homeostatic hormonal changes.[103]

Iron

The fetus effectively parasitizes the mother's iron stores regardless of the state of her iron homeostasis. At birth the hemoglobin level appears to be unrelated to anemia in the mother.

Iodine

The iodine-deficient woman who is pregnant may fail to provide sufficient mineral to the fetus.[104] The fetus suffers the same pathologic consequences of the deficiency as the mother and can be born with goiter and signs of cretinism (Fig. 7–9). Features of cretinism, retarded bone growth and ossification, epiphyseal dysgenesis, myxedema, constipation, umbilical hernias, and cutaneous mottling will be present at birth or soon after in the untreated infant. If the condition is untreated, mental retardation is the most important sequela.

Oxygen

Chronic intrauterine hypoxia occurs in a number of circumstances. Cigarette smoking and certain pulmonary, cardiovascular, and hematologic disorders prevent the mother's blood from being consistently and completely oxygenated.[105–108] Chronic hypoxemia also occurs in women who

live at altitudes greater than 2000 m.[109,110] These situations limit the mother's delivery of adequate oxygen to the fetus. Chronic fetal hypoxia can also result from placental dysfunction, preeclampsia, and nontoxemic hypertension.

Impairment of intrauterine growth results from chronic mild hypoxemia, regardless of the cause. In several circumstances a direct correlation has been demonstrated between the degree of hypoxia and the severity of growth impairment. For pregnancies at high altitude, birth weights decrease 100–200 g for every 1000 m above sea level. Alzamora et al.[111] also found an increased incidence of patent ductus arteriosus and atrial septal defects among infants born at high altitudes. A progressive decrease in birth weight has also been directly correlated with diastolic blood pressure in hypertensive mothers and with the degree of oxygen desaturation in mothers with cyanotic heart disease.[112] Neill et al.[107] noted dramatic intrauterine growth retardation among infants of mothers with cyanotic heart disease whose hemoglobin level was greater than 18 g/dl, hematocrit greater than 65%, and oxygen saturation less than 65%. Infants of mothers with less severe cyanotic heart disease had less severe intrauterine growth retardation. Neill et al. also noted an increased risk of abortion, fetal death, and preterm delivery of pregnancies complicated by maternal cyanotic heart disease.

Acute intrauterine hypoxemia can cause fetal death or neurologic impairment. This outcome may follow umbilical cord occlusion and premature placental separation.

Excess of essential metabolites

Hyperparathyroidism

Since most hormones and tropic substances cross the placenta with difficulty, if at all, hyperfunctioning endocrine glands exert their influence indirectly. Less than 100 cases of maternal hyperparathyroidism, usually due to parathyroid adenomas, have been reported.[113] The excessive production of parathyroid hormone results in maternal hypercalcemia, which is reflected transplacentally in fetal hypercalcemia that in turn depresses the fetal parathyroid gland. This simplistic schema may in fact be much more complicated, involving 1,25-dihyroxyvitamin D_3 synthesis, hypomagnesemia, and/or end-organ responsiveness to parathyroid hormone as well. Maternal hyperparathyrodism results in excessive abortion and stillbirth and, because of suppression of the fetal parathyroid gland, predisposes the newborn to hypocalcemia and tetany.

Hyperthyroidism

Transfer of maternal thyroxin to the fetus is negligible during early pregnancy. Free thyroxin can cross the placenta, but the relative thyroid-binding globulin capacity favors the mother. During the final weeks of pregnancy fetal thyroid-binding globulin may compete more favorably and thyroxin may be transferred to the fetus. Triiodothyronine is less bound by thyroid-binding globulin and can more freely cross the placenta in all stages of pregnancy. Thyroid-stimulating hormone does not cross the placenta. Immunoglobulins that stimulate the thyroid gland do cross the placenta and may potentially stimulate the fetal thyroid gland.[114–116]

Most cases of hyperthyroidism during pregnancy are due

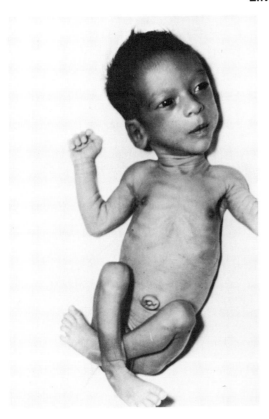

Fig. 7-10. Small for gestational age infant born of a mother with hyperthyroidism. Infant had transient signs of hyperthyroidism: agitation, tachycardia, tachypnea, and excessive hunger.

to Graves disease. In untreated state, fetal death often follows. The presence of thyroid-stimulating globulins in Graves disease places the fetus at risk for thyrotoxicity regardless of the treatment status of the maternal disease. When maternal hyperthyroidism is treated, two contrasting influences can affect the fetus. If thyroid-stimulating globulins are present, hyperthyroidism can be induced in the fetus. Alternatively, the fetal gland can be suppressed by transplacental passage of antithyroid medications.

Neonatal thyrotoxicosis induced by transplacental thyroid-stimulating globulins usually is a transient phenomenon, commonly lasting several months.[117,118] Most affected infants have goiter, exophthalmos, restlessness, and tachycardia (Fig. 7-10). Less than one-half will show periorbital edema, ravenous appetite, temperature elevations, cyanosis or cardiac failure, and hepatosplenomegaly. Craniosynostosis has been reported in several infants.[119] In some instances the neonatal thyrotoxicity persists, suggesting in these cases a heritable thyroid dysfunction rather than a transient influence of exposure to thyroid-stimulating globulin(s).[120] Goiter, hypothyroidism, and scalp defects have resulted from the use of antithyroid medications during pregnancy.

Cushing syndrome

Hyperfunction of the adrenal gland during pregnancy may be caused by tumor or hyperplasia.[121] One-half of the pregnancies will result in abortion or perinatal death. Maternal overproduction of adrenocortical steroids can suppress the fetal adrenal gland, which becomes manifest in the neonatal period as adrenal insufficiency.

Sex hormones

During pregnancy, the serum concentrations of progesterone and estrogen are higher than at any other time during life. Transplacental hormones can cause breast engorgement, neonatal vaginal bleeding, and the cutaneous eruption herpes gestationis. Breast engorgement occurs in male and female fetuses during the final 4-6 weeks of gestation. At term the usual breast nodule measures 5 mm more and regresses over the first postnatal month. Some infants have excessive breast enlargement and may produce a few drops of milk. Vaginal bleeding related to estrogen and progesterone withdrawal may occur during the neonatal period, beginning in the first week of life and rarely lasting beyond a couple of days.

Androgens produced by arrhenoblastoma or luteoma of pregnancy can masculinize female fetuses. The full extent of masculinization, usually some degree of clitoral hypertrophy and labial adhesion, will be apparent at birth. Androgen-secreting adrenocortical adenomas have also resulted in masculinization of female fetuses. Although overproduction of androgens also occurs in the adrenogenital syndrome, fetuses born of such pregnancies have not shown masculinization or other ill effects.

Herpes gestationis

A curious erythematobullous eruption associated with pregnancy, herpes gestationis causes intense pruritis, its major symptom.[1,122] The natural confinement of the condition to pregnancy and the artificial induction of lesions with progestational steroids provide justification for considering it a hormonally induced entity. The name *herpes gestationis* is inaccurate since it incorrectly suggests that the eruption is asssociated somehow with herpesvirus. Herpes gestationis occurs once in every 10,000 pregnancies and can recur in consecutive or nonconsecutive pregnancies. Lesions usually erupt at 4-5 mo gestation but can appear as late as 2 weeks after delivery. About 10%-20% of infants born of affected mothers will have lesions at birth or will develop lesions within the first 48 hr of life. The bullous lesions clear spontaneously within 1 week.

Aminoacidopathies

Phenylketonuria

Prior to treatment with a phenylalanine-limited diet, most phenylketonurics became severely mentally retarded during childhood, and few reproduced. The offspring of those women who did become pregnant were also mentally impaired. Substantial experience with pregnancy in phenylketonuric women has confirmed that the metabolic derangements in untreated maternal phenylketonuria almost invariably injure the offspring.[123-125]

Infants born of mothers with untreated phenylketonuria have intrauterine and postnatal growth retardation, microcephaly, mental retardation, and cardiac defects, the frequencies of these impairments being directly related to the maternal phenylalanine level (Fig. 7-11). When the mater-

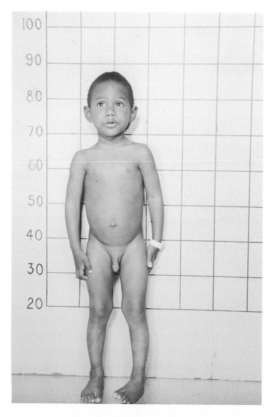

Fig. 7–11. Three-year-old male with microcephaly, mental retardation (IQ 55), short stature, and seizures. Born of a PKU woman who received no treatment during pregnancy. Her three other pregnancies resulted in one abortion and two microcephalic infants.

nal phenylalanine level exceeds 20 mg/dl, 92% of infants have mental retardation; 73%, microcephaly; 40%, intrauterine growth retardation; and 12%, cardiac malformations. One-fourth of pregnancies are spontaneously aborted. Rigid compliance with dietary treatment beginning prior to conception offers the only hope of decreasing this high incidence of malformation and other impairments among the offspring of phenylketonuric women.

Other aminoacidopathies

Only limited data exist concerning pregnancies in women with various aminoacidopathies. With the exception of hydrocephaly in two infants born of mothers with homocystinuria and Hartnup aminoaciduria, adverse affects on pregnancy outcome have not been reported.[126,127]

Myotonic dystrophy

An unknown factor appears instrumental in augmenting the severity of myotonic dystrophy in infants born of women with this disease.[128,129] During intrauterine life, affected infants grow slowly and have decreased movements, and pregnancies are complicated by malposition and polyhydramnios. At birth the infants show generalized weakness and experience difficulty in respiration and feeding. The facies characteristically show tenting of the upper lip, ptosis, absence of movement, and anterior cupping of the pinnae (Fig. 7–12). Clubfoot is often present. Postnatal growth continues

to be slow, and developmental impairment becomes obvious. These features do not occur in infants with myotonic dystrophy who inherit the mutant gene from their fathers.

The myotonic dystrophy gene has been shown to contain a segment of CTG repeats which tends to amplify in each generation.[129] On this basis, some increase in severity of phenotypic expression might be anticipated in successive generations. It has not been determined that this is the only factor responsible for the marked involvement in infants of women with myotonic dystrophy. Maternal imprinting of the myotonic gene has been suggested as an alternative hypothesis.[130]

Vitamin and mineral excess

Calcium

Maternal hypercalcemia due to parathyroid hyperplasia or adenoma can result in fetal hypercalcemia that in turn suppresses the fetal parathyroid gland.[113] While the hypercalcemia causes no difficulty in utero, once delivered the infant may experience transient hypocalcemia and tetany until parathyroid function is restored.

Vitamin A

See Isotretinoin, etretinate, vitamin A, below.[131]

Vitamin D

Although it has not been proven that vitamin D is harmful, circumstantial evidence has linked excessive maternal vitamin D intake and the idiopathic hypercalcemia syndrome (Williams syndrome).[132–134] In the hypercalcemia syndrome multiple systems are involved, intrauterine and postnatal growth retardation occurs, and mental retardation becomes apparent during childhood.

Severely affected infants generally have multiple system involvement. Intrauterine growth is reduced, and delayed development and mental retardation become obvious. The facies is characterized by broad forehead, prominent and widely spaced eyes, reticular pattern to the stroma of the iris, strabismus, depressed nasal bridge with anteverted nostrils, rounded cheeks, and prominent lips. The cornea may contain calcium deposits. The usual cardiovascular abnormality is supravalvular aortic stenosis, but infants with coarctation, stenosis, or hyperplasia of systemic and peripheral pulmonary arteries have been noted. Renal impairment and nephrocalcinosis may be present. Patients have decreased muscle tone, but deep tendon reflexes are usually brisk. Skeletal changes consist of dense calcifications of the skull, vertebrae, pelvic bones, and metaphyses of the long bones. Craniosynostosis can occur. Dental abnormalities include enamel hypoplasia, malocclusion, and caries.

The idopathic hypercalcemia syndrome was noted in Europe at a time when large supplements of vitamin D were given during pregnancy and infancy. Most infants born after pregnancy supplementation, however, showed no evidence of hypocalcemia syndrome, and excessive pregnancy intake could not be documented in those infants with features present at birth. The cause of this sporadically occurring syndrome remains elusive. The possibility that abnormal maternal, fetal, or placental metabolism of vitamin D, calcitonin,

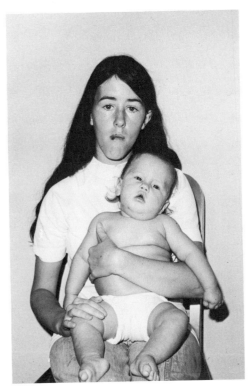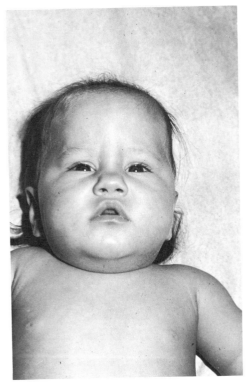

Fig. 7–12. Mother and daughter with myotonic dystrophy. Mother has characteristic elongated and expressionless facies. Daughter has elevated upper lip ("cupid's bow" lip).

or calcium plays a causative role cannot be excluded.[113] Alternatively, the syndrome may prove to be a heritable entity.

Drugs and environmental chemicals

Cigarette smoking

Increased pregnancy loss accompanies maternal cigarette smoking.[135,136] Abruptio placenta and placenta previa account for most fetal and neonatal deaths, although the specific mechanism by which smoking causes fetal loss is not known. Uterine ischemia with secondary decidual necrosis results from smoking and offers a plausible explanation for the increased risk of abruptio placenta.

The fetus grows more slowly when the mother smokes.[135,137,138] The growth impairment parallels the amount of smoking; infants of mothers who smoke more than one pack (20 cigarettes) per day weigh up to 300 g less than expected. The growth-retarding properties of smoking probably act throughout pregnancy. Certainly weight reduction can be seen in infants born at any time during the third trimester. Altered caloric distribution to the fetus, placental dysfunction, fetal hypoxia, and direct chemical toxicity of compounds in tobacco smoke can contribute to prenatal growth impairment. Postnatal catch-up growth occurs during the first year of life.

Alcohol

In 1973, Jones et al.[139] called attention to the effects of prenatal exposure to alcohol, renewing concerns about alcohol

use during pregnancy that had existed since the early Greek city-states.[140,141] They described a pattern of malformations and other morphologic changes, growth impairment, and cognitive defects among infants of chronic alcoholics. This prenatal alcohol syndrome is now recognized as one of the most common causes of birth defects among patients with mental retardation.

Reduced head circumference, length, and weight present at birth persists postnatally. Facial characteristics, largely reflecting impaired brain growth, consist of small eyes and short palpebral fissures, ptosis, epicanthus, midface hypoplasia, long and smooth philtrum, and thin upper lip (Fig. 7–13). Atrial and ventricular septal defects are the most common of a wide variety of cardiac defects. Radioulnar and cervical vertebral fusions, camptodactyly and other joint contractures, hip dislocation, deformations of the feet, hypoplastic distal phalanges and nails, and altered palmar creases are skeletal components of the full syndrome. Less common defects include protuberant ears, cleft lip/palate, hydrocephaly, neural tube defects, urogenital abnormalities, hemangiomas, and radial ray deficiencies.[142]

Frank mental retardation occurs in one-half of children with prenatal alcohol syndrome. Mental retardation can be accompanied by muscle weakness, poor coordination, tremors, hyperactivity, reduced attention span, speech impairment, strabismus, and sensorineural and conduction hearing deficits. Structural and functional impairments occur in up to one-half of infants born of alcoholic women who drink heavily ($\geq$3 oz absolute alcohol daily) during pregnancy. Functional and growth disturbances without other morphologic changes can occur in infants whose mothers drink moderately (1–2 oz absolute alcohol daily). No adverse effects

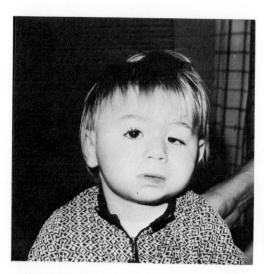

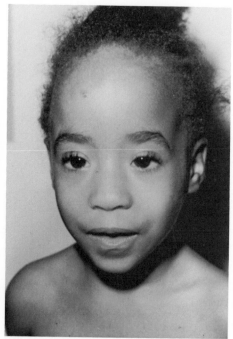

Fig. 7–13. Prenatal alcohol syndrome. The 3-yr-old boy at left has microcephaly, left ptosis, short palpebral fissures (<3rd percentile), smooth philtrum, thin upper lip, fingernail hypoplasia, and devel-opmental delay. The 27-mo-old girl at right has short stature, mi-crocephaly, midface hypoplasia, short palpebral fissures (<3rd per-centile), smooth philtrum, thin upper lip, and developmental delay.

have been documented in infants of mothers who drink less than 1 oz absolute alcohol daily. The possibility that subclin-ical damage may be reflected later in school and work per-formance cannot be excluded. Because of our limited under-standing of the effects of prenatal exposure to alcohol, total abstinence from alcohol during pregnancy is a wise precau-tion.

Cocaine

During the 1980s, cocaine became one of the most com-monly used recreational street drugs among pregnant women. One in 10 women in the United States use cocaine during pregnancy. Among the wide range of abnormalities now being reported in infants of cocaine users, most appear related to the propensity of the drug to affect the cardiovas-cular system.[143-146] A 10-fold increased risk of stillbirth re-lates almost exclusively to abruptio placenta. Vascular-based disruptions, skull defects, cutis aplasia, porencephaly, ileal atresia, visceral infarcts, genitourinary abnormalities, and limb reductions constitute most of the structural defects. In-trauterine growth impairment and cardiac defects have also been reported. Collectively these defects affect less than 10% of infants. A similar low percentage of infants exhibit with-drawal symptoms during the neonatal period. Necrotizing enterocolitis has been reported as a possible postnatal vas-cular complication. The incidence of sudden infant death syndrome appears to be increased.

Marijuana

Although a dose-related reduction in birth weight has been found in infants of mothers who used marijuana, neither major malformations nor patterns of malformations have been identified among these infants.[147]

Lysergic acid diethylamide (LSD)

Chromosome breakage of leukocytes has been induced in vitro and in vivo by LSD.[1,148] The breakage appears transitory and has not been implicated as a cause of malformations or other ill health in infants of mothers who ingested LSD dur-ing pregnancy. Several infants of mothers who used LSD have had malformations.[1] While these infants have had no single characteristic malformation, limb and other skeletal anomalies have predominated. The evidence remains insuf-ficient to implicate LSD as a cause of human malformations.

Anticonvulsant drugs

Diphenylhydantoin (Dilantin)

Seizure disturbances affect 1 in 300 pregnant women. The majority of affected women require continuous anticonvul-sant therapy during pregnancy. Diphenylhydantoin, the an-ticonvulsant used most commonly, was the first to be sus-pected of causing intrauterine damage.[149,150]

After initial studies linked diphenylhydantoin with cleft lip and cleft palate, a broader syndrome of malformations, other morphologic changes, and functional impairments were attributed to prenatal exposure.[149-154] Affected infants have some combination of intrauterine and postnatal growth impairments, microcephaly, hypertelorism, depressed nasal bridge, ptosis, wide mouth, hypoplasia of the distal phalanges and nails, and developmental impairment (Fig. 7–14). Cleft lip and palate and cardiac defects are the most common

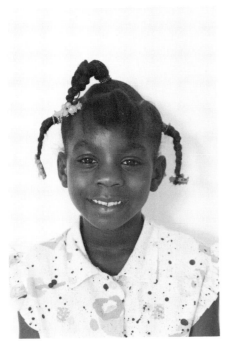
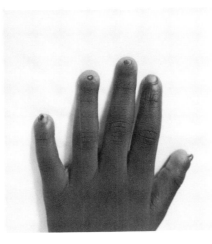
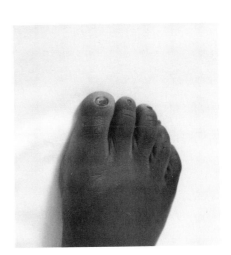

Fig. 7–14. Prenatal hydantoin exposure. A 7-yr-old female with prenatal exposure to hydantoin. Fingernails and toenails show marked hypoplasia. Facial appearance and school performance in first grade were normal.

major malformations. Colobomas, glaucoma, and other ocular abnormalities have been reported, as have diaphragmatic, umbilical, and inguinal hernias.

It has been suggested that about 10% of exposed infants will have significant malformations or mental defect, with a somewhat higher percentage having one or more minor features.[154] Exposed infants may also have an increased risk of developing tumors of neural tissue during childhood.

Trimethadione, paramethadione

Of the anticonvulsants, trimethadione and paramethadione pose the greatest prenatal hazard.[155] One-fourth of pregnancies are spontaneously aborted. One-third of those born die during the first year of life. The majority of liveborn infants have prenatal and postnatal growth deficiency, developmental delay, malformations, and distinctive facies, including V-shaped eyebrows with or without synophrys, broad nasal bridge, arched or cleft palate, and malpositioned ears, with anterior cupping and/or excessive folding of the superior helices (Fig. 7–15). A wide variety of major and minor defects in virtually all systems has been reported. Cardiovascular defects, renal malformations, tracheoesophageal anomalies, hernias, and hypospadias are most common. Survivors often have mild to moderate mental retardation and speech impairment.

Valproic acid

Reports of an association between valproic acid and spina bifida prompted concern that this anticonvulsant might be an important teratogen.[156] The risk for meningomyelocele, primarily lumbar or lumbosacral, appears to be about 1%–2% following first-trimester exposure (two- to fourfold higher than the population frequency). Intrauterine growth proceeds normally, but developmental delay, a pattern of craniofacial features, and other malformations have been described.[157,158] Bitemporal narrowing, tall forehead with metopic prominence, shallow orbits with epicanthus and infraorbital creases, small nose with flattened bridge, long and flat philtrum, small mouth with thin upper vermilion, rotated pinnae, and micrognathia form a more or less distinctive craniofacial morphology. Cardiovascular defects, oral

Fig. 7–15. Prenatal trimethadione exposure. Facial appearances of two brothers aged 10 yr (left) and 13 yr (right) exposed prenatally to trimethadione. Both have V-shaped eyebrows, broad nasal bridge, epicanthus, and low-set retroverted ears with excessively folded superior helices. Both had borderline intellectual function. Courtesy Dr. Elaine Zackai, Children's Hospital of Philadelphia.

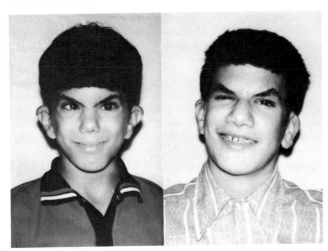

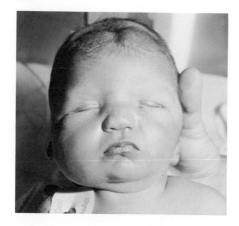 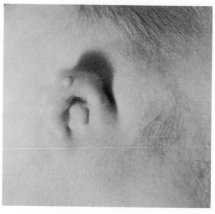 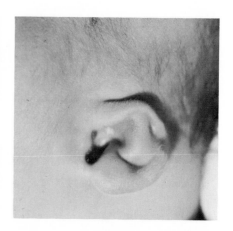

Fig. 7–16. Malformation in an infant exposed to retinoic acid during the first 18 weeks of gestation. Features include hypertelorism, downslanting palpebral fissures, microtia, cleft palate, hydrocephalus, hypoplasia of the cerebellum, and a heart defect. Courtesy Dr. Paul M. Fernhoff, Emory University School of Medicine, Atlanta, GA.

clefts, inguinal hernias, hypospadias, clubfoot, dolichostenodactyly, strabismus, and nystagmus occur in a minority of infants. An overall risk cannot yet be given.

Carbamazepine (Tegretol)

Once considered to be the drug of choice for seizure management during pregnancy, carbamazepine has recently been incriminated as the cause of minor facial and skeletal abnormalities.[159] In retrospective and prospective observations, Jones et al.[159] have found a small percentage of exposed infants to have growth retardation, abnormal facies, nail hypoplasia, and developmental delay. Craniofacial features include microcephaly, narrow bitemporal diameter, upslanted palpebral fissures, epicanthus, short nose, and long philtrum. Cardiac defects were found in 2 of 8 cases ascertained retrospectively and 1 of 35 cases ascertained prospectively.

Thioureas

Propylthiouracil and other thiourea compounds interrupt thyroxin production by blocking both the iodination of tyrosine and the coupling of diiodotyrosine. They are widely and effectively used in the therapy of hyperthyroidism. Niswander and Gordon[160] found hyperthyroidism in 1 of every 500 pregnancies. Thioureas readily cross the placenta and can cause goiter and hypothyroidism in the fetus.[90,160,161] Thiouracil goiters are usually mild to moderate in size and do not compromise the respiratory and alimentary tracts in otherwise normal infants. With the exception of umbilical hernias, any of the signs of hypothyroidism can be present. Goiter and other signs of hypothyroidism spontaneously regress over a 2–6 week period, and regression can be hastened by thyroxin supplements.[161] Limited follow up has not shown residual growth or mental impairments.

Carbimazole, methimazole

Aplasia cutis congenita of the scalp has been noted among infants born of hyperthyroid women treated during pregnancy with carbimazole or methimazole.[162] Typically the lesions are single, well-circumscribed, midline scalp defects, but multiple defects have occurred as well. Among the nine cases reviewed by Milham,[162] two also had umbilical defects.

Isotretinoin, vitamin A

Within 1 yr of the release of isotretinoin for the treatment of cystic acne, malformations were linked to its use during pregnancy.[163] That isotretinoin would affect the developing human was not unexpected because of its known teratogenicity in animals and because of the teratogenicity of the related compounds etretinate and vitamin A in humans. Isotretinoin (Accutane) used during the embryonic period causes an increased risk for spontaneous abortion (40%) and for malformations (25%) among survivors.[131,164,165] Anomalies of the central nervous system, cardiovascular system, and craniofacial structures predominate (Fig. 7–16). Most affected infants have central nervous system defects. Hydrocephaly with or without other structural abnormalities of the cerebrum and cerebellum occurs. The ears are usually small, malformed, or misplaced with atresia of the external auditory canal and underdevelopment of the middle ear. Less common alterations of the craniofacial structures include sloping or narrow forehead, accessory parietal sutures, depressed and wide nasal root, micrognathia, and cleft palate. One-third of the affected infants have cardiovascular anomalies, usually affecting the aortic arch or conotruncal area of the heart. Thymic agenesis, hypogenesis, or ectopia may accompany these cardiovascular defects. Isotretinoin defects have been attributed to a disturbance of the migration and influence of the cranial neural crest cells. Lammer et al.[166] have also found craniofacial alterations in fetuses exposed only after 60 days postovulation. These infants have prominent metopic sutures, epicanthus, and dimples or creases on the posterior aspect of the ears. Since isotretinoin has a serum half-life of 16–20 hr and is not stored in tissue, use prior to conception carries little if any risk during a subsequent pregnancy.

Vitamin A intake in excess of 25,000 IU daily during the first trimester has been associated with malformations. Single cases of sirenomelia and oculo-auriculo-vertebral syndrome and several cases of genitourinary abnormalities have been reported.[167,168] Although these are insufficient data to conclude that vitamin A is teratogenic, there exists no com-

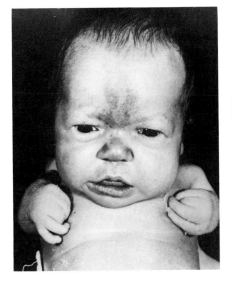 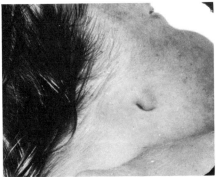 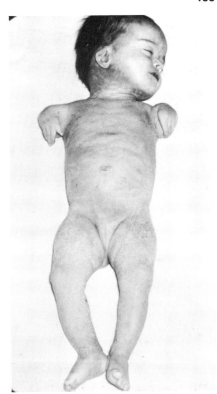

Fig. 7–17. Prenatal thalidomide exposure. Left: midline facial hemangioma and upper limb reduction malformation. Middle: mi-crotia. Right: upper limb reduction malformation. Courtesy Dr. Helen Taussig, Johns Hopkins Hospital, Baltimore.

pelling reason for use of such extraordinary doses during pregnancy.

Etretinate

Like its congener isotretinoin, etretinate can cause central nervous system, cardiovascular, and skeletal malformations. It is used primarily in the treatment of psoriasis. In contrast to isotretinoin, etretinate is predominantly bound to lipoproteins and persists in the circulation for years after use. Grote et al.[169] have reported unilateral limb defects in a fetus conceived 4 mo after the mother's last dose of etretinate.

Thalidomide

More than any other event, the thalidomide tragedy alerted the world to the teratogenic potential of drugs. A chemical with sedative properties, thalidomide was marketed alone or in various compounds for a wide variety of ailments beginning in 1956. The most extensive distribution was in West Germany, but substantial use occurred throughout Europe and in certain Asian and American countries.[170] Thalidomide was available for only 4 yr before its teratogenicity was recognized and distribution was halted. Only the unusual and dramatic nature of the malformations accounts for the drug's teratogenic properties being recognized that quickly. Over 4000 infants are known to have been injured by prenatal exposure.

Thalidomide produced malformations limited to tissues of mesodermal origin, primarily limbs, ears, cardiovascular system, and gut musculature.[171,172] The types of malformations could be related to the age of the embryo at the time of

ingestion. Malformations resulted from repeated use and from single ingestions during the critical period of 20–40 days postovulation.

Abnormal development of the long bones produced an almost endless and striking variety of limb reduction malformations (Fig. 7–17). Typically the upper limbs were more severely involved than the lower limbs. Of the long bones of the upper limbs, the radius was most frequently involved. However, any of the bones could be defective or, in severe cases, totally absent. The hands in some cases were normally formed, in other cases lacked thumbs or other fingers, and in still other cases were totally absent. Oligodactyly, syndactyly, and polydactyly occurred. Lower extremities could be similarly affected, but less frequently and less severely.

The head and neck escaped gross malformation, and mentation appeared normal. Characteristically, a midline hemangioma extended from the frontal area over the tip of the nose and ended on the upper lip. Ear malformations ranging from agenesis to preauricular tags occured in one-fifth of cases. Some infants had facial or abducens palsy, usually unilateral.

A wide variety of cardiovascular defects were seen, affecting about 10% of infants. Visceral anomalies included agenesis of spleen, gallbladder, and appendix and atresias or stenoses of the esophagus, duodenum, and anus. The mechanism by which thalidomide produced malformations is entirely unknown.

Warfarin

Anticoagulants are used prophylactically following cardiac valve transplantation and in the treatment of thrombophle-

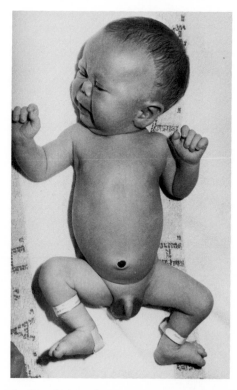

Fig. 7-18. Prenatal warfarin exposure. Infant was exposed throughout pregnancy. He has marked nasal and midface hypoplasia, narrow nasal passages, brachydactyly, and nail hypoplasia. Development was normal at age 7 mo. Courtesy Dr. J.M. Pettifor, Johannesburg, South Africa.

bitis, thrombosis, embolus, and polycythemia. Warfarin and other related vitamin K antagonists cross the placenta and can cause spontaneous abortion, malformations, and fetal anticoagulation.[173-175] The sentinel signs of embryonic pathology, nasal hypoplasia, and skeletal stippling depend on exposure during the critical period of 4–6 weeks postovulation (Figs. 7–18, 7–19). Midtrimester exposure can result in optic atrophy, brain anomalies, and mental impairment. Third-trimester exposure can anticoagulate the fetus, predisposing to perinatal hemorrhage.

In warfarin embryopathy, the nose appears small, with depression of the nasal bridge and accentuated demarcation between the alae nasi and the tip of the nose. Choanal stenosis may coexist. Prenatally, the restricted nasal airway may contribute to the increased frequency of polyhydramnios and postnatally to respiratory embarrassment and death. Calcific stippling occurs primarily in the tarsals, proximal femurs, and paravertebral processes but may be present in other areas of the skeleton and in the laryngeal and tracheal cartilages. Brachydactyly and small nails, with greater severity in the upper limbs, have been present in about one-half of affected infants. Optic atrophy, microphthalmia, and blindness can apparently result from exposure during the first or second trimester. Mortality is high (20%) among affected infants, and one-third of survivors will be mentally retarded.

A variety of structural anomalies of the brain, microcephaly, optic atrophy, visual impairment, seizures, hypotonia, and mental retardation have been noted among infants exposed throughout pregnancy and among infants exposed only after the first trimester. Others with intracranial hemorrhage in the perinatal or postnatal periods have developed hydrocephaly and mental retardation.

Methotrexate, aminopterin

The folic acid antagonists are used primarily in the treatment of psoriasis and certain malignant diseases. Their potent teratogenic properties have been known since the 1950s, when the drug was also used as an abortifacient.[176] The folic acid antagonists produce cranial and skeletal malformations (Fig. 7–20).[177,178] Bony malformations of the skull include absent or defective ossification, misshapen bones, sutural synostosis, and anencephaly. The globular head, wide-spaced and prominent eyes, depressed nasal bridge, micrognathia, malformed ears, and underdeveloped supraorbital ridges compose a somewhat characteristic facies. Cleft lip and/or cleft palate have been present in several cases. Further skeletal anomalies, including mesomelic shortening of the limbs, dislocated hips and elbows, coalescence of carpals and tarsals, clubfoot, and delayed bone maturation, have been reported. Prenatal and postnatal growth have been severely impaired, but mental development in survivors is only mildly affected.[179]

Fig. 7-19. Prenatal warfarin exposure. Radiographs show irregular ossification (stippling) of the tarsal bones (left) and articular or periarticular calcification along the vertebral column (right).

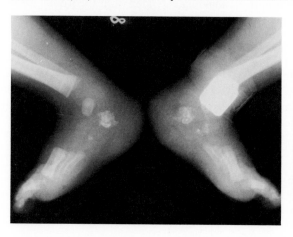
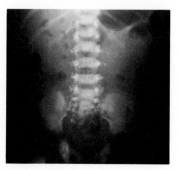

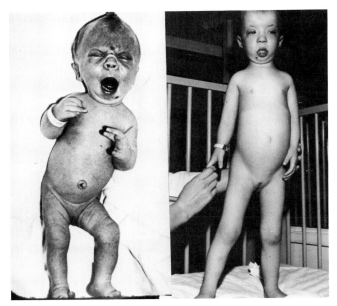

Fig. 7-20. Prenatal aminopterin exposure. Photographs (at birth and at age 18 mo) of a girl exposed to aminopterin during the first trimester. Features included globular skull with deficient calcification, low-set ears, ocular hypertelorism, micrognathia, cleft palate, dislocated hips, short forearms, and other minor skeletal anomalies. Reprinted with permission from Shaw EB, Steinbach HL: Am J Dis Child 115:477, 1968, American Medical Association, copyright 1969.[177]

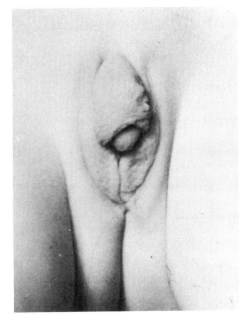

Fig. 7-21. Virilization of a female fetus caused by an androgen-producing maternal tumor.

Corticosteroids

Long-standing concern has existed regarding two potential prenatal effects of exogenous corticoids, cleft palate and adrenal atrophy.[180,181] One percent or less of infants of mothers receiving corticosteroids will have either of these effects. Importance must be attached, however, to even a low incidence of adrenal atrophy, since it may be life-threatening in the neonatal period. Additionally, the risk of stillbirth appears increased severalfold, perhaps to an adverse effect of corticoids on placental function.

Androgens

Masculinization of the female infant results from exposure to excessive androgen during pregnancy.[182–186] Androgens have been used during pregnancy for a variety of reasons, including prevention of abortion. There are currently no acceptable uses of androgens during pregnancy. Contemporary exposures to androgens are more likely to be from endogenous production by maternal tumors or from the use of progestational agents having androgenic activity.

Masculinization due to prenatal androgen exposure does not progress after birth, and some measure of regression may occur. Enlargement of the clitoris and labia majora results from androgen stimulation following formation of the genitalia; labial fusion and inhibition of uterovaginal descent to the perineum requires exposure prior to 10 weeks postfertilization (Fig. 7-21). The severity of these changes depends on the potency of the androgens and on the duration and period of gestation when used. Females exposed to androgen prenatally do not generally experience excessive growth but they may have advanced bone age. The possibility that changes in

genital development and bone maturation occur in males has not been investigated.

Progestins

Exogenous sex hormones have been used purposely and inadvertently during pregnancy. Progestin–estrogen combinations have been administered for several days in early gestation as a pregnancy confirmation test, and progesterone and various synthetic progestins have been given on a prolonged basis in an attempt to protect against abortion. Neither use is currently recommended. Estrogen and progestins, used sequentially or in combination as oral contraceptives, may be used for variable periods of time before pregnancy is recognized.

While progesterone lacks androgenic properties, certain synthetic progestins have sufficient androgenic activity to cause mild virilization in the user and, when used in pregnancy, to masculinize the female fetus.[183,184] Prenatal masculinization is not unlike that caused by maternally administered androgens, that is, manifested by labial fusion, persistence of the urogenital sinus, and enlargement of the clitoris and labia majora. The incidence of masculinization varies with the drug, dosage, timing, and duration of usage. Progestational agents that have been associated with fetal masculinization are listed in Table 7-3. The frequency of masculinization following norethindrone (Norlutin) exposure has been reported to be 18%; following ethisterone (Pranone) exposure, 13%; and following medroxyprogesterone (Provera) exposure, 1%.[1,183,184]

Considerable controversy has surrounded the question of whether progestins cause other malformations.[187–192] Several studies have demonstrated an association between progestins and conotruncal cardiac defects,[187,188,190,191] neural tube defects,[193] limb reduction defects,[187,189,194] esophageal atresia,[192] and the VACTERL malformations.[191] In general, these studies have shown a two- to fourfold increase in these malfor-

Table 7–3. Progestational agents that have been associated with fetal masculinization

17α-Ethynyltestosterone (ethisterone, Pranone)

17α-Ethynyl-19-nortestosterone (norethisterone, norethindrone, Norlutin)

17α-Ethynyl-19-nortestosterone acetate

17α-Ethynyl-17-hydroxy-4-estren-3-one + ethynylestradiol 3-methyl ether (norethindrone + mestranol, Ortho-Novum)

17α-Ethynyl-17-hydroxy-5(10)-estren-3-one + ethynylestradiol 3-methyl ether (norethynodrel + mestranol, Enovid)

17α-Hydroxy-6α-methyl-4-pregnene-3,20-dione acetate (medroxy-progesterone acetate, Provera)

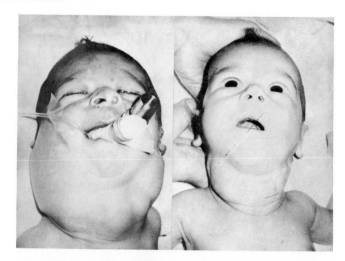

Fig. 7–22. Immense goiter (left) in infant born of mother taking iodides during pregnancy. The firm goiter compromised respiration. The infant also had hypothyroidism and cardiac failure but responded to thyroxin therapy. Goiter had greatly resolved by age 2 mo (right). Reprinted with permission from Senior B, Chernoff HL: Pediatrics 47:510, 1971.[201]

mations among infants born of pregnancies in which progestins were used as a pregnancy test, as protection against abortion, or as a birth control measure. Other studies have failed to find such associations.[195–197] Further experience is required to determine if there is a causal relationship between progestins and any malformation or whether the associations found in some studies are due to other factors.

Diethylstilbestrol

As many as 2–3 million pregnant women received the synthetic estrogen diethylstilbestrol over a 25 yr period prior to 1971.[198] In early pregnancy it was used primarily as prophylaxis against pregnancy loss in women who had experienced recurrent abortions. Alarm about prenatal diethylstilbestrol exposure came with the Herbst and Scully[199] report of vaginal adenocarcinoma in young women whose mothers had received the drug. Further studies have documented structural changes in the genital tract and abnormalities of menses; reproductive impairment may also be related to prenatal diethylstilbestrol exposure.

Over one-half of women exposed prenatally to diethylstilbestrol will have vaginal adenosis in which Müllerian mucosa persists over the cervix and upper vagina. Disorganization of the fibromuscular structure of the cervix produces irregular surface anatomy with ridges, protuberances, and sulci. The uterus may be hypoplastic with abnormal configuration and synechiae of the cavity. The Fallopian tubes are short and narrow, with short ostia and absent fimbria. These abnormalities contribute in part to excessive menstrual irregularities, impaired fertility, ectopic pregnancies, and preterm deliveries.

Approximately one-third of males exposed prenatally to diethylstilbestrol have some abnormality of the reproductive system.[200] These include small penis with hypospadias or meatal stenosis, cryptorchidism, small testes with induration of the capsule, and epididymal cysts. Impaired sperm production accompanies these structural changes.

Iodides

Inorganic iodides have been used as a mucolytic agent for various respiratory ailments and to suppress hyperfunction of the thyroid gland. Iodides readily cross the placenta and in excess can interfere with fetal thyroid function. Inhibition of organification, coupling of iodotyrosines, and release of thyroxin by the thyroid gland all contribute to the iodides' goitrogenic effect.

The massive fetal thyromegaly produced by iodides is unequaled by any other goitrogenic agent or disease.[201] The goiter may be sufficiently large to cause polyhydramnios prenatally and respiratory and alimentary obstruction postnatally (Fig. 7–22). Although no permanent thyroid dysfunction should be anticipated, transient hypothyroidism or, less commonly, hyperthyroidism can occur in the neonatal period.

Lithium

The major use of lithium salts in medicine is in the treatment of manic–depressive illness. Of 166 infants exposed to lithium during pregnancy (cases reported to the international Registry of Lithium Babies prior to 1976), 18 (10.8%) had malformations.[202] Thirteen of the malformed infants had cardiovascular malformations, and four of these were the Ebstein anomaly. Additionally, one of six stillborn infants in the series had tricuspid atresia. Thus there appears to be an increased risk of cardiovascular malformations, specifically those involving the tricuspid valve. Additionally, infants exposed to lithium may experience transient lethargy, hypotonia, cyanosis, poor feeding, and poor respiratory efforts during the early neonatal period.[203]

Mercury

Two serious incidents of food contamination with alkylated mercury, a potent neurotoxin, have occurred during the past three decades.[204,205] In both instances disturbances of neurologic function were documented in infants who were exposed prenatally. In the 1950s, methylmercury sulfide and methylmercury chloride were discharged in the Minamata Bay (Japan) by a vinylchloride and acetaldehyde plant.[204] Residents of the area who consumed large amounts of fish and shellfish from the polluted waters accumulated toxic levels of

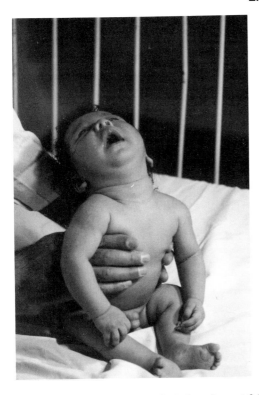

Fig. 7–23. Infant with marked neurologic impairment following prenatal exposure to the fungicide, methylmercury. Courtesy Dr. Sami Elhassani, Mary Black Hospital, Spartanburg, SC.

Table 7–4. Selected drugs and chemicals reported to have teratogenic effects.[a]

Drug/chemical	Reported effect on the fetus	Status
Agent Orange	Neural tube defects, various other anomalies	Unlikely
Angiotensin converting enzyme (ACE) inhibitors	Hypoplasia of skull, dysgenesis of renal tubules	Likely
Amphetamines	Cardiac defects, exencephaly, biliary atresia	Uncertain
Bendectin	Limb defects, pyloric stenosis, diaphragmatic hernia	Doubtful
Chlordiazepoxide	CNS defects	Doubtful
Clomiphene	Down syndrome, neural tube defects	Doubtful
Corticosteroids	Cleft lip/palate	Disproven
D-penicillamine	Connective tissue defects	Likely
Diazepam	Cleft lip/palate	Likely
Haloperidol	Limb reduction defects	Uncertain
Imipramine	Limb defects	Disproven
Lysergic acid diethylamide (LSD)	Limb, CNS, spine and renal defects	Disproven
Marijuana	Limb defects	Disproven
Meclizine	Clefting, limb defects	Doubtful
Meprobamate	Heart defects	Doubtful
Salicylates	Limb and cardiac defects, cleft lip/palate, anencephaly	Doubtful
Spermicides	Trisomies, limb reduction defects, hypospadias	Doubtful
Sulfonylureas	Limb, cardiac, diaphragmatic, ear, and other anomalies	Doubtful
Tetracycline	Limb reduction defects	Disproven

[a]From multiple sources.[1,2,4,208–212]

mercury and suffered neurologic impairments. Similar widespread exposure occurred in 1972 among rural Iraqis who ingested bread prepared from wheat treated with the fungicide methylmercury.[205] Prenatally exposed infants exhibited a wide range of neurologic abnormalities: mental retardation, speech and language delays, visual and hearing impairments, weakness, ataxia, gait disturbance, involuntary movements, swallowing dysfunction, hyperreflexia, and emotional lability (Fig. 7–23). Morphologic changes of the central nervous system included microcephaly, heterotropias, and other abnormalities of cytostructure. Irregular tooth size and malocclusions were also found in affected children.

Chlorobiphenyls

Epidemics of reversible skin eruptions due to the ingestion of cooking oil contaminated with polychlorinated biphenyls have occurred in Japan and Taiwan.[206,207] The persistence of these chemicals in tissues for a number of years has resulted in the prenatal exposure of many infants. Affected infants have lower birth weights, cutaneous and mucosal hyperpigmentation, gum hypertrophy, natal teeth, nail dystrophy, acne, and conjunctivitis. The generalized increase in mucocutaneous pigmentation (cola-colored babies) appears accentuated over the face and gums, digits and nails, and genitals. Neonatal acne resolves with or without scarring, but the hyperpigmentation persists. A minority of affected infants have ocular hypertelorism, flaring of the eyebrows, cranial hair loss, scalp calcifications, hirsutism, chipping of the teeth, clinodactyly, chronic respiratory infections, and developmental delay.

Other drugs

Questions about the safety of a number of drugs and other chemicals during pregnancy have been raised by retrospective studies and isolated case reports.[208–213] Some further investigations have failed to confirm any association between certain of these substances and adverse pregnancy outcome (Table 7–4). For other substances, the body of information remains insufficient to form reliable conclusions.

Mechanical forces

The maternal pelvis, abdominal wall, uterus, and amniotic fluid participate in protecting the conceptus against mechanical injury. Each becomes less protective as pregnancy advances. By midtrimester, the fetus lies outside the safety of the pelvis. The abdominal wall and the uterus become progressively thinner as the conceptus grows, and the ratio of amniotic fluid to mass of fetus decreases steadily. Prior to 8 weeks fertilization age, amniotic fluid makes up 95% of intraamniotic volume. The amniotic fluid component of in-

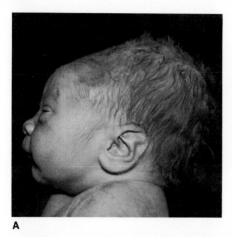
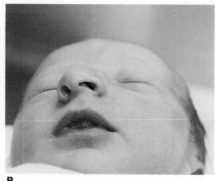
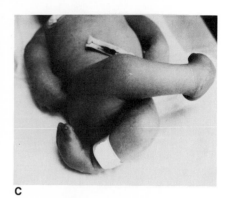

A   B   C

Fig. 7–24. Deformations caused by intrauterine mechanical forces. Cephalic molding (A) and nasal deformation (B) can occur from prolonged constraint in a malformed uterus or from the forces of delivery. Clubfoot and other limb deformations (C) occur from prolonged constraint. Fetuses with neuromuscular impairments are at greater risk for such deformations.

traamniotic volume decreases to one-half by 14 weeks and to one-third by 36 weeks. Some degree of intrinsic protection against mechanical injury may also be provided by the plasticity of embryonic and early fetal tissues and by their capacity to repair local damage.

Mechanical forces can alter prenatal development by direct trauma to tissues, by interruption of blood supply, by constraint, and by damaging the placenta or cord. About 6%–7% of women sustain physical injury during pregnancy.[214,215] Vehicle accidents account for the majority of such injuries, with falls, gunshots, stabbings, and physical abuse constituting other significant causes. Little role has been demonstrated for these external forces as a cause of malformation. Penetrating and blunt trauma can cause death by damaging the fetus, placenta, or cord. Rare instances of similar injury have resulted from amniocentesis.

A greater potential for mechanical alteration of morphology comes from within the mother. The same structures that surround and protect the conceptus against mechanical injury can, in certain circumstances, impose constraints detrimental to development.

Malformations of the uterus

The size of the intrauterine cavity and its ability to accommodate the growing conceptus may be limited by malformations of the uterus. Pregnancies in such cases are associated with greater risks of spontaneous abortion, malpresentation, stillbirth, and premature delivery. One-third of liveborn infants have craniofacial or limb deformations, evidence of late intrauterine constraint (Fig. 7–24).[216,217] Craniofacial asymmetry, excessive folding and flattening of the ears, flattening of the nose, joint contractures, and limb edema have been reported. Compression earlier in pregnancy can impair peripheral circulation, particularly in the limbs. Graham and associates[217] have attributed limb hypoplasia and various limb reduction abnormalities to early constraint caused by malformations of the uterus.

Fibroids

Because they occupy space in the uterine cavity, fibroids limit space for placentation and growth of the conceptus. Growth deficiency, deformations, and disruption of the limbs similar to those caused by compression in the malformed uterus have been reported.

Amnion

The amniotic system provides the innermost and perhaps the most substantial of the safeguards against prenatal mechanical injury. Within the amniotic membrane, the developing organism is suspended in an aqueous medium by a mobile and elastic cord, free of impingements that could impair symmetric growth or limit movement. Failure of this system can be catastrophic, causing a striking array of structural anomalies.

Inadequate production or chronic loss of amniotic fluid allows the uterus to compress the more pliable parts of the external fetal anatomy. Typically the facies are flattened, with depression of the tip of the nose and abnormal folding of the ears (Potter facies), the feet and hands are malpositioned, and the skin is excessively wrinkled (Fig. 7–25).[218–221] In the absence of amniotic fluid, the lungs remain underdeveloped and ill-prepared for neonatal respiratory function.

The amniotic membrane participates directly in the production of abnormalities through several mechanisms.[219–221] Strips of amnion may separate partially or completely from the amniotic membrane and become suspended in the amniotic fluid. These amniotic bands may encircle digits or entire limbs, eventually compromising blood supply to the distal part. Growth and development of limbs thus entangled may become disrupted, with residual constriction rings, syndactyly, and amputations (Fig. 7–26).

Bands of amnion may also be swallowed. If the band is attached to the amniotic membrane, the fetus becomes tethered and through continued swallowing efforts pulls itself to the point of attachment. The strong amniotic tether can cut into orofacial structures, leaving clefts unrelated to lines of embryonic fusion (Fig. 7–27). Bizarre lobation of the cranium can result from twisting of the fetus, and cranial tissues can fuse to the amnion and placenta.

In other circumstances, the amnion may rupture, collapsing more or less in toto about the embryo or fetus. This blanket of amnion deprives the developing organism of free

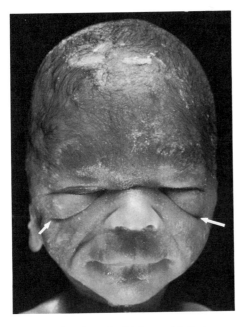
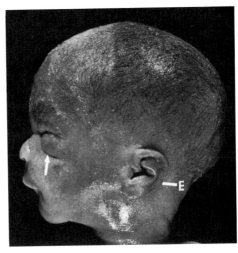

Fig. 7-25. Facial features of a 23-week-old fetus with Potter syndrome secondary to type IIB cystic dysplasia. Note the prominent lower palpebral folds (arrows), flattening of the nose, and low-set and flattened ears (E). Courtesy Dr. Will Blackburn and N. Reede Cooley, Jr, University of South Alabama College of Medicine, Mobile.

movement and holds it close to its placental attachment. Anomalies related to amnion rupture depend on the time of rupture, the presence of amniotic bands, the degree of compression exerted by surrounding structures, and the occurrence of adhesions. Amnion rupture during the period of embryogenesis presumably causes malformations through adhesions and compression of the gelatinous embryonic tissues. Later amnion rupture disrupts structures already formed through direct compression and vascular compromise of exposed parts. Graham and associates[217] include limb reduction defects, body wall deficiencies, neural tube defects, postural deformations, scoliosis, and growth deficiency among the effects of acute or prolonged compression related to amnion rupture. Affected infants may also have band-related anomalies and short umbilical cords.

Twins

The human uterus has a limited capacity to accommodate twins and other multiple pregnancies. Mechanical forces undoubtedly contribute in some measure to the increased risk of growth deficiency, prenatal and postnatal mortality, malformations, disruptions, deformations, and premature delivery in such pregnancies (see Volume II, Chapter 36).[222,223] Fetal growth is influenced by the number of fetuses present. The growth deceleration that occurs at about 36 weeks in sin-

Fig. 7-26. Amniotic bands. Left and middle: fetus with ring constrictions, digital fusions, and amputations secondary to amniotic bands. Note string of amnion attached to dorsal aspect of digits. Right: ring constrictions and amputations in a 27-yr-old man.

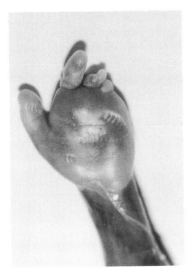
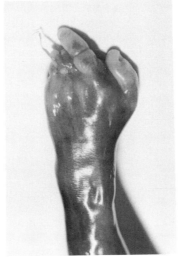
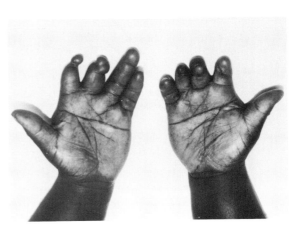

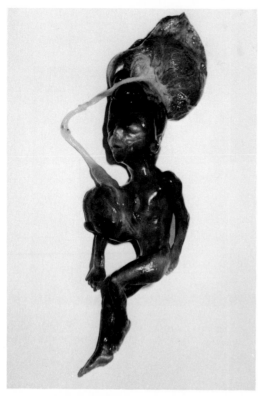

Fig. 7–27. Amniotic rupture and bands in two fetuses. Left: unusual cranial lobation, fusion of cranium to placenta, and ompha-locele. Right: cleft lip, cranial fusion to placenta, and digital amputations with amniotic bands between right hand and placenta.

gletons takes place at about 30 weeks in twins, 27 weeks in triplets, and 26 weeks in quadruplets (Fig. 7–28).[224] Some contribution to growth deficiency in twins may be related to mechanical constraint, but the greater influence must be assigned to placental function. Constraint is likely the major contributor to craniofacial and limb deformations in twins. Although there is increased risk of malformations and dis-

Fig. 7–28. Growth curves from 24 weeks to term for singletons, twins, triplets, and quadruplets. Adapted from McKeown and Record.[224]

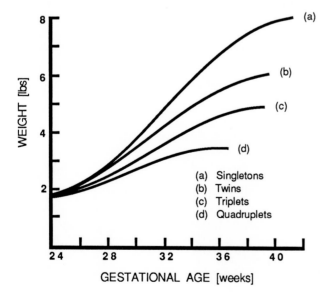

ruptions in twins, these have been related to other factors, usually vascular, rather than mechanical, forces.

Immunologic influences

The extent to which immunologic processes influence human development is not known. A growing body of information implicates immune mechanisms as an important cause of infertility.[225–227] Certain maternal immunologic diseases, notably lupus erythematosus, are associated with excessive pregnancy wastage. The possibility that subclinical disease contributes in some substantial way to pregnancy loss overall cannot be dismissed. Maternal antibodies transferred transplacentally can interfere with a wide variety of systemic functions in the fetus and continue for variable periods postnatally. The role of immune processes in causing congenital anomalies is less clear. Prenatal immunologic influences may be mediated by direct attack on tissues of the conceptus, particularly the placenta, by transplacental transfer of globulins that may attack fetal cells from within, and by transfer of immunocompetent cells that provide a nidus for initiating graft versus host disease.

Rh isoimmunization

Hydrops fetalis is the end result of severe fetal involvement by Rh isoimmunization. The preceding cascade of events is initiated by Rh-positive fetal erythrocytes gaining entry into the circulation of a previously sensitized Rh-negative mother (Fig. 7–29).[228] Maternal IgG antibodies to the Rh antigens

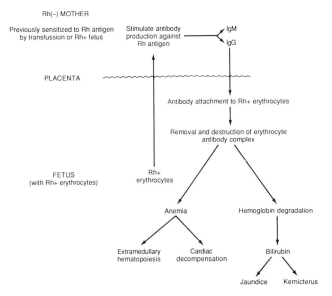

Fig. 7-29. Schematic showing events leading to Rh disease of the fetus (erythroblastosis fetalis).

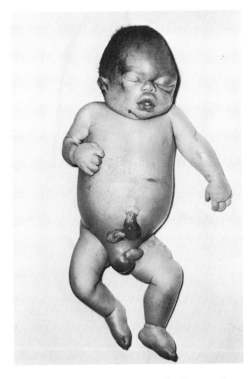

Fig. 7-30. Newborn infant with hydrops fetalis secondary to Rh incompatibility.

cross the placenta and attach to fetal erythrocytes. Destruction of these erythrocytes, primarily by the spleen, causes anemia. When the fetal hematopoietic response cannot compensate for the anemia, cardiac failure and universal edema ensue (Fig. 7-30). Fetomaternal incompatibility for erythrocyte antigens other than the Rh and ABO antigens can also cause hemolytic disease, but prenatal hemolysis sufficient to produce hydrops fetalis is distinctly uncommon.[229]

ABO incompatibility

Fetomaternal incompatibility for ABO antigens is the most common blood group incompatibility, occurring in 20% of pregnancies.[1] Only a small percentage of ABO incompatible pregnancies results in fetal hemolysis, this occurring most commonly in A or B fetuses of mothers with blood group O. Fetal hemolysis is rarely sufficient to stress the cardiovascular system and never leads to hydrops fetalis.

Platelet isoimmunization

Maternal antibodies against fetal platelets can lead to prenatal and transient postnatal thrombocytopenia.[230] The hazard of hemorrhage, particularly intracranial, appears to be greatest during the perinatal period. Prenatal hemorrhage and infarction can occur, however, with residual hydrocephaly and porencephaly.

Thyroid antibodies

A number of thyroid antibodies have been described and are widely used for diagnostic purposes.[231,232] At least two types of thyroid antibodies can influence fetal thyroid function. Thyroid-stimulating immunoglobulins bind the thyroid-stimulating hormone receptor and stimulate thyroid function. These antibodies are present in Graves disease, are 7S in size, cross the placenta, and can stimulate the fetal thyroid.

Affected fetuses develop goiter and hyperthyroidism, which may persist for several weeks or months postnatally.

A second type of thyroid antibody is inhibitory in nature. This antibody also binds to the thyroid-stimulating hormone receptor but blocks thyroid function, producing hypothyroidism. This blocking immunoglobulin also crosses the placenta and may cause cretinism in the fetus. Although the thyroid gland may not be visible on radioactive scanning during the early months of life, thyroid function will return once the antibodies have dissipated, generally a matter of several months.

Lupus erythematosus

A potentially serious disorder may be seen at birth or soon thereafter in a minority of infants of mothers with systemic lupus erythematosus. Congenital heart block, hepatosplenomegaly, lupus erythematosus rash, and pancytopenia are the major features.[233,234] The hematologic findings resolve over the first couple of months and the rash by 6 months. Heart block becomes manifest by bradycardia before or after delivery and is permanent. One-third of infants with heart block also have cardiac malformations and endocardial fibroelastosis. An excessive frequency of abortion and stillbirth also occurs in women who have lupus erythematosus.

Although two-thirds of mothers of affected infants are asymptomatic, Ro antibodies (antibody to Sjögren syndrome A antigen) will usually be present in mothers and infants. Antinuclear antibody and La antibody (antibody to Sjögren syndrome B antigen) may be present as well. Some individuals with this self-limited syndrome in the neonatal period develop other signs of systemic lupus erythematosus in adolescence or early adulthood.

Pemphigus vulgaris

Infants of mothers with pemphigus vulgaris may have bullous or erosive lesions at birth, presumably the result of transplacentally acquired pemphigus antibodies.[235] Skin lesions are typical of pemphigus vulgaris, having acantholytic cells, neutrophils, eosinophils, and blisters above the basal layer and leukocyte infiltrates deeper in the dermis. IgG and C3 are deposited in the intercellular spaces of the dermis. Some infants are small for gestational age, and the risk of stillbirth appears to be increased. Liveborn infants generally have a benign course, with spontaneous and permanent resolution of the skin lesions within the initial couple of weeks of life.

Myasthenia gravis

Ten percent of infants born of mothers with myasthenia gravis will exhibit signs of myasthenia during the initial weeks of life.[1,236] These infants are inactive, have hypotonia, and suck, cry, and swallow poorly. Although the face is expressionless, ptosis and ocular motor palsies do not usually occur. Most infants have no structural anomalies, although deformations due to fetal inactivity have been reported. Transplacental passage of antimuscle antibodies or other humoral factors have been suspected but not proven to be the cause of transient neonatal myasthenia gravis.

Engraftment of foreign cells

Three possibilities exist for fetal exposure to foreign immunocompetent cells. Maternal cells may gain access to the fetal circulation through leaks in the villous membrane or through fetomaternal vascular anastomoses. In twin pregnancies, vascular anastomoses in the placenta may allow sharing of bood cells. This usually occurs only in monozygotic twins; hence the admixing of cells is with the same genotype. Intrauterine transfusion in the treatment of fetal anemia can also be the source of foreign cells. Establishment of the viable grafts from each of these sources has occurred.[237-241] Although immunodeficiency of the fetal host has been documented or suspected in most cases of intrauterine engraftment with foreign cells, viable grafts have occurred in apparently normal fetuses. Graft versus host disease has occurred only in instances of intrauterine engraftment of maternal cells. Ill effects from graft versus host disease usually develop after birth, but some affected infants are growth deficient, with pancytopenia and scaling dermatitis at birth. Malformations have not been associated with intrauterine engraftment of foreign cells.

References

1. Stevenson RE: The Fetus and Newly Born Infant, ed 2. CV Mosby, St. Louis, 1977.
2. Shepard TH: Catalog of Teratogenic Agents, ed 6. Johns Hopkins University Press, Baltimore, 1989.
3. Kalter H, Warkany J: Congenital malformations: etiologic factors and their role in prevention. N Engl J Med 308:424, 491, 1983.
4. Sever JL, Brent RL: Teratogen Update: Environmentally Induced Birth Defect Risks. Alan R Liss, Inc, New York, 1986.
5. Wilson JG: Current status of teratology: general principles and mechanisms derived from animal studies. In Handbook of Teratology, vol 1. JG Wilson, FC Fraser, eds. Plenum, New York, 1977, p 47.
6. Trasler DG: Strain differences in susceptibility to teratogenesis: survey of spontaneously occurring malformations in mice. In Teratology. JG Wilson, J Warkany, eds. University of Chicago Press, Chicago, 1965, p 38.
7. Fraser FC: The genetics of cleft lip and cleft palate. Am J Hum Genet 22:336, 1970.
8. Brent RL: Radiation teratogenesis. Teratology 21:281, 1980.
9. Penfil RL, Brown ML: Genetically significant dose to the United States population from diagnostic medical roentgenology, 1964. Radiology 90:209, 1968.
10. Goldstein L, Murphy DP: Etiology of the ill-health in children born after maternal pelvic irradiation. Part II. Defective children born after postconception pelvic radiation. Am J Roentgenol 22:322, 1929.
11. Dekaban A: Abnormalities in children exposed to X-radiation injury to the human fetus. Part 1. J Nucl Med 9:471, 1968.
12. Murphy DP: The outcome of 625 pregnancies in women subjected to pelvic radium or roentgen irradiation. Am J Obstet Gynecol 18:179, 1929.
13. Mayer MD, Harris W, Wimpfheimer S: Therapeutic abortion by means of X-ray. Am J Obstet Gynecol 32:945, 1936.
14. Neel JV, Satoh C, Goriki K, et al.: Search for mutations altering protein charge and/or function in children of atomic bomb survivors: final report. Am J Hum Genet 42:663, 1988.
15. Russell KP, Rose H, Starr P: Maternal and fetal thyroid function during pregnancy. Surg Obstet Gynecol 104:560, 1957.
16. Fisher WD, Voorhess ML, Gardner LI: Congenital hypothyroidism in infant following maternal I-131 therapy. J Pediatr 62:132, 1963.
17. Tabuchi A: Fetal disorders due to ionizing radiation. Hiroshima J Med Sci 13:125, 1964.
18. Brent RL: The effect of embryonic and fetal exposure to X-ray, microwaves, and ultrasound: counseling the pregnant and nonpregnant patient about these risks. Semin Oncol 16:347, 1989.
19. Brent RL: Radiations and other physical agents. In Handbook of Teratology, vol 1. JG Wilson, FC Fraser, eds. Plenum, New York, 1977, p 153.
20. Goldhaber MK, Polen MR, Hiatt RA: The risk of miscarriage and birth defects among women who use video display terminals during pregnancy. Am J Indust Med 13:695, 1988.
21. Carstensen EL, Gates AH: The effects of ultrasound on the fetus. J Ultrasound Med 3:145, 1984.
22. McLeod DR, Fowlow SB: Multiple malformations and exposure to therapeutic ultrasound during organogenesis. Am J Med Genet 34:317, 1989.
23. Miller P, Smith DW, Shepard TH: Maternal hyperthermia as a possible cause of anencephaly. Lancet 1:519, 1978.
24. Clarren SK, Smith DW, Harvey MAS, et al.: Hyperthermia—a prospective evaluation of a possible teratogenic agent in man. J Pediatr 95:81, 1979.
25. Pleet H, Graham JMJ, Smith DW: Central nervous system and facial defects associated with maternal hyperthermia at four to 14 weeks' gestation. Pediatrics 67:785, 1981.
26. Edwards MJ: Congenital defects in guinea pigs: fetal resorptions, abortions, and malformations following induced hyperthermia during early gestation. Teratology 2:313, 1969.
27. Supernau DW, Wertelecki W: Brief clinical report: similarity of effects—experimental hyperthermia as a teratogen and maternal febrile illness associated with oromandibular and limb defects. Am J Med Genet 21:575, 1985.
28. Lipson AH, Webster WS, Brown-Woodman PDC, et al.: Mobius syndrome: animal model—human correlations and evidence for a brainstem vascular etiology. Teratology 40:339, 1989.
29. Krugman S, Gershon AA: Infections of the Fetus and the Newborn Infant. Alan R Liss, Inc., New York, 1975.
30. Monif GRG: Viral Infections of the Human Fetus. Macmillan, London, 1969.
31. Hanshaw JB, Dudgeon JA: Viral Diseases of the Fetus and Newborn. WB Saunders, Philadelphia, 1978.
32. Kurent JE, Sever JL: Infectious diseases. In Handbook of Teratology. JG Wilson, FC Fraser, eds. Plenum, New York, 1977, p 225.
33. Medearis DN: Observations concerning human cytomegalovirus infection and disease. Bull Johns Hopkins Hosp 114:181, 1964.
34. Reynolds DW, Stagno S, Stubbs KG: Inapparent congenital cytomegalovirus infection with elevated cord IgM levels. N Engl J Med 290:291, 1974.
35. Stern H, Tucker SM: Prospective study of cytomegalovirus infection in pregnancy. Br Med J 1:268, 1973.

36. Schaffer AJ: Diseases of the Newborn, ed 2. WB Saunders, Philadelphia, 1966.

37. South MA, Thompkins WAF, Morris CR, et al.: Congenital malformation of the central nervous system associated with genital type (type 2) herpes virus. J Pediatr 75:13, 1969.

38. Alkalay AL, Pomerance JJ, Rimoin DL: Fetal varicella syndrome. J Pediatr 111:320, 1987.

39. Paryani SG, Arvin AM: Intrauterine infection with varicella-zoster virus after maternal varicella. N Engl J Med 314:1542, 1986.

40. Abler C: Neonatal varicella. Am J Dis Child 107:492, 1964.

41. Coffey VP, Jessop WJE: Maternal influenza and congenital deformities: a prospective study. Lancet 2:935, 1959.

42. Shone JD, Armas SM, Manning JA: The mumps antigen test in endocardial fibroelastosis. Pediatrics 37:423, 1966.

43. Cooper LZ, Ziring PR, Ockerse AB, et al.: Rubella: clinical manifestations and management. Am J Dis Child 118:18, 1969.

44. Monif GRG, Hardy JB, Sever JL: Studies in congenital rubella, Baltimore 1964–65. Bull Johns Hopkins Hosp 118:85, 97, 1966.

45. Desmond MM, Wilson GS, Melnick JL, et al.: Congenital rubella encephalitis. J Pediatr 71:311, 1967.

46. Chiriboga-Klein S, Oberfield SE, Casullo AM, et al.: Growth in congenital rubella syndrome and correlation with chemical manifestations. J Pediatr 115:251, 1989.

47. Gregg NM: Congenital cataract following German measles in the mother. Trans Ophthalmol Soc Aust 3:35, 1941.

48. Rodis JF, Hovick TJJ, Quinn DL, et al.: Human parvovirus infection in pregnancy. Obstet Gynecol 72:733, 1988.

49. Oleske J, Minnefor A, Cooper RJ, et al.: Immune deficiency syndrome in children. JAMA 249:2345, 1983.

50. Rubinstein A, Sicklick M, Gupta A, et al.: Acquired immunodeficiency with reversed T4–T8 ratios in infants born to promiscuous and drug-addicted mothers. JAMA 249:2350, 1983.

51. Scott GB, Buck BE, Leterman JG, et al.: Acquired immunodeficiency syndrome in infants. N Engl J Med 310:76, 1984.

52. Marion RW, Wiznia AA, Hutcheon RG, et al.: Human T-cell lymphotropic virus type III (HTLV-III) embryopathy. Am J Dis Child 140:638, 1986.

53. Iosub S, Bamji M, Stone RK, et al.: More on human immunodeficiency virus embryopathy. Pediatrics 80:512, 1987.

54. Brown GC, Evans TN: Serologic evidence of coxsackievirus etiology of congenital heart disease. JAMA 199:183, 1967.

55. Gauntt CG, Gudvangen RJ, Brans YW, et al.: Coxsackievirus group B antibodies in the ventricular fluid of infants with severe anatomic defects in the central nervous system. Pediatrics 76:64, 1985.

56. Gear J: Coxsackie virus infections in Southern Africa. Yale J Biol Med 34:289, 1961.

57. Manson MM, Logan WPD, Loy RM: Rubella and other virus infections during pregnancy. In Ministry of Health: Reports on Public Health and Medical Subjects. No. 101. Her Majesty's Stationery Office, London, 1960.

58. Green DM, Reid SM, Rhaney K: Generalized vaccinia in the human fetus. Lancet 1:1296, 1966.

59. Moss PD, Heffernan CK, Thurston JG: Enteroviruses and congenital abnormalities. Br Med J 1:110, 1967.

60. Siegel M, Greenberg M: Poliomyelitis in pregnancy. Effect on fetus and newborn infant. J Pediatr 49:280, 1956.

61. Lin HH, Lee TY, Chen DS, et al.: Transplacental leakage of HBeAg-positive maternal blood as the most likely route in causing intrauterine infection with hepatitis B virus. J Pediatr 111:877, 1987.

62. Ryan GMJ, Abdella TN, McNeeley SG, et al.: *Chlamydia trachomatis* infection in pregnancy and effect of treatment on outcome. Am J Obstet Gynecol 162:34, 1990.

63. Naessens A, Foulon W, Breynaert J, et al.: Postpartum bacteremia and placental colonization with genital mycoplasmas and pregnancy outcome. Am J Obstet Gynecol 160:647, 1989.

64. Braun P, Lee Y-H, Klein JO, et al.: Birth weight and genital mycoplasmas in pregnancy. N Engl J Med 284:167, 1971.

65. Monif GRG: Infectious Diseases in Obstetrics and Gynecology. Harper & Row, Hagerstown, MD, 1974.

66. Ewing CI, Roberts C, Davidson DC, et al.: Early congenital syphilis still occurs. Arch Dis Child 60:1128, 1985.

67. Centers for Disease Control: Summary of notifiable diseases, United States, 1988. MMWR 37:38, 1989.

68. Harter CA, Benirschke K: Fetal syphilis in the first trimester. Am J Obstet Gynecol 124:705, 1976.

69. Putkonen T: Does early treatment prevent dental changes in congenital syphilis? Acta Derm Venereol (Stockh) 43:240, 1963.

70. Bulova SI, Schwartz E, Harrer WV: Hydrops fetalis and congenital syphilis. Pediatr 49:285, 1972.

71. Murphy FK, Patamasucon P: Congenital syphilis. In Sexually Transmitted Diseases. KK Holmes, P-A Mardh, PF Sparling, PJ Wiesner, eds. McGraw-Hill, New York, 1984, p 352.

72. Lindsay S, Luke IW: Fatal leptospirosis (Weil's disease) in a newborn infant. J Pediatr 34:90, 1949.

73. MacDonald AB: Gestational Lyme borreliosis. Rheum Dis Clin North Am 15:657, 1989.

74. Bruner JP, Elliott JP, Kilbride HW, et al.: *Candida* chorioamnionitis diagnosed at amniocentesis with subsequent fetal infection. Am J Perinatol 3:213, 1986.

75. Sever JL, Ellenberg JH, Ley AC, et al.: Toxoplasmosis: maternal and pediatric findings in 23,000 pregnancies. Pediatrics 82:181, 1988.

76. Eichenwald HF: A study of congenital toxoplasmosis. In Human Toxoplasmosis. Ejnar Munksgaards Forlag, Copenhagen, 1960, p 41.

77. Saxon SA, Knight W, Reynolds DW, et al.: Intellectual deficits in children born with subclinical congenital toxoplasmosis: A preliminary report. J Pediatr 82:792, 1973.

78. Covell G: Congenital malaria. Trop Dis Bull 47:1147, 1950.

79. Farquhar JW: The child of the diabetic woman. Arch Dis Child 34:76, 1959.

80. North AFJ, Mazumdar S, Logrillo VM: Birthweight, gestational age, and perinatal deaths in 5,471 infants of diabetic mothers. J Pediatr 90:444, 1977.

81. Naeye RL: Infants of diabetic mothers: a quantitative, morphologic study. Pediatrics 35:1980, 1965.

82. Farquhar JW: Prognosis for babies born to diabetic mothers in Edinburgh. Arch Dis Child 44:36, 1969.

83. Pedersen LM, Tygstrup I, Pederson J: Congenital malformations in newborn infants of diabetic women: correlation with maternal diabetic vascular complications. Lancet 1:1124, 1964.

84. Lucas MJ, Leveno KJ, Williams ML: Early pregnancy glycosylated hemoglobin, severity of diabetes, and fetal malformations. Am J Obstet Gynecol 161:426, 1989.

85. Mills JL: Malformations in infants of diabetic mothers. In Teratogen Update: Environmentally Induced Birth Defect Risks. JL Sever, RL Brent, eds. Alan R Liss, Inc, New York, 1986, p 165.

86. Lowett RM, Schwartz R: The infant of the diabetic mother. Pediatr Clin North Am 29:1213, 1982.

87. Becerra JE, Khoury MJ, Cordero JF, et al.: Diabetes mellitus during pregnancy and the risks for specific birth defects: a population based case–control study. Pediatrics 85:1, 1990.

88. Siegler AM: Pregnancy and cretinism: report of a case and review of the literature. Obstet Gynecol 8:639, 1956.

89. Jones WS, Man EB: Thyroid function in human pregnancy. VI. Premature deliveries and reproductive failures of pregnant women with low serum butanol-extractable iodines. Maternal serum TBG and TBPA capacities. Am J Obstet Gynecol 104:909, 1969.

90. Burrow GN, Bartsocas C, Klatskin EH, et al.: Children exposed in utero to propylthiouracil: subsequent intellectual and physical development. Am J Dis Child 116:161, 1968.

91. Sutherland JM, Esselborn VM, Burket RL, et al.: Familial nongoitrous cretinism apparently due to maternal antithyroid antibody. N Engl J Med 263:336, 1960.

92. Landing BH, Kamoshita S: Congenital hyperparathyroidism secondary to maternal hypoparathyroidism. J Pediatr 77:842, 1970.

93. Smithells RW, Sheppard S, Schorah CJ: Vitamin levels and neural tube defects. Arch Dis Child 51:944, 1959.

94. Smithells RW, Nevin NC, Seller MJ, et al.: Further experience of vitamin supplementation for prevention of NTD recurrences. Lancet 1:1027, 1983.

95. Smithells RW, Sheppard S, Wild J, et al.: Prevention of neural tube defect recurrence in Yorkshire: Final report. Lancet 2:498, 1989.

96. Laurence KM, James N, Miller MH, et al.: Double-blind randomised controlled trial of folate treatment before conception to prevent recurrence of neural tube defects. Br Med J 282:1509, 1981.

97. Mulinare J, Cordero JF, Erickson JD, et al.: Periconceptional use of multivitamins and the occurrence of neural tube defects. JAMA 260:3141, 1988.

98. Milunsky A, Jick H, Jick SS, et al.: Multivitamin/folic acid supplementation in early pregnancy reduces the prevalence of neural tube defects. JAMA 262:2847, 1989.

99. Mills JL, Rhoads GG, Simpson JL, et al.: The absence of a relation between the periconceptional use of vitamins and neural-tube defects. N Engl J Med 321:430, 1989.

100. Pritchard JA, Scott DE, Whalley PJ, et al.: Infants of mothers with megaloblastic anemia due to folate deficiency. JAMA 211:1982, 1970.

101. MRC Vitamin Study Research Group: Prevention of neural tube defects: results of the Medical Research Council Vitamin Study. Lancet 338:131, 1991.

102. Maxwell JP: Further studies in adult rickets (osteomalacia) and foetal rickets. Proc R Soc Med 28:265, 1934.

103. Pitkin RM: Calcium metabolism in pregnancy and the perinatal period: a review. Am J Obstet Gynecol 151:99, 1985.

104. Held KR, Cruz ME, Moncayo F: Clinical pattern and genetics of the fetal iodine deficiency disorder (endemic cretinism): results of a field study in highland Ecuador. Am J Med Genet 35:85, 1990.

105. Bureau MA, Shapcott D, Berthiaume Y, et al.: Maternal cigarette smoking and fetal oxygen transport: a study of P50, 2,3-diphosphoglycerate, total hemoglobin, hematocrit and type F hemoglobin in fetal blood. Pediatrics 72:22, 1983.

106. Gordon M, Niswander KR, Berendes H, et al.: Fetal morbidity following potentially anoxigenic obstetric conditions. VII. Bronchial asthma. Am J Obstet Gynecol 106:421, 1970.

107. Neill CA, Swanson S, Hellegers AE: Cyanotic congenital heart disease in pregnancy. In Intrauterine Development. AC Barnes, ed. Lea & Febiger, Philadelphia, 1968.

108. Anderson M, Went LN, MacIver JE, et al.: Sickle-cell disease in pregnancy. Lancet 2:516, 1960.

109. Ballew C, Haas JD: Hematologic evidence of fetal hypoxia among newborn infants at high altitude in Bolivia. Am J Obstet Gynecol 155:166, 1986.

110. Yip R: Altitude and birth weight. J Pediatr 111:869, 1987.

111. Alzamora V, Rotta A, Battilana G, et al.: On the possible influence of great altitudes on the determination of certain cardiovascular anomalies. Pediatr 12:259, 1953.

112. Johnson GT: Comments in Non-toxaemic Hypertension in Pregnancy. NF Morris, JCM Browne, eds. Churchill, London, 1958, p 60.

113. Jacobson BB, Terslev E, Lund B, et al.: Neonatal hypocalcemia associated with maternal hyperparathyroidism. Arch Dis Child 53:308, 1978.

114. Green WL: Humoral and genetic factors in thyrotoxic Graves disease and neonatal thyrotoxicosis. JAMA 235:1449, 1976.

115. Burrow GN: The management of thyrotoxicosis in pregnancy. N Engl J Med 313:562, 1985.

116. Davis LE, Lucas MJ, Hankins GDV, et al.: Thyrotoxicosis complicating pregnancy. Am J Obstet Gynecol 160:63, 1989.

117. Sunshine P, Kusumoto H, Kriss JP: Survival time of circulating long-acting thyroid stimulator in neonatal thyrotoxicosis: implications for diagnosis and therapy of the disorder. Pediatrics 36:869, 1965.

118. Nutt J, Clark F, Welch RG, et al.: Neonatal hyperthyroidism and long-acting thyroid stimulator protector. Br Med J 2:695, 1974.

119. Stevenson RE, Trent HW III: Maternal hyperthyroidism and congenital craniosynostosis. Proc Greenwood Genet Center 9:3, 1990.

120. Hollingsworth DR, Mabry CC, Eckerd JM: Hereditary aspects of Graves' disease in infancy and childhood. J Pediatr 81:446, 1972.

121. Koerten JM, Morales WJ, Washington, SR III, et al.: Cushing's syndrome in pregnancy: a case report and literature review. Am J Obstet Gynecol 154:626, 1986.

122. Kolodny RC: Herpes gestationis. Am J Obstet Gynecol 104:39, 1969.

123. Mabry CC, Denniston JC, Coldwell JG: Mental retardation in children of phenylketonuric mothers. N Engl J Med 275:1331, 1966.

124. Stevenson RE, Huntley CC: Congenital malformations in offspring of phenylketonuric mothers. Pediatr 40:33, 1967.

125. Lenke RR, Levy HL: Maternal phenylketonuria and hyperphenylalaninemia. N Engl J Med 303:1202, 1980.

126. Mahon BE, Levy HL: Maternal Hartnup disorder. Am J Med Genet 24:513, 1986.

127. Stevenson RE, Taylor HA: Pregnancy and pyridoxine-responsive homocystinuria. Proc Greenwood Genet Center 3:47, 1984.

128. Harper PS, Dyken PR: Early-onset dystrophia myotonica: evidence supporting a maternal environmental factor. Lancet 2:53, 1972.

129. Brook JD, McCurrach ME, Harley HG, et al.: Molecular basis of myotonic dystrophy: expansion of a trinucleotide (CTG) repeat at the 3' end of a transcript encoding a protein kinase family member. Cell 68:799, 1992.

130. Hall JG: Genomic imprinting. Arch Dis Child 65:1013, 1990.

131. Rosa FW, Wilk AL, Kelsey FO: Teratogen update: vitamin A congeners. Teratology 33:355, 1986.

132. Black JA: Review—idiopathic hypercalcemia and vitamin D. Ger Med Monthly 9:290, 1964.

133. Daeschner GL, Daeschner CW: Severe idiopathic hypercalcemia of infancy. Pediatr 19:362, 1967.

134. Antia AU, Wiltse HE, Rowe RD, et al.: Pathogenesis of the supravalvular aortic stenosis syndrome. J Pediatr 71:431, 1967.

135. Werler MM, Pober BR, Holmes LB: Smoking and Pregnancy. In Teratogen Update: Environmentally Induced Birth Defect Risks. JL Sever, RL Brent, eds. Alan R Liss, Inc, New York, 1986, p 131.

136. Naeye R, Harkness W, Utts J: The duration of maternal cigarette smoking, fetal and placental disorders. Early Hum Dev 3:229, 1979.

137. MacMahon B, Alpert M, Salber EJ: Infant weight and parental smoking habits. Am J Epidemiol 82:247, 1966.

138. Underwood P, Hester LL, Lafitte TJ, et al.: The relationship of smoking to the outcome of pregnancy. Am J Obstet Gynecol 91:270, 1965.

139. Jones KL, Smith DW, Ulleland CN, et al.: Pattern of malformation in offspring of chronic alcoholic mothers. Lancet 1:1267, 1973.

140. Warner RH, Rossett HL: The effects of drinking on offspring: an historical survey of the American and British literature. J Stud Alcohol 36:1395, 1975.

141. Lemoine P, Harousseau H, Borteyru J, et al.: Children of alcoholic parents: abnormalities observed in 127 cases. Quest Med 21:476, 1968.

142. Jones KL: The fetal alcohol syndrome. Growth Gen Horm 4:1, 1988.

143. Hadeed AJ, Siegel SR: Maternal cocaine use during pregnancy: effect on the newborn infant. Pediatrics 84:205, 1989.

144. Chasnoff IJ, Chisom GM, Kaplan WE: Maternal cocaine use and genitourinary tract malformations. Teratology 37:201, 1988.

145. Fulroth R, Phillips B, Durand DJ: Perinatal outcome of infants exposed to cocaine and/or heroin in utero. Am J Dis Child 143:905, 1989.

146. Bingol N, Fuchs M, Diaz V, et al.: Teratogenicity of cocaine in humans. J Pediatr 110:93, 1987.

147. Hingson R, Alpert JJ, Day N, et al.: Effects of maternal drinking and marijuana use on fetal growth and development. Pediatrics 70:539, 1982.

148. Long SY: Does LSD induce chromosomal damage and malformations? A review of the literature. Teratology 6:75, 1972.

149. Melchior JD, Svensmark O, Trolle D: Placental transfer of phenobarbitone in epileptic women, and elimination in newborns. Lancet 2:860, 1967.

150. Meadow WR: Congenital abnormalities and anticonvulsant drugs. Proc R Soc Med 63:48, 1970.

151. Kelly TE: Teratogenicity of anticonvulsant drugs. Am J Med Genet 19:413, 435, 445, 451, 1984.

152. Hill RM, Verniaud WM, Horning MG, et al.: Infants exposed in utero to antiepileptic drugs: a prospective study. Am J Dis Child 127:645, 1974.

153. Hanson JW, Smith DW: The fetal hydantoin syndrome. J Pediatr 87:285, 1975.

154. Hanson JW, Myrianthoupoulos NC, Harvey MAS, et al.: Risks to offspring of women treated with hydantoin anticonvulsants with emphasis on the fetal hydantoin syndrome. J Pediatr 89:662, 1976.

155. Zackai EH, Mellman WJ, Neiderer B, et al.: The fetal trimethadione syndrome. J Pediatr 87:280, 1975.

156. Robert E: Valproic acid and spina bifida: a preliminary report—France. MMWR 31:565, 1982.

157. DiLiberti JH, Farnon PA, Dennis NR, et al.: The fetal valproate syndrome. Am J Med Genet 19:473, 1984.

158. Hardinger HH, Atkin JF, Blackston RD, et al.: Verification of the fetal valproate syndrome phenotype. Am J Med Genet 29:171, 1988.

159. Jones KL, Lacro RV, Johnson KA, et al.: Pattern of malformations in the children of women treated with carbamazepine during pregnancy. N Engl J Med 320:1661, 1989.

160. Niswander KR, Gordon M: The Women and Their Pregnancies. WB Saunders, Philadelphia, 1972, p 246.

161. Refetoff S, Ochi Y, Selenkow HA, et al.: Neonatal hypothyroidism

and goiter in one infant of each of two sets of twins due to maternal therapy with antithyroid drugs. J Pediatr 85:240, 1974.

162. Milham SJ: Scalp defects in infants of mothers treated for hyperthyroidism with methimazole or carbimazole during pregnancy. Teratology 32:321, 1985.

163. Rosa FW: Teratogenicity of isotretinoin. Lancet 2:513, 1983.

164. Fernhoff PM, Lammer EJ: Craniofacial features of isotretinoin embryopathy. J Pediatr 105:595, 1984.

165. Lammer EJ, Chen DT, Hoar RM, et al.: Retinoic acid embryopathy. N Engl J Med 313:837, 1985.

166. Lammer EJ, Schunior A, Holmes LB: Retinoic acid fetopathy. Proc Greenwood Genet Center 9:68, 1990.

167. von Lennep E, El Khazen N, De Pierreux G, et al.: A case of partial sirenomelia and possible vitamin A teratogenesis. Prenat Diagn 5:35, 1985.

168. Mounoud RL, Klein D, Weber F: A propos d'un cas de syndrome de Goldenhar: intoxication aigue a la vitamine A chez la mere pendant la grossesse. J Genet Hum 23:135, 1975.

169. Grote W, Harms D, Janig U, et al.: Malformation of a fetus conceived 4 months after termination of maternal etretinate treatment. Lancet 1:1276, 1985.

170. Lenz W: A short history of thalidomide embryopathy. Teratology 38:203, 1988.

171. Quibell EP: The thalidomide embryopathy: an analysis from the UK. Practitioner 225:721, 1981.

172. Taussig HB: A study of the German outbreak of phocomelia: the thalidomide syndrome. JAMA 180:1106, 1962.

173. Hall JG: Embryopathy associated with oral anticoagulant therapy. BDOAS:XII(5):33, 1976.

174. Stevenson RE, Burton M, Ferlauto GJ, et al.: Hazards of oral anticoagulants during pregnancy. JAMA 243:1549, 1980.

175. Hall JG, Pauli RM, Wilson KM: Maternal and fetal sequelae of anticoagulants during pregnancy. Am J Med 68:122, 1980.

176. Thiersch JB: Therapeutic abortions with a folic acid antagonist, 4-amino pteroylglutamic acid, administered by the oral route. Am J Obstet Gynecol 63:1298, 1952.

177. Shaw EB, Steinbach HL: Aminopterin-induced fetal malformation. Am J Dis Child 115:477, 1968.

178. Milunsky A, Fraef JW, Gaynor MF: Methotrexate-induced congenital malformations. J Pediatr 72:790, 1968.

179. Shaw EB, Rees EL: Fetal damage due to aminopterin ingestion: follow-up at 17½ years of age. Am J Dis Child 134:1172, 1980.

180. Bongiovanni AM, McPadden AJ: Steroids during pregnancy and possible fetal consequences. Fertil Steril 11:181, 1960.

181. Grajwer LA, Lilien LD, Pildes RS: Neonatal subclinical adrenal insufficiency: result of maternal steroid therapy. JAMA 238:1279, 1977.

182. Grumbach MM, Ducharme JR: The effects of androgens on fetal sexual development: androgen-induced female pseudohermaphrodism. Fertil Steril 11:157, 1960.

183. Wilkins L: Masculinization of female fetus due to the use of orally given progestins. JAMA 172:1028, 1960.

184. Burnstein R, Wasserman HC: The effect of Provera on the fetus. Obstet Gynecol 23:931, 1964.

185. Jewelewicz R, Perkins RP, Dyrenfurth I, et al.: Luteomas of pregnancy, a cause of maternal virilization. Am J Obstet Gynecol 109:24, 1971.

186. Verhoeven AT, Mastboom JL, van Levsden HA: Virilization in pregnancy coexisting with an (ovarian) mucinous cystadenoma—a case report and review of virilizing ovarian tumors in pregnancy. Obstet Gynecol Surv 28:597, 1973.

187. Janerich DT, Piper JM, Glebatis DM: Oral contraceptives and congenital limb-reduction defects. N Engl J Med 291:697, 1974.

188. Heinonen OP, Slone D, Monson RR, et al.: Cardiovascular birth defects and antenatal exposure to female sex hormones. N Engl J Med 296:67, 1977.

189. Kricker A, Elliott JW, Forrest JM, et al.: Congenital limb reduction deformities and use of oral contraceptives. Am J Obstet Gynecol 155:1072, 1986.

190. Nora JJ, Nora AH, Wexler PL: Exogenous sex hormones and birth defects: continuing the dialogue. Am J Obstet Gynecol 144:860, 1982.

191. Nora JJ, Nora AH: Birth defects and oral conraceptives. Lancet 1:941, 1973.

192. Lammer EJ, Cordero JF: Exogenous sex hormone exposure and the risk for major malformations. JAMA 255:3128, 1986.

193. Gal I, Kirman B, Stern J: Hormonal pregnancy tests and congenital malformation. Nature 216:83, 1967.

194. Czeizel A, Keller S, Bod M: An etiological evaluation of increased occurrence of congenital limb reduction abnormalities in Hungary, 1975–1978. Int J Epidemiol 12:445, 1983.

195. Oakley GP, Flynt JW, Falek A: Hormonal pregnancy tests and congenital malformations. Lancet 2:256, 1973.

196. Mulvihill JJ, Mulvihill CG, Neill CA: Congenital heart defects and prenatal sex hormones. Lancet 1:1168, 1974.

197. Harlap S, Prywes R, Davies AM: Birth defects and oestrogens and progesterones in pregnancy. Lancet 1:682, 1975.

198. Stillman RJ: In utero exposure to diethylstilbestrol: adverse effects on the reproductive tract and reproductive performance in male and female offspring. Am J Obstet Gynecol 142:905, 1982.

199. Herbst AL, Scully RE: Adenocarcinoma of the vagina in adolescence: a report of seven cases including clear cell carcinomas (so-called mesonephromas). Ca 25:745, 1970.

200. Mills JL, Bongiovanni AM: Effect of prenatal estrogen exposure on male genitalia. Pediatrics 62(Suppl):1160, 1978.

201. Senior B, Chernoff HL: Iodide goiter in the newborn. Pediatrics 47:510, 1971.

202. Weinstein MR: The international registry of lithium babies. Drug Infect J 10:94, 1976.

203. Warkany J: Teratogen update: lithium. Teratology 38:593, 1988.

204. Murakami U: The effect of organic mercury on intrauterine life. Adv Exp Med Biol 27:301, 1971.

205. Amin-zaki L, Majeed MA, Elhassani SB, et al.: Prenatal methylmercury poisoning: clinical observations over five years. Am J Dis Child 133:172, 1979.

206. Rogan WJ, Gladen BC, Hung K-L, et al.: Congenital poisoning by polychlorinated biphenyls and their contaminants in Taiwan. Science 241:334, 1988.

207. Miller RW: Cola-colored babies: chlorobiphenyl poisoning in Japan. Teratology 4:211, 1971.

208. Friedman JM, Little BB, Brent RL, et al.: Potential human teratogenicity of frequently prescribed drugs. Obstet Gynecol 75:594, 990.

209. Wilson JG; Embryotoxicity of drugs in man. In Handbook of Teratology, vol 1. JG Wilson, FC Fraser, eds. Plenum, New York, 1977, p 309.

210. Holmes LB: Teratogen update: bendectin. Teratology 27:277, 1983.

211. Carter MP, Wilson F: Antibiotics in early pregnancy and congenital malformations. Dev Med Child Neurol 7:353, 1965.

212. Mjolnerod OK, Rasmussen K, Dommerud SA, et al.: Congenital connective-tissue defect probably due to D-penicillamine treatment in pregnancy. Lancet 1:673, 1971.

213. Doll DC, Ringerberg S, Yarbro JW: Antineoplastic agents and pregnancy. Semin Oncol 16:337, 1989.

214. Stafford PA, Biddinger PW, Zumwalt RE: Lethal intrauterine fetal trauma. Am J Obstet Gynecol 159:485, 1988.

215. Franger AL, Buchsbaum HJ, Peaceman AM: Abdominal gunshot wounds in pregnancy. Am J Obstet Gynecol 160:1125, 1989.

216. Miller ME, Dunn PM, Smith DW: Uterine malformation and fetal deformation. J Pediatr 94:387, 1979.

217. Graham JMJ, Miller ME, Stephen MJ, et al.: Limb reduction anomalies and early in utero limb compression. J Pediatr 96:1052, 1980.

218. Thomas IT, Smith DW: Oligohydramnios, cause of the non-renal features of Potter's syndrome, including pulmonary hypoplasia. J Pediatr 84:811, 1974.

219. Torpin R: Fetal Malformations Caused by Amnion Rupture During Gestation. Charles C Thomas, Springfield, IL, 1968.

220. Higginbottom MC, Jones KL, Hall BD, et al.: The amniotic band disruption complex: timing of amnion rupture and variable spectra of consequent defects. J Pediatr 95:544, 1979.

221. Miller ME, Graham JMJ, Higginbottom MC, et al.: Compression-realted defects from early amnion rupture: evidence for mechanical teratogenesis. J Pediatr 98:292, 1982.

222. Bryan EM: The intrauterine hazards of twins. Arch Dis Child 61:1044, 1986.

223. Phelan MC, Stevenson RE: Adverse outcomes of twin pregnancies. Proc Greenwood Genet Center 8:3, 1989.

224. McKeown T, Record RG: Observations and fetal growth in multiple pregnancies in man. J Endocrinol 8:386, 1952.

225. Gleicher N, El-Roeiy A: The reproductive autoimmune failure syndrome. Am J Obstet Gynecol 159:223, 1988.

226. Sargent IL, Wilkins T, Redman CWG: Maternal immune responses to the fetus in early pregnancy and recurrent miscarriage. Lancet 2:1099, 1988.

227. McIntyre JA, Faulk WP: Recurrent spontaneous abortion in human pregnancy: results of immunogenetical, cellular, and humoral studies. Am J Reprod Immunol 4:165, 1983.

228. Cohen F, Zuelzer WW, Gustafson DC, et al.: Mechanisms of iso-immunization. I. The transplacental passage of fetal erythrocytes in homospecific pregnancies. Blood 23:621, 1964.

229. Scanlon JW, Muirhead DM: Hydrops fetalis due to anti-Kell iso-immune disease: survival with optimal long-term outcome. J Pediatr 88:484, 1976.

230. Palchak AE, Aster RH, Gottschall J, et al.: Effect of maternal–fetal platelet incompatibility on fetal development. Pediatr 74:570, 1984.

231. Matsuda T, Momoi T, Akaishi K, et al.: Transient neonatal hyperthyroidism and maternal thyroid stimulating immunoglobulins. Arch Dis Child 63:205, 1988.

232. Connors MH, Styne DM: Transient neonatal "athyreosis" resulting from thyrotropin-binding inhibitory immunoglobulins. Pediatrics 78:287, 1986.

233. Doshi N, Smith B, Klionsky B: Congenital pericarditis due to maternal lupus erythematosus. J Pediatr 96:699, 1980.

234. Olson NY, Lindsley CB: Neonatal lupus syndrome. Am J Dis Child 141:908, 1987.

235. Merlob P, Metzker A, Hazaz B, et al.: Neonatal pemphigus vulgaris. Pediatrics 78:1102, 1986.

236. Oosterhuis HJGH, Feltkamp TEW, van der Geld HRW: Muscle antibodies in myasthenic mothers and their babies. Lancet 2:1225, 1966.

237. Borzy MS, Magenis E, Tomar D: Bone marrow transplantation for severe combined immune deficiency in an infant with chimerism due to intrauterine-derived maternal lymphocytes: donor engraftment documented by chromosomal marker studies. Am J Med Genet 18:527, 1984.

238. Stevenson RE, Sorell M, Kapoor N, et al.: Chimerism in an infant with severe combined immunodeficiency. Proc Greenwood Genet Center 3:30, 1984.

239. Bastian JF, Williams RA, Ornelas W, et al.: Maternal isoimmunization resulting in combined immunodeficiency and fatal graft-versus-host disease in an infant. Lancet 1:1435, 1984.

240. Turner JH, Hutchinson DL, Petricciani JC: Chimerism following fetal transfusion. Scand J Haematol 10:358, 1973.

241. Parkman R, Mosier D, Umansky I, et al.: Graft-versus-host disease after intrauterine and exchange transfusions for hemolytic disease of the newborn. N Engl J Med 290:359, 1974.

8

Human Anomalies and Cultural Practices

JOHN M. GRAHAM, Jr., KATHERINE C. DONAHUE, and JUDITH G. HALL

Humankind has always been fascinated by its own form. The human face is the first image infants learn to recognize and one of the first children learn to draw. Advertisements and other types of propaganda utilize the human form to convey messages of beauty, virility, and power. The human body is a favorite subject of sculptors and painters. Many cultures have selected the human form as the image of their god(s).

Abnormalities of the human anatomy are common, being detected in 2%–5% of newborn infants.[1] Additional anomalies are found in the following years. Anomalies constitute the major reason for genetic evaluation during the first year of life and remain one of the major reasons in all age groups.[2] Dysmorphologists are trained to associate facial features, variations in growth, and other anomalies to arrive at a diagnosis in those presented for evaluation. Diagnosis serves as the basis for developing management strategies and counseling.

Human morphology conveys strong messages—immediate, nonverbal, lasting, powerful. No people are immune to malformations or other distinctive features; hence all cultures have faced variations in human morphology and dysmorphology in particular. How have various cultures dealt with structural defects, facial differences, and variations in growth? Why did some past cultures purposefully distort the human body and cranium? How do the various cultures of today view congenital anomalies?

It appears that the feelings of, impact on, and responses of cultures relative to malformations have not been extensively studied. If so, this taboo to scientific scrutiny in this area matches the taboo on discussion of defects by individual families and society.

A society's views regarding morphology and dysmorphology form the basis for the care afforded to affected members. In many circumstances, the response bears some relationship to the prevailing concepts about causation (see Volume I, Chapter 1). Approaches toward humans with malformations have varied through the ages. Some cultures eliminated individuals with anomalies. After a malformed infant was killed, the infant's likeness was sometimes set up as an idol. Conversely, other cultures adored the malformed. Warkany[3] has suggested that when human deities were worshiped, it was the unusual human who was accorded divine status. This is apparent in the Greek gods and some of the crests found among Northwest Coast native American Indians.

Sterilization and euthanasia of individuals with malformations or retardation were practiced under the eugenics policies of the United States and the European states during the first half of the twentieth century. Discrimination based on morphologic features was extended politically, resulting in restriction of movement by certain groups and ethnic genocide.[4,5]

Currently there is a robust effort worldwide to prevent the birth of infants with anomalies. The effort incorporates carrier detection, prenatal screening and diagnostic testing, and counseling. Abortion of fetuses with anomalies has become a widespread practice. With understanding of the underlying pathogenesis and natural history of many structural defects, it has also become possible to correct some anomalies. In many instances, the same principles used by primitive societies to alter human structures in the pursuit of beauty can be used to reshape deformations into a more normal or functional shape.

Cultural concepts of beauty

In the pursuit of beauty, many cultures have developed ways of altering various parts of the body. Hippocrates mentions the practice of cranial deformation among a race he called the *Macrocephali:*

> There is no other race of men which have heads in the least resembling theirs. At first, usage was the principal cause of the length of their head, but now nature cooperates with usage. They think those the most noble who have the longest heads. It is thus with regard to the usage: immediately after the child is born, and while its head is still tender, they fashion it with their hands, and constrain it to assume a lengthened shape by applying bandages and other suitable contrivances whereby the spherical form of the head is destroyed, and it is made to increase in length.[6]

Postnatal methods of altering body structures attest to the plasticity of the body's soft tissues and, to a lesser degree, of the skeleton. The cranium, facial structures, umbilicus, and feet are most commonly manipulated. Soft tissues may be altered at virtually any time in life. Skeletal structures must be altered during the period of most rapid growth.

Growth has a major influence on form. Thus the rate and direction of growth in a given tissue will determine the magnitude of the forces it exerts on adjacent tissues. The plasticity of a tissue affects its susceptibility to alteration by mechanical forces. Fetal tissues are more pliable than those of the infant, which in turn are more pliable than those of the child or adult. Localized constraint can be used to reshape pliable structures in the infant much more successfully than similar techniques in older children.[7]

Collagen fibers align themselves in the direction of stress. Their underlying strength and integrity, and the form into which their growth is channeled, is under genetic control. Variations in the expressions of these genes determine differences within and between species. The alignment of collagen fibrils in the extracellular space appears to be determined predominantly by mechanical forces. With no consistent direction to these mechanical forces, collagen strands become ar-

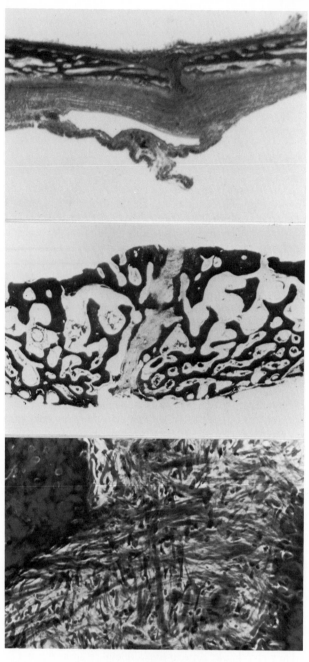

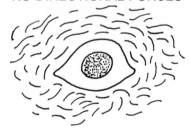

NO DIRECTIONAL FORCES

DIRECTIONAL FORCES

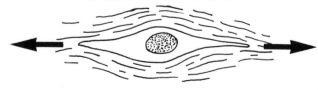

ranged in a haphazard fashion. With sustained direction of the forces, the strands become organized and woven in relation to those forces (Fig. 8–1).

Cranial deformation

Deformation is the alteration of form in response to mechanical forces. Archaeological and ethnographic evidence shows that artificial deformation of infant crania has been practiced worldwide for thousands of years.[8] In some societies, constraint forces were used to mold infant heads into a characteristic recognizable shape. In other cultures, swaddling or papoose-board immobilization of infants may have inadvertently increased the likelihood of certain head shapes.

Deformation of the infant skull was usually initiated shortly after birth and the process maintained for varying lengths of time. Application of a deforming apparatus was usually concluded by the end of the first year. In East Asia and Australia, the practice of cranial deformation may extend back to the late Pleistocene era.[9] In Europe, skulls from the fourth and fifth centuries show evidence of deformation[8] as do skulls from ancient Crete and from the Hittite Empire.[10] Egyptian sculptures and reliefs from the time of Nefertiti and Akhenaten reveal unusual head shapes (similar to those seen with extensive vertex molding), but Dingwall[8] was unable to find any Egyptian skulls that confirmed the practice of artificial deformation.

The excellent preservation of skulls from ancient Peru provides evidence of the widespread use of a variety of deforming techniques throughout the pre-Columbian period. Highland Peruvians applied circumferential bandages to elongate the calvarium. By combining banding with the application of occipital boards, the cranium could be molded into either a bilobed shape or a "tower skull" configuration (Figs. 8–2, 8–3).

Paintings and photographs of coastal Northwestern American Indians demonstrate the use of deforming practices well after the arrival of white Europeans (Fig. 8–4). The Kwakiutl Indians of British Columbia utilized cedar boards and leather thongs to mold their infants' foreheads into a sloping configuration. Similar practices were used by the Chinook Indians to achieve a slightly different head shape.

The Chinook tribe lived along the Columbia River in the Pacific Northwest. They intentionally deformed their infants' crania by placing the infant on a board and attaching another board over its forehead at roughly a 25° angle (Fig. 8–4). The forehead board was used to apply steady pressure to the forehead by tightening a cord. The process was not painful. It slowly redirected the growth of the infant's cranium into a sloping configuration with a flat occiput and pointed vertex. The Chinook believed that this head shape was a mark of distinction.[11] The Kwakiutl thought that a flat forehead was a mark of beauty and referred to a person with such a head shape as being *well cradled.*[12]

Fig. 8–1. Craniosynostosis histology. The top photomicrograph shows a normal sagittal suture from a 2-week-old infant. The lower two photomicrographs show low- and high-power views of a synostotic sagittal suture from a young infant whose craniostenosis was attributed to fetal head constraint. Note the disorganized sutural connective tissue pattern in the high-power view (bottom).

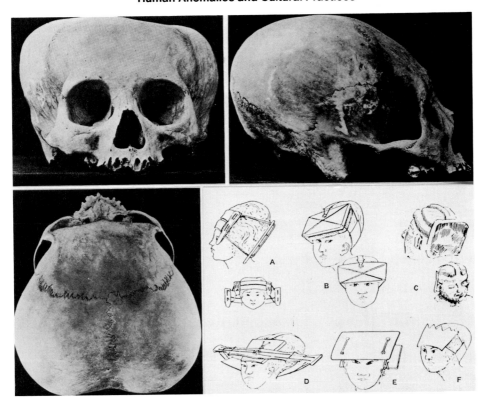

Fig. 8–2. This bilobed skull from highland Peru was created by application of a board to the occiput and a band over the sagittal suture and around the head. Other techniques of cranial molding are depicted in the drawing. (From Dingwall.[8])

In some instances, deformation may have been unintentional, as in the occipital flattening that occurred when cradleboards were used for long periods of time. Among the Lebanese Maronites, infants were left swaddled on their backs in cradles with flat wooden bottoms.[10] Some Native Indian tribes bound their infants onto cradleboards a few days after birth. The infant spent most of the next 6 months bound to the cradleboard, which was generally discarded when the infant began to walk. Many groups padded the boards with sphagnum moss or shredded reeds; however, if the infant's head was kept in direct contact with a hard cradleboard, occipital flattening resulted. Many Southwest Native American Indian tribes, and the historic tribes of Wisconsin, thought that such padding was not necessary.[11]

Similar deformations occur today, when infants are left reclining in flat-backed infant seats for prolonged periods of time. The end result is a brachycephalic headshape with broadening and widening of the face. If the infant has torticollis, with a head turned to one side or the other, then plagiocephaly (a rhomboid head shape) is likely to result.

Deformations severe enough to be considered congenital anomalies occur in 3% of newborns, and the limbs and head are especially susceptible.[7] Plagiocephaly occurs in 1 of 300 neonates and is often the result of external forces. When unusual head shapes result from deformation, corrective forces can be used to reshape the cranium into a more normal shape.[7,13,14]

Helmet therapy is currently used to correct cosmetic deformations of the cranium. A mold is made of the deformed cranium at around age 6 mo, and from this mold a bust is made out of plaster of Paris. The bust duplicates the size and shape of the deformed cranium. Where the head is prominent, the bust is left alone, but where the bust is recessed or flattened, plaster of Paris is added to achieve a symmetrically round head shape. Then a plastic helmet is fashioned around the corrected bust in a vacuum oven. A foam liner is positioned between the bust and the plastic helmet prior to placing it in the oven, so that the inside of the helmet is lined. With use of the custom-designed helmet over a period of several months, the infant's cranium grows within the symmetric contours of the helmet (Fig. 8–5).

This reshaping is accomplished by application of external molding in conjunction with normal brain growth and therefore must be completed during the first year or so of life. This is exactly analogous to the cranial deformation practices of primitive cultures. Such reshaping does not result in premature closure of sutures or in brain compression. Likewise, it is not successful in correcting headshapes that are caused by premature closure of sutures or aberrant brain growth.

Facial deformation

Among many cultures, facial structures were altered and adorned to enhance beauty and to indicate social standing. Earrings and ear plugs were used by a variety of cultures (Fig. 8–6). The South American Incas used cylinders of wood or gold to expand holes placed in their earlobes. Young boys had their lobes pierced when they first began to wear breech cloths, and only men of Incan royalty were allowed to wear ornaments of prestige and beauty.[12]

Other cultures inserted decorative objects into holes pierced into their lips. The Alaskan Eskimos pierced the lips

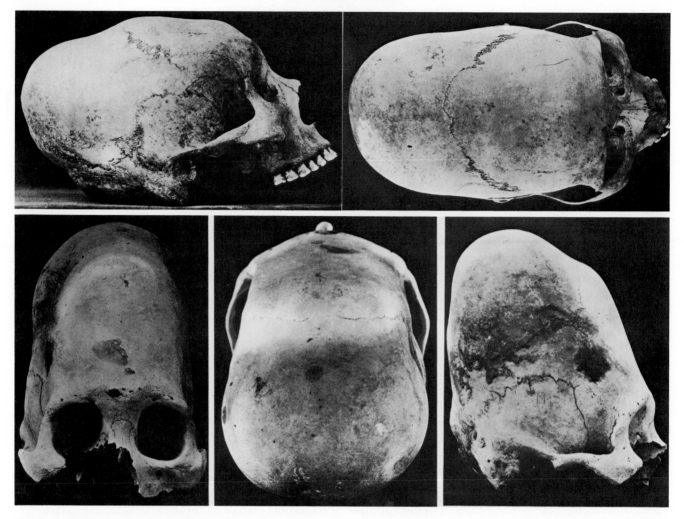

Fig. 8–3. Peruvian head molding. Highland Peruvians applied circumferential bandages to the calvarium to achieve the headshape of the top skull, while Coastal Peruvians applied boards to the occiput and pads to the frontal region along with circumferential banding. (From Dingwall.[8])

of the adolescent boy with a small pin and gradually dilated the hole until it could accommodate a decorative plug about 1 cm in diameter, called a *labret.* Labrets were made from polished stone, bone, ivory, beads, and, after contact with white traders, glass or bottle stoppers. Among the Bororo Indians of Brazil, the quill end of a feather was inserted through the nasal columella or the lip. Northwest Coast Indians, Eskimos, and the San Blas Indians of Panama were all known to use nose rings.[12]

Other deformations

Purposeful injury or irritation of the skin to produce patterns of scars or reaction nodules on the face or trunk is inflicted in many primitive cultures (Fig. 8–6).[15–18] Deformation of other body structures has been practiced in certain cultures but appears to be distinctly less common than deformation of craniofacial structures. Augmentation of the size of the umbilicus has been artificially achieved in African tribes who consider large umbilical hernias a sign of female beauty. It is a nonsurgical method analogous to augmentation mammoplasty in other contemporary cultures. For close to 1,500 years, certain young Chinese girls were subjected to extensive foot molding in order to produce the desired small feet that were considered sexually attractive.[19] The form into which the feet were molded is demonstrated in Figure 8–7.

Painting

The use of various pigments to camouflage or to accentuate various human features can be found in most cultures. Body painting is used for many purposes: to enhance, to amuse, to frighten (Fig. 8–6). Facial and nail painting are common in most contemporary cultures; full-body painting is generally restricted to aboriginal or underdeveloped areas.

Anomalies of the face: examples in the crests of Northwest Coast Native American Indians

The study of masks used by Northwest Coast Native American Indians provides some insight into their view of congenital anomalies of facial structures. The face provides important nonverbal messages in human communication. Why did some societies choose certain facial characteristics to portray magical or ritualistic concepts? Northwest Coast Indian

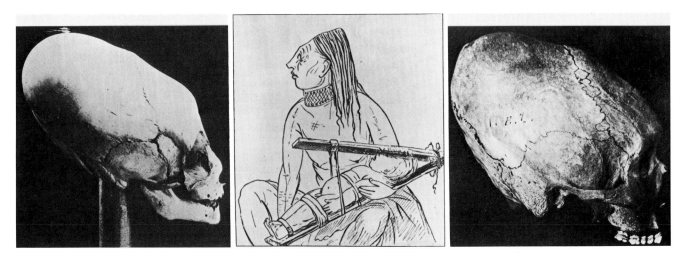

Fig. 8–4. Northwest Coast Indian head molding. The Kwakiutl Indians bound cedarboards to their infants' heads for 5–7 mo to achieve the sloping foreheads depicted in the skulls. (From Dingwall.[8])

Fig. 8–5. When conservative measures proved unsuccessful in correcting this child's asymmetric head shape by age 6 mo, a stockinette cap was placed over the head (A) to prevent hair from becoming embedded in rapidly drying plaster splint material (B). Plaster of Paris was poured into the mold, and the bust was placed on a base (C) so that the plaster bust could be augmented where the skull had been flattened and the cranium needed to fill out. In areas that were too prominent, the bust was left unchanged. Foam layers were placed around the bust (D), and three-eighths inch polypropylene plastic was molded around the bust in a vacuum oven. The helmet was then cut away from the bust with one foam lining attached to it. The infant wore the helmet constantly for the next 3 months, and the head grew into a symmetric shape. The head shape before helmet therapy (E) and 3 months later (F). (From Graham.[7])

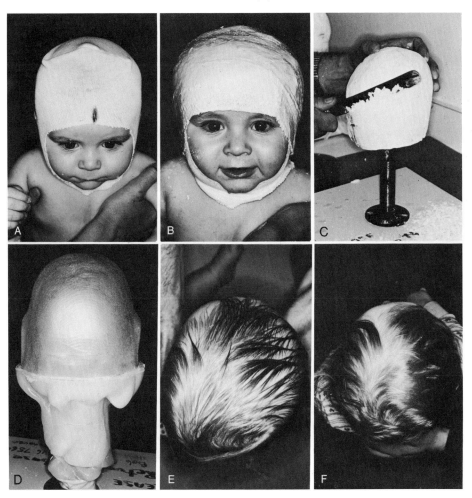

173

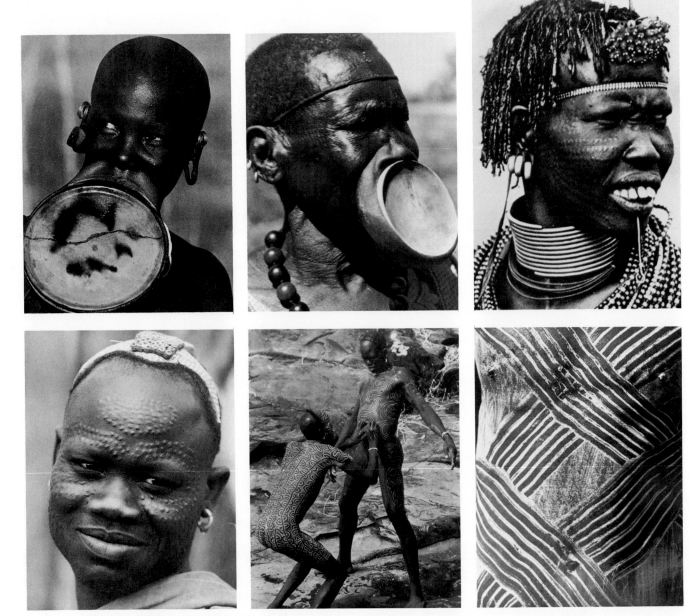

Fig. 8–6. Adornments used in African tribes. Top left: large lower lip plate, earrings, and earplugs worn by a Surma woman. Top center: upper lip plate and earrings worn by a Lobi woman. Top right: Toposa woman with scarified markings on face, a lower lip wire, earrings, and a neck coil. Bottom left: Bumi man with scarified designs on face indicating tribal identity. Bottom center and right: Body painting by Surma men in preparation for stick fights. (Courtesy of Angela Fisher. Top left and bottom center and right from Beckwith C, Fisher A: The Eloquent Surma of Ethiopia, Natl Geog 179:77, 1991. Top center from Beckwith C, Fisher A: African Ark, Harry N. Abrams, New York, 1990. Top right and bottom left from Fisher A: Africa Adorned, Harry N. Abrams, New York, 1984.)

families each had a specific set of crests or totems that represented certain spirits or powers. These were often displayed on poles (i.e., totem poles), ornaments, or masks during ceremonies. Certain of these crests demonstrate physical characteristics that appear to resemble known human congenital anomalies or malformation syndromes.[20]

Native Indians recognized a close relationship between man and animal, and humans with congenital anomalies may have been regarded as a transition between man and animal with special powers. When a mask was worn portraying a certain crest, it was thought that this provided the wearer with some protection or power. Why were certain congenital anomalies represented in certain crests? What is it about these particular anomalies or syndromes that led to the elaboration of a cultural myth?

Three crests from the Northwest Native Indians have particular interest to the dysmorphologist. Tsonaqua ("Zo-na-kwa"), the old woman of the woods, was a large bear-like creature who roamed the forest and was especially fond of devouring children who wandered off into the woods alone. She was a spirit concerned with fertility and power, who moved slowly and had a heavy brow, sunken cheeks, pursed lips, and droopy eyelids. She was hairy with claw-like hands and long nails that deviated laterally (Fig. 8–8). The pursed

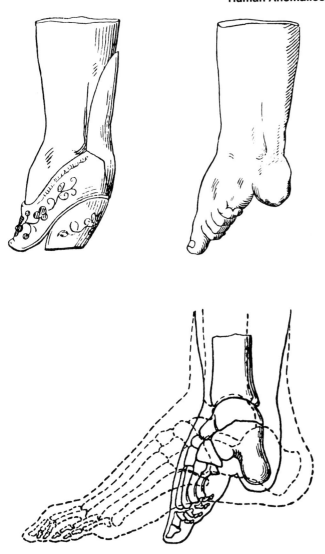

Fig. 8-7. Chinese footbinding was practiced in China for much of the past 15 centuries. The drawings show how shoes were used to remold feet into a smaller form. (From Graham.[7])

lips and ptosis of Tsonaqua resemble the puckered mouth of Freeman-Sheldon syndrome. Individuals with this syndrome can have joint contractures, including clubbed feet and clubbed hands, which in a primitive culture could slow movement and result in a bear-like gait. They may have speech abnormalities due to palatal abnormalities. It is possible that an individual with this syndrome could survive to roam slowly through the woods on deformed feet as an outcast.

A second spirit, Nhoomal ("Nuh-mal") plays the part of a fool but is very clever. His is dirty, with long hair, large nose, and mucus streaming out of his nose and across his cheeks. He is unable to speak and has outbursts of outrageous, bizarre behavior. He often cries out in pain and hits himself and others around him. Nhoomal masks usually demonstrate downslanting palpebral fissures, midface hypoplasia, underdeveloped zygoma, and micrognathia with a highly placed, prominent nose (Fig. 8-9). These features resemble the midface hypoplasia and flattened cheekbones of Treacher Collins syndrome. One-third of patients with Trea-cher

Collins syndrome have a cleft palate, and even without a cleft palate the speech is nasalized. These individuals usually have associated chronic otitis media with deafness due either to chronic otitis media or to malformed ossicles. Thus an individual with Treacher Collins syndrome who might be born into a primitive society would have a very unusual appearance with chronic ear infections and poor speech quality. Such a person might show outbursts of bizarre behavior due to otitis media and the associated pain. This might also lead to chronic nasal discharge and unusual speech.

Northwest Coast Native Indians also used a globular rattle with a face demonstrating a large midline cleft lip and eyes that were either widely or closely set (Fig. 8-10). It emitted a high-pitched sound and was used on ceremonial occasions to mark major transitions in life, particularly birth or death. This rattle resembles the lethal holoprosencephaly malformation sequence and may have taken its origin from the birth of such a child. These examples of crests probably reflect the chance occurrences of new mutations for recognizable monogenic syndromes. These conditions have not been found to have an increased incidence among Northwest Coast Native Indians today.

Anomalies of growth

Individuals with short stature can be found in the works of art of Egyptian, Oceanic, Mayan, Peruvian, European, and other cultures.[21-25] Because of their unusual appearance, short people were valued and viewed as having special wisdom and powers. They were among the few courtiers who were allowed to offer guidance to rulers, often through their roles as jesters.

The archaeologic record does not permit a complete interpretation of prehistoric treatment of humans with congenital anomalies or growth deficiency. However, the recent finding of a dwarf buried during the Upper Paleolithic in Italy suggests that particular care was given to this individual.[26] The Egyptians depicted dwarfs in their art works. A stone statue of a dwarf was excavated at Saqqarah in the nineteenth century. The dwarf was apparently a man of some importance, since he had an elaborate tomb.[22] A caravan leader, one Harkhuf, wrote on one of his journeys to Pharaoh Pepy II, around 3000 BC, that he had a dancing dwarf whom he planned to bring to the court. The Pharaoh answered that he "desired to see the dwarf more than the products of Sinai and Punt."[22]

The Mayans depicted individuals with growth deficiency on their reliefs. Frequently such individuals were pictured presenting a ruler with offerings or members of the underworld. The Moche people of northern Peru made a remarkable variety of pots, many representing human and animal forms. These people, whose civilization was at its peak around the years AD 300 to 700, before the Incas expanded their domination over much of Peru, depicted diseases and deformities in realistic form in their art. Among the human variations represented in the pots are those caused by growth disorders, leprosy, and malformations.[24,25]

Persons with growth abnormalities were commonly displayed in fairs throughout Europe during earlier centuries. Those with short stature were particularly popular. Many of the royal families also kept short people in their courts as attendants or jesters. Short people appear in Italian frescoes at

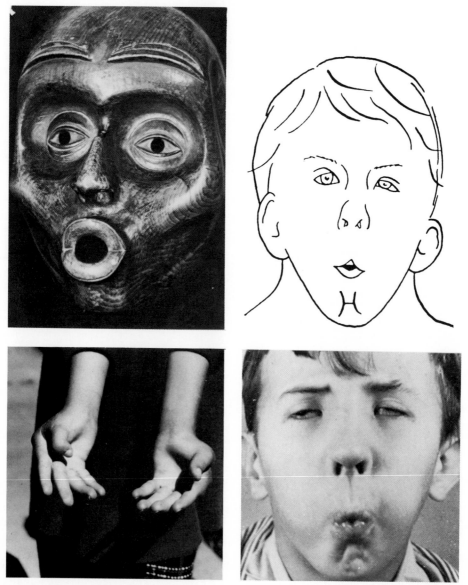

Fig. 8–8. The Northwest Indian mask of Tsonaqua (top left) is from the Kwakiutl tribe (University of British Columbia Museum of Anthropology, Catalog No. 2601). She was a female giantess who roamed the forest in search of children, whom she carried away in the basket on her back. Compare to the child who has Freeman-Sheldon syndrome (top right, bottom left, bottom right). (Schematic at top right is from Goodman and Gorlin.[43] Bottom figures are from Jones.[44])

ducal courts, and Spanish paintings show them as finely dressed court attendants (Fig. 8–11).[22]

Other anomalies

Interest in a wide range of human anomalies can be found in the folklore, literature, and art of most cultures. Perhaps nowhere is that interest more evident than in the popularity of circuses, sideshows, and "freak shows" of the eighteenth and nineteenth centuries.[27–30] Individuals with extremes in growth—little people, giants, fat ladies, and living skeletons—were the mainstays of these exhibitions. Equally popular were individuals with features that could be compared with animals: elephant man, fishskin boy, monkey-faced child, mermaids, and the like. Rubber men, conjoined twins, amelics, and hermaphrodites might round out the troupe.

Most of the individuals exhibited had bona fide anomalies, although hoaxes were not unheard of.

Exhibitions were popular among all classes. People of wealth would often arrange for private shows as an evening of entertainment in their homes. The most famous of the persons exhibited in America and Europe during the nineteenth century included the Siamese twins Eng and Chang Bunker and the midget Tom Thumb.

Cultural views of the placenta

Within the ethnographic literature there is described a rich mythology surrounding the placenta. In some ways, anthropologists have devoted more attention to the placenta than to other aspects of childbearing. The placenta is an integral part of the birth process. Passage of the placenta was of grave

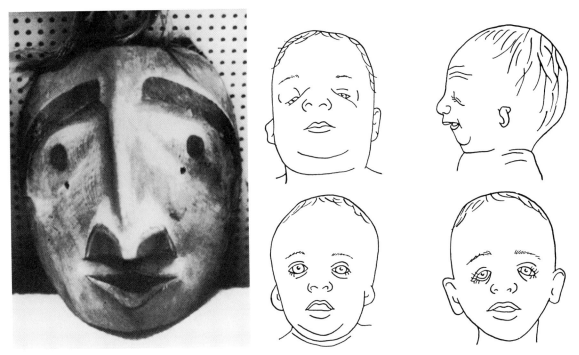

Fig. 8–9. The Northwest Indian mask of Nhoomal (left) is compared with schematic representations of children with Treacher Collins syndrome. (From Goodman and Gorlin.[43])

concern to many societies, and retention of the placenta was the most dreaded complication of childbirth. Practices related to disposal of the placenta may reflect wider cultural values within a society. Either the placenta was imbued with magical powers and therefore subjected to a variety of rituals, or it was considered disgusting and quickly discarded. Among a survey of more than 300 cultural groups in the Human Relations Area Files, no culture characteristically ate the placentas after birth, though this currently occurs in up to 5% of home births in the United States.[31,32] Among 200 cultures that described disposal practices for the placenta, only seven threw it away without regard; another 130 cultures buried it, often in a special place.[32]

In Ganda, Africa, the placenta was considered to be the second (twin) child, with a spirit that rapidly became a ghost. If the child was a male, the placenta was placed at the root of

Fig. 8–10. The Northwest Indian transition rattle (left) is compared with a schematic representation of a child with holoprosencephaly. (From Goodman and Gorlin.[43])

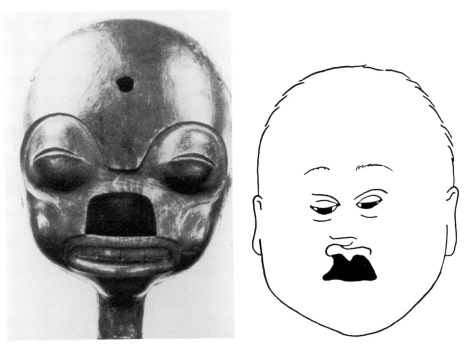

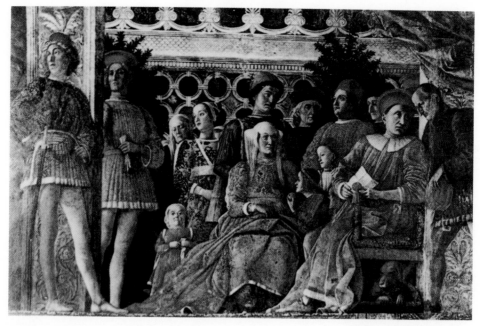

Fig. 8–11. This fresco by Andrea Mantegna from 1474 depicts an achondroplastic dwarf with the Duchess of Mantua. (From Kunze and Nippert.[21])

a plantain tree from which beer was made. If the child was female, it was also placed at the root of a plantain tree, but the fruit was eaten as a vegetable. The tree was guarded by older women from the clan, because if anyone outside the clan drank beer or ate fruit from this plantain tree, then the living child would die in order to follow its twin ghost. Other cultures had similar views of the placenta as being related in some spiritual way to the living child. The placenta was also considered to be the younger sibling of the birth child in the cultures of Malasia, Jordan, Java, and among the Fellahin.[32]

Consequences for failure to dispose of the placenta properly affected the health of the mother and her infant, and these ranged from minor to severe (i.e., death). The Kwakiutl safeguarded their infants' health by burying the placenta where it could be walked over. A boy's placenta was buried in front of the house door, while a girl's placenta was buried at the high water mark, as this was thought to make her a good clam-digger. Sometimes, a boy's placenta would be exposed where ravens could eat it and endow the boy with the ability to see into the future.[33]

Among Tikopian Islanders in Oceania, the placenta was also buried under some well-trodden path so that if the child developed hiccups a caretaker could go out to the place where the placenta was buried and step on it, thereby rendering a cure. Afterbirths from male children were buried right after birth on the nonsacred side of the house, but placentas from females were left for morning so that their spiritual component could be observed and removed. It was thought that if these manifestations of the god Feke (the octopus deity) were not removed, it might cause the girl to die or to become insane. In Okinawa, children were expected to laugh as the placenta was buried so that the child would be happy. The Thai washed the placenta and placed it in a pot with salt, so that the baby would not get pimples.[32]

Many cultures treated placentas from males and females

differently, and some regarded the treatment as helping to determine the future career of the child. The Aymara buried the placenta with miniature farm implements if the child was male and with cooking utensils if it was female. In the Marshall Islands, a boy's placenta was thrown into the sea so that he would be a great fisherman, whereas a girl's was hung in a pandanus tree so that she would be a great weaver. Trobrianders buried the placenta in the garden so that the child would be a good gardener, and Iranians stuffed the placenta into a mousehole so that the child would be smart. In parts of Mexico, placing the placenta in a tree was thought to endow the child with the ability to climb trees, while the Nootka sprinkled the placenta with down and spun a top on it to make the child a good dancer.[32]

The Copper Eskimos allowed the newborn infant to look through the placental membranes so as to endow it with second sight. They thought that this ritual would help to determine the child's career as a shaman. In other cultures, disposal of the placenta was related to family planning. The Tzeltal buried the placenta deeply if they did not want more children. Among the Cherokee, spacing between children (in years) was related to the number of mountain ridges the father crossed before burying the placenta.[32]

In cultures with no magical beliefs about the placenta, it was usually considered dirty or unclean and was quickly disposed of through burial, burning, hanging on a tree, or being tossed onto a trash pile or into a river. Burial appeared to be the most common method of disposal. There appears to be a great variability in how different cultures viewed the placenta. No instances have been found in which the placenta was thought to be a cause for birth defects, though this is a commonly held belief in our own culture, e.g., the etiology for amniotic band defects. It seems quite unusual that there has not been more recorded about the placenta as a cause for birth defects. It is almost as if the subject of birth defects itself was regarded as taboo and was not to be discussed.

Current views of congenital anomalies in relation to ethnic background

The great diversity of views regarding congenital anomalies noted in earlier cultures can be found in today's cultures as well. Contemporary societies vary greatly in their perceptions of congenital anomalies, their access to and reception of medical information, their resources, and their mechanisms for coping with the stresses that accompany the birth of a malformed infant. Cultural traditions, religious beliefs, and position in society all influence their views of congenital anomalies. For today's medical providers, these differences are more than sociologic curiosities, since they affect the effectiveness of genetic evaluation, counseling, and medical care in general.

To some, having a child with an anomaly may be seen as a blessing, but to others it is a curse. Access to genetic services and counseling is a service to some, a threat to others. New information and new technology may be eagerly accepted in one culture, viewed with reservation in another, and rejected in another. In dysmorphology and genetics, the pace of discovery and the technologic advances may be faster than many cultures can immediately accommodate.

Effective communication between care providers and families requires an understanding of the family's cultural background. The manner in which information is presented may be all important in the reception and usefulness of the information. A sensitive, compassionate, and knowledgeable demeanor is a fundamental asset to geneticists and counselors in any culture. Appropriate concern for the well-being of the affected family is universally received.

Given the mixing of people from many different ethnic backgrounds in our current society it is important for genetic counselors to be aware of certain cultural biases so as to present information in the most effective and compassionate manner. A number of cultures are mentioned briefly as examples that may be encountered by the medical team dealing with congenital anomalies.

In places where racial discrimination and oppression have made certain ethnic groups more sensitive about their cultural status, the birth of a child with congenital anomalies may heighten feelings of guilt, shame, anger, or depression for the parents. Lack of information or misunderstanding of information can cause such individuals to emphasize the role of karma, fate, or an "evil eye." Discussions regarding prevention may be interpreted as genocidal in intent.

In traditional Hispanic and Asian cultures, the maintenance of family honor is of supreme importance. The Chinese use the term *face* to indicate family honor. The birth of an infant with congenital defects may be viewed as a threat to the honor or status of the traditional family. A clear understanding of the nature of the disorder, its etiology and management, can help the family to deal with guilt and grief. Since there may be a reluctance to express feelings freely to outsiders, it is important for such parents to know that other families have experienced the same feelings after the birth of an infant with anomalies. Many Chinese and Japanese families cope with their "loss of face" by calling upon the support of their extended family.

Certain nonverbal cues can lead to misunderstanding during communication surrounding the birth of a child with congenital anomalies. People differ in the amount of eye contact they exchange during speaking and listening. For instance, blacks make eye contact 80% of the time when speaking, but only 50% of the time when listening. Middle-class whites make eye contact 50% of the time when speaking and 80% of the time when listening. Among Southeast Asian cultures, extensive eye contact is considered rude, especially if it is uninterrupted.[34]

The respect and deference to authority in Asian cultures may call for a more directive and structured approach to counseling than in other cultures. Presentation of an array of options in a totally nondirective setting may only increase the difficulty in decision making. During the presentation of disease information to Asian parents, it is important that everyone else who is included in the family decision making also be present. It is particularly important to include elders if the parents are young.

Many Asians value restraint as part of their preference for moderation and balance. For this reason, excessive emotion or gesturing should be avoided so that one does not create an impression of being out of control.

To convey respect upon greeting a Southeast Asian, the head should be bowed slightly. The head of the household should always be addressed first (even if another family member is being counseled). If something is handed to an elder, it should be held with both hands. The head is considered to be the resting place of a person's soul and hence is considered to be sacred. For this reason, it is wise to minimize touching the head during physical examination. If the head is to be touched, preliminary explanation is most important.[34]

Among Asian cultures, individual nations vary in their approaches to family life. Among Filipinos, parents are greatly respected, living in their children's homes during their senior years. Children are expected to be obedient and submissive, and relationships are expected to be harmonious. Filipinos believe that illness arises from spiritual and moral imbalance and that evil spirits or spells cast by persons with supernatural powers cause disease.[35]

Chinese children are expected to be quiet and obedient, with a strict hierarchy of respect that is accorded to older siblings. Extended families tend to take care of their own problems, and it is considered shameful to discuss problems with a stranger. Politeness is uppermost in Asian interpersonal relations, and emotions are seldom displayed in public. Metaphors are used to avoid hurting or embarrassing others and to maintain harmonious human relations. Respect for age and the reluctance to voice disagreements can make decision making very difficult for young parents. Consequently, there may be reluctance to seek help until advanced stages of personal problems. Most Asian cultures do not emphasize verbal communication, and they may not be able to discuss feelings or personal information.

Among the Chinese, pregnant women are expected to eat certain foods (chicken cooked in wine, certain soups, and herbs) and to avoid others (shellfish and duck). Some activities may be curtailed during pregnancy for fear of causing birth defects (e.g., the use of scissors may cause cleft lip and palate). Because of such beliefs, it is important that rapport be established early and that the counselor know the family's beliefs regarding birth defects. Medical explanations should be clear and illustrated with visual aids and analogies.

Hispanic Americans likewise differ in their approach to problems based on their country of origin. Mexican Americans often manifest a passivity or fatalism that revolves around a belief in the will of God. Large families are valued due to high rates of morbidity and mortality in many rural villages. Children are expected to care for their parents during their elder years, and large numbers of children provide social security for elderly parents.

Caribbean Hispanics may consider a child with a handicap to be a gift from God that indicates that the parents are special people. The burden or blessing may not be shared equally by the parents. Women are often expected to "carry their cross" alone, since men may not accept responsibility for the child's problems. This lack of acceptance may lead to discord within the family and cause the father to isolate himself. Unlike Asians, Hispanics like to touch and be touched.

Black Americans also have strong family bonds and value extended family members. Because eugenics has been linked with racism, blacks may be very suspicious of geneticists. These feelings of mistrust can undermine a counseling situation, as can variation in educational levels. West Indian blacks often stress high educational goals, while American blacks have a strong achievement orientation. Black American children are taught respect for their elders. They are taught religion and family pride and to keep personal matters within the family. They may be used to working problems out within their own family or religious group, and it may be difficult for some blacks to be open with anyone but family members. Because of this intricate network of support, it may be important to establish communication with these members.[36]

The Sikh people from East India have yet another set of cultural perspectives. The Sikh religion is an offshoot of Hinduism, and Sikhs believe in reincarnation. Women are considered the mainstay of the family unit, and the family is the most important element in their society.

Despite the celebrated status of the family, male children are much more valued than females because the marriage system requires the bride's family to provide a dowry. Women who cannot produce male offspring are not viewed favorably by their in-laws, and the birth of twins is considered a bad omen.[37]

When a child is born with birth defects, Sikhs often attribute this occurrence to fate, the evil eye, karma, retribution for sins of the mother in a previous life, or sins in the present life. In the past, such children were neglected or killed, and the mother was stigmatized. The seeking of help from outside agencies may serve to enhance the shame and guilt of the family, and showing grief or mourning is considered contrary to Sikh teaching. To North American health care workers, this reluctance to share feelings may be misinterpreted as a lack of caring.[37]

Certain food practices are adhered to by the Sikh people during pregnancy. Food intake may be decreased to prevent the fetus from becoming so large as to make delivery difficult. Protein-rich foods are avoided early in the pregnancy and after the fifth month. Fruits and milk products are often avoided after delivery. Often the mother will miss meals because she is so busy caring for the rest of the family.[37] Neural tube defects are common among the Sikhs, and they have a high recurrence risk. Despite this fact, they are reluctant to seek genetic counseling, particularly if the child is female.

Highly religious Jews often consult rabbis for scriptural interpretations to aid in making complex and difficult decisions.[38] Often guidance based on Jewish law is combined with advice to help people make actions coincide with values inherent in Talmudic law. Birth defects are recognized within religious texts as potentially stigmatizing, and there are instances in which parental influences are considered to have affected the unborn child.

In a study of 18 highly religious Israeli families who had a child with Down syndrome or an oral cleft, Strauss[38] found that families who interpreted their child's defect as punishment for wrongdoing or atonement for a sin were less likely to involve their children in community recreation and other activities. All families were encouraged by their rabbi to keep their disabled child in the home, and children with disabilities were included in family religious life. When the need to place the child outside the home arose, the rabbi handled the process through religious social service agencies and an informal network of contacts with interested Jewish families. Treatment decisions were often influenced by how the child was expected to fit into community life. In general, girls were expected to attend to family and home matters, while boys were expected to lead a life of religious scholarship and employment.

Male children are particularly valued in Arab cultures; they bring status to the family and help to keep the wealth within the family. Families are patrilinear, and upon the death of the family head, sons get a full share of the family wealth, while daughters get half a share. Females are expected to be quiet and submissive, and marriages are often arranged between cousins. Females are breastfed 4 months longer than their brothers because the males inherit most of the property and wealth.[39]

Infertility is considered a major disgrace in Arab cultures and often leads to divorce. Childless women are not allowed to visit a mother and her new baby for fear that an evil eye will be cast and the new mother will be unable to bear further children. A malformed child is considered to be punishment for a previous wrongdoing or to be representative of the power of the "evil eye." Divorce was previously accomplished very easily, and under traditional laws the husband needed only to say "I divorce you" three times and the transaction was considered complete. Divorced women are considered stigmatized and can only remarry a man who has been divorced.[39]

Among the Moslems, a premium is placed on the pursuit of knowledge, and for this reason prenatal diagnosis is considered generally acceptable. Abortion may be possible up to the nineteenth week of pregnancy. If an abnormality is found during prenatal diagnosis, a committee of Islamic jurisprudence (the Fikh Committee) may help the couple to arrive at a decision that is in accord with Islamic law. Contraception and gamete selection are considered acceptable, but adoption, artificial insemination, and ovum donation are not acceptable reproductive options. In cases of neonatal death, it is acceptable for couples to hold the baby and to pursue postmortem studies, if these alternatives are handled in a sensitive way. Funeral arrangements can be made in the usual ways, but baptism and cremation are prohibited.[40]

Congenital anomalies are expected in all populations. Knowledge of cultural differences enables the medical team to be sensitive to the wide range of concepts and emotions that can be encountered. Respect and empathy for the individual and the family will help the team members through even the most difficult counseling sessions.

Acknowledgments—We appreciate the assistance of the Field Museum of Natural History (Chicago, IL) and the University of British Columbia Museum of Anthropology (Vancouver, B C). This research was supported in part by a Saul Blatman Clinical Fellowship Award to J.M.G., who is also partially supported by grant HO24580017 from the U.S. Department of Education, Office of Special Education and Rehabilitative Services, and by SHARE's Child Disabilities Center. We also express our thanks to Sheilah Levin for secretarial assistance.

References

1. Graham JM: Clinical approach to human structural defects. Semin Perinatol 15(Suppl 1):2, 1991.

2. Stevenson RE, Dean JH: Malformations as a cause of referral for genetic evaluation. Proc Greenwood Genet Center 11:3, 1992.

3. Warkany J: Congenital Malformations: Notes and Comments. Year Book Medical Publishers, Chicago, 1971.

4. Stevenson RE: Reproductive fitness. Semin Perinatol 9:263, 1985.

5. Mitscherlich A, Mielke F: The Death Doctors [tr by J Cleugh]. Elek Books, London, 1962.

6. Hippocrates: The Hippocratic Writings. On Airs, Waters, and Places [tr by F Adams], Encyclopedia Britannica, 1952, p 15.

7. Graham JM, Jr: Smith's Recognizable Patterns of Human Deformation, ed 2. WB Saunders, Philadelphia, 1988.

8. Dingwall EJ: Artificial Cranial Deformation: A Contribution to the Study of Ethnic Mutilation. John Bale, Sons, London, 1931.

9. Brothwell D: Possible evidence of a cultural practice affecting head growth in some lage cases—Pleistocene East Asian and Australasian populations. J Arch Sci 2:75, 1975.

10. Ewing JF: Hyperbrachycephaly as influenced by cultural conditioning. Papers of the Peabody Museum of American Archeology and Ethnology. Harvard Universtiy, Cambridge, vol 23(2), 1950.

11. Ritzenthaler RE: Indian cradles. Lore 1(2):1, 1967.

12. Niehoff A: For beauty's sake. Lore 3(2):1, 1969.

13. Clarren S, Smith DW, Hanson JW: Helmet therapy for plagiocephaly and congenital muscular torticullis. J Pediatr 94:43, 1979.

14. Clarren S: Plagiocephaly and torticollis: etiology, natural history and helmet treatment. J Pediatr 98:92, 1981.

15. Gillison G, Gillson D: Living theater in New Guinea's highlands. Natl Geographic 164:147, 1983.

16. Fisher A: Africa adorned. Natl Geographic 166:600, 1984.

17. Jeffrey D, Magubane P: Pioneers in their own land. Natl Geographic 169:262, 1986.

18. Beckwith C, Fisher A: The eloquent Surma of Ethiopia, Natl Geographic 179:76, 1991.

19. Lery HS: Chinese Footbinding. Walton Rawls, New York, 1966.

20. Hall JG: Recognizable human congenital anomaly syndromes in the masks of Northwest Coast Native American Indians. Unpublished data.

21. Kunze J, Nippert I: Genetics and Malformations in Art. Grosse Verlag, Berlin, 1986.

22. Clair C: Human Curiosities. Abelard Schuman, London, 1968.

23. Stuart GE, Stuart GS: The Mysterious Maya. National Geographic Society, Washington, DC, 1977.

24. Benson ER: The Mochica. Praeger, New York, 1972.

25. Donnan C: Moche Art of Peru. Museum of Cultural History (UCLA), Los Angeles, 1978.

26. Frayer DW, Macchiarelli R, Mussi M: A case of chondrodystrophic dwarfism in the Italian Late Upper Paleolithic. Am J Phys Anthropol 75:549, 1988.

27. Fiedler L: Freaks: Myths and Images of the Secret Self. Simon and Schuster, New York, 1978.

28. Drimmer F: Very Special People. Amjon Publishers, New York, 1973.

29. Monestier M: Human Oddities: a book of Nature's Anomalies. Citadel Press, Secaucus, NJ, 1987.

30. Wallace I, Wallace A: The Two. Simon and Schuster, New York, 1978.

31. Human Relations Area Files, Yale University, HRAF, Inc, New Haven, CT.

32. Trevathan WR: Human Birth: An Evolutionary Perspective. Aldine de Gruyter Publishers, Berlin, 1987.

33. Boas F: In: Kwakiutl Ethnography. H Codere, ed. University of Chicago Press, Chicago, 1966, p 362.

34. Lum RG: The patient–counselor relationship in a cross-cultural context. BDOAS XXIII(6):133, 1987.

35. Yuen J: Asian Americans. BDOAS XXIII(6):164, 1987.

36. Smith SC: Barriers to cross-cultural counseling: the American black perspective. BDOAS XXIII(6):183, 1987.

37. Keena BA, Jawanda M, Hall JG: Cultural influences and neural tube defects in the East Indian Sikh population of British Columbia. BDOAS XXIII(6):245, 1987.

38. Strauss RP: Genetic counseling in the cross cultural context: the case of highly observant Judaism. Patient 11:43, 1988.

39. Young M, Lieber C: Vitiligo in an Arab family. BDOAS XXIII(6):249, 1987.

40. Swinford AE, El-Fouty MH: Islamic religion and culture: principles and implications for genetic counseling. BDOAS XXIII(6):253, 1987.

41. Beckwith C, Fisher A: African Ark. Harry N. Abrams, New York, 1990.

42. Fisher A: Africa Adorned, Harry N. Abrams, New York, 1984.

43. Goodman RM, Gorlin RJ: The Malformed Infant and Child: An Illustrated Guide. Oxford University Press, New York, 1983.

44. Jones KL: Smith's Recognizable Patterns of Human malformations, ed 4, WB Saunders Co, Philadelphia, 1988.

9

Congenital Anomalies: Providing Information to the Family

JUDITH G. HALL

Talking with a family after the birth of an infant with congenital anomalies is rarely easy. Families are often distraught, the information may be quite technical, and it is always difficult to give bad news. However, it is the responsibility of health professionals to provide family members with as much information as possible so that they can make decisions that are appropriate for them. Frequently, the geneticist is the person to provide this information, but it could also be a family physician, a pediatrician, a pathologist, or an obstetrician. In many medical centers, there is a team of individuals who work together to provide information to families.

Genetic counseling is actually a process of information exchange: the medical geneticist needs to obtain information regarding the family history, review medical records, determine the concerns and questions of the family, and deal with many other details in order to provide the family with the information they require to make informed decisions regarding health care and reproductive planning. Furthermore, the process of providing information is usually an ongoing one. Rarely are all the details of the evaluation of an infant with anomalies available at the first contact with the family. Findings that come to attention during the course of the evaluation may require changes in the information initially given. Furthermore, as new discoveries occur, new diagnostic techniques are developed, and it may become possible to provide a specific diagnosis or other important information about the anomaly at a later date.

The type of information provided to a family at a particular time often depends on the urgency of the situation, the need to make decisions, or the need to collect additional information. However, a general outline of the information to be conveyed at some point during the course of the evaluation is provided below.

The need for information falls into three general time frames. The first occurs following the prenatal diagnosis of a congenital anomaly. At this time a family must decide whether to continue the pregnancy. If the pregnancy is continued, they must decide on the extent of usual or extraordinary support to be provided for the pregnancy and for the infant after delivery. Concerns for the mother's health must also be considered. The second situation in which there is an urgent need for information occurs when a child is born with unexpected congenital anomalies and decisions must be made immediately regarding how aggressively to support the child. Equally important in this situation are the fears and concerns of the parents. They will naturally wonder why the problem occurred, what should have been done differently, and who is to blame. In most such cases the family physician or pediatrician also urgently needs information on which to base therapy and prognosis. The third situation in which a family needs information arises a bit later, as they are trying

to make life-planning and reproductive decisions. This is usually in a calmer milieu, but the emotions and unresolved anxieties experienced by the family may be no less intense than in the two more urgent situations.

Clearly each of these three situations requires a slightly different approach. More importantly, though, each is unique. The family brings to the counseling session a unique set of personal and cultural experiences. Each disorder has a unique set of complications, diagnostic possibilities, and natural history. The health professionals involved also bring to the case their own set of values. These values may affect the way in which counseling is provided if great care is not taken to avoid judgmental or directive advice.

Frequently it is necessary to have several meetings with the family, since all of their concerns and questions cannot usually be addressed at one time. For example, long-term planning is not an appropriate topic for discussion in a life and death situation involving a critically ill newborn. Nevertheless, there are several general areas that need to be covered at some point, and the art of counseling lies in determining the best time and circumstances in which to convey complex but essential information. In acute situations, family members generally will not retain complicated details, and the information they receive will often be colored by their own anxieties or feelings of guilt. Families and individuals will usually go through predictable stages of emotional response when a child is found to have congenital anomalies: first there is denial, then a sense of loss and grieving, then anger and seeking someone to blame, followed by resignation, acceptance, and the search for meaningful and useful action (see chapter 10). Depending on which stage they are experiencing, information will be received in very different ways. In addition, different family members will often be at different stages, so it is important to consider individual members of the family.

Guidelines to providing information

As a rule, there are five basic principles to follow in providing information.

Education process

The provision of information is intended to be an educational process for the patient and/or family. Thus it is essential that it be provided in a way that is understandable to the family. Translators may be present, booklets written in lay language can be given, and a letter to the family summarizing the information discussed is a good follow-up procedure. Reviewing the information with the family or gently quizzing them on what they understood helps to determine whether in fact the educational goal has been met. To provide information on rare anomalies may require prior literature searches, use of computerized diagnostic programs, and extensive reading on the part of the counselor.

Exchange of information

As indicated earlier, a great deal of information is needed *from* the family in order to make an accurate diagnosis and to provide them with the information and counseling they need. Many elements of the family history are required, including ethnic origin, consanguinity, parental age, history of abortions and stillbirths, number of children with congenital anomalies, causes of any deaths, and so forth. All of these pieces of information from the family play a role in determining what information that particular family needs to receive during the genetic counseling session. Obtaining a proper family history usually takes at least one full hour, if carried through to third-degree relatives. Often it is necessary to send for records in order to confirm suspected diagnoses in family members. Without this type of detailed family history the information provided can be misleading or entirely erroneous. Further information about the pregnancy, delivery, and clinical course are also extremely important. If biopsies or autopsies have been done, those results must also be reviewed to confirm the accuracy of the current diagnosis.

Concerns and questions of the family

It is essential to determine what questions the family members have. The health care provider may believe they need to know one thing, while family members actually wish to know something entirely different. It may be appropriate to start any discussion with the family by asking them to list the questions they want to have answered. They can be encouraged actually to write their questions down as they think of them at home and to bring the list to appointments. They should be reassured that no matter how simple the question may seem, if it is important to them it needs to be answered.

Ongoing process

Providing information to a family is almost always an ongoing process. Often the medical geneticist will need to meet with the family on more than one occasion, initially because of critical medical circumstances and then later to obtain additional information or to discuss test results. However, even when all available information has been provided, it is appropriate for the family to keep in touch on a regular basis because of the possibility that there is a new development in diagnostic and management techniques, new methods of prenatal diagnosis or carrier detection, and so forth. Even in disorders that are thought to be environmental or due to a genetic predisposition to environmental influence, tests may be developed in the future to screen those individuals at risk.

Nondirective approach

Genetic counselors in North America agree that a nondirective approach is the preferred way to deal with families in the counseling as well as in the clinical setting. In other words, it is not the health professional's job to tell the family what to do, and it is ethically appropriate to support whatever decision they make. Nevertheless, this is a rather idealistic approach, since health professionals are likely to have personal or scientific values that may color their approach. It is important at least to attempt to recognize one's own biases and to present information in such a way that there are many alternative choices of action available to the family. Most families feel very lost at the time of diagnosis and assume that there are only one or two options available to them. The health professional should be aware that there are usually multiple options and multiple "appropriate" responses to the same situation. Part of the job, then, is to normalize for the family their reactions and to validate their emotions. They should be reassured that others facing the same situation would decide as they have. In addition, support should be provided so that each family can work through making the decisions that will be right for them.

The legal and ethical issues surrounding the question of individual rights versus the rights of society are very complex. The rights of the unborn are currently the subject of extensive discussion and debate. At present in North America, the consensus among health professionals is that a baby born after twenty-four weeks gestation with a functional central nervous system should be given every possible means of medical support to help insure its survival.

Topics to be covered during genetic counseling

There are five main areas that need to be covered in the provision of information during genetic counseling.[1-3] These are diagnosis, natural history, recurrence risk, available therapies, and prevention. The order in which these topics are covered will vary with different situations and different families as well as with different genetic counselors. Most often the best order in which to provide information will be determined by the details of the situation. However, it is important to make certain that each family has been given information in all of these areas before communication is ended.

Frequently, a family will not know what questions to ask. Therefore, the health professional may determine the family's background and knowledge and then place himself in the position of the family member by asking, "if I were in this situation, what kinds of information would I want to know?" It is important to remember that most families are fairly naive with regard to biology and medicine and that they do not have sufficient background to ask all of the questions that may have significant impact on their decisions.

Diagnosis

The diagnosis of the affected individual is the primary factor that determines the course of the counseling. Each type of congenital anomaly is relatively rare. The diagnosis should be written down for the family, and there should be some indication as to whether this is a specific diagnosis or a general category of related disorders and whether the diagnosis has been determined by a laboratory test or made on clinical grounds. Families will tolerate ambiguity surprisingly well, and the fact that a diagnosis is a clinical rather than a laboratory one is usually quite acceptable. What will not be well tolerated, however, are paternalistic reassurances that trivialize the family's need for information. The family needs to know the medical name of the disorder, what category it falls into, and what the different causes of this particular problem can be. Most families will raise the issue of blame at this point, wanting to know whether someone did something wrong or whether a specific drug or other agent might have caused the disorder. Care needs to be taken at this point not to encourage litigation or an inappropriate search for someone to blame. If it is a genetic condition, every effort needs to be made to avoid "finger-pointing."

The specific diagnosis needs to be put in perspective with regard to the frequency of congenital anomalies in the general population. Five percent of all individuals (2%–3% are obvious in newborns) have an abnormality of embryonic or fetal development that will require extensive hospitalization, major surgery, and long-term therapy or will alter the ability of the individual to function as an independent adult. Many anomalies are individually rare, but, when taken together, they represent a major source of morbidity and mortality in the general population. It has been estimated that each human being carries three to five recessive genes that could lead to a lethal disorder in a homozygous offspring. Since the carrier state for most recessive genes cannot be recognized, it is basically a matter of chance whether a spouse or partner also carries the same recessive genes.

Natural history

Frequently, the family is as much concerned about what to expect in the future of an affected child as they are about whether the disorder will recur in other offspring. Thus the natural history of the disorder needs to be discussed and the spectrum, from the most severe to the mildest variants, of the disorder explained. Changes anticipated over time and whether there will be deterioration or improvement, should be discussed, including a description of the various organ systems that may become involved, the usual age of incapacitation or death if that is probable, the likelihood that the individual will be able to live independently, and specific changes that will be necessary in terms of school and life planning for the affected child. It is important that the family have some perspective regarding where their child lies in the spectrum of involvement, i.e., whether it is a relatively mild or a relatively severe case. It is also important to be honest and forthright with the family, but it is not necessary to overwhelm or frighten them by overemphasizing negative details.

Recurrence risk

The recurrence risk for offspring of the patient, the parents, and other family members needs to be discussed with the family. In single gene disorders the recurrence risk may be straightforward. In complex or multifactorial disorders the risk may be uncertain, but it is unwise to say that a disorder can never recur. However, the relative frequency is important, and the family needs to have the risk of recurrence put into laymen's terms. In addition, the specific recurrence risk should be defined for all members of the pedigree. All members of the family may have concern regarding their risk when a relative is born with a congenital anomaly even though they may not seek medical advice directly. Thus it is usually a good idea to tell the family that other family members will probably be somewhat worried and information on their specific risk should be made available to them. It may help to explain that family members usually do not want to

upset the parents further and therefore may well not ask about their own personal risk. This reticence to ask difficult or painful questions usually stems from a concern for the feelings of the family, but it is important that specific risks for all family members be discussed.

Therapies

Depending on the particular disorder, a number of therapies may be available. If the natural history of the disorder is known, appropriate referral to specialists can be provided at the proper time. Much can be done in the way of preventive therapy, e.g., if a particular complication is common in that disorder, screening for that complication can be conducted at regular intervals. It is also important to indicate to the family what types of problems will not arise, e.g., patients with this disorder do not have an increased risk of developing cancer, mental retardation, and so forth. Because many individuals with congenital anomalies did not survive in the past, the long-term natural histories of some disorders are not known and data on the long-term effects of therapy are not yet available.

Planning for the future: prevention

Planning for the future involves preventing the birth of additional affected offspring when possible and appropriate. This may take the form of carrier detection, use of birth control or sterilization, utilization of prenatal diagnosis, and a variety of other modes of genetic diagnosis or therapy. It is important to be certain that the family has information about the current status of prevention and that prevention strategies not available today may become available very soon in this rapidly changing field. Thus families should try to keep up to date, either by joining specific disease-related lay groups or by regular consultation with their physician or genetic counselor, or both.

Anticipation of future needs for insurance, management of the family estate, and special care provisions may require additional planning by the family. If the child is severely disabled, it is important that the parents plan for that child in later life when the school system no longer provides appropriate care or when the parents can no longer care for the child at home. Considerations of birth control or sterilization may be important for the child who will be mobile, independent, and sexually active.

Many families have difficulty in knowing how to let friends and other family members know about the problems the affected child has. In general, it is important to help the family find the language to deal with their particular situation. This may include mention of a congenital anomaly on the birth announcement, such as, "We have been told by the doctor that baby Estelle has Down syndrome. She is very healthy, however, and we are feeling very fortunate that she doesn't seem to have some of the life threatening problems that many children with Down syndrome have." It is also important to help the family find ways to break the silence that their friends often maintain because of their own discomfort regarding the problems of the child or their concern over embarrassing the family. If the child has obvious physical abnormalities the family needs to prepare themselves to deal with the curiosity and rudeness of strangers. They should be encouraged on their "good days" to smile and be interactive, while on their "bad days" they should feel free to respond to rudeness by identifying it as rudeness. Discussing these feelings and experiences with other parents who have a similarly affected child can be extremely helpful to a family in normalizing and validating their feelings and in finding alternative ways to deal with difficult situations.

It is important to remind the family that the decisions and plans they have made need to be discussed regularly among the family members, since many things can change over time. For instance, the family of a child with Down syndrome may find it helpful to sit down each year and ask how each member is coping. Are the normal children being neglected? Does all the activity of the family center around the disabled child? Is the marital relationship suffering because the parents have little time alone together? By recognizing that such problems could or do exist, a family can plan changes for the coming year, making sure that time is set aside for the entire family, and that each family member receives special attention. This type of formal reassessment will help maintain the cohesion of the family and allow members to cope with the stresses of disability without totally sacrificing their own needs.

The parents of a child with a congenital anomaly need to become experts on that anomaly. Frequently, their experience will provide them with more information and knowledge than most physicians have, particularly in the case of a rare congenital anomaly. They need to be encouraged to develop their knowledge through appropriate reading (which can be provided through most hospital libraries under the guidance of their physician or counselor) and to seek out other parents or a lay support group for families of children with their particular disorder. It will be extremely important in the long run that they develop such knowledge and support, as it will aid in obtaining the best possible care for their child, as well as helping to realize the child's full potential. In reading medical information, a family will probably need a certain amount of interpretation. It is also important that they not "go off on tangents" that have no scientific basis. Again, being part of a lay support group is often the most useful way to direct such interest and energy.

Talking with families can be an extremely rewarding experience for the health professional, even when bad news must be given. The family needs information they can understand in order to make appropriate decisions, and a physician or counselor can provide invaluable support during a difficult time. In general, families need to be aware that there are many options available to them in any given situation and that it is appropriate to take the broad view. This will allow them time to consider alternatives that they might not have felt were right for them initially but that turn out to be the best choice for their present situation. Ideally, they will not need to make instant decisions and will therefore have the opportunity to weigh the various options. It is important that a family not feel "backed into a corner," but rather are helped to recognize that negative emotions and reactions are normal and natural. It is important, also, that they be helped to progress emotionally and not get "hung up" on one feeling or solution, since the evolution of feelings is a normal process for families of children with congenital anomalies.

References

1. Kelly TE: Clinical Genetics and Genetic Counselling. Year Book Medical Publishers, Chicago, 1980.
2. Garver KL, Marchese SG: Genetic Counselling for Clinicians. Year Book Medical Publishers, Chicago, 1986.
3. Berini RY, Kahn E, eds: Clinical Genetics Handbook. National Genetics Foundation, Medical Economics Books, Oradell, NJ, 1987.

10

Implications of the Child with Malformations for the Family and Society

PATRICK M. MACLEOD

> ... then the paediatrician arrives; she examines the baby very carefully which appears to last for hours. She slowly crosses the delivery room, her head slightly bent forward and the mother senses her worried expression. She takes the mother's hand and, in a vibrating somewhat low voice says "there is some problem, your baby has a significant handicap." Although these words do not tell much about the baby's condition, the mother does perceive the seriousness of the situation—and slowly, very slowly tears begin to flow. What has happened to the wonderful dreams of these parents? The dream is gone, it is gone forever, and a nightmare begins to unfold: the world crumbles and folds around them.[1]

Throughout history, congenital anomalies have been observed in all nations and in all branches of the human family. They are the common legacy of mankind. In all cultures, birth defects have claimed a fascination difficult to explain on a purely rational basis.

They have attracted disproportionate attention and elicited astonishment or fright. The question of cause and meaning emerged and has been answered in various ways, mostly by attributing malformations to God's inscrutable plans or to malevolent spirits.[2]

There is a close correlation between body image and self-esteem. We look to see if other people approve or disapprove of us (and ours) in our activities, dress, and appearance.[3] Physical disfigurement, deformities, disabilities, and diseases constitute major stigmas. Stigma is an attribute, an undesirable differentness, that discredits or disqualifies the individual from full social acceptance.[4] The degree of discrimination depends on the extent and forms of social interaction and acceptance in the culture involved.[5]

The central feature of the stigmatized individual's situation in life ... is a question of what is often, if vaguely, called "acceptance."... although each individual is born belonging to the human community, he or she soon questions whether there is a place for them in the group. All of us devalue ourselves early in our existence. It is for this reason, universal to us all, that the birth of a child who is different, other than "normal," affects each and every family member. Having questioned his or her belonging and most likely decided that acceptance is conditional—"I belong only if . . ."—each family member assimilates the fact of the birth of an abnormal child and draws a conclusion about his or her own value and acceptance. The actual difference of the child is not as important as the conclusion of each person about the impact of the event. It is the individual perception of each relative of the child that will affect how he or she adjusts to the birth of that child. . . .[6]

Implications for the individual

Impact on life span

Fetal loss (as stillbirths) during the late second and the third trimesters of pregnancy occurs once in 80–120 births, with malformations accounting for approximately 25% of the

loss. The majority of deaths are the result of multifactorial, chromosomal, and single gene disorders.[7] Congenital anomalies have become the leading cause of infant mortality during the first week and the first year of life. They are the fifth leading cause of years of potential life lost.[8]

The increased mortality during the perinatal period of infants born with congenital anomalies carries over into early childhood and beyond. The fourth edition of *Smith's Recognizable Patterns of Human Malformation*[9] gives as part of the natural history of each condition a reference to life span and cognitive function in 278 conditions that have one or more anomalies. Thirty-five percent of these conditions are associated with death in the neonatal period, early infancy, or childhood. The increased mortality associated with congenital anomalies is summarized in Table 10-1. In addition, mental retardation occurs in roughly 32% of those children with malformations who survive their first year of life. This monograph further shows that the malformation syndromes have various etiologies, and many of them are hereditary (Table 10-2). In general, chromosomal anomalies produce the most severe forms of disability with the greatest proportion of early death.

The natural history of malformations

Research into the long-term outcome of hereditary disorders including malformations has begun to provide useful insights into the natural history of individuals with birth defects. Costa et al.[10] have completed one study using the McKusick catalog[11] as a source for a description of single

Table 10-1. Perinatal and postnatal mortality associated with 278 conditions with congenital anomalies

Period of lethality	No.	Percent
Perinatal period	40	14
Infancy	15	6
Childhood	24	8
Adolescence	19	7
Total	98	35

From Jones.[9]

Table 10-2. The etiology in 278 recognizable patterns of human malformations

Etiology	No.	Percent
Autosomal recessive	83	30
Autosomal dominant	74	27
Unknown	34	12
Chromosomal	31	11
Sporadic	24	8
X-linked	19	7
Teratogenic	13	5
Total	278	100

From Jones.[9]

gene disorders. The fifth edition listed 1489 dominant, 1117 recessive, and 205 X-linked conditions. Costa et al.[10] calculated that two-thirds of all entities caused impairment, disability, or handicap. A malformation phenotype was present in 42% of cases. The authors went on to quantify the impact of life span, reproductive capability, and psychosocial characteristics. Life span was reduced in 57% of the conditions, particularly in those with congenital or preadolescent onset. Reproductive capability was impaired in two-thirds of the phenotypes, and most conditions caused psychosocial handicap and resulted in limited access to schooling and employment. They also studied the effects of treatment on life span and reproductive capability. Their findings are summarized in Table 10-3.

The outlook for children born with a malformation of the heart has improved considerably in the past twenty years with the recognition that the infant with congenital heart disease is frequently normally developed and well nourished and can stand operation well, provided the diagnosis and decisions have been made before any deterioration in the condition has occurred.[12] Children with many types of congenital heart lesions are now reaching adulthood. It has been estimated that in the United States in 1995 there will be nearly 300,000 children under the age of 21 yr with congenital heart disease.[13] Of these, at least one-third will have had one or more surgical procedures. Previously, without effective treatment, at least 40% of such children died within the first 5 yr of life.[12]

Table 10-3. The effects of treatment on hereditary diseases

Aspect	Untreated: reduced or impaired	Treated		
		Restored to normal	Improved	Unchanged
Life span	86ᵃ	24	29	47
Reproduction	91	17	30	53
Somatic growth	66	41	18	41
Intelligence	54		37	63
Schooling	67		36	64
Ability to work	86			71
Cosmetic integrity	78		41	59

ᵃValues are percentages of cases studied.

From Costa et al.[10]

Much less dramatic progress has been achieved for children born with defects in closure of the neural tube. Despite the early assessment and intervention of a multidisciplinary team composed of a pediatrician, neurologist, neurosurgeon, urologist, physiatrist, social worker, clinical psychologist, pharmacist, and dietician using the most sophisticated forms of diagnosis and treatment, fewer than one-half of babies born with neural tube defects survive their third birthday. Of those who do, 50% have two or more major disabling complications as they grow into adolescence and young adulthood.[14]

Chronic illness

Although cumulatively congenital anomalies represent a significant fraction of the chronic diseases of childhood, they are individually rare. So rare in fact are individual anomalies that most family physicians have little or no previous experience in dealing with the multiplicity of problems posed by affected infants and children. In many cases there is little specific information available, and there are generally few local medical experts to help the family gain access to specialized diagnostic and treatment opportunities. Often these goals are achieved through the intervention of parent support networks such as the National Organization of Rare Diseases. Therefore, the treatment implications for the individual with a malformation are best viewed from the perspective of the child with a chronic disease.

An estimated 1 million children in the United States have serious chronic conditions, including juvenile-onset diabetes mellitus, muscular dystrophy, cystic fibrosis, spina bifida, sickle cell anemia, congenital heart disease, hemophilia, leukemia, cleft palate, and severe asthma. Another 9 million children have less severe conditions. Put another way, about 10%–15% of the childhood population has a chronic illness. Among chronically ill children, about 10% (or 1%–2% of the total childhood population) have a severe disability, which places heavy demands on general pediatric practice.

Baird et al.[15] estimate the incidence of genetic diseases, including congenital anomalies, in British Columbia to be 60.7 per 1000 live births. However, the prevalence of most individual congenital anomalies is still low. The rarity of many of these conditions may serve as a disincentive for a physician to become involved with affected children, because they pose special problems.

Because of the physiologic diversity of anomalies, the varying life expectancy of affected children, and the range of treatment options, there has been a tendency for individual corps of specialists to develop around specific malformations. Medical professionals become affiliated with specialty clinical centers, and advocacy groups and lobbyists in the various governmental assemblies also become highly specialized. The net result is competition for funding rather than cooperation and fragmentation of what could otherwise be a potent political lobby.

In addition, the rehabilitation efforts, so much a part of the program of the young disabled child, tend to falter as the child moves into adolescence. Numerous studies have shown that beginning in adolescence there is a rapid decline in contact with the health care system. It has been estimated that 90% of handicapped young adults do not receive physiotherapy and occupational therapy, which are usually considered integral to treatment programs.[16]

Education and employment

The three areas with the least success in treatment—intelligence, learning, and the ability to work—deserve additional attention. In the majority of cases, chromosome and monogenic disorders perturb early embryonic development, especially of the nervous system, and commonly produce a static condition characterized by irreversibly impaired intelligence. In many of the remaining cases, however, the potential for normal intellectual development is intact.

Education

The problems confronting the physically disabled children who are being educated in ordinary schools, variously described as a "national disgrace" or a chronic backlog of unmet needs, have been the subject of two decades of heated debate. One estimate is that less than one fourth of the children who have a physical handicap and who are in need of special educational services are being helped.[17]

A recent Health and Limitation Survey in Canada indicates perhaps an encouraging trend toward integration of the physically handicapped into the educational mainstream. Approximately 25% of the total population of Canada are between the ages of 0 and 14 yr, and of these 5.2% are classified as disabled. Of those who are disabled and between the ages of 5 and 14 yr, 51% attend regular schools and an additional 30% are enrolled in special classes; only 6% attend special schools. Eight percent do not attend any type of school. Data for the remaining 5 percent are unavailable.[18] Greater than 95% live within private households, and fewer than 1% are in institutions. The remainder live in group home settings.

Employment

The opportunities for people who are physically disabled to receive vocational training are limited. Despite the development of incentives within the workplace to hire the handicapped and despite modern medical treatment, most people with major anomalies do not work.

The employability of people with moderate-to-severe physical handicaps is receiving increased attention. It is now recognized that handicapped people can enjoy the normalizing attributes of a nonsheltered workplace and the prospects of advancement, increased wages, and benefits that competitive employment offers. It has been determined that these social benefits outweigh any advantages of segregated adult programs.[19] Alliances between special education and vocational teachers, rehabilitation and placement counselors, administration representatives from the business community, and advocacy groups representing the handicapped have bound together to foster job placement. A variety of programs funded by state, provincial, and federal agencies are now in place to develop equal work opportunities for the disabled.

Psychosocial development

The interplay of such factors as family functioning, school competence, social support, self-perception, and the microstressors of everyday life in the determination of self-esteem and the development of the adaptable and compensatory attitude necessary for psychosocial development is now beginning to be understood in the context of the malformed child.[20] Similarly, behaviorial research is being directed toward understanding the elements of the psychosexual development of young adults with handicapping conditions. Counseling on these issues for individuals and families is becoming integrated into comprehensive treatment programs.[21]

Implications for the family

We now recognize that the majority of all women who conceive lose their babies through abortion, stillbirth, or infant death. Data from a number of studies demonstrate that two-thirds of human ova, embryos, and fetuses fail to reach birth. It has been estimated that about 30% of human ova perish at the time of fertilization. Fully 50% of spontaneously aborted embryos in the first trimester have an abnormal karyotype. In addition, approximately 25% of the estimated 8/1000 fetuses that are stillborn have multiple congenital malformations. Until very recently we seem to have been unwilling to accept stillbirth as a tragedy that could seriously affect the mental health of the bereaved mother and family. Bourne[22] has shown that physicians are (surprisingly) reluctant to know or remember anything about the patient who had a stillbirth. The conspiracy of silence surrounding the issue has only now been breached with the acknowledgement of a generalized abhorrence of stillbirths[23] and with the subsequent development of protocols for the evaluation and postmortem examination of stillbirths with the emphasis on suspected genetic disease.[24,25]

> Every year those who have suffered childbearing loss are joined by millions of new mourners: 600,000 to 800,000 who miscarry, 60,000 with ectopic pregnancy, the parents of almost 250,000 victims of perinatal death, 5,000 SIDS [sudden infant death syndrome] parents, 1.5 million women who abort, and over 3 million who cannot conceive.[29]

> Is it any wonder we have a country of grieving women? And if the women are grieving, can we not expect their babies, their children—society itself—to be in pain?[26]

The birth of a child with a major congenital anomaly is every parent's fear. However, troublesome thoughts are usually suppressed, and most parents are therefore totally unprepared when confronted by the reality of an afflicted child.

Parental reactions

The tasks of parenting a child with a defect are similar to those of parenting a normal child. Effective parenting requires empathy, learning the infant's cues, organizing and expanding alert periods, and supporting the infant in the gradual development of a tolerance for frustration.[27]

> If a child can grow up in a loving and caring environment where the parents have an understanding of basic issues of child development and the wisdom and sensitivity to make use of such knowledge then this child's future is not in jeopardy. If parents respond positively to their child, the child will gain self-confidence and trust. These principles hold true for families with both normal as well as handicapped children.[1]

To accomplish all this, parents must be self-assured and positive in their role. Parents who must face the reality that their newborn is less than perfect suffer a blow to their self-esteem that puts them off balance.

There is no reason to expect that mothers [parents] are automatically equipped for the specialized task of bringing up such a child in a manner calculated to minimize the handicap. On the contrary, the mother's natural hurt and despair concerning her child's defect, the injury to her pride and pleasure in her child, will all work toward estranging her from the task of mothering thereby increasing the initial damage. . . . There are a whole host of emergency situations of this kind in which the normal mother will feel helpless without guidance. . . .[29]

No one can directly enhance another person's self-esteem, but clinicians and medical support staff can indirectly affect it by targeting the determinants of general self-esteem. A major determinant is the need for strong social support. This is provided by the most significant persons in the parent's life, especially the immediate family members—spouse, parents, and siblings.[20,28]

Often disturbing events that may further undermine parental adaptation and attempts at coping include cesarean section, premature birth, separation from the infant because of the need for special tests, a mother's hospital discharge without her infant, and specific difficulties in arranging caretaker needs.

There is a complex interplay of factors that affect parental reactions to the birth of a handicapped child. These include the severity and correctibility of the defect, how they were told about it, the infant's temperament and capacity to interact and be organized, the uncertainty about the short-range and long-range implications of the defect, the nature of the medical treatment required, and previous expectations for the child. The parent's views of themselves as parents, their prior means of coping with stress, the nature of the marital relationship, their experiences in parent–child relationships, and the presence or absence of environmental supports also influence their reactions.[27]

During the past twenty years some research has focused on the reactions of parents to the birth of a handicapped child. Various authors[30–35] have reviewed this work and conceptualized what has become to be known as the *bereavement response*. This is defined as the psychological work that has to be done to come to terms with the loss of a significant object or loved person.[36] Similar to the stages of death and dying formulated by Elisabeth Kübler-Ross, the bereavement response occurs in stages as the physical, emotional, mental, and spiritual aspects of childbearing loss are dealt with.

Grief is a gift . . . it is a pure, natural emotion—the infinite sadness of missing a loved one or losing something cherished. When grief is unfiltered, it is right and good and healthy. It needs no work or change or therapy . . . it heals itself. But when we begin to filter our grief through sieves of guilt, anger, resentment, bitterness or self-pity, then we need to work. . . .[37]

Grieving

The "stages of grieving" model describes the initial crisis response as shock, denial, and disbelief. This is quickly followed by a period of what has been termed *emotional disorganization,* during which the parents experience guilt, disappointment, anger, and lowered self-esteem. Eventually, the parents reach the stage characterized by emotional organization, adjustment, and acceptance. This is a time of diminishing self-preoccupation and of movement toward realistically addressing the problems of the child and the family.[38] Proponents of this model have been criticized for

stereotyping parents,[39] but it is now the case that more objective data are being collected.[40]

In my experience, grieving is ongoing over many months, with the adjustment and acceptance commonly appearing in the first 6 months. This stage has been conceptualized as a series of disappointments associated with adjustments to the limitations posed by the malformation(s). I view the parents' psychological responses as a series of crises that continue beyond the first year and that can be anticipated and dealt with by timely recall and reinforcement. As new feelings emerge they must be understood in terms of causation. The work of rebuilding self-esteem must be supported and encouraged; an environment of understanding, concern, and acceptance must be fostered; and the support of partners, relatives, and friends must be developed. Genetic counseling must continue, sometimes over a period of several years, until the task is completed,[41] and any succeeding pregnancy must be planned differently to include the prospects of prenatal diagnosis and the choices which that brings.[42]

The initial response to the news that the baby is malformed is generally one of disbelief, followed by panic. This slowly gives way to heart-wrenching sorrow felt by both parents because they have brought a sick or damaged child into the world.

Do you know that when I was told that my baby was handicapped, something died in me . . . something that I know will never live again. A part of me had died, a part that will never live again.[28]

During the first few days and weeks these feelings give way to more personal and frightening aspects as the aftershocks begin. Guilt in all its forms takes its toll.

I did this to her . . . she can never have kids and its my fault. . . .

Please God, make him better, take this away and I promise I will never . . . again.

As time passes and a new, brighter day has begun, then rage begins to fill up the few remaining places in an already overburdened spirit. These are hellish days.

I still have not come to terms with it, . . . and I don't know if I ever will. I went through the why-me phase, wondering why people who have perfect children give them away, and here I am with everything to give a child and I have *him.*[43]

Damn it I knew I should have had a C-section then none of this would be happening.

Jim says that there is no one on his side of the family with this spina bifida, it must be on ours.

Such anger is directed as much against oneself as against a self-absorbed world made up of people and events that seem to conspire to attack the family's self-esteem and to isolate their grief.

Friends stopped calling, and when I walked down the corridor to the Nursery everybody stopped talking.

There were no congratulations . . . just nothing.

The first time I took Adam out in the stroller to the market a lady came up behind me in the line. When she noticed I had caught her looking at the baby she put her hand on my arm and said "there, there my dear, you are so brave."

But eventually, in the coming days and weeks that slowly, like a dream, pass into months and then years, the spirit responds with new vigor as resignation gives way to hope.

. . . but you can't go on feeling that way. He's six months old. He's a person now, not some creature who comes into your life and destroys everything. . . . [34]

I don't know what my reasons for living were before—they don't seem important any more. . . . Now we have people to educate, letters to write, special teachers to see. It makes us feel we are doing something to help Kimberly. [33]

Maladaptive responses

If for whatever reason the family does not work through these stages to completion, they become sidetracked and mired in maladaptive responses.

Ours is a death denying culture, and an emotion denying culture. It is this denial which immobilizes us in our attempts to reach out to others in open acceptance of real grieving. . . . We say to one another, "Oh, it happened for a reason," or "It could have been worse," or "Everything will be all right." Statements like these close the door on communication, minimize the intensity of grief and give us the message that our feelings are not all right, cannot be understood or shared and thus we are blocked from releasing them. . . . [44]

In the case of congenital anomalies, the bereavement response may involve mourning the loss of the perfect child who was stillborn or who died in the perinatal period. Alternatively it may involve the continued presence of the malformed child in the family group, forcing a constant awareness of the imperfections and the causes and consequences of the imperfections, the extra work, and the recurring sense of disappointment. [36]

Some parents of malformed infants become fixed in a chronic state of denial. One consequence is that they go "doctor shopping," an expensive, disruptive, and oftentimes counterproductive journey. Denial is part of the human repertoire of primitive psychological defenses. The function of denial is to protect against painful truths. Denial of reality is illogical and therefore cannot be overcome by logic. [45]

For the psychodynamically oriented counselor, Leon's recent book *When a Baby Dies* [46] is a primer for developing a psychotherapeutic understanding of and treatment strategies for an individual or couple trapped in a maladaptive response. The counselor must guard against any natural tendency to argue or to become angry, resentful, or rejecting or otherwise to contribute to the perpetuation of denial. This is the time for empathy, understanding, and patience. The consequences of unresolved maladaptive responses can be a brief relationship between parents and child that ends in the nursery with overt rejection and placement of the child in foster care or, rarely, up for adoption. It can also lead to a lifetime of overprotection.

For the most part, however, the immediate and short-term impact of the birth of a child with a congenital anomaly is absorbed by the couple, if not by other members of the extended family. This is in part due to the innate capacity of each individual to adapt to change. Exactly how this adaptation evolves is rooted in the individual's upbringing, maturity, emotional stability, and general philosophy of life. With sympathy, compassion, and the tincture of time, denial ultimately gives way to acceptance, perhaps the most complicated response, made up as it is of fantasy, duty, resignation, and love.

Whenever I hear James cry, I hear his cry, but I also hear the perfect cry, of the perfect baby I never had.

Acceptance is the death of an imaginary ideal child, and the redirection of parental love to the newly perceived child as he is in reality. [36]

Mothers, at least, appear to undergo an adjustment process that results in the perception of a somewhat lesser burden than what they would have envisioned prior to having an affected child. [47] They begin to make complex decisions to achieve an acceptable solution rather than an optimal one. [48]

As acceptance is reached the process of restitution begins, but occasionally a family can become sidetracked if they are unable to make the transition as parents of a handicapped baby to the parents of a handicapped child, or young adult. Efforts to maintain the status quo or becoming overly mobilized, a crusader for the child, are manic defense mechanisms against grief and anger and a frantic obscuring of chronic sorrow. [28]

Chronic sorrow

There are occasions (important milestones; the child's entering puberty, the 21st birthday, unforeseen medical complications such as the development of seizures, or social concerns such as the establishment of guardianship) when for even the best-adjusted parents the intense grieving feelings are re-evoked and re-experienced. The negative feelings—the shock, the guilt, and the bitterness—never disappear; they remain part of each parent's emotional life as an enduring, chronic sorrow. [49] The findings of Wikler et al. [58] suggest that parents' responses showed no decrease in the intensity of the emotions experienced with the passage of time. Chronic sorrow does not seem to be an abnormal response; rather, it is a normal reaction to an abnormal situation, and periodic grieving should be considered a coping strength rather than a neurotic reaction.

Self-esteem

It is important to recognize the magnitude of the assault to the family's self-esteem that occurs with the birth of a malformed infant. One of the psychological tasks of any birth is to view the infant as part of the self and partner and family, but also as a separate person. When a child is born with a defect, this task is more difficult to accomplish because the child may represent the negative or defective part of the self. [51] During the initial period of disequilibrium both parents' capacity to assume the parenting role is compromised if they view the infant as a negative part of themselves rather than as a separate person.

It is important to identify positive aspects of the infant and to view the infant as a separate person if the grief-work is to occur. . . . The parents' injured self-esteem needs to be addressed prior to the successful initiation of the process of grieving. [27]

The marriage

Much of the literature suggests that the birth of a malformed infant is accompanied by deterioration in the marriage relationship. For example, Gath [52] found in her prospective study that the marriages of couples who had a child with Down syndrome were significantly more likely to be unhappy 1 year after the birth of the child. In a study of 107 families with a child with spina bifida, Walker et al. [53] found that more than one-third of the parents were in relationships that they thought had deteriorated; in three cases the marriage had broken down completely. In a second study of families with a spina bifida child, Tew et al.[54] found that the quality of the marital relationship in the index families deteriorated over the years, and the divorce rate was twice that among controls and the general population.

Among the less-educated and younger families, and among those from the lower socioeconomic class, the burden of caring for a child with a severely disabling condition such as cystic fibrosis, muscular dystrophy, or hemophilia has an additive negative effect on the family. More marital difficulties were reported by couples whose affected child was their only child or one who required special home care.[55] Some couples, by virtue of their own social isolation, inadequate support system, marital maladjustment, financial problems, and inadequate child care arrangements, are at high risk for becoming abusing parents of the child with congenital anomalies.[56,57]

On the other hand, there are many anecdotes in the literature attesting to the positive effects of parenting a child with a birth defect.

> . . . but if you work at it, this special child can be the opportunity for better communication, for finding new courage and love in your partner. . . . Personally, I have never appreciated my husband so much; the feeling of mutual support has enhanced our marriage.[1]

Marriages that are based on firm foundation of love and care usually are enhanced and become stronger.

> In marriage, as in other realms, the rich get richer and the poor get poorer.[1]

The siblings' adjustment

Only a very few studies have been designed to measure the impact of a handicapped child on the siblings, and the results have been difficult to interpret. For example, in one study the siblings of patients with spina bifida were four times more likely to exhibit maladjustment in school than were the siblings of healthy control subjects, and the siblings of the children with slight handicaps were the most disturbed.[58] As with marital discord, deviant behavior in siblings of mentally retarded children was related to family size and social class, with the larger and poorer families exhibiting the greatest susceptibility to stress.[59]

Being the sibling of a handicapped child can be a frustrating, unhappy, and anxious experience filled with jealousy, insecurity, and resentment, particularly if there is competition for parental support, attention, and financial resources or if the siblings become burdened with domestic responsibility or the prospect of becoming a long-term primary caregiver. A lack of understanding of the cause or the familial nature of the birth defect can add to the bruden. On the other hand, there are as many opportunities for the siblings to experience positive feelings from their participation in caring and support of the affected sibling, and of their support during times of parental adjustment, an enhanced appreciation of human frailty and the learning of compassion.

The grandparents' reactions

Grandparents bring their own unique life experiences, approaches, and biases to the situation of the family of a child born with a congenital anomaly or genetic disorder. Their views of life and spirituality often represent shared family values and attitudes and can be a source of immediate and steadfast support. However, these interrelationships may also be affected by private views. For example, a lack of acceptance of their child's choice of marriage partner may be further exacerbated by the birth of a child with a defect.[6] Having to deal with the expectations, blame, guilt, or over-protectiveness of the grandparents only adds to the burden of the parents.

> Each family member and the family as a whole desires to belong, to be connected to the larger community of humankind. . . . The birth of a child with a genetic disorder (or malformation) challenges this sense of belonging.[6]

The parents' awareness, knowledge, and understanding of their child's condition, together with support from parent groups, extended family, and friends; having more than one child; economic security; ongoing professional services for the child; and personal faith and religion appear to be the most important factors in the positive adjustment of parents.[60] The 1980s was a decade in which parent support groups developed for most if not all types of malformation syndromes. A public-supported coalition representing well over 100 organizations, foundations, and self-help groups has formed the National Organization of Rare Disorders, which is dedicated to the prevention, control, and cure of over 5000 rare "orphan" diseases and to the welfare of people afflicted by these devastating illnesses.[61]

The implications for society of congenital anomalies

Congenital anomalies have the notable ability to arouse and hold people's interest and attention. The oldest word in our language to denote an individual with a malformation, *monster,* has obscure origins, but whether it derives from *moneo,* meaning *to warn,* or *monstro,* meaning *to show forth,* the implications are the same: congenital malformations are the products not of a whim of nature but of the design of Providence.[62]

Perceived by society as unfortunate messengers, afflicted children and adults have always suffered at the hands of their brothers, whether as part of the ritual sacrifices of priestly executioners or as part of what Benno Muller-Hill[63] terms the "destructive symbiosis between science and government" represented by the New Order that the Nazis imposed on Germany and most of Europe. Between these epochs the malformed found a home of sorts in sideshows and circus tents. This too is disappearing.

> That the respect, the devotion, the time and the means required to help handicapped persons, those who are gravely lacking in their mental faculties, is the price society must generously pay to live truly as human.[64]

Economic implications

The impact of congenital anomalies on society can be measured in part by studying the economics of meeting the special needs of a family with an affected child and of maintaining those social programs that have evolved in response to these needs.

The social costs

With the development of prenatal diagnostic procedures, the prevention of some birth defects has become possible at reasonable cost. As a result, data have been collected in an attempt to determine how much to invest in preventing birth defects. The most detailed analyses have concentrated on Down syndrome because it is the most common handicapping condition for which reliable prenatal diagnosis is available. A cost-of-condition analysis takes into consideration a myriad of factors, including prevalence, loss of output, and the costs of prevention, education, residential care, day care, and homemaking services, as well as any other unpaid help received. One such analysis estimated that the aggregate social cost of Down syndrome in the United States is in excess of $4.5 billion.[65]

Family expenses

Parenting, variously described as "a mixture of love, anger, inspiration and obstinacy,"[66] universally involves monetary expenses as well as the emotional ones. Although society shares in the financial cost through the provision of preschool, education, and youth services, public housing and subsidies, direct financial transfers to children in the form of family allowances and tax credits, or benefits when parental care breaks down, it is the parents who carry the major costs of feeding, clothing, and providing housing, education, medical care, and recreation. Parenting is increasingly associated with a reduction in the total family income when the mother of a handicapped child must leave the workforce for extended periods of time without financial reimbursement; at the same time, the mother may lose opportunities to pursue a career, to compete for a promotion, or to make contributions to personal benefit programs.[67]

The actual measurement of the lifetime care costs is complicated and seldom complete. However, it is known that for these families costs are disproportionately high. To give some perspective of the potential ruinous financial implications, Table 10–4 lists some of the medical costs that have been reported in various reviews.

Insurance

While the majority of children with anomalies are now covered by some form of private health insurance, either as beneficiaries of programs provided their employed parents or by private subscription, the benefits are for the most part limited to the reimbursement of medical costs and there are often additional premiums and specific exclusions or limited coverage for nonmedical costs. When the costs of transportation, special applicances, medications, counseling, and custodial care are added to the lost wages for time away from work, the "out-of-pocket" expenses are substantial; for many families they range from 10% to 30% of the family income.[68]

For a significant minority of parents who are chronically unemployed or living below the poverty line, private insurance coverage is not a possibility. For these families, and to some extent for all families, the financing of the special health care needs of their children is a particularly complex and often frustrating exercise in searching through a maze of federal, provincial, state, and voluntary programs. In any community, families with disabled children are a tiny minority of those seeking assistance because of unemployment, marriage breakdown, or poverty. There is little opportunity for social agencies to gain experience with the special needs of these families. Their plight is made more poignant by the misguided attempts of some third party agencies to deny insurance or to insist that they take steps to avoid the conception or birth of another affected child.[69]

As a result, caring for handicapped children can become an isolating experience. The parents feel that they are left alone to cope, to learn what help is available, and to obtain it often after considerable frustration and delay and that their concern is unrecognized and unshared. When approached, these parents are likely to request services and support; they are looking for skilled, informed, and prompt help, advice, encouragement, and recognition, rather than money.

Our society seems to lack anything like a tradition for raising reasonably happy, reasonably self-fulfilling handicapped children. Few parents have had the experience of being handicapped themselves, and there is no cultural tradition that tells a parent how to raise a handicapped child.[66]

In the absence of such a tradition and in these increasingly constrained economic times, with governments cutting public expenditure and sweeping away the so-called dependency culture,[67] we have turned to "prevention" as a socially sanctioned means of dealing with risks. As we observed the Decade of the Disabled, we were poised on the verge of the twenty-first century with its unprecedented promises of highly refined conventional therapies, including organ transplantation, gene manipulation, and even gene replacement. With respect to congenital anomalies, however, there is the growing appreciation of another reality. Because so many of the diseases with onset before birth are congenital anomalies, and since the most severely affected phenotypes are those with the earliest onset, prevention—some would say, avoidance—rather than treatment is likely to be the most efficient, cost-effective and humanitarian strategy for dealing with this burdensome issue.

An array of prenatal screening and diagnostic strategies are being developed and implemented. The routine monitoring of at-risk pregnancies in women aged 35 yrs or older by chorionic villus biopsy or genetic amniocentesis is now being supplemented by population-based measurement of material serum α-fetoprotein to screen for neural tube defects and measurement of estriol and β-human chorionic gonadotropin to screen for autosomal trisomies. The widespread use of obstetric ultrasound is providing early diagnosis of congenital anomalies at an unprecedented rate. As a result some congenital anomalies such as neural tube defects are "a vanishing nightmare."[70]

However, about 20% of families will not use pregnancy termination to deal with a prenatally detected malformation.

Table 10–4. Average costs of care for selected chronic childhood illnesses

Condition	Average cost per year
Cystic fibrosis	$ 6,191
Congenital heart disease	13,000
Hemophilia	10,238
Chronic renal disease	6,729–16,520
Spina bifida	10,850–22,405

From Perrin and Ireys.[68]

The scarcity of follow-up data on these families leaves the medical profession poorly prepared to deal with their plight. Among parents of children with Down syndrome there is an extreme range of opinions regarding such controversial issues as amniocentesis and abortion. The extremes are indicative of a lack of consensus about the appropriateness of such procedures.[71] By comparison, the agenda for mothers at risk for the fragile X syndrome is more concerned with the availability of treatment, the risk for having an affected grandchild, expectations for future functioning of affected children, and the availability of prenatal diagnosis.[72] The broad range of reported priorities underscores the need for data to enable informative multivariate analyses of the factors that shape attitudes toward prenatal diagnosis.

In the meantime, the counselor is forewarned that hostility is frequently and personally experienced in association with discussions of amniocentesis because, it has been suggested, the counselor is seen by many women as holding the power to permit or prevent their children being born.[72] There was a time when prenatal diagnosis was denied women if they would not agree in advance to terminating the pregnancy if the fetus proved to be affected, a policy that ran counter to the prevailing credo of genetic counseling as being nondirective and supportive of the reproductive decision of the consultand.

Social programs and the imperiled newborn

Another significant event that occurred during the Decade of the Disabled was the development of a consensus regarding the care of the malformed newborn. The airing of the "pseudosecret"[63] of the deliberate withholding of life-saving surgery for infants with Down syndrome and duodenal atresia gave way to an open discussion of the selective withholding of intensive care for approximately 15% of infants admitted to special care facilities. This candid reporting led to increasingly frequent interventions, comments, and criticisms from various sources outside the health profession that added a new facet to what was at one time a very personal and private dilemma.

The recognition that the "quality of life" of the infant patient was being considered by the physicians triggered a political controversy over the legality and morality of passive euthanasia in the neonatal intensive care unit. An uneasy alliance between right-to-life groups and several advocacy groups for the handicapped were successful in bringing this issue to the political forefront and having the federal government respond by issuing regulations that defined nontreatment of the malformed as discrimination against the handicapped. The initial Baby Doe regulations had the effect of making neonatal intensive care an absolute right for every child and promised prosecution of any health care worker or institution failing to comply. The dominant themes in the debate became questions of law and politics, with ethics placing a distant third.[74]

The events that led to this historic legislation and to the subsequent developments are important to recall if one is to understand the social evolution that has occurred during the past century, culminating in a working consensus of how we as a society will treat malformed individuals for our own mutual benefit and protection.

During the 3 years that followed the initial Baby Doe rulings there was mounting concern that the prolongation of life would become the sole end, irrespective of the havoc it would wreak on other persons or desirable goals.[75] The parents, who were not an organized political force during this time, stood to suffer the most.

> Much of the discussion . . . has centered round the rights of handicapped infants to medical treatment. Little has centered round the question of how far one person can rightly be required to sacrifice her life for another, when she has not been consulted beforehand. This may be due to the fact that most of the discussants are men, while nearly all the carers are women. . . .[76]

Subsequently the regulations were invalidated by the Supreme Court on procedural grounds, and new legislation was prepared. The American Academy of Pediatrics drafted a statement of policy indicating that the "best interest of the child" should be the determining factor in nontreatment decisions, and legislators working with a coalition of 19 groups representing disabled persons, right-to-life advocates, and the medical profession produced a proposal to amend the Child Abuse Prevention and Treatment Act. This amendment was passed by both houses of Congress and signed into law in late 1985. This legislation provided for the development of a "child-centered best interest standard" to be used for evaluating decisions with respect to malformed newborns and for the establishment of Infant Care Review Committees to scrutinize the process.[77]

The "best interest of the child" assessment now includes consideration of both the clinical state (such as brain death or persistent vegetative state, irreversible progression, imminent death, or intractable pain and suffering) and the potential for self-consciousness and relations with others. Gone are such considerations as mental retardation or disability.

The paradox of congenital anomalies and the ethics of ambiguity

The final impact of congenital anomalies on society is their creation of a fundamental state of ambivalence.

> On the one hand we rush to defend the infant denied treatment, praise the courage of the parents who care for such a child at home and we celebrate disabled individuals who achieve. On the other hand we tremble at the possibility that we might have a seriously disabled child ourselves, we make scattered and poorly funded efforts to help disabled children and their families, and we balk at removing barriers to disabled adults.[64]

We are also finding that the commitments of principle taken in recent years to ensure services for all who need them call for much greater financial commitment than the public is ready to support.[78]

Consider the public outcry against passive euthanasia of the imperiled newborn with the increasing acceptance of prenatal diagnosis and selective abortion for congenital anomalies. Fletcher[79] has shown that there are different moral features that characterize the two situations and that allow parents to make a decision for abortion after prenatal diagnosis without committing themselves to euthanasia in the management of a seriously malformed infant. The liberalization of policies that allow for the selective abortion of potentially disabled fetuses comes at a time when legislation has been drafted to improve the plight of the disabled. This philosophically paradoxical development attests to a certain degree of sophistication in our society that advocates both abortion of genetic disease, most notably malformations, while at the same time promoting maximum care and rights for those living with these disorders.[80] Left unanswered is the moral claim on society by the families of these disabled children, a claim that the state has an obligation to help support these families realistically for the remainder of the child's life.

The risks of having a disabled child are common risks. Society needs women to have babies in order to survive. We make collective provision for many other contingencies—unemployment, industrial injuries, sickness, widowhood and retirement. Why not recognize the contingent risks of bearing a disabled child who after all is sometimes injured by and often kept alive by advances in technology that benefit us all. Indeed in some circumstances their impairments could have been prevented if the state had arranged better maternity, child health and preventive services.[67]

The diagnosis, treatment, and prevention of congenital anomalies should be an integral part of every health care system. In developing countries it is probably realistic to train the primary health worker in the elements of diagnosis of congenital anomalies in order to identify the individual who requires further evaluation.[81]

Perception of needs in international health range from the sublime to the pragmatic, from reflection on our responsibility for the destiny of mankind and a commitment, individually and collectively, to transform health into a bridge for peace and understanding, among all peoples and all nations.[82]

Conclusion

This chapter has reviewed the impact of congenital anomalies on the individual, the parents, and society. In most instances a major anomaly and disability are synonymous. A United Nations expert group has estimated that at least 25% of any population are people whose lives are influenced by disability, whose time and energy are to some degree deflected by the requirements of people who are impaired.[78] Persons concerned with the total problem of congenital anomalies must accept that the area of responsibility is a closely knit continuum of prevention, rehabilitation, and social action.

References

1. Pueschel SM: The impact on the family: living with the handicapped child. Issues Law Med 2:171, 1986.
2. Kunze J, Nippert I: Genetics and Malformations in Art. Grosse Verlag, Berlin, 1986.
3. Schechter MD: The orthopaedically handicapped child: emotional reactions. Arch Gen Psychol 42:247, 1961.
4. Goffman E: Stigma: Notes on the Management of Spoiled Identity. Prentice-Hall, Englewood Cliffs, NJ, 1963.
5. Boutte MI: "The stumbling disease": a case study of stigma among Azorean-Portuguese. Soc Sci Med 24:209, 1987.
6. Fairfield B, Quinton B: Concerns of unaffected relatives. BDOAS XX(6):150, 1984.
7. Opitz JM, FitzGerald JM, Reynolds JF, et al.: The Montana fetal genetic pathology program and a review of prenatal death in humans. Am J Med Genet Suppl 3:93, 1987.
8. Centers for Disease Control: Premature mortality due to congenital anomalies. MMWR 37:505, 1988.
9. Jones KL: Smith's Recognizable Patterns of Human Malformation, ed 4. WB Saunders Co, Philadelphia, 1988.
10. Costa T, Scriver CR, Childs B: The effect of mendelian disease on human health: a measurement. Am J Med Genet 21:231, 1985.

11. McKusick VA: Mendelian Inheritance in Man: Catalogs of Autosomal Dominant, Autosomal Recessive and X-linked Phenotypes, ed 5. Johns Hopkins University Press, Baltimore, 1978.
12. Survival in severe congenital heart disease. Br Med J 2:723, 1971.
13. Roberts NK, Cretin S: The changing face of congenital heart disease. Med Care 18:930, 1980.
14. Cushing D, MacLeod P: The genetic epidemiology and natural history of neural tube defects in southeastern Ontario. Unpublished data from Thesis for M.S. degree at Queen's University (D. Cushing), 1991.
15. Baird PA, Anderson TW, Newcombe HB, et al.: Genetic disorders in children and young adults: a population study. Am J Med Genet 42:677, 1988.
16. Benjamin C: The use of health care resources by young adults with spina bifida. Z Kinderchir 43:12, 1988.
17. Wehman P, Hill JW: Competitive employment for moderately and severely handicapped individuals. Pediatr Clin North Am 31:221, 1984.
18. Health and Activity Limitation Survey. Government of Canada, Ottowa, 1990.
19. Wehman P, Hill JW: Competitive employment for moderately and severely handicapped individuals. Except Child 47:338, 1981.
20. Varni JW, Rubenfeld LA, Talbot D, et al.: Determinants of self-esteem in children with congenital/acquired limb deficiencies. Dev Behav Pediatr 10:13, 1989.
21. Rucker B: Legal, ethical and religious issues related to fertility enhancement of men with spinal cord injuries. Can J Rehabil 1:225, 1988.
22. Bourne S: The psychological effects of stillbirths on women and their doctors. J R Soc Genet Pract 16:103, 1968.
23. Lewis E: The management of stillbirth: coping with unreality. Lancet 2:619, 1976.
24. Mueller RF, Sybert VP, Johnson J, et al.: Evaluation of a protocol for post-mortem examination of stillbirths. N Engl J Med 309:586, 1983.
25. Kronick JB, Scriver CR, Goodyer PR, et al.: A perimortem protocol for suspected genetic disease. Pediatrics 71:960, 1983.
26. Cohen S: Introduction. In: Ended Beginnings. C Panuthos, C Romeo, eds. Bergin & Garvey, South Hadley, MA, 1984.
27. Punch L: Hospitals frequently end up carrying handicapped infants' treatment costs. Mod Health Care 14:94, 1984.
28. Pope AW, McHale SM, Craighead WE: Self-Esteem Enhancement With Children and Adolescents. Pergamon Press, Elmsford, NY, 1988.
29. Freud A: The child guidance clinic as a center of prophylaxis and enlightenment. In: The Writings of Anna Freud, vol 5. International Universities Press, New York, 1960, p 281.
30. Boyd D: The three stages of the growth of a parent of the mentally retarded child. Am J Ment Defic 55:608, 1951.
31. Drotar DA, Baskiewicz A, Irwin N, et al.: The adaptation of parents to the birth of an infant with a congenital malformation: A hypothetical model. Pediatrics 56:710, 1975.
32. Emde RN, Brown C: Adaptation to the birth of a Down's syndrome infant. J Am Acad Child Psychiatry 17:299, 1978.
33. Kennedy JF: Material reactions to the birth of a defective baby. Soc Casework 51:410, 1970.
34. MacKeith R: The feelings and behavior of parents of handicapped children. Dev Med Child Neurol 15:524, 1973.
35. Mercer RT: Mothers' responses to their infants with defects. Nurs Res 23:133, 1974.
36. Bicknell J: The psychopathology of handicap. Br J Med Psychiatry 56:167, 1983.
37. Panuthos C, Romeo C: Ended Beginnings. Bergin & Garvey, South Hadley, MA, 1984.
38. Blacher J: Sequential stages of parental adjustment to the birth of a child with handicaps: Fact or artifact? Ment Retard 22:58, 1984.
39. Allen DA, Affleck G: Are we stereotyping parents? A postscript to Blacher. Ment Retard 23:200, 1985.
40. Sorenson JR, Scotch NA, Swazey JP, et al.: Reproductive Past, Reproductive Futures: Genetic Counseling and Its Effectiveness. Alan R. Liss, New York, 1981, p 99.
41. Antley RM, Bringle RG, Kinney KL: Down's syndrome. In: Psychological Aspects of Genetic Counseling. AEH Emery, I Pullen, eds. Academic, London, 1984, p 75.
42. Lippman-Hand A: Genetic counseling—the postcounseling period: I. Parents' perceptions of uncertainty. Am J Med Genet 4:51, 1979.
43. Zwarum S: The birth of a disabled child. Chatelaine 61:78, 1988.

44. McMahon PO: Foreword. In: Ended Beginnings. Panuthos C, Romeo C, eds. Bergin & Garvey, South Hadley, MA, 1984, p viii.

45. Emery A, Pullen I: Psychological Aspects of Genetic Counseling. Academic, London, 1984.

46. Leon IG: When a Baby Dies. Yale University Press, New Haven, 1990.

47. Meryash DL: Perception of burden among at-risk women of raising a child with fragile-X syndrome, Clin Genet 36:15, 1989.

48. Lippman-Hand A, Fraser FC: Genetic counseling: parents' responses to uncertainty. BDOAS XV(5C):325, 1979.

49. Olshansky S: Chronic sorrow: a response to having a mentally defective child. Soc Casework 43:190, 1962.

50. Wikler L, Wasow M, Hatfield E: Chronic sorrow revisited: parent vs. professional depiction of the adjustment of parents of mentally retarded children. Am J Orthopsychiatry 51:63, 1981.

51. Bibring GL: Some considerations of the psychosocial processes of pregnancy. Psychoanal Study Child 14:113, 1959.

52. Gath A: Down's Syndrome and the Family. Academic, London, 1978, p 58.

53. Walker JH, Thomas M, Russell JT: Spina bifida—and the parents. Dev Med Child Neurol 13:462, 1971.

54. Tew BJ, Payne H, Laurence KM: Must a family with a handicapped child be a handicapped family? Dev Med Child Neurol 16(Suppl 32):95, 1974.

55. Sultz HA, Schlesinger ER, Mosher WE: Long-term Childhood Illness. University of Pittsburgh Press, Pittsburgh, 1972.

56. Friedrich WN, Boriskin JA: The role of the child in abuse: a review of the literature, Am J Orthopsychiatry 46:580, 1976.

57. Lynch MA, Roberts J: Predicting child abuse: signs of bonding failure in the maternity hospital. Br Med J 1:624, 1977.

58. Tews BJ, Laurence KM: Mothers, brothers and sisters of patients with spina bifida. Dev Med Child Neurol 15(Suppl 9):69, 1973.

59. Gath A: Sibling reaction to mental handicap: a comparison of the brothers and sisters of mongol children. J Child Psychol Psychiatry 15:187, 1974.

60. Weber G, Parker T: A study of family and professional views of the factors affecting family adaptation to a disabled child. In: Roots of Well Being. N Stinnett, J DeFrain, K King, eds. University of Omaha Press, Omaha, 1980.

61. National Organization of Rare Diseases. P.O. Box 8923, New Fairfield, CT 06812.

62. Fiedler L: Freaks: Myths and Images of the Secret Self. Simon and Schuster, New York, 1978.

63. Muller-Hill B: Murderous Science. Oxford University Press, Oxford, 1988.

64. Document of Saint-Siege for the International Year of the Handicapped Person. Catholic Documentation 1807:428, 1981.

65. Conley RW: Down syndrome: economic burdens and benefits of prevention. Basic Life Sci 36:35, 1985.

66. Gleidman J, Roth W: The Unexpected Minority—Handicapped Children in America. Harcort Brace Jovanovich, New York, 1980.

67. Bradshaw J: The social impact of childhood disablement. Z Kinderchir 43:5, 1988.

68. Perrin JM, Ireys HT: The organization of services for chronically ill children and their families. Pediatr Clin North Am 31:235, 1984.

69. Taylor P: Genetic crystal-ball gazing opens up a Pandora's box of social, moral issues. The Globe and Mail April 14, 1990, p 1A.

70. Lorber J: Spina bifida—a vanishing nightmare. In: Spina Bifida–Neural Tube Defects. D Voth , P Glees, eds. Walter de Gruyter, New York, 1986, p 3.

71. Elkins TE, Stovall TG, Wilroy S, et al.: Attitudes of mothers of children with Down syndrome concerning amniocentesis, abortion, and prenatal genetic counseling techniques. Obstet Gynecol 68:181, 1986.

72. Meryash DL, Abuelo D: Counselling needs and attitudes toward prenatal diagnosis and abortion in fragile-X families. Clin Gen 33:349, 1988.

73. Silvestre D, Fresco N: Reactions to prenatal diagnosis. Am J Orthopsychiatry 50:610, 1980.

74. Murray TH: The final, anticlimatic rule on Baby Doe. Hastings Center Rep 17:5, 1984.

75. Bioethics Committee: Treatment decisions for infants and children. Can Med Assoc J 135:447, 1986.

76. Simms M: Informed dissent: the views of some mothers of severely mentally handicapped young adults. J Med Ethics 12:72, 1986.

77. Lantos J: Baby Doe five years later: implications for child health. N Engl J Med 317:444, 1987.

78. Acton N: The world's response to disability: evolution of a philosophy. Arch Phys Med Rehabil 63:145, 1982.

79. Fletcher J: Abortion, euthanasia, and care of defective newborns. N Engl J Med 292:75, 1975.

80. Motulsky AG, Murray J: Will prenatal diagnosis with selective abortion affect society's attitude toward the handicapped. Prog Clin Biol Res 128:277, 1983.

81. Bochkov NP, Bulyzhenkov VE: Trends in managing hereditary diseases. In: Issues in Contemporary International Health. TA Lambo, SB Day, eds. Plenum, New York, 1990, p 253.

82. Day SB, Lambo TA: Issues in Contemporary International Health. Plenum, New York, 1990, p 1.

11

Prenatal Diagnosis

DAGMAR BAUER-HANSMANN and MITCHELL S. GOLBUS

With the demonstration more than two decades ago that chromosome analysis could be performed on cultured human amniotic fluid cells, prenatal diagnosis was formally introduced into medical practice.[1] The technical improvement of diagnostic ultrasound, the revolution in molecular biology, and the newer developments of noninvasive screening and early diagnostic procedures have ushered in a new era in reproductive genetics. In most developed countries, genetic counseling and prenatal monitoring are an integral part of maternal care and family planning.

Noninvasive procedures for prenatal diagnosis

Clinical assessment of fetal well-being

It remains important not to overlook the status of the mother when determining fetal welfare. Maternal health and weight gain are crucial to fetal development; maternal blood pressure may provide a clue to subtle circulatory compromise; and fundal height measurements, particularly in the third trimester, may uncover fetal growth retardation. Assessment of the fetal heart rate and the biophysical profile offer insight into fetal well-being. Manual assessment of fetal size and position allows recognition of an abnormal lie, which, if it persists into late pregnancy, suggests abnormal placentation, uterine anomalies, or fetal problems. Failure to palpate fetal parts easily suggests polyhydramnios and should initiate further investigation.

Ultrasonography

For fetal anomalies

Since the introduction of ultrasound to obstetrics by Ian Donald in the 1950s, the dramatic improvements in ultrasonic instrumentation, particularly the high-resolution real-time scanners, have established ultrasound as the most successful method of noninvasive monitoring of pregnancy, without known deleterious short-term or long-term side effects.[2-4]

The ability of sonography to survey multiple organ systems rapidly and sequentially makes it indispensible to the geneticist. Its flexibility allows fetal movements to be viewed directly, enabling rapid reorientation of the transducer to the desired plane of interest. An ever-increasing number of birth defects can be assessed prenatally by visualization of the fetal anatomy to confirm or to rule out malformations in an at-risk fetus.

In contrast to the National Institutes of Health consensus that routine antenatal ultrasound had no favorable influence on fetal outcome, prospective randomized studies conducted in Europe have demonstrated that antenatal ultrasound screening can reduce the perinatal death rate and can decrease morbidity, particularly by earlier recognition of fetal growth retardation.[5,6] A basic obstetrics ultrasound examination should follow the guidelines of the American College of Obstetrics and Gynecology Task Force on Ultrasound, which are similar to the recommendations of the Section on Obstetric/Gynecologic Ultrasound of the American Institute of Ultrasound in Medicine and include:

1. Fetal number and survey for gross anomalies
2. Fetal cardiac activity (after 7 weeks)
3. Fetal lie (after 12 weeks)
4. Placental location
5. Gestational age (by multiple parameters when possible)
6. Amount of amniotic fluid
7. Maternal pelvic survey (with special attention to detecting the presence of clinically significant uterine pathology or large pelvic masses)

Table 11–1 lists the major human anomalies that can be detected in the midtrimester with ultrasound. The benefit of routine ultrasound for congenital malformation detection is hard to assess because of the low incidence of positive findings. The patient found to have a fetus with a congenital anomaly such as diaphragmatic hernia, abdominal wall defect, or obstructive uropathy should be referred to a specialized ultrasound center with a well-coordinated perinatal care and neonatal surgical unit.[10] Even more important than the mode of delivery (cesarean section vs. vaginal delivery) is good perinatal care.[11-13]

If the fetal condition is incompatible with life or is associated with severe retardation or anatomic disease, the parents can elect termination of the pregnancy within the legal limits. When the fetal condition seems to be treatable prenatally or postnatally, a search for associated malformations or a cytogenetic abnormality is mandated. Because polyhydramnios, oligohydramnios, growth retardation, and multiple congenital malformations are all associated with chromosomal anomalies, a fetal karyotype needs to be done in such situations before the parents can be counseled about the fetal/neonatal prognosis.[14]

As a guide to invasive techniques for prenatal diagnosis

Ultrasonography has been well established as a method to guide the accurate placement of a needle into the amniotic cavity, the placenta, the cord, or the fetus for diagnostic and therapeutic purposes. In utero sampling of fetal blood, skin, or liver has become an important tool in prenatal diagnosis and pregnancy management.

Table 11-1. Anomalies detected by ultrasound examination during the second trimester[a]

Nervous system	Cardiovascular	Gastrointestinal	Genitourinary	Musculoskeletal	Other
Anencephaly	Septal defects	Bowel atresias and obstructions	Renal agenesis	Facial clefting	Tumors
Encephalocele	Valve atresias, malpositions		Renal cysts	Limb reduction	
Microcephaly	Hypertrophic cardiomyopathy	Omphalocele	Obstructive	Skeletal dysplasias	
Macrocephaly	Hypoplastic aortic arch	Gastroschisis	Horseshoe kidney	Bladder exstrophy	
Holoprosencephaly	Interrupted aortic arch	Umbilical hernia	Nephroblastoma	Cloacal exstrophy	
Hydrocephaly	Hydrops			Ectopia cordis	
Cerebellar agenesis	Cystic hygromas			Diaphragmatic hernia	
Dandy-Walker malformation					
Choroid plexus cyst					
Porencephalic cyst					
Iniencephaly					
Spina bifida					
Caudal regression					

[a]Data are from Escobar et al.,[7] Nicolaides and Campbell,[8] and Fermont et al.[9]

The value of ultrasound in enhancing the safety of amniocentesis is well recognized. To avoid fetal and placental injury, the needle should be introduced aseptically into a pocket of amniotic fluid under continuous ultrasound visualization. For chorionic villus sampling (CVS) a consistent and high success rate is needed, and reports of success rates of blind CVS varied from 0–78%. Localization of the implantation site and ultrasonographic guidance of the sampling instrument are of the utmost importance and have contributed to a high success rate with safety.

Maternal serum α-fetoprotein (MS-AFP)

Human α-fetoprotein (AFP) was recognized as a fetal-specific protein in 1956 and was isolated and characterized in 1970.[15–17] AFP is synthesized by the yolk sac and later by the fetal liver. It normally enters the amniotic fluid through fetal urination and appears in maternal circulation through direct transfer across fetal membranes. Serum AFP is found in very low concentrations (1–2 ng/ml) except in fetuses (fetal plasma AFP concentration peaks at 10–13 menstrual weeks, with a level of about 3000 μg/ml), pregnant women (peak concentration of MS-AFP between 28 and 32 menstrual weeks is 200 ng/ml), and patients with hepatomas and germ cell tumors. The AFP concentration gradient between fetal plasma and amniotic fluid is about 200:1, and the gradient between fetal and maternal serum at 15–20 weeks is almost 50,000:1. This is why fetal blood contamination will give misleadingly high amniotic fluid AFP values.

In 1972, Brock and Sutcliffe[18] reported elevated amniotic fluid alpha-fetoprotein (AF-AFP) concentrations in fetuses with open neural tube defects (NTDs). Elevated AF-AFP is also observed in fetal anomalies that lack normal skin integrity such as ventral wall defects, and in sacrococcygeal teratomas, cystic hygromas, and fetal demise. One year later, they reported an association between raised MS-AFP concentrations and fetuses with open NTDs.[19] A subgroup of pregnancies with elevated MS-AFP levels have normal fetal findings initially, but pregnancy is later complicated by intrauterine growth retardation, abruptio placenta, placenta previa, premature labor, postmaturity, or fetal loss. More than a decade of experience has supported the decision to use routine MS-AFP screening in obstetric practice. During this time refinements have included the adjustment of MS-AFP levels for weight, ethnic background, and the presence of insulin-dependent diabetes. MS-AFP screening is a standard part of obstetric care in the United States.[20–22]

In most AFP screening programs, MS-AFP is measured at 16 to 18 menstrual weeks. The cut-off value chosen to necessitate further evaluation depends on the desired level of detection and the false-positive rate but is usually 2.0 or 2.5 multiples of the median (MoM) for singleton pregnancies and 4.0 or 4.5 MoM for twins.[23] If the MS-AFP level lies above the upper limit and the patient is less than 18 weeks, then the patient's blood is drawn again, because 45%–50% of women with initially elevated MS-AFP values will have a normal value on the second test.[24] If the second level is also raised or if the pregnancy is beyond week 18 of gestation, a level I ultrasound is done to rule out incorrect dating, twins, fetal demise, anencephaly, or other abnormalities. If no abnormalities can be detected and the gestational age is accurate, amniocentesis is performed for AF-AFP and acetylcholinesterase (AChE). If both ultrasound and amniocentesis results are normal, the pregnancy still should be considered high risk, with antepartum testing as appropriate. Whether antepartum testing will avoid the poorer outcome of these pregnancies remains to be proved.

In 1984, Merkatz et al.[25] observed, and Cuckle et al.[26] and Fuhrmann et al.[27] confirmed, a highly significant association between low MS-AFP concentrations and Down syndrome, an important finding for women under 35 yr who bear, in spite of their average risk of 1:1000, about 80% of the infants with Down syndrome. In a prospective study in 1987, Di Maio et al.[28] showed that a low MS-AFP value in women under 35 yr is as effective at detecting chromosomal anomalies as maternal age screening. Among the 5% of pregnancies with a low MS-AFP value (below 0.5 multiples of the median), 20% of fetal chromosomal abnormalities would be detected.[29–32]

Usually a sliding scale related to maternal age is used for the AFP cut-off. MS-AFP levels below the cut-off require level I ultrasound for confirmation of gestational dating. If gestational age was correctly defined, amniocentesis for karyotyping is recommended. A repeat MS-AFP test should be perfomed only if the original test was found to have been performed before 15 weeks.

Milunsky et al.[33] prospectively studied 13,486 women with high and low MS-AFP levels in singleton pregnancies. A high MS-AFP value (3.9% of the study group) was associated with NTDs (relative risk = 224), other major congenital defects (relative risk = 4.7), fetal deaths (relative risk = 8.1), neonatal death (relative risk = 4.7), low birth weight (relative risk = 4.0), newborn complications (relative risk = 3.6), oligohydramnios (relative risk = 3.4), abruptio placenta (relative risk = 3.0), and preeclamptic toxemia (relative risk = 2.3). A low MS-AFP value was associated with chromosomal defects (relative risk = 11.6) and fetal death (relative risk = 3.3). Either high or low MS-AFP values were associated with 34.2% of all major congenital defects, 19.1% of all perinatal deaths, 11.0% of major pregnancy complications, and 15.9% of serious newborn complications.

Other maternal circulatory placental hormones and fetal proteins

Human chorionic gonadotropin

Low levels of the placental protein human chorionic gonadotropin (hCG) during early pregnancy are predictive of an abnormal outcome, usually a spontaneous abortion.[34] As at least 50% of first-trimester spontaneous abortions are due to chromosomal abnormalities, one might expect decreased levels of hCG to be a potential predictor of chromosomally abnormal pregnancies.[35] Serum hCG levels rise rapidly soon after conception to peak between 8 and 11.5 weeks, then decline to a nadir at 18 weeks. As hCG levels plateau between 18 and 25 weeks, no gestational age-related adjustments are necessary for hCG screening during this period.[36]

According to Bogart et al.[37] 65% of chromosomally abnormal pregnancies can be identified, with a false-positive rate of 4.05% by measuring second-trimester total β-hCG level with cut-off rates below 0.25 MoM and above 2.5 MoM. Alternatively, by measuring both total β-hCG and α-hCG with a cut-off rate of greater than 2.5 MoM, 76% of the abnormal pregnancies can be detected, with a false-positive rate of 4.05%. Using a cut-off level of 2.0 MoM for α-hCG, the detection rate for aneuploidies increases to 84%, with a false-positive rate of 6.75%. The combined detection rate for their two studies (in 1987 and 1989), using cut-offs for total β-hCG of below 0.25 and greater than 2.5 and an α-hCG cut-off of 2.0 MoM, is 80%, including 83% (25 of 30) of trisomy 21 cases.[37,38] Total β-HCG and α-hCG level determination is superior to AFP determination for detection of the chromosomally abnormal fetus in the second trimester. Unfortunately, total hCG or α-hCG evaluation at 9–11 weeks does not appear to be useful for detection of pregnancies at risk for trisomy 21.[38]

Unconjugated estriol (UE₃)

A relationship between low maternal serum UE$_3$ and a fetus with Down syndrome has been reported, but the explanation for the decreased level in the second trimester is still unknown.[39] The synthesis of UE$_3$ is dependent on the fetal adrenal cortex, the fetal liver, and the placenta. Low concentra-

tions of maternal serum UE$_3$ in pregnancies involving a Down syndrome fetus could result from immaturity of one or all of these organs.

Combination of markers

According to Wald et al.[40,41] low unconjugated estriol levels combined with maternal age has a detection rate of 35% for Down syndrome. Thus unconjugated estriol plus maternal age is slightly more efficient than MS-AFP plus maternal age (30%).[33] The use of unconjugated estriol, MS-AFP, and maternal age to select women with a 1:250 risk for fetal Down syndrome would yield a 45% detection rate, with 5.2% false-positive results.

Wald et al.[40,41] described a mechanism for the combination of four measurements: MS-AFP, MS-hCG, MS-UE$_3$, and maternal age, to develop a combined risk factor. This combination yielded a detection rate of 60%, with a false-positive rate of 5%. However, higher detection rates (with a 5% false-positive rate) have been reported with the use of just the three measurements MS-AFP, MS-hCG, and maternal age.[42,43]

Schwangerschaftsprotein-1, human placental lactogen, progesterone

Because other placental products might be informative in a pregnancy with Down syndrome, Knight et al.[44] examined maternal serum Schwangerschaftsprotein-1 (SP1), human placental lactogen (hPL), and progesterone (pro). Average concentrations for all the placental markers were elevated in cases of fetal Down syndrome, but hCG proved to be most consistently elevated. SP1, hPL, and pro do not significantly improve the detection rate achieved with hCG, AFP, and UE$_3$.

Fetal cells in the maternal circulation

An alternative method of population fetal screening depends on the ability to recover fetal cells from maternal blood. The presence of fetal cells in the maternal circulation and the transplacental migration of fetal cells into the mother are based on many positive observations.[45–48] In 1969, Walknowska et al.[45] found fetal XY cells in the maternal circulation by means of partial karyotyping. The proportion of fetal cells ranges from less than 0.1% to 4%[43] between 6 weeks gestation and term.[48] Schwinger et al.[49] could not prove the presence of a Y-specific sequence after amplifying the Y-chromosome sequence via the polymerase chain reaction (PCR).

Monoclonal antibodies have been made against first-trimester human placental cytotrophoblasts and are available against potentially paternally inherited antigens. After no cross-reactivity with maternal peripheral blood is proved, fetal labeled cells can be detected and sorted by means of a fluorescence-activated cell sorter and used for prenatal diagnosis.[50] The enrichment by cell sorting has allowed recovery of male fetal cells in a ratio of 1 to 1000 maternal cells.[51] Although Selypes and Lorencz[52] purported to show fetal cells in the maternal circulation by the "air-culture" cytogenetic technique, this work has not been confirmed.[53]

Fluorescence in situ hybridization (FISH) can identify interphase trisomic cells with chromosome-specific probes. Y-specific probes can be used for rapid identification of fetuses at risk for X-linked disorders.[54] X-specific probes can be used for rapid identification of fetuses at risk for Turner or Kline-felter syndromes and of triple X females.[55] The PCR can be used for in vitro DNA amplification of specific parts of the genome in fetal cells obtained from the maternal circulation.

A number of serious problems are still unresolved, including presence of twin fetuses, of fetal cells from previous pregnancies, and of cells from a vanishing twin, that can lead to erroneous diagnoses.[56] Although this method of screening is theoretically attractive, it is still in the earliest experimental stages.

Invasive procedures for prenatal diagnosis

Amniocentesis

Over the last 20 years amniocentesis undoubtedly has become the most widespread invasive method of prenatal diagnosis. It can be performed as early as 10 menstrual weeks and as late as the end of the pregnancy. The indications for amniocentesis are age-related risk of having a fetus with a trisomy, parental translocation, prior offspring with a chromosome abnormality or NTD, or fetus at risk for a biochemical or single gene disorder diagnosable by enzymatic or recombinant DNA techniques (Table 11–2).

Amniocentesis at the "traditional" time of 15–16 menstrual weeks is performed after the ideal area for puncturing the abdominal wall is sonographically located, the abdomen is sterilely prepped, and local anesthetic (if desired) is applied. The amniotic sac is entered with a 22 gauge 3.5 inch spinal needle (in some centers 20 gauge needles are used) under sonographic guidance. A volume of 20–25 cc amniotic fluid is routinely drawn for karyotyping and for measuring AFP.

The overall rate of fetal losses that are possibly procedure related was found in national and single-center studies to be 1% or less.[57] At the University of California, San Francisco (UCSF), among the first 3000 amniocenteses there was a 1.5% total loss rate following amniocentesis.[58] We counsel our patients that the added risk of causing a fetal loss attributable to amniocentesis is 0.5% or less, that the maternal risk appears minimal, that the risk of major fetal injury consistent with pregnancy continuation is very remote, and that needle scarring is rare. If the first 1–2 cc sample of amniotic fluid obtained is discarded, the risk of maternal cell contamination is very low, and the incidence of true mosaicism is below 0.5%.[59,60]

Early amniocentesis is performed between 10 and 14 menstrual weeks, and approximately 1 cc of amniotic fluid per week is withdrawn. In the study by Evans et al.[61] 227 early amniocenteses and 3439 traditional amniocenteses were performed. Although the number of pregnancy losses after early amniocentesis was low (0.4%) and was similar to the loss rate after traditional amniocenteses (0.3%) by 4 weeks postam-

niocentesis, it appears that there may be a slightly higher risk with the early procedure.

Chorionic villus sampling

More than 70,000 CVS procedures have been reported. It can now be considered a reasonable alternative to amniocentesis.[62,63] CVS can be performed at almost any stage of pregnancy and is applicable to the same diagnostic situations addressed by amniocentesis except for previous NTD. Two common sampling techniques are utilized, the transabdominal and the transcervical approaches.

For the transabdominal approach, we use a 20-gauge needle, as do most other groups. Under ultrasound guidance, the needle traverses the abdominal wall and is directed to the villi. With about 10 cc of negative pressure on a 20 cc syringe, the needle is moved back and forth in the placenta and then withdrawn. The needle is rinsed in tissue culture medium and the aspirate examined under a dissecting microscope to see that sufficient villi have been obtained. This approach can be utilized anytime after 9 menstrual weeks.

For transcervical CVS, chorionic villi are aspirated under ultrasound guidance through a 16 gauge catheter with a stainless steel stylet. After the vagina is prepped with betadine, the catheter is bent appropriately to be passed to the area of the villi. A syringe is used to create a vacuuming action as the catheter is slowly withdrawn through the villi. The material obtained is washed out of the catheter with tissue culture medium and observed under a dissecting microscope. We do not put anything in our syringe; some centers use heparinized media in their syringe.

Two major studies published in 1989, the U.S. and the Canadian collaborative studies, reported 0.8% and 0.6% higher risks of spontaneous abortion after transcervical CVS than after amniocentesis.[64,65] Neither of these differences was statistically significant. Procedures that required more than one attempt, especially those requiring three or four passes, were associated with an increased loss rate. For counseling purposes, we add this additional risk to the amniocentesis risk and quote a 1.0%–1.2% procedure-related risk. At UCSF, we have not found a significant difference between the total loss rates to delivery of patients undergoing transcervical (3.3%) and transabdominal (3.5%) CVS. A summary of data from other centers also indicates no difference between the total loss rates to delivery of the two approaches. Most anterior placentas are preferably approached via the abdominal route and most of the posterior placentas via the cervix.

Successful cytogenetic diagnosis was achieved in 97.8% of CVS versus 99.4% of amniocentesis procedures.[60] Additionally, 17 of 2235 CVS patients (0.8%) had to undergo amniocentesis because of ambiguous cytogenetic results.

As placental biopsy can be performed at any gestational stage, late transabdominal CVS might be a substitute for amniocentesis or percutaneous umbilical blood sampling (PUBS) in the last half of pregnancy. Combined data on 774 late transabdominal CVS procedures included 30 therapeutic abortions (3.9%), 4 social abortions (0.5%), 15 spontaneous abortions (2.03%), and 3 stillbirths (0.4%), for a total unintended loss rate of 2.4%.[66]

Percutaneous umbilical blood sampling

Since 1973, fetal blood has been sampled via fetoscopy. Because the procedure-related fetal loss rate of 3%–4% in skilled

Table 11–2. Indications for genetic amniocentesis

Maternal age >35 yr at term gestation
Parental chromosomal rearrangement
Previous pregnancy with chromosomal anomaly
Maternal carrier of X-linked disease
Both parents carriers of recessive gene for metabolic disease or hemoglobinopathy
Increased risk of neural tube defect

Table 11-3. Indications for fetal blood sampling

Indication	Fetoscopy (n = 90)		Percutaneous umbilical blood sampling (n = 77)	
	No. of pregnancies	Percent	No. of pregnancies	Percent
Cytogenetic	5	6[a]	37	48
Hemoglobinopathies	47	52	12	16
β-Thalassemia	28		4	
α-Thalassemia	3		2	
Sickle cell anemia	9		4	
Compound/double heterozygotes	7		2	
Sickle β-thalassemia	4		2	
Sickle hemoglobin C disease	2		0	
Hemoglobin E β-thalassemia	1		0	
Erythrocyte isoimmunization	0		10	13
Coagulopathies	24	27	9	12
Hemophilia A	24		4	
Hemophilia B	0		5	
Immunologic	7	8	5	6
Severe combined immunodeficiency	1		5	
Chédiak-Higashi syndrome	1		0	
Chronic granulomatous disease	3		0	
Wiskott-Aldrich syndrome	2		0	
Miscellaneous	7	8	4	5
Duchenne muscular dystrophy	3		0	
Paternity	1		0	
Abetalipoproteinemia	1		0	
α₁-Antitrypsin	1		0	
Nonimmune hydrops	1		2	
Rubella infection	0		1	
Alloimmune thrombocytopenia	0		1	

[a]Percentages exceed 100 because of rounding.

hands was unavoidable with the use of a trocar of 2.2 mm diameter, fetoscopy is no longer performed at most centers. PUBS, because of its simplicity and safety, has paved the way for more routine fetal blood testing.[67-71] PUBS has three major advantages: it can be performed from menstrual week 18 until the end of pregnancy, it can be repeated as often as necessary during pregnancy, and it is performed on an outpatient basis. Medication is generally not necessary for this procedure, although some patients might need a sedative.

The cord insertion site is localized by means of real-time ultrasound. With regard to preparing the abdomen and using local anesthetic and a 22-gauge 3.5 inch spinal needle, PUBS is very similar to amniocentesis. If the placenta is anterior, it is traversed, and the cord is punctured without entering the amniotic cavity. With a posterior placenta, the amniotic cavity is entered and the cord punctured 1-2 cm from its insertion into the placenta. Longer needles are available for cases of posterior implantation, polyhydramnios, or extreme obesity. Up to 3 ml of fetal blood, depending on the gestational age and quantity required for the specific analysis, is withdrawn into a heparinized syringe or into syringes containing specific anticoagulants used for special assays (e.g., sodium citrate for clotting factors). The presence of fetal blood is immediately confirmed using a ZBI Coulter Counter and chan-

nelyzer that differentiates fetal from maternal erythrocytes by their size. A modified Betke-Kleihauer method can be used to verify quickly the presence of fetal cells when the Coulter Counter is not available.[72]

Indications for fetal blood sampling have changed as PUBS replaced fetoscopy because of both the improved safety of the procedure and the new DNA techniques that replaced the need for fetal blood sampling for diagnosing certain conditions.[73-77] Prior to 1985, the most common indication for fetal blood sampling at UCSF was a fetus at risk for a hemoglobinopathy (52%) or a coagulopathy (27%). Since 1985, 48% of the PUBS have been performed for fetal rapid karyotyping after fetal abnormalities were found sonographically, because karyotype results from fetal lymphocytes are available in 48-72 hours. Other indications for PUBS now include hemoglobinopathies (16%), red cell isoimmunization (13%), and coagulopathies (12%). Miscellaneous indications include severe combined immunodeficiency, Chédiak-Higashi disease, Wiskott-Aldrich syndrome, chronic granulomatous disease, α₁-antitrypsin deficiency, abetalipoproteinemia, paternity identification, nonimmune hydrops, fetal infection, and alloimmune thrombocytopenia (Table 11-3).[71,77-83]

Purity of the fetal blood sample is of utmost importance,

because even a very little maternal contamination can mistakenly provide the presence of IgM and lead to the incorrect diagnosis of congenital infection or provide amniotic fluid dilution falsely leading to the diagnosis of fetal anemia. A pure fetal specimen was obtained at the first attempt in 97% of PUBS at UCSF. The uncorrected risk of fetal demise after PUBS was 10% (corrected to 2% for the presence of lethal fetal anomalies or disease).[71]

Fetal liver biopsy

Some inherited enzyme deficits are only expressed in hepatic cells. As long as the gene defect has not been detected, prenatal diagnosis of such diseases is only possible by fetal liver biopsy. Fetal liver biopsy has been performed at UCSF in eight pregnancies of six patients between June 1982 and May 1986. The procedure is performed with a 16.5 gauge thin-walled needle entering the fetal abdomen immediately below the right costal margin under ultrasound guidance. The samples are centrifuged immediately to separate liver tissue from blood contamination. Indications included ornithine transcarbamylase deficiency,[84] von Gierke glycogen storage disease type IA,[85] and carbamylphosphate synthetase deficiency. Satisfactory results were obtained in six out of eight cases and all diagnoses were confirmed after delivery. No losses or preterm deliveries occurred (Table 11–4).

Fetal skin biopsy

By 18–20 menstrual weeks, dermis, epidermis, and junctional areas of skin are fully differentiated, and the diagnosis of inherited dermatoses is possible by histopathologic analysis of a fetal skin fragment. Fetal skin biopsies, initially performed under fetoscopy, are now performed under direct ultrasound guidance. Indications for the 15 procedures performed at UCSF between January 1979 and December 1987 included harlequin ichthyosis,[86] epidermolysis bullosa,[87] and autosomal dominant ichthyosiform erythroderma.[88] Satisfactory results were obtained in 14 cases. One pregnancy resulted in a spontaneous abortion with chorioamnionitis 2 days after sampling. One biopsy performed for ichthyosiform erythroderma gave a false-negative result, as the newborn was mildly affected. All other diagnoses were confirmed after birth. Worldwide, a 3%–4% spontaneous abortion rate after fetal skin biopsy has occurred (Table 11–5).

Methods of studying fetal samples

Chromosome analysis of cultured amniocytes

Cells present in the amniotic fluid are of fetal origin; therefore cytogenetic analysis of cultured amniotic fluid cells (amniocytes) reflects the fetal chromosome constitution. The first successful karyotype analysis of cultured amniocytes was reported by Steele and Breg[1] in 1966. Cytogenetic diagnosis was obtained in 4% of the samples studied. With improved culture methods and banding techniques, chromosome analysis of cultured amniocytes now can be achieved in over 99% of cases.

Generally, about 20 cc of amniotic fluid is obtained for prenatal chromosome analysis. This allows for parallel cultures to be established so that a diagnosis can be obtained in

Table 11–4. Fetal liver sampling indications

Indication	Results		
	Normal	Affected	No results
Ornithine carbamylase deficiency (4 cases)	0	3	1[a]
Glycogen storage disease type IA (3 cases)	2	1	0
Nonketotic hyperglycinemia (1 case)	0	0	1[a]

[a]Normal at delivery.

the event of growth failure or contamination in one batch of cultures. Amniotic fluid to be used for chromosome analysis must be obtained in a sterile vessel and transported to the laboratory as soon as possible, preferably within 24 hr of sampling. The fluid is centrifuged, the supernatant removed, and the cell pellet resuspended and transferred to culture flasks or petri dishes. One week or more is generally required to obtain a sufficient quantity of cells for chromosome analysis.

Chromosome analysis of amniotic fluid cells may be complicated by the finding of mosaicism, two different cell lines within a single individual. Chromosome mosaicism is difficult to interpret, and it is important to distinguish between true fetal mosaicism and pseudomosaicism. True fetal mosaicism is the presence of two or more cells with the same chromosome aberration in at least two independent cultures from one amniotic fluid. Pseudomosaicism is the presence of two or more cells with the same chromosome aberration in only one culture from an amniotic fluid sample. Pseudomosaicism is presumed to be a clonal artifact that does not reflect the fetal karyotype, while true mosaicism is considered to represent constitutional mosaicism in the fetus. Difficulties in interpretation arise concerning the proportion of normal and abnormal cells in the fetus and the possible effects on the baby's phenotype.

Another rare complication of prenatal chromosome analysis is maternal cell contamination. The growth and analysis of maternal cells in an amniotic fluid culture may lead to the misdiagnosis of a male fetus as female, the misdiagnosis of a chromosomally abnormal fetus as normal, or the prediction of an XX/XY sex chromosome mosaicism in the fetus.

The most frequent indication for prenatal chromosome analysis is advanced maternal age. It is well known that women over age 35 yr are at increased risk of producing offspring with trisomy 21 and other chromosome aneuploidies. Other indications include a previous child with a chromo-

Table 11–5. Fetal skin sampling indications

Indication	Results		
	Normal	Affected	No results
Epidermolysis bullosa (8 cases)	8	0	0
Harlequin ichthyosis (5 cases)	3	1	1
Ichthyosiform erythroderma (2 cases)	1	1[a]	0

[a]The results of fetal skin sampling were normal; after delivery, the infant was found to be mildly affected.[88]

some abnormality, mosaicism or chromosome rearrangement in a parent, a history of multiple spontaneous pregnancy loss, fetal sex determination for carriers of X-linked disorders, and increased risk of trisomy 21 based on maternal screening.

Cytogenetics by in situ hybridization

It has now become possible to directly hybridize a fluorescently labeled human chromosome–specific probe to genomic DNA of cells on slides. This allows detection of constitutional chromosome aberrations. The target DNA on the slides has been denatured to single strands. The probe has to be nick translated, biotinylated, denatured, and hybridized to the DNA on the slides. As avidin has a high affinity to biotin, avidin bound to a fluorescent molecule is added. To amplify the signal, a biotinylated goat antiavidin antibody can be added that binds more fluorescein-labeled avidin. The advantage of in situ hybridization compared with karyotyping is that all cells, not exclusively metaphases, can be used. Utilizing multiple specific probes with different fluores raises the possibility of simultaneous detection of multiple nucleic acid sequences.[89] Specific repetitive probes for chromosomes 13, 18, and 21 are available and have been successfully tested in our laboratory.[90]

In situ hybridization with biotinylated chromosome-specific DNA probes has the potential to complement prenatal diagnosis in an unforeseen dimension, particularly when single gene probes are available. It has been found to be a time-efficient and cost-efficient method. It can be applied with equal success to fetal blood, amniocytes, and chorionic villus cells.[91]

Amniotic fluid biochemistry

Hexosaminidase A for Tay-Sachs disease. Tay-Sachs disease, or G_{M2} gangliosidosis, a lysosomal storage disease, is characterized by the onset in infancy of severe developmental retardation that progresses to dementia, blindness, paralysis, and death by age 2–4 yr. The disease is caused by an autosomal recessive gene on chromosome 15. A disease prevalence of 1:4000 in Ashkenazi Jews (compared with 1:400,000 in the non-Jewish population) led to establishment of a screening program in this high-risk group. The carrier frequency is 1:30 in Ashkenazi Jews and 1:300 in others. Hexosaminidase A is normally present in serum, leukocytes, and cultured fibroblasts. The activity is diminished to 40%–60% in heterozygotes and is almost absent in homozygotes; thus the disease is a suitable candidate for population screening and prenatal diagnosis.

In Tay-Sachs disease, the hexosaminidase A deficiency manifests in the amniotic fluid.[92–94] The possibility of maternal blood contamination suggests that enzyme assays should be performed on chorionic villi or cultured amniocytes and not only on cell-free amniotic fluid.

21-Hydroxylase for virilizing congenital adrenal hyperplasia (CAH). By far the most common cause of female pseudohermaphroditism is CAH, an autosomal recessive disorder due to 21-hydroxylase deficiency. The disease frequency ranges from 1:500 births in Yupik Eskimos to 1:5000–13,000 among various Caucasian populations. The enzyme defect blocks cortisol synthesis, resulting in adrenocortical hyperplasia with overproduction of metabolites occurring

before the block, including androgens. This results in virilization in the female fetus and sexual precocity in the male. Glucocorticoid administration to the mother must start as soon as 5 menstrual weeks to decrease virilization in the female.[95] In approximately two-thirds of the cases of classic CAH there is also deficiency of aldosterone (salt-wasting type), and the infant may present between 1 and 4 weeks of age with life-threatening hyponatremia.

Elevated levels of 17-hydroxyprogesterone were found in second-trimester amniotic fluid of fetuses with the salt-wasting classic form of CAH.[96–98] Raux-Demay et al.[99] showed that the clear-cut difference between normal and pathologic 17-hydroxyprogesterone values is even more striking in first-trimester fluids. Determinations of other steroid levels did not improve the accuracy of diagnosis.

Because both classic and nonclassic CAH are HLA linked (the gene for steroid 21-hydroxylase is located on chromosome 6p21.3 within the HLA complex), HLA typing offers an additional means of carrier detection and prenatal diagnosis by identifying a fetus as HLA concordant or HLA discordant from an index case.[100,101] When specific 21-hydroxylase probes became available, direct prenatal diagnosis was theoretically possible if preliminary family studies showed that the index case is homozygous for a deletion.[102] The routine use of RFLPs has not been successful due to a lack of polymorphisms in this area.

Amniotic fluid alpha-fetoprotein. Antenatal diagnosis of NTDs can be accomplished by either high-quality ultrasound or AF-AFP assay combined with AChE testing.[103] Because few ultrasound centers are aware of the sensitivity and specificity for finding such lesions, AF-AFP analysis has remained the standard method of testing for NTDs since the mid-1970s. By means of AF-AFP and AChE analysis, a diagnosis of NTD is possible in all except the 5% of lesions that are skin covered. Hence both amniocentesis and ultrasound should be recommended to couples at a higher risk for NTD.

The association between an open NTD and a high AFP level is nonspecific, and increased levels of AFP reach the amniotic fluid by diffusion from fetal serum or cerebrospinal fluid across open or leaking membranes. For this reason, other "open" fetal malformations, such as omphalocele or gastroschisis, can also produce elevated levels of amniotic fluid AFP. Additionally, because of decreased swallowing and AFP absorption by the fetus, elevated AF-AFP can occasionally be observed in the presence of intestinal atresias. Elevated AF-AFP can also be found in fetuses affected with congenital nephrosis and other renal lesions due to increased loss in the fetal urine. Finally, contamination of amniotic fluid with fetal blood might be the reason for elevated AF-AFP in a normal fetus.

Amniotic fluid Acetylcholinesterase (AF-AChE). At present, AChE gel electrophoresis is widely used as a secondary diagnostic test when AF-AFP levels are elevated.[104] This system has proved highly reliable for identifying both true- and false-positive AFP results. AF-AChE, an enzyme presumably derived from the fetal nervous system, is not detectable in maternal serum and is normally not present in amniotic fluid after gestational week 12. The neural tube is closed after day 28 of development.[105] AChE results are positive in 99.4% of cases with an open NTD and are negative at least 90% of the time when an elevated AFP value occurs with an unaffected pregnancy.[106]

Elevated AF-AFP levels occur in unaffected pregnancies at

the rate of approximately 8 per 1000 samples tested.[107] Therefore, a conservative estimate would place about 1 per 1000 AF samples from unaffected pregnancies as being associated with both elevated AFP values and a visible AChE band.[104]

In association with elevated AF-AFP, AF-AChE is present in 80% of open ventral wall defects (VWDs), because intestinal nerve plexuses may be exposed to the amniotic fluid. A densitometric scan ratio of AChE to pseudocholinesterase is useful for the differential diagnosis of NTD and VWD.[108]

Kelly et al.[109] found an AChE/pseuodcholinesterase ratio above 0.13 in samples from fetuses with open NTDs (62 of 65) or cystic hygroma. All cases of ventral wall defects (n = 29), fetal blood contamination (n = 16), or fetal ascites (n = 2) had ratios below 0.13. All patients with normal outcomes but positive AChE had ratios below 0.12. AChE/pseudocholinesterase ratios are a valuable part of accurately diagnosing fetal abnormalities. An immunochemical technique for measuring AChE in AF utilizing 4F9 monoclonal antibody has also proven capable of distinguishing between affected and unaffected pregnancies with reasonable reliability and might provide additional information.[104]

Microvillar intestinal enzymes (MIE) for cystic fibrosis (CF). Cystic fibrosis is one of the most common recessively inherited diseases in the Caucasian population, with a disease frequency of 1:2000 live births and a calculated carrier frequency of about 5%. It affects a number of organs including the lung, pancreas, and sweat glands. Traditionally, the sweat test in infants and children and the immunoreactive trypsin on blood for neonatal screening were the only available tests, each with some margin of error.

When no abnormality was detected in cultured fibroblasts of CF patients, investigators began looking for a protein marker in amniotic fluid. Because many of the affected organ systems have epithelial cell surfaces specialized in the form of microvilli, and because amniotic fluid cells have a high content of epithelioid-like cells, microvillar enzymes such as gamma-glutamyltranspeptidase (GGTP), aminopeptidase M (APM), and alkaline phosphatase (ALP) were tested and found to be decreased in the fluid of CF fetuses.

According to Muller et al.,[110] the optimal time for MIE-based prenatal diagnosis of CF was from 17 to 18 gestational weeks. As the distributions of MIEs are non-Gaussian, the cut-off line was taken as 0.5 times the median for the relevant gestational week.[111] Scoring the three enzymes simultaneously on each sample followed by multivariate analysis gave the most acceptable result. If two or more enzymes were below 0.5 times the median for its distribution at the relevant gestational week, the pregnancy would be classified as affected. Conversely, if one or none were below 0.5, it would be classified as normal. With the MIE approach there were 4.4% false negatives (3/68) and 2.3% (3/131) false positives.[112] Prenatal diagnosis was restricted to pregnancies with a clearly defined 1 in 4 risk of recurrence of CF. However, recently the CF gene, previously localized to chromosome 7, was cloned and characterized, thus making the molecular diagnosis of CF and detection of gene carriers possible (vide infra).[113,114]

Prenatal diagnosis by DNA analysis

For all disorders due to a defect in a single gene, the possibility of diagnosis at the DNA level theoretically exists.[115] Most mutations are "point mutations," or changes in one or a few nucleotides. These changes can be in the form of substitutions, deletions, or insertions. Only 1%–5% of gene mutations involve gross gene alterations such as insertions or deletions of relatively large pieces of genetic material. One exception is the α-globin cluster where most of the mutations causing α-thalassemia involve deletion of one or more entire genes.

Despite the impressive list of cloned genes, prenatal diagnosis is not yet available for most of these disorders. Sickle cell disease is the only one of the testable heritable conditions for which one mutation gives rise to all affected cases. For each of the other disorders, DNA markers must be found that distinguish the affected (mutant) gene from the normal genes. In the optimal situation, the sequences of both the normal and mutant gene are known and precise DNA probes or markers can be used. These DNA markers are short sequences of nucleotides (oligonucleotides) that are synthesized to be exactly complementary to the gene sequence in question so that they will selectively recognize the affected or normal gene. Unfortunately, the applicability of oligonucleotide probes is limited because the exact sequences of the mutant and normal gene are often not known. For a given disease, different families usually have different mutations. In some cases, as in β-thalassemia, knowledge of the ethnic group points to the likely mutations and therefore which DNA probes to utilize.

In other cases, when the exact molecular defect is not known, the recognition of abnormal genes is accomplished indirectly through the use of DNA polymorphisms that are linked to the abnormal gene. Polymorphisms are differences in DNA base sequences due to normal variability. These may be recognizable after the DNA is cut by a restriction endonuclease (an enzyme that recognizes and cleaves DNA at a specific nucleotide sequence). Because 1 in 500 nucleotides differs between two randomly selected alleles and about 5% of this variability can be recognized by a restriction endonuclease, the human genome contains a large number of such DNA polymorphisms.[115] The polymorphism is not the mutation that causes the disorder, but distinguishes the chromosome carrying the mutant gene from the chromosome carrying the normal gene. In a given family, an "informative" polymorphism occurs when an affected member has a polymorphism in the DNA that is closely linked to the affected gene. In this way, the affected gene can be traced and its inheritance determined without knowledge of the precise disease causing mutation in the gene.

A new technique, the polymerase chain reaction, has contributed a third way to detect genes.[116,117] It allows one to use a very small amount of genomic DNA (theoretically the amount found in a single cell) to make hundreds of thousands of copies of a sequence of interest in a matter of hours. Human genomic DNA is rendered single stranded (denatured), and a heat-stable polymerase (Taq polymerase) is used to synthesize the strands complementary to the original single-stranded DNA. A requirement for amplification of DNA, in addition to free nucleotides, is short starting pieces of DNA called *oligonucleotide primers.* The primers (usually around 20 nucleotides long) are synthesized so that they are complementary to the gene of interest; therefore the sequence of the gene must be known. The primers flank the area of genomic DNA that is to be studied after amplification. This technique can be used to diagnose quickly the presence or absence of the sickle cell mutation. It has also proved to be reliable as a rapid sex test for prenatal diagnosis by detecting the presence of the Y chromosome.

At the end of 1985, the CF locus was assigned to the middle of chromosome 7.[118-120] With the discovery of RFLPs tightly linked to the CF gene, a new approach was available.[121] Very tightly linked probes (XV-2c and KM-19) have been informative in 98% of cases.[122,123] The first mutation of the CF gene, detected in 68% of CF patients, has been cloned: a deletion of 3 bp that results in the omission of a phenylalanine residue at amino acid position 508.[113,114] Forty-six percent of CF patients will be homozygous for this deletion, while another 43% will be compound heterozygotes for this deletion and another mutation. The time for mass population screening is close, but not yet here. In addition to the Δ508 mutation, 60 other mutations in the CF gene have been identified.[124] The frequency of the most common of these mutations is usually only 2%–5%.[125] Thus any mass population screening for detection of CF carriers appears to be a difficult task, requiring numerous tests to gain a reasonable percentage of CF mutations. Such a program awaits the identification of the most common mutations (probably 8–10) that when combined with the Δ508 mutation will be capable of detecting >90% of all CF mutations.[126]

Currently, prenatal diagnosis of CF can be performed for families at risk for producing an affected child due to a family history positive for CF. By combining direct testing for the Δ508 mutation and a few other CF mutations a detection rate of about 85% can be achieved. Direct detection in combination with linkage analysis employing XV-2c and KM-19 can identify virtually all fetuses carrying a CF mutation. This testing can be performed using the PCR, allowing rapid analysis. Because the PCR uses minute amounts of DNA, it is also an ideal technique.

Genetic counseling

Genetic counseling has been defined by an ad hoc committee of the American Society of Human Genetics as a communication process dealing with the occurrence, or risk of recurrence, of a genetic disorder. This process includes helping the individual or family (1) to understand the medical facts, including diagnosis, prognosis, and therapy; (2) to understand the role of genetics in the disorder and the risk of recurrence; (3) to understand the reproductive options; (4) to choose an appropriate course of action; and (5) to adjust as well as possible to the disorder or to the risk of its recurrence. Basically, genetic counseling should be viewed as a special type of instruction and advice given by physicians to patients.

The unit of clinical genetic practice should be the family, not the individual. This represents an extension of the physician–patient relationship to a physician–family relationship. Genetic counseling has three components. The first is the obtaining and presentation of the relevant medical and genetic information. Appropriate counseling requires accurate facts, starting with the diagnosis of the affected member(s) of the family. The counselor must be sure of the accuracy of the diagnosis before proceeding further. Estimating the risk of occurrence or recurrence involves the use of three types of information: modular information, arrived at by the rational use of Mendelian principles; empirical information,

obtained from the analysis of data from population surveys; and particular information, derived from analysis of the pedigree of the family in question. Laboratory information and age of onset relevant to the genetic condition also can be incorporated into the risk estimate using Bayesian calculations. Once obtained, the medical and genetic information must be presented to the family in the manner they are most likely to comprehend.

The second component of genetic counseling is aiding those being counseled to consider the information in light of the reproductive options available and to formulate a course of action appropriate to their individual circumstances. To enable an informed choice, a variety of viewpoints must be presented objectively. The extent to which guidance toward a particular decision is given varies greatly among counselors. It is virtually impossible to present information in a totally neutral fashion. Quoting a 10% risk of abnormality may not have the same psychological impact as quoting a 9-to-1 probability of a normal outcome. There may be no solution to this problem, but it is one of which the counselor should be aware in order that the choice of words can be made precisely rather than randomly.

The major concerns weighed by families considering their reproductive options are the risk of occurrence of a disorder and the burden of the disorder in terms of its severity and its duration (survival time of the affected individual). There are many other considerations in parental genetic decision-making, however, including the couple's capacity to withstand adversity, the status of their marital relationship, their perceived impact of an affected child on existing or prospective children, their financial status, and their individual and joint moral commitments.

The third component of genetic counseling is psychological. It is important to gain insight into the family's emotional state. They are often anxious, hostile, and depressed about the situation bringing them to the genetic counselor. The educational aspects of counseling will be ineffective unless these feelings are dispelled or reduced. Feelings of guilt, denial, grief, and mourning are associated with giving birth to a child with a genetic disorder, and they must be brought to the surface and dealt with.

In spite of the specialized nature of genetic counseling, it is neither desirable nor possible that it be carried out only by medical geneticists. For many problems the ideal counselor is the family physician, who knows the family's physical, emotional, and financial resources. For physicians who feel unsure about the matter, or in situations requiring specialized skills in diagnosis, risk ascertainment, or counseling, a referral can be made to a medical genetics service equipped with personnel trained to fill these needs.

Success in genetic counseling can be measured in terms of whether the counselee understood and learned the diagnostic and risk information, whether the information presented by the counselor entered into the reproductive decisions made, and whether the counseling influenced actual reproductive outcomes. Genetic counseling appears to have limited success in educating the subjects. About 60% of patients improve their "diagnostic accuracy," and 40 percent are still completely inaccurate after counseling. The risk figures quoted in counseling are remembered better, with various studies indicating that 65%–95% of those counseled recall the numerical risk correctly.[127] There is some tendency to under-

Table 11–6. Reproductive attitudes and outcomes after genetic counseling[a]

	Genetic risk >10%	Genetic risk <10%
Number of couples	333	381
No further pregnancies desired	225 (67)	99 (26)
Further pregnancies desired	86 (26)	265 (70)
Undecided	22 (7)	17 (4)
Actual pregnancies that occurred	132	257
Number of pregnancies per couple	0.40	0.67

[a]Values in parentheses are percentages. From Bobrow.[128]

estimate the risk: patients at high risk remember their risk figures more accurately than do patients at low risk.

The attitudes toward further reproduction are influenced by genetic counseling, as indicated by the results of one study[128] which are listed in Table 11–6. Approximately two-thirds of couples to whom a high risk (more than 10%) was quoted intended to have no further pregnancies; 70 percent of couples to whom a low risk (less than 10%) was quoted did plan further pregnancies. The actual number of pregnancies that occurred after counseling was 0.40 per couple in the high-risk group and 0.67 per couple in the low-risk group. Approximately one-half the families reported that they believe genetic counseling to have influenced their reproductive planning. There is a strong relationship between a couple's concept of the burden of the disorder and their reproductive attitudes. If one assumes that those patients and families receiving genetic counseling will turn their intentions into reproductive reality, the net reproductive effect of counseling would be a 15% increase in the number of pregnancies in the counseled population. This is so because many couples are actually at less risk than they believed before they received counseling.

More recently, efforts have been made to understand how families perceive their risks and arrive at their reproductive decisions.[129] Couples have been found to develop a perception of the problem facing them while assessing their ability to cope with different aspects of it. This decision-making in a situation of uncertainty leads to focusing on a binary outcome of any future pregnancy—the infant will or will not be affected with the disorder. Couples often considered their options by creating scenarios in which one of the binary outcomes was conceptualized as having occurred, and then imagining the consequences. They then appeared to select the option that would result in the least loss and in which none of the outcomes would be beyond their ability to cope.[130]

Although this section has dealt with genetic counseling as an established entity, there are still many unanswered questions about it. Who is the best counselor—those with an M.D., a Ph.D., or M.A. degree in counseling? How well do lay counselors function? Should counseling be exclusively verbal? If not, what other media should be used? Would a written summary of the counseling session help the family? When and how often should counseling be repeated? What is the magnitude of the need for genetic counseling? How should these services be funded? These questions are posed so that the reader will realize that, although we are moving forward, we do so with some uncertainty regarding the direction in which we are traveling.

References

1. Steele MW, Breg WR Jr: Chromosome analysis of human amniotic-fluid cells. Lancet 1:383, 1966.
2. Donald I, MacVicar J, Brown TG: Investigation of abdominal masses by pulsed ultrasound. Lancet 1:1188, 1958.
3. American Institute of Ultrasound in Medicine Bioeffects Committee: Bioeffects considerations for the safety of diagnostic ultrasound. J Ultrasound Med 7(Suppl):S1, 1988.
4. Cartwright RA, McKinney PA, Hopton PA, et al.: Ultrasound examinations in pregnancy and childhood cancer. For the Inter-Regional Epidemiological Study for Childhood Cancer Group. Lancet 2:999, 1984.
5. Eik-Nes SH, Okland O, Aure JC, et al.: Ultrasound screening in pregnancy: a randomized controlled trial. Lancet 1:1347, 1984.
6. Waldenstroem U, Axelsson O, Nilsson S, et al.: Effects of routine one-stage ultrasound in pregnancy: a randomized controlled trial. Lancet 2:585, 1988.
7. Escobar LF, Bixler D, Weaver DD, et al.: Bone dysplasias: the prenatal diagnostic challenge. Am J Med Genet 36:488, 1990.
8. Nicolaides KH, Campbell S: Diagnosis of fetal abnormalities by ultrasound. In: Genetic Disorders and the Fetus, ed 2. A Milunsky, ed. Plenum, New York, 1986, p 521.
9. Fermont L, de Geeter B, Aubry MC, et al.: A close collaboration between obstetricians and paediatric cardiologists allows antenatal detections of severe cardiac malformations by 2D echocardiography. In: Second World Congress of Paediatric Cardiology. Springer-Verlag, New York, 1985, p 10.
10. Harrison MR, Golbus MS, Filly RA: The Unborn Patient. Prenatal Diagnosis and Treatment. Grune & Stratton, Orlando, FL, 1984.
11. Hutson JM, McNay M, McNay MB, et al.: Antenatal diagnosis of surgical disorders by ultrasonography. Lancet 1:621, 1985.
12. Kirk EP, Wah RM: Obstetric management of the fetus with omphalocele or gastroschisis: a review and report of one hundred and twelve cases. Am J Obstet Gynecol 146:512, 1983.
13. Grundy H, Anderson RL, Filly RA, et al.: Gastroschisis: prenatal diagnosis and treatment. Fetal Ther 2:144, 1987.
14. Bauer D, Golbus MS: Fetal obstructive uropathies. In: Fetal Physiology and Pathology (Proceedings of The 12th World Congress of Obstetrics and Gynecology, Rio de Janeiro, 1988). P Belfort, JA Pinotti, TKAB Eskes, eds. Parthenon, Lancaster, 1989, p 97.
15. Bergstrand CG, Czar B: Demonstration of a new protein fraction in serum from the human fetus. Scand J Clin Lab Invest 8:174, 1956.
16. Halbrecht, Klibanski C: Identification of a new normal embryonic hemoglobin. Nature 178:794, 1956.
17. Nishi S: Isolation and characterization of a human fetal-alpha-globulin from the sera of fetuses and a hepatoma patient. Cancer Res 30:2507, 1970.
18. Brock DJH, Sutcliffe RG: Alpha-fetoprotein in the antenatal diagnosis of anencephaly and spina bifida. Lancet 2:197, 1972.
19. Brock DJH, Sutcliffe RG: Prental diagnosis of anencephaly. Biochem Soc Trans 1:149, 1973.
20. UK Collaborative Study on Alpha-Fetoprotein in Relation to Neural-Tube-Defects: Maternal serum-alpha-fetoprotein measurement in antenatal screening for anencephaly and spina bifida in pregnancy. Lancet 1:1323, 1977.
21. Fersguson-Smith MA: The reduction of NTDs by MS-AFP screening. Br Med Bull 39:365, 1983.
22. Milunsky A, Alpert E: Results and benefits of a M-AFP screening program. JAMA 252:1438, 1984.
23. Knight GJ: Survey of the participants in the Foundation for Blood Research External Quality Assessment Scheme, 1990. unpublished data.
24. Wald NH, Cuckle HS: Open neural tube defects. In: Antenatal and Neonatal Screening. NJ Wald, ed. Oxford University Press, New York, 1984, p 39.
25. Merkatz IR, Nitowsky HM, Macri JM, et al.: An association between low maternal serum alpha-fetoprtein and fetal chromosome abnormalities. Am J Obstet Gynecol 148:886, 1984.

26. Cuckle HS, Wald NJ, Lindenbaum RH: Maternal alpha-fetoprotein measurement: a screening test for Down syndrome. Lancet 1:926, 1984.

27. Fuhrmann W, Wendt P, Weitzel H: Maternal serum AFP as screening test for Down syndrome. Lancet 2:413, 1984.

28. DiMaio MS, Baumgarten A, Greenstein RM, et al.: Screening for fetal Down's syndrome in pregnancy by measuring maternal serum alpha-fetoprotein levels. N Engl J Med 317:342, 1987.

29. Doran TA, Cadeskey K, Wong PY, et al.: MS-AFP and fetal autosomal trisomies. Am J Obstet Gynecol 154:277, 1986.

30. Palomaki GE, Haddow IE: Maternal serum-alpha-fetoprotein, age, and Down syndrome risk. Am J Obstet Gynecol 156:460, 1987.

31. Hook EB: Down syndrome: frequency in human populations and some factors pertinent to variation in rates. In: Trisomy 21 (Down Syndrome): Research Perspectives. FF de la Cruz, PS Gerald, eds. University Park Press, Baltimore, 1981, p 3.

32. Hook EB, Cross PK, Schreinemachers DM: Chromosomal abnormality rates at amniocentesis and in live-born infants. JAMA 249:2034, 1983.

33. Milunsky A, Jick SS, Bruell CL, et al.: Predictive values, relative risks, and overall benefits of high and low maternal serum alpha-fetoprotein screening in singleton pregnancies: New epidemiologic data. Am J Obstet Gynecol 161:291, 1989.

34. Brody S, Carlstrom G: Human chorionic gonadotropin in abnormal pregnancy. Serum and urinary findings using various immunoassay techniques. Acta Obstet Gynaecol Scand 44:32, 1965.

35. Boue J, Boue A, Lazar P: The epidemiology of human spontaneous abortions with chromosome anomalies. In: Aging Gametes, RJ Blandau, ed., Karger, Basel, 1975, p 330.

36. Braunstein G, Rasor J, Adler D, et al.: Serum human chorionic gonadotropin levels throughout normal pregnancy. Am J Obstet Gynecol 126:678, 1976.

37. Bogart MH, Pandian MR, Jones OW: Abnromal maternal serum chorionic gonadotropin levels in pregnancies with chromosome abnormalities. Prenat Diagn 7:623, 1987.

38. Bogart MH, Golbus MS, Sorg ND, et al.: HCG levels in pregnancies with aneuploid fetuses. Prenat Diagn 9:379, 1987.

39. Canick JA, Knight GJ, Palomaki GE, et al.: Low second trimester maternal serum unconjugated oestriol in pregnancies with Down's syndrome. Br J Obstet Gynaecol 95:330, 1988.

40. Wald NJ, Cuckle MS, Densem JW, et al.: Maternal serum screening for Down's syndrome in early pregnancy. Br Med J 297:883, 1988.

41. Wald NJ, Cuckle HS, Densem JW, et al.: Maternal serum unconjugated oestriol as an antenatal screening test for Down's syndrome in early pregnancy. Br J Obstet Gynaecol 95:334, 1989.

42. Petrocik E, Wassman ER, Kelly JC: Prenatal screening for Down syndrome with maternal serum and human chorionic gonadotropin levels. Am J Obstet Gynecol 161:1168, 1989.

43. Suchy SF, Yeager MT: Down syndrome screening in women under 35 with maternal serum hCG. Obstet Gynecol 76:20,1990.

44. Knight GJ, Palomaki GE, Haddow JE, et al.: Maternal serum levels of the placental products hCG, hPL, SP1, and progesterone are all elevated in cases of fetal Down syndrome. Am J Hum Genet 45:A263, 1989.

45. Walknowska J, Conte FA, Grumbach MM: Practical and theoretical implications of fetal/maternal lymphocyte transfer. Lancet 1:1119, 1969.

46. Schroeder J: Fetal cells in the blood of pregnant mothers. J Med Genet 18:321, 1981.

47. Kulozik A, Pawlowitzke IH: Fetal cells in the maternal circulation: detection by direct AFP-immunofluorescence. Hum Genet 62:221, 1982.

48. Covone AE, Mutton D, Johnson PM, et al.: Trophoblast cells in peripheral blood from pregnant women. Lancet 2:841, 1984.

49. Schwinger E, Hillers M, Vosberg HP: No identification of Y-chromosomal DNA in blood from pregnant women bearing a male fetus? Am J Hum Genet 45(Suppl):A268, 1989.

50. Lebo RV: Chromosome sorting and DNA sequence localization. Cytometry 3:145, 1982.

51. Herzenberg LA, Bianchi DW, Schroder J, et al.: Fetal cells in the blood of pregnant women: detection and enrichment by fluorescence-activated cell sorting. Proc Natl Acad Sci USA 76:1453, 1979.

52. Selypes A, Lorencz R: A noninvasive method for determination of the sex and karyotype of the fetus from the maternal blood. Hum Genet 79:357, 1988.

53. Youssef M, Tharapel AT, Shulman LP, et al.: Attempted documentation of fetal cells in maternal circulation using the "air-culture" cytogenetic technique. Am J Hum Genet 45(Suppl):A274, 1989.

54. Lau YF, Huang JC, Dozy AM, et al.: A rapid screening test for antenatal sex determiantion. Lancet 1:14, 1984.

55. Gray J, Pinkel D, Yu LC, et al.: Fluorescence in situ hybridization (FISH) applied to prenatal diagnosis. Am J Hum Genet 43:A235, 1988.

56. Schindler A, Graf E, Martin-Du-Pan L: Prenatal diagnosis of fetal lymphocytes in the maternal blood. Obstet Gynecol 40:340, 1972.

57. Tabor A, Madsen M, Obel EB, et al.: Randomised controlled trial of genetic amniocentesis in 4,606 low-risk women. Lancet 1:1287, 1986.

58. Golbus MS, Loughman WD, Epstein CJ, et al.: Prentatal genetic diagnosis in 3000 amniocenteses. N Engl J Med 300:157, 1979.

59. Benn PA, Hsu LYF: Maternal cell contamination of amniotic fluid cell cultures: result of a U.S. nationwide survey. Am J Med Genet 15:297, 1983.

60. Gosden C, Nicolaides KH, Rodeck CH: Fetal blood sampling in investigation of chromosome mosaicism in amniotic fluid cell culture. Lancet 1:613, 1988.

61. Evans MI, Drugan A, Koppitch FC III, et al.: Genetic diagnosis in the first trimester: the norm for the 1990s. Am J Obstet Gynecol 160:1332, 1989.

62. Jackson LG: CVS Newsletter. No. 29, January 18, 1990.

63. Medical News and Perspectives: Trial appears to confirm safety of chorionic villus samples procedures. JAMA 259:3521, 1988.

64. Canadian Collaborative CVS–Amniocentesis Clinical Trail Group: Multicentre randomized clinical trial of chorion villus sampling and amniocentesis. Lancet 1:1, 1989.

65. Ledbetter DH, Martin AO, Verlinsky, Y et al.: Cytogenetic results of chorionic villus sampling: high success rate and diagnostic accuracy in the United States collaborative study. Am J Obstet Gynecol 162:495, 1990.

66. Holzgreve W: personal communication, 1990.

67. Hobbins JC, Grannum P, Romero R, et al.: Percutaneous umbilical blood sampling. Am J Obstet Gynecol 152:1, 1985.

68. Nicolaides KH, Rodeck CH, Gosden CM: Rapid karyotyping in non-lethal malformations. Lancet 1:283, 1986.

69. Weiner CP: Cordocentesis for diagnostic indications: two years experience. Obstet Gynecol 70:664, 1987.

70. Daffos F, Capella-Pavlovsky M, Forestier F: Fetal blood sampling during pregnancy with use of a needle guided by ultrasound: a study of 606 consecutive cases. Am J Obstet Gynecol 153:655, 1985.

71. Golbus MS, McGonigle KF, Goldberg JD, et al.: Fetal tissue sampling: the San Francisco Experience with 190 pregnancies. West J Med 150:423, 1989.

72. Wang ZQ, Gilliam AL, Golbus MAS: A modified elution method for determining the presence of fetal red blood cells. Prenat Diagn 8:555, 1988.

73. Harper K, Winter RM, Pembrery ME, et al.: A clinically useful DNA probe closely linked to haemophilia A. Lancet 2:6, 1984.

74. Gianelli F, Anson DS, Choo KH, et al.: Characterization and use of an intragenic polymorphic marker for detection of carriers of haemophilia B (factor IX deficiency). Lancet 1:239, 1984.

75. Embury SH, Scharf SJ, Saiki RK, et al.: Rapid prental diagnosis of sickle cell anemia by a new method of DNA analysis. N Engl J Med 316:656, 1987.

76. Rubin EM, Kan YW: A simple sensitive prenatal test for hydrops fetalis caused by alpha-thalassaemia. Lancet 1:75, 1986.

77. Kidd VJ, Golbus MS, Wallace RB, et al.: Prenatal diagnosis of alpha-1 antitrypsin deficiency by direct analysis of the mutation site in the gene. N Engl J Med 310:639, 1984.

78. Durandy A, Oury C, Griscelli C: Prenatal testing for inherited immune deficiencies by fetal blood sampling. Prenat Diagn 2:109, 1982.

79. Holmberg L, Gustaavii B, Jonsson A: A prenatal study of fetal platelet count and size with application to fetus at risk for Wiscott-Aldrich syndrome. J Pediatr 102:773, 1983.

80. Matthay KK, Golbus MS, Wara DWW, et al.: Prental diagnosis of chronic granuloomatous disease. Am J Med Genet 17:731, 1984.

81. Kidd VJ, Fainaru M, Deckelbaum R, et al.: Apolipoproteins in

human fetal blood and amniotic fluid in mid-trimester pregnancies. Prenat Diagn 1:125,1981.

82. Golbus MS, Stephens JD, Cann HM: In utero paternity testing utilizing fetal blood obtained by midtrimester fetoscopy. Am J Hum Genet 32:88, 1980.

83. Daffos F, Forestier F, Capella-Pavlovsky M, et al.: Prenatal management of 746 pregnancies at risk for congenital toxoplasmosis. N Engl J Med 318:271, 1988.

84. Holzgreve W, Golbus MS: Prenatal diagnosis of ornithine transcarbamylase deficiency utilizing fetal liver biopsy. Am J Hum Genet 36:320, 1984.

85. Golbus MS, Simpson TJ, Koresawa M, et al.: The prenatal determination of glucose-6-phosphatase activity by fetal liver biopsy. Prenat Diagn 8:401, 1988.

86. Elias S, Mazun M, Sabbagh R, et al.: Prenatal diagnosis of harlequin ichthyosis. Clin Genet 17:275, 1980.

87. Rodeck CH, Eady RA, Gosden CH: prenatal diagnosis of epidermolysis bullosa lethalis. Lancet 1:949, 1980.

88. Golbus MS, Sagebiel RW, Filly RA, et al.: Prenatal diagnosis of congenital bullous ichthysiform erythroderma (epidermolytic hyperkeratosis) by fetal skin biopsy. N Engl J Med 302:93, 1980.

89. Nederlof PM, Robinson D, Aubknesha R, et al.: Three-colour fluorescence in situ hybridization for the simultaneous detection of multiple nucleic acid sequences. Cytometry 10:20, 1989.

90. Lichter P, Cremer T, Tang CJ, et al.: Rapid detection of human chromosome 21 aberrations by in situ hybridization. Proc Natl Acad Sci USA 85:9664, 1988.

91. Guyot B, Bazin A, Sole Y, et al.: Prenatal diagnosis with biotinylated chromosome specific probes. Prenat Diagn 8:485, 1988.

92. Friedland J, Perle G, Saifer A, et al.: Screening for Tay-Sachs disease in utero using amniotic lfuid. Proc Soc Exp Biol Med 136:1297, 1971.

93. O'Brien JS, Okada S, Fillerup DL, et al.: Tay-Sachs disease: prenatal diagnosis. Science 172:61, 1971.

94. Harzer K. Erste erfahrunge bei der praenatalen diagnose der Tay-Sachsschen erkrankung durch isoelektrische fokussierung der hexosaminidase A aus amnion-fluessigkeit. Klin Wochenschr 52:145, 1974.

95. David M, Forest MG: Prenatal treatment of congential adrenal hyperplasia resulting from 21-OH deficiency. J Pediatr 105:799, 1984.

96. Forest M: Pitfalls in prenatal diagnosis of 21-OH deficiency by amniotic fluid steroid analysis, six years experience in 102 pregnancies at risk. Ann NY Acad Sci 458:130, 1985.

97. Pang S, Pollack MS, Loo M, et al.: Pitfalls in prenatal diagnosis of 21-OH deficiency congenital adrenal hyperplasia. Ann NY Acad Sci 458:111, 1985.

98. Couillin P, Raux-Demay MC: Conseil genetique et diagnostic prenatal du deficit en 21 hydroxylase. In: Le Diagnostic Prenatal. F Mattei, V Dumez, eds. Doin, Paris, 1986, p 99.

99. Raux-Demay M, Mornet E, Boue J, et al.: Early prenatal diagnosis of 21-OH deficiency using amniotic fluid 17-OHP determination and DNA probes. Prenat Diagn 9:457, 1989.

100. White PC, New MI, Dupont B: Cloning and expression of cDNA encoding a bovine adrenal cytochrome P-450 specific for steroid 21-hydroxylation. Proc Natl Acad Sci USA 81:1986, 1984.

101. Mornet E, Boue J, Raux-Demay M, et al.: First trimester prenatal diagnosis of 21-hydroxylase deficiency by linkage analysis to HLA-DNA probes and by 17-OHP determination. Hum Genet 74:358, 1986.

102. Werkmeister JW, New MI, Dupont B: Frequent deletion and duplication of the steroid 21-hydroxylase genes. Am J Hum Genet 39:461, 1984.

103. Hogge WA, Thiagarajah S, Ferguson J II, et al.: The role of ultrasonograpy and amniocentesis in the evaluation of pregnancies at risk for neural tube defects. Am J Obstet Gynecol 161:520, 1989.

104. Goldfine CH, Knight GJ, Haddow JE, et al.: Amniotic fluid acetylcholinesterase measurements: comparing immunochemical and polyacrylamide gel techniques. Prenat Diagn 9:167, 1989.

105. Muller F, Oury JF, Boue A: First trimester amniotic fluid acetylcholinesterase electrophoresis. Prenat Diagn 9:173, 1989.

106. Report of the Collaborative AChE Study: Amniotic fluid acetylcholinesterase electrophoresis as a secondary test in the diagnosis of anencephaly and open spina bifida in early pregnancy. Lancet 2:321, 1981.

107. Second Report of the U.K. Collaborative Study on AFP in Relation to NTDs: AF-AFP measurement in antenatal diagnosis of anencephaly and open spina bifida in early pregnancy. Lancet 2:651, 1979.

108. Wald NJ, Barlow RD, Cuckle HS, et al.: Amniotic fluid gel cholinesterase density ratios in fetal open defects of the neural tube and ventral wall. Br J Obstet Gynaecol 90:238, 1983.

109. Kelly JC, Petrocik E, Wassmann ER: Amniotic fluid acetylcholinesterase ratios in prenatal diagnosis of fetal abnormalities. Am J Obstet Gynecol 161:703, 1989.

110. Muller F, Berg S, Frot JF, et al.: Alkaline phosphatase isoenzyme assays for prenatal diagnosis of cystic fibrosis. Lancet 1:572, 1984.

111. Brock DJH, Bedgood D, Barron L, Hayward C: Prospective prenatal diagnosis of cystic fibrosis. Lancet 1:1175, 1985.

112. Brock DJH, Clarke HAK, Barron L: Prenatal diagnosis of cystic fibrosis by microvillar enzyme assay on a sequence of 258 pregnancies. Hum Genet 78:271, 1988.

113. Kerem BS, Rommens JM, Buchanan JA, et al.: Identification of the cystic fibrosis gene: genetic analysis. Science 245:1073, 1989.

114. Riordan JR, Rommens JM, Kerem BS, et al.: Identification of the cystic fibrosis gene: cloning and characterization of complementary DNA. Science 245:1066, 1989.

115. Antonarakis SE: Diagnosis of genetic disorders at the DNA level. N Engl J Med 320:153, 1989.

116. Embury SH, Scharf SJ, Saiki RK, et al.: Rapid prenatal diagnosis of sickle cell anemia by a new method of DNA analysis. N Engl J Med 316:656, 1987.

117. Kogan SC, Doherty M, Gitschier J: An improved method for prenatal diagnosis of genetic diseases by analysis of amplified DNA sequence. N Engl J Med 317:985, 1987.

118. Knowlton RG, Cohen-Haguenauer O, vanCong N, et al.: A polymorphic DNA marker linked to cystic fibrosis is located on chromosome 7. Nature 318:380, 1985.

119. Wainwright B, Schambler, P, Schmidtke J, et al.: Localization of cystic fibrosis locus to human chromosome 7cen-q22. Nature 318:384, 1985.

120. White R, Woodward S, Leppert M, et al.: A closely linked genetic marker for cystic fibrosis. Nature 318:382, 1985.

121. Farrall M, Rodeck CH, Stanier P, et al.: First trimester prenatal diagnosis of cystic fibrosis with linked DNA probes. Lancet 1:1402, 1986.

122. Estivill X, Farrall M, Scambler PJ, et al.: A candidate for the cystic fibrosis locus isolated by selection for methylation free islands. Nature 326:840, 1987.

123. Beaudet AL, Spence JE, Montes M, et al.: Experience with new DNA markers for diagnosis of cystic fibrosis. N Eng J Med 318:50, 1988.

124. Davis K: Complementary endeavors. Nature 348:110, 1990.

125. Cutting GR, Latsch LM, Rosenstein BJ, et al.: A cluster of cystic fibrosis mutations in the first nucleotide-binding fold of the cystic fibrosis conductance regulator protein. Nature 346:366, 1990.

126. Beaudet A: Invited editorial: carrier screening for cystic fibrosis. Am J Hum Genet 46:603, 1990.

127. Evers-Kiebooms G, van den Berghe H: Impact of genetic counseling: a review of published follow-up studies. Clin Genet 1:465, 1979.

128. Bobrow M: Genetic counseling: a tool for the prevention of some abnormal pregnancies. J Clin Pathol 10(Suppl):145, 1976.

129. Leonard CO, Chase GA, Childs B: Genetic counseling: a consumer's view. N Engl J Med 287:433, 1972.

130. Lippman-Hand A, Fraser FC: Genetic counseling: parents' responses to uncertainty. BDOAS XV (5C):325, 1979.

12

An Approach to Postnatal Diagnosis

RICHARD J. SCHROER and ROGER E. STEVENSON

If all conceptuses with structural anomalies were to survive, the demands on society would be overwhelming, to the extent that little could be accomplished beyond caring for those affected. The vast majority of conceptuses with anomalies, however, are eliminated by spontaneous abortion or stillbirth.[1-4] Yet many anomalies are compatible with live birth, and, of these, most are compatible with longevity. Each year in the United States approximately 80,000 newly born infants will have major malformations.[5-7] This constitutes 2% of all liveborn infants. An equal number of infants initially believed to be normal will have anomalies diagnosed prior to age 5 years.[8]

Structural anomalies are the most common reason for genetic evaluation during the first year of life (Table 12-1). They constitute as well the major cause of death in infants (Table 12-2). After the first year of life the reasons for genetic evaluation become more diverse. Growth and developmental impairments assume an increasingly important role during the childhood years. Thereafter, reproductive matters, including prenatal diagnosis, become the major reason for genetic consultation.

Annually in the United States, 160,000 infants will be born with anomalies, 40,000 infants will be stillborn, and 120,000 infants will have mental retardation.[4-7,9] To these can be added lesser numbers of individuals with growth problems, impairments of the special senses, failure of sexual maturation and function, and metabolic disturbances. In total, those who might appropriately have genetic evaluation exceed 10% of those born each year. In addition, 235,000 couples seek prenatal diagnosis each year.[10] With less than 600 board-certified clinical geneticists in the United States, it is clear that all persons who might seek genetic services cannot be seen by these specialists. In fact, most infants with anomalies are evaluated by other medical specialists. Structural anomalies present most commonly during infancy and childhood. It is thus appropriate that neonatologists, pediatricians, and family physicians have developed considerable skills in the diagnosis and management of anomalies. Many other specialists who deal with infants and young children—ophthalmologists, neurologists, plastic surgeons, orthopedists, cardiologists—likewise become experienced in the evaluation of birth defects. Specialists responsible for the evaluation of birth defects must have a working knowledge of the principles of heredity, embryogenesis, and teratogenesis.

Nowhere in medicine is a sympathetic and discerning ear more important than in the evaluation of the infant with a birth defect. The family may be devastated by the announcement that the "perfect baby" anticipated has or may have a significant defect. The evaluation must begin at the time the defect is recognized or suspected, although full evaluation may be postponed in some infants with anomalies that are not life threatening. This permits parent–infant bonding to proceed without interruption and the infant to be discharged from the hospital with the mother. In other circumstances, evaluation must be carried out more urgently. Certain anomalies, particularly cardiac and gastrointestinal anomalies, are potentially lethal if not treated immediately. Others with lethal conditions for which no treatment is available need urgent diagnosis in order to plan appropriate management with the family. Some anomalies may not be life threatening, but evaluation is no less urgent. Chief among these is the infant with ambiguous genitalia.

The infant with anomalies who dies poses another emergency situation. All parties wish for a speedy disposition and, because of this, adequate evaluation of such an infant may be neglected. Only with a diagnosis can correct information regarding the cause of death and the risk of recurrence be provided for the family. A preplanned protocol to evaluate the infant with anomalies who dies should include complete examination, storage of appropriate samples (serum, urine, tissues), photographs, radiographs, and necropsy.[11,12] These procedures can be efficiently carried out with little interruption of the family plans. The same applies to abortions and stillbirths.

The nature of anomalies

Anomalies can become apparent at any age. Most significant anomalies are found during infancy and early childhood years.[8] Anomalies of the genital system may become obvious only at puberty. Genetic males with female external genitals may be diagnosed only because of the failure of menorrhea. Females with uterine anomalies may be diagnosed because

Table 12-1. Percentage of referrals at various ages for genetic evaluations due to structural anomalies[a]

Reason for referral	Age (years)					
	0–1	1–3	3–5	5–12	12–20	>20
Malformations	47	22	20	24	24	14
Dysmorphic feature(s)	18	13	8	7	12	4
Cutaneous feature(s)	6	5	6	8	8	11
Subtotal	71	40	34	39	44	29
Family history of physical defect	1	1	2	<1	2	5

[a]Based on 1500 referrals to a general genetics clinic during the years 1981–1991. Excludes referrals for prenatal diagnosis and postmortem examination. See introduction for a full listing of reasons for referrals.

Table 12–2. Causes of death in singleton births

	Neonatal deaths (<28 days)		Infant deaths (<365 days)	
	Birth weight <2500 g (n = 18,109)	Birth weight >2500 g (n = 6723)	Birth weight <2500 g (n = 21,509)	Birth weight >2500 g (n = 16,133)
Prematurity, low birth weight	28[a]	1	23	<1
Respiratory distress syndrome	19	3	18	2
Other respiratory disorders	8	9	7	4
Birth trauma, hypoxia	7	11	6	5
Other perinatal disorder	17	9	15	4
Infection	4	8	5	11
Congenital anomalies	15	48	16	30
Sudden infant death syndrome	<1	5	4	26
Circulatory arrest	<1	<1	<1	2
Other causes	2	5	5	16

[a]All values are percentages. Data are from the Centers for Disease Control[43] and are for the United States (1980).

of difficulties in reproduction. Other anomalies, such as polycystic kidneys, may become symptomatic only during adult life. Still others never become symptomatic and may be discovered incidentally. Unilateral renal agenesis is an example.

Major and minor anomalies

Major anomalies are those that require medical or surgical treatment and those with serious cosmetic impact. Minor anomalies do not generally require medical intervention. Minor defects are thus of less significance and may be normal variations or familial features (Table 2–2).[13–15] Multiple minor defects increase the risk of an associated major defect, may be associated with later appearance of functional deficits, and, in the composite, may be helpful in reaching a diagnosis of a dysmorphic condition.

Isolated anomalies

Anomalies may be isolated or one of a composite of features in the patient. Isolated anomalies are relatively common (Table 12–3) and are often multifactorial in etiology. When this is the case there is a 2%–5% risk of recurrence. The same defect, however, as a part of multiple anomaly syndromes, may have quite different recurrence risks. Isolated cleft lip and palate has a 2%–5% recurrence risk. When it is a feature of the amniotic band syndrome, it has a negligle recurrence risk; when a feature of trisomy 13, a 1% recurrence risk; when a part of Roberts syndrome, a 25% recurrence risk; and when a feature of Van der Woude syndrome, a 50% recurrence risk. Hence determination of the etiology is fundamental to providing recurrence risk estimates.

Composite of anomalies

Multiple anomalies may in some cases be pathogenetically linked to a single preceding event, factor, or anomaly.[16–18] Lung hypoplasia, contractures, and deformation of the facial structures may result from oligohydramnios. A defect in fibrillin may result in lens dislocation, ligamentous laxity, medial necrosis of the aorta, floppy mitral valve, and dolichostenomelia found in Marfan syndrome. Amniotic bands may

produce digit amputation, ring constrictions, syndactyly, and facial clefting. In other cases, multiple anomalies may have a common cause, but the pathogenetic mechanism linking the anomalies may not be known at present. In the chromosomal defect trisomy 21, the heart defect, brachycephaly, flat facies, duodenal atresia, hypogenitalism, and short stature cannot be linked to a single pathogenetic process. Nor is a single mechanism recognized to cause the heart defect, short stature, and polydactyly found in the single gene defect, Ellis-van Creveld syndrome. The same is true for the microtia, limb reduction defects, heart defects, and gut anomalies in the teratogenic syndrome caused by exposure to thalidomide in early pregnancy.

Individual anomalies in a composite may suggest a specific diagnosis, but this is the exception. Facial angiofibromas are pathognomonic of tuberous sclerosis, Lisch nodules of neurofibromatosis, and ring constrictions of amniotic band syndrome, but rarely is a diagnosis made on the basis of one of these single features alone. Usually it is the composite of features that suggests a diagnosis and gives direction to the evaluation.

Table 12–3. Incidence of common isolated anomalies

Anomaly	Incidence
Undescended testes	1:30 (M only)
Heart defect	1:150
Club foot[a]	1:300 (M > F)
Pyloric stenosis	1:300 (M > F)
Neural tube defects	1:500 (F > M)
Umbilical hernia	1:500[b]
Cleft lip ± cleft palate	1:1000 (M > F)
Hypospadias	1:1000 (M only)
Hip dislocation[a]	1:1500 (F > M)
Polydactyly	1:1500 (M > F)[b]
Cleft palate	1:2000 (F > M)
Craniosynostosis	1:2000 (M > F)
Syndactyly	1:2000 (M > F)

[a]Deformations.

[b]Incidence tenfold greater in blacks.

Malformations, disruptions, deformations

Anomalies are commonly divided into malformations, disruptions, and deformations, depending on the presumed pathogenesis (see Chapter 2).[19] Malformations arise during the formation of body structures and are hence caused by intrinsic or extrinsic insults during embryogenesis. Disruptions arise after formation of structures by destructive processes. They are for the most part due to vascular causes. Deformations usually arise late in gestation because of mechanical pressure on various structures.[20] Pressure from within (edema) or without (constraint, oligohydramnios) causes malalignment, malposition, or misshaping of structures but without substantial tissue destruction. Intrinsic defects such as nervous system anomalies, poorly ossified bones, or muscle disease may permit deformities to be produced by normal intrauterine pressures.

Major anomalies are being diagnosed prenatally with increased frequency. This results from the use of pregnancy screening tests (primarily maternal serum α-fetoprotein, human chorionic gonadotropin, and estriol analyses), ultrasound scanning, and prenatal testing via amniocentesis, chorionic villus sampling, and percutaneous umbilical blood sampling. Depending on the suspected anomaly, the place and method of delivery may be altered if it offers a greater opportunity for prompt evaluation and treatment.

Evaluation

The goal of evaluation of the individual with a structural anomaly is to arrive at a specific diagnosis, following which the prognosis can be projected, a management plan formulated, and recurrence risks discussed with the family. If the pathogenesis can be determined, it may be helpful in understanding the anomaly and in explaining the defect to the family.

History

The agenda in evaluating the infant with a birth defect is little different from that used in general medical evaluations. In most medical diagnoses, history-taking plays an extraordinarily powerful role. The diagnosis is suggested by the history more often than by any other diagnostic adjunct. In the case of anomalies, the diagnosis may be immediately obvious to parents and physician alike because of prior occurrence in the family. Often, however, the history is less revealing. Nevertheless, attention must be given for clues in the history that help establish a diagnosis. Advanced maternal age suggests an increased risk of a chromosomal cause for the anomaly, advanced paternal age suggests an increased risk for a new dominant single gene defect, kinship between the parents signals the possibility of an autosomal recessive gene defect. Prior history of abortions or stillbirths suggests the possibility of recurrence of a heritable defect—chromosomal, single gene, or multifactorial.

Pregnancy history may likewise yield subtle clues to diagnosis. Fetuses that move poorly in utero may signal brain anomalies, other neuromuscular defects, limb malformations, or short limb skeletal dysplasias. Breech position may indicate constraint or a neuromuscular abnormality that impaired the ability to achieve cephalic presentation. Excessive low back pain associated with lack of movement may indi-

Table 12–4. Findings in the newborn that prompt a search for occult anomalies

Older parents

Family history of anomalies, abortions, or stillbirths

History of teratogenic exposures

History of oligohydramnios or polyhydramnios

History of decreased fetal movement

Prematurity or postmaturity

Breech presentation

Overgrowth or undergrowth for gestational age

Discordance of measurements

Three or more minor anomalies

Failure of neonatal adaptation

cate constraint. Polyhydramnios indicates lack of fetal swallowing or gastrointestinal absorption of the amniotic fluid because of central nervous system or gastrointestinal anomalies. Oligohydramnios may signal obstructive urinary tract anomalies or anomalies of the kidneys. Certain maternal diseases and exposures during pregnancy alert the clinician to the possibility of particular anomalies; maternal diabetes and alcohol ingestion are the two most frequently encountered.

When evaluation for congenital anomalies is requested, the defect may be obvious or there may only be circumstances that suggest the possibility of an anomaly. The latter is often the case in the neonatal period. Table 12–4 lists findings in the newborn infant that may prompt a search for occult anomalies.

The manner in which the newborn adapts to postnatal life often suggests the possibility of an occult anomaly. The infant who experiences difficulty with respirations and feeding and with maintenance of muscular tone is particularly suspect. Anomalies of the central nervous system, other neuromuscular impairments, and cardiac defects may create problems in transition to postnatal life. In the older infant and child, developmental progress becomes a more important clue to the possibility of occult anomalies, particularly those involving the nervous system and special senses.

In spite of the powerful role of history taking in establishing a diagnosis, the clinician must always be aware that historical clues and familial features may be misleading. The history of prenatal distress may incline one to think of hypoxia or physical injury but may occur in the fetus with an intrinsic defect as well. Facial features that appear unusual may be familial rather than a sign of a syndromic complex. A negative history of drug exposure does not preclude drug ingestion during the pregnancy. Likewise, a history of exposure to a chemical during pregnancy does not mean that the exposure caused the fetal defect. Only when the pregnancy history is congruous with the physical defects can one accept the cause-and-effect relationship.

Examination

Major anomalies that affect topographic anatomy become obvious on physical examination. Minor anomalies may require more careful attention, including measurements and comparisons to normal growth charts, but can provide equally important clues to diagnosis. Evaluation of the volar

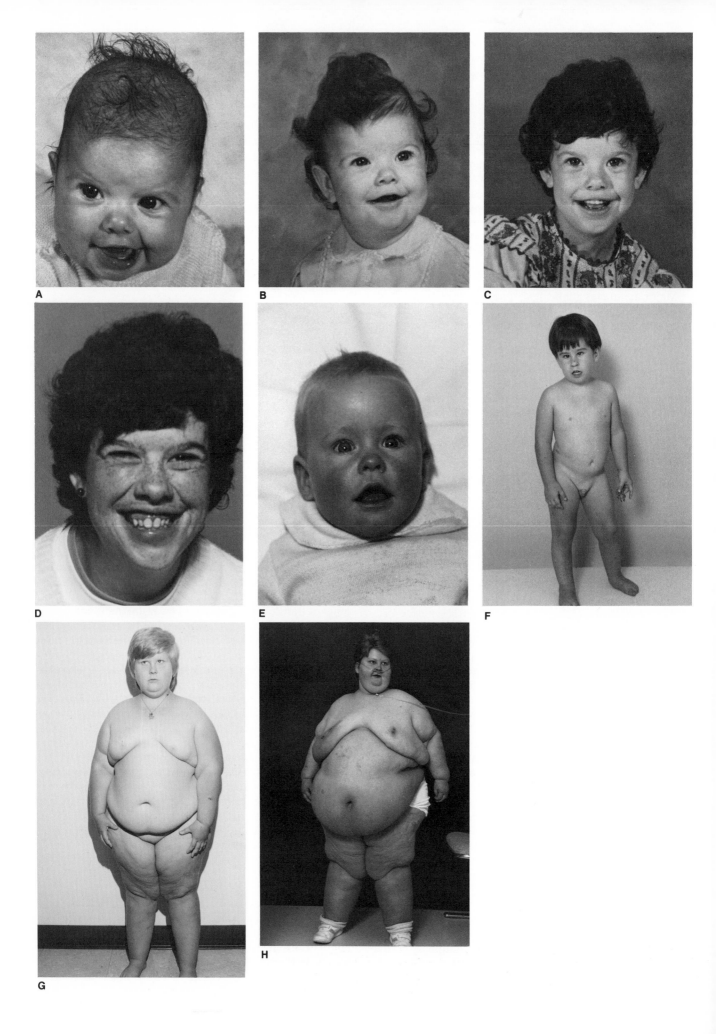

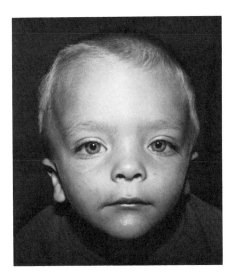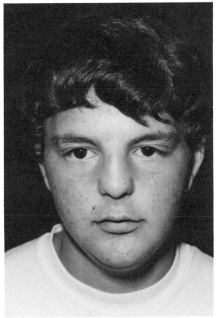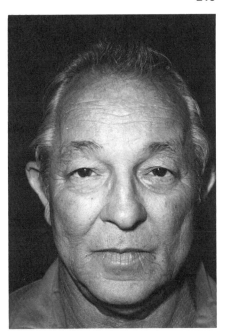

Fig. 12–2. Aarskog syndrome in 3 males at ages 2 yr, 18 yr, and 60 yr. The triangular facial configuration with prominence of the forehead and hypertelorism becomes less apparent with increasing age.

dermal ridges and creases may be helpful in certain syndromes (see Chapter 33). Both the nature of the anomalies and the composite of anomalies have diagnostic importance. When three or more minor anomalies are found, the evaluator should search for occult major malformations.

Childhood is marked by rapid changes in topographic features, growth, and developmental abilities. Features diagnostic at birth may not have been apparent in the midtrimester fetus, and they will not remain the same throughout childhood and adolescence.[21–25] Many conditions with diagnostic facial features in late childhood, adolescence, or adult life can appear entirely normal at birth. Numbered among these are individuals affected with Williams syndrome, fragile X syndrome, storage disorders, Angelman syndrome, Prader-Willi syndrome, and muscular dystrophy (Fig. 12–1). Conversely, infants with distinctive features may become less distinctive as the years pass. This is the case with Aarskog syndrome (Fig. 12–2).

At different ages, diagnosis depends on different features (Figs. 12–3,12–4). At birth, infants with 45,X Turner syndrome have lymphedema, excess nuchal skin, and coarctation of the aorta; during childhood they have stunted growth; and at adolescence they fail to mature sexually.[26] In the fragile X syndrome, one expects large size at birth; developmental delay, particularly in speech, during the early years; and facial characteristics and macroorchidism in the postpubertal years.[25] Infants with certain storage diseases may exhibit excessive growth, umbilical hernia, and hepatosplenomegaly

at birth. During childhood they develop contractures or other skeletal abnormalities, eye abnormalities, and developmental impairment.

Physical observations should include detection of major anomalies, notation of minor defects and variations, assessment of growth (head circumference, weight and height or length), measurement of individual features that appear abnormal, and an estimate of developmental status. Repeated observations over a period of years may ultimately lead to a diagnosis not initially obvious or to revision of an incorrect diagnosis. Comparison of minor features, particularly facial characteristics, with those of the parents and siblings often permits separation of family features from those that may be of diagnostic importance. Review of photographs of family members taken at the same age as the patient can be helpful.

Laboratory testing and imaging

Diagnostic technology has received considerable attention during the past few decades. Radiographs and other imaging procedures are used to define anomalies; cytogenetic, molecular, and biochemical testings screen for underlying chromosomal and gene errors; and computer data banks synthesize information. It may seem that the clinician's role in the evaluation may be displaced by these techniques. To the contrary, the physician geneticist remains central to the evaluation process. Of equal importance to the clinician's roles in

Fig. 12–1. A–D: Williams syndrome showing evolution of facial features at 6 mo (A), 12 mo (B), 4 yr (C), and 20 yr (D). E–H: Prader-Willi syndrome with 15q interstitial deletion. (E) 9-month-old female with hypotonia and feeding difficulties requiring tube feedings. Slight cupid's bow configuration to the upper lip is present but the facies appear normal otherwise. (F) 3-year-old male with history of

hypotonia, feeding difficulties requiring tube feedings until age 6 mo, and developmental delay. He has esotropia, cupid's bow configuration to upper lip, and short stature. (G) 9-year-old girl with moderate obesity, short stature, small hands and feet, and (H) same girl at age 16 yr showing morbid obesity.

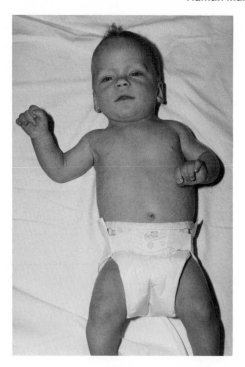
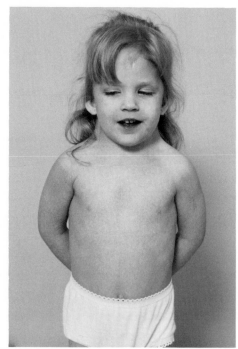
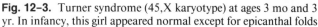

Fig. 12–3. Turner syndrome (45,X karyotype) at ages 3 mo and 3 yr. In infancy, this girl appeared normal except for epicanthal folds and puffiness of the hands and feet. By age 3 yr she had short stature and webbing of the neck had become prominent.

arriving at a correct diagnosis and providing information for the family, is the development of a long-term relationship with the family. This has particular importance because of the pace at which new knowledge, diagnostic techniques, and prevention strategies are being devised. The sensitive clinician also orchestrates the evaluation in such a manner as to be most efficient and least stressful to the emotions and finances of the family.

Laboratory and imaging technologies play important roles in the diagnosis of the infant with anomalies. These roles will likely increase as an understanding of the molecular basis for anomalies is gained. Testing is appropriately used, first, to confirm a suspected diagnosis and, second, as a diagnostic probe. Most genetic testing is noninvasive. Selection of tests should be made judiciously, nonetheless, if for no other reason than the costs involved.

In most cases laboratory testing involves blood samples, urine specimens, or tissue biopsy. The ability to perpetuate genotypically stable cell lines (as fibroblasts or lymphoblasts) has been of great utility in the study of infants with anomalies and other heritable disorders. Cells from these cultures may be frozen and later thawed and subcultures reestablished for analysis. This has been particularly helpful in those cases where the patient has died and in situations where there is the need to transport diagnostic materials to some distant site.

Chromosomes

Chromosome preparations may be made from cultures of lymphocytes, skin and other solid tissues, amniotic fluid cells, and chorionic villi. Chromosome preparations can also be made on bone marrow and chorionic villus cells without culture. The quality of such preparations is less satisfactory than that of preparations from cell culture. Table 12–5 lists many conditions in which chromosome analysis may be indicated. None of these conditions always has a chromosomal etiology, but this possibility may need to be excluded when another etiology has not been established.

Biochemical tests

Biochemical testing of infants with anomalies gives only limited yield. Usually, infants and children with metabolic disorders do not have structural anomalies or other dysmorphic features. Important exceptions do occur. Some infants with metabolic disorders have structural anomalies or distinctive anatomic features at birth, and others develop distinctive features with the progression of the metabolic disorder (Table 12–6).[27–31] Glutaric acidemia is accompanied by agenesis of the corpus callosum and renal cysts; I cell disease by coarsening of the facial features, hernias, and hepatosplenomegaly; Zellweger syndrome by distinctive facies and renal cysts.

The peroxisomal disorders in particular may be accompanied by anomalies at birth.[29] Persons with lysosomal storage diseases typically develop abnormal features with the passage of time. Infants with Hurler disease (MPS 1-H) may have excessive weight, macrocephaly, hernias, macroglossia, and hepatosplenomegaly at birth or during the very early months of life. During childhood they develop gibbous deformation, stiffness of the joints, corneal clouding, and short stature. Other storage diseases appear entirely normal at birth but develop many of the same features during early childhood.

Traditionally the study of hormones and enzymes, metabolism has expanded to the study of gene products that are involved in the structure of various tissues. These gene prod-

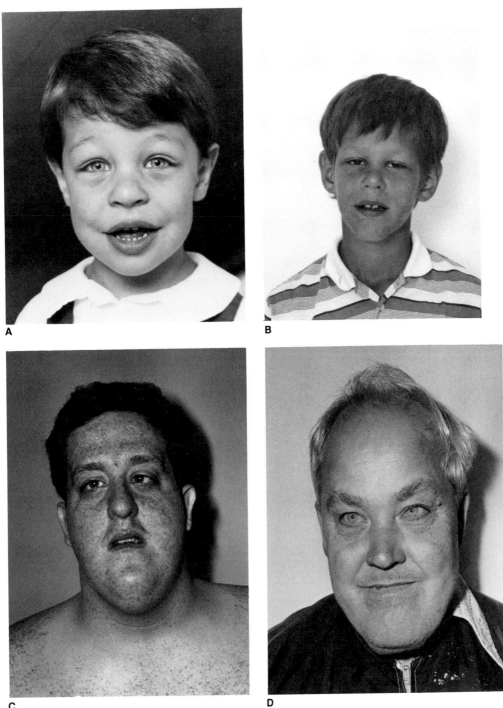

Fig. 12–4. Four males with fragile X syndrome at ages 3 yr (A), 7 yr (B), 23 yr (C), and 41 yr (D). Prominence of the forehead is evident from early childhood, but enlargement of the lower jar develops in late adolescence or adult life.

ucts, collagen, fibrillin, elastin, and others, are certain to prove important in the pathogenesis of some anomalies. Collagen defects have been demonstrated in osteogenesis imperfecta, Stickler syndrome, and spondyloepiphyseal dysplasias, and defective fibrillin has been found in Marfan syndrome.[32–35]

A battery of simple biochemical tests can be performed on urine specimens to screen for a variety of metabolic disorders.[36] These tests are not specific and should be used only as screening tests. Most laboratories include the following tests: Benedict's test (detects reducing sugars), dinitrophenylhydrazine (detects ketoacids), toluidine blue spot test (detects mucopolysaccharides), the nitroprusside test (detects cystine and homocystine), nitrosonaphthol test (detects tyrosine metabolites), and ferric chloride (detects phenylalanine and histidine metabolites). These tests have only limited use in the evaluation of the child with congenital anomalies. With the exception of the mucopolysaccharidoses, the conditions de-

Table 12–5. Indications for chromosome analysis

Individual with

Features of recognizable chromosomal syndrome

Mental retardation of unknown cause

Unexplained major and minor anomalies

Multiple congenital anomalies

Abnormalities of sexual development, including ambiguous or hypoplastic genitalia and failure of sexual maturation at puberty

Unexplained abnormalities of growth

Certain malignancies

Unexplained failure of neonatal adaptation

Features of mosaicism (hypomelanotic spots, streaky pigmentary disturbance, asymmetry)

Couples with

Repeated spontaneous abortions

Infertility

Offspring with a chromosomal duplication, deletion, or other rearrangement

Family members of

An individual with an inherited chromosome duplication, deletion or other rearrangement

Pregnancy products

Abortions

Unexplained stillborns

Hydropic placentas

---

exception of the mucopolysaccharidoses, the conditions detected by these screening tests do not commonly have anomalies. Some laboratories include an oligosaccharide screen in their metabolic battery.[37] This test may be positive in several lysosomal storage diseases (mucolipodosis II, G_{M1} gangliosidosis, G_{M2} gangliosidosis, fucosidosis, mannosidosis, glycogen storage disease type II, galactosialidoses, sialic acid storage diseases, and aspartylglucosaminuria), conditions that, like the mucopolysaccharidoses, may have hernias, hepatosplenomegaly, and excessive intrauterine growth. Urine screening tests may be performed on random specimens or timed collections.

Table 12–6. Features that suggest the presence of an underlying metabolic defect

Excessive intrauterine growth

Corneal clouding

Cataracts

Macroglossia

Hepatosplenomegaly

Hernias (inguinal or umbilical)

Dysplasia of the bone on radiographs

Limb curvature or fracture

Poor ossification of the cranium

Blue sclerae beyond infancy

Developmental regression

Molecular analysis

A number of conditions with structural anomalies have now been localized to more or less discrete regions of the genome (Table 14–16). The recombinant DNA technologies are now being employed in the diagnosis, carrier testing, and prenatal detection of many of these conditions. Expansion of the utility of molecular diagnostics will be a certain result of the effort in progress to delineate the entire human genome.

Imaging

Sonographic and magnetic resonance imaging are to the soft structures of the body what X-ray imaging has been to the skeleton. The anatomy of internal soft tissues, previously hidden to a large degree, can now be studied with noninvasive techniques. Heart anatomy can be defined without catheterization; spine and brain anatomy can be outlined without pneumoencephalography or vascular imaging; the kidneys can be seen without contrast infusions. Most imaging of nonskeletal internal structures can now be done without radiation exposure by using sonography and magnetic resonance. Radiographs are necessary in the evaluation of the skeletal dysplasias.

Photography

Photography provides an easy means of documenting distinctive anatomic features and recording changes that take place over time. Features of interest should be photographed against a neutral backdrop. A scaled background can be used to give an estimate of size. Measurements of various features can be taken from photographs made under standardized conditions. Elimination of shadows that obscure details of various features may be achieved by indirect illumination. It may be desirable to remove clothing, jewelry, or makeup that cover the feature(s) of interest.

Discussions with the family

Communication of information to the affected individual and family is perhaps the most important responsibility of the physician. The physician must be comfortable in the explanation of the heritable or environmental basis of anomalies when an etiology is established and knowledgeable about the potential for prevention through various pregnancy alternatives, including prenatal diagnosis. The accuracy of the information provided by the physician must be assured by careful attention to the details of the case and by a continual awareness of new knowledge. The physician responsible for determining the cause of anomalies must become accustomed to the use of the phrase, "I don't know." Search for the cause of human anomalies fails in about one-half of the cases (Table 12–7).[38,39] Even without knowing the cause, information gained during the evaluation may benefit the family. Based on experience with similar cases, the prognosis may be reasonably stated and the recurrence risk given. In the course of the evaluation, the physician and coworkers develop an interest in the affected individual and family, gain a feeling for the impact that the defect may have on family members, and assume a position of trust and confidence

Table 12-7. Causes of structural anomalies in humans

	Wilson[a] (1973)[39]	Nelson and Holmes[b] (1989)[38]
Genetic causes		
Chromosome aberrations	3–5	10.1
Single gene mutation	20	3.1
"Familial"		14.5
Multifactorial cause	?	23.0
Teratogens	8.5	3.2
Uterine factors	—	2.5
Twinning	—	0.4
Unknown	65–70	43.2

[a]Estimates based on multiple literature sources.
[b]Findings in 1549 malformed infants of at least 20 weeks gestation.

from which continuing support can be given. Sensitivity assists the physician in relating to the family.

Much has been said in favor of having a team of specialists from different disciplines participate in the evaluation and management of certain anomalies.[40–42] One advantage is bringing the various medical, surgical, and paramedical personnel to one site. When the availability of specialists and the logistics make this impractical, it is optimal for one physician to assume responsibility for coordinating all aspects of the complex evaluation.

Attention should be given to support of the family unit and amelioration of the guilt that often develops in one or both parents. Paramount among the questions asked by the affected individual or parents are what is the defect, why did it happen, and will it happen again? In the best of circumstances, all these questions can be answered. In the worst, none can be answered completely. In any circumstance, an approach to management of the anomaly must be worked out with the family. The family may elect to have the support and advice of family members, friends, clergy, or others. When appropriate, members of the extended family may also be brought into the evaluation.

When a diagnosis cannot be made, the physician or family may wish to consult other geneticists and dysmorphologists. This may be accomplished by direct consultation in another center or by correspondence. If done by correspondence, the sharing of photographs of features is a tremendous asset to the consultant.

References

1. Kajii T, Ferrier A, Niikawa N, et al.: Anatomic and chromosomal anomalies in 639 spontaneous abortuses. Hum Genet 55:87, 1980.
2. Shepard TH, Fantel AG, Fitzimmons J: Congenital defect rates among spontaneous abortuses: twenty years of monitoring. Teratology 39:325, 1989.
3. Pitkin RM: Fetal death: diagnosis and management. Am J Obstet Gynecol 157:583, 1987.
4. Angell PM, Sandison A, Brain AD: Chromosome variation in perinatal mortality: a survey of 500 cases. J Med Genet 21:39, 1984.
5. Van Regemorter N, Dodion J, Druart C: Congenital malformations in 10,000 consecutive births in a university hospital: need for genetic counseling and prenatal diagnosis. J Pediatr 104:386, 1984.
6. Chung CS, Myrianthopoulos NC: Congenital anomalies: mortality and morbidity, burden and classification. Am J Med Genet 27:505, 1987.
7. Källén B: Population surveillance of multimalformed infants—experience with the Swedish registry of congenital malformations. J Genet Hum 35:205, 1987.
8. Graham JM: Clinical approach to human structural defects. Semin Perinatol 15(Suppl 1):2, 1991.
9. Moser HW, Wolf PA: The nosology of mental retardation: including the report of a survey of 1378 mentally retarded individuals at the Walter E. Fernald State School. BDOAS VII(1):117, 1971.
10. Association of Cytogenetic Technologists: International Cytogenetic Laboratory Directory. Assoc Cytogen Tech, 1990, p 2.
11. Blackburn W, Curtiss JR, Cooley NR Jr: The role of dysmorphogenesis in perinatal morbidity and mortality: a perinatal pathologist's view. Proc Greenwood Genet Center 9:89, 1990.
12. Mattos TC, Giugliani R, Haase HB: Congenital malformations detected in 731 autopsies of children aged 0 to 14 years. Teratology 35:305, 1987.
13. Leppig KA, Werber MM, Cann CI, et al.: Predictive value of minor anomalies. I. Association with major malformations. J Pediatr 110:531, 1987.
14. Méhes K, Stalder G: Minor Malformations in the Neonate. Akadémiae Kiadó, Budapest, 1983.
15. Marden PM, Smith DW, McDonald MJ: Congenital anomalies in the newborn infant, including minor variations. J Pediatr 64:357, 1964.
16. Smith DW: Classification, nomenclature, and naming of morphological defects. J Pediatr 87:162, 1975.
17. Gilbert-Barness E, Opitz JM, Barness LA: The pathologist's perspective of genetic disease: malformations and dysmorphology. Pediatr Clin North Am 36(1):163, 1989.
18. International Nomenclature of Constitutional Diseases of Bone. Revision, May 1983. Ann Radiol 26:457, 1983.
19. Spranger JW, Opitz JM, Smith DW, et al.: Errors of morphogenesis: concepts and terms. Recommendations of an international working group. J Pediatr 100:160, 1982.
20. Dunn PM: Congenital postural deformities. Br Med Bull 32:71, 1976.
21. Morris CA, Demsey SA, Leonard CO, et al.: Natural history of Williams syndrome, physical characteristics. J. Pediatr 113:318, 1988.
22. Allanson JE, Hall JG, Hughes HE, et al.: Noonan syndrome: the changing phenotype. Am J Med Genet 21:507, 1985.
23. Butler MG, Meaney FJ, Palmer CG: Clinical and cytogenetic survey of 39 individuals with Prader-Labhart-Willi syndrome. Am J Med Genet 23:793, 1986.
24. DeBusk FL: The Hutchinson-Gilford progeria syndrome: review of 4 cases and review of the literature. J Pediatr 80:697, 1972.
25. Stevenson RE, Prouty LA: Fragile X syndrome. VI. A subjective assessment of the facial features in blacks and whites. Proc Greenwood Genet Center 7:103, 1988.
26. Simpson JL: Disorders of Sexual Differentiation: Etiology and Clinical Delineation. Academic, New York, 1976, p 260.
27. Costa T, Scriver CR, Childs B: The effect of mendelian disease on human health: a measurement. Am J Med Genet 21:231, 1985.
28. Leroy JG, Demars RI, Opitz JM: I-cell disease. BDOAS V(4):174, 1969.
29. Singh I, Johnson GH, Brown FR III: Peroxisomal disorders: biochemical and clinical diagnostic considerations. Am J Dis Child 142:1297, 1988.
30. Mitchell G, Saudubray JM, Gubler MC et al.: Congenital anomalies in glutaric aciduria type 2. J Pediatr 104:961, 1984.
31. Applegarth DA, Dimmich JE, Toone JR: Laboratory detection of metabolic disease. Pediatr Clin North Am 36(1):49, 1989.
32. Tsipouras P, Ramirez F: Genetic disorders of collagen. J Med Genet 24:2, 1987.
33. Knowlton RG, Weaver EJ, Struyk AF, et al.: Genetic linkage analysis of hereditary arthro-ophthalmopathy (Stickler syndrome) and the type II procollagen gene. Am J Med Genet 45:681, 1989.
34. Lee B, Vissing H, Ramirez F, et al.: Identification of the molecular defect in a family with spondyloepiphyseal dysplasia. Science 244:978, 1989.
35. Pyeritz RE: Marfan syndrome. N Engl J Med 323:987, 1990.
36. Thomas GH, Howell RR: Selected Screening Tests for Genetic Metabolic Diseases. Year Book Medical Publishers, Chicago, 1973.
37. Sewell AC: Urinary oligosaccharides. In: Techniques in Diagnostic Human Biochemical Genetics. FA Hommes, ed. Wiley-Liss, New York, 1991, p 219.

38. Nelson K, Holmes LB: Malformations due to presumed spontaneous mutations in newborn infants. N Engl J Med 320:19, 1989.

39. Wilson JG: Environment and Birth Defects. Academic, New York, 1973.

40. Thompson GH, Bilenker RM: Comprehensive management of arthrogryposis multiplex congenita. Clin Orthop Rel Res 194:6, 1985.

41. Salyer KE, Munro IR, Whitaker LA, et al.: Difficulties and problems to be solved in the approach to craniofacial malformations. BDOAS XI(7):315, 1975.

42. Lee PA, Mazur T, Danish R, et al.: Micropenis. I. Criteria, etiologies and classification. Johns Hopkins Med J 146:156, 1980.

43. Centers for Disease Control: National Infant Mortality Surveillance (NIMS), 1980. MMWR 38(SS-3):43, 1989.

13

The Importance of Measurements

ROBERT A. SAUL

From ancient times quantitative assessments have been used in virtually every human endeavor—from the "cubits" of the ark builders to the "angstroms" of the electron microscopists, from the "hands" of the breeders of thoroughbred horses to the "stories" of the designers of modern-day skyscrapers, and from the "centiMorgans" of molecular biologists to the "Dow Jones averages" of the stockbrokers. Measurements assure observers that their eyes are not deceiving them. They assure those who depend on the observation that subjectivity or guesswork has been limited and that the observation can be confirmed by others.

Measurements are widely used in all branches of medicine. Virtually every patient evaluation includes measurements of topographic features. Pediatricians are perhaps most diligent in obtaining topographic measurements. During infancy and childhood, the years of rapid growth, these measurements are used in composite as a sign of overall health and for the purpose of gaining clues to constitutional, nutritional, and other environmental insults. They can also be used to monitor the progress of various treatments.

Clinical geneticists and dysmorphologists are likewise attentive to measuring topographic features to aid in the diagnosis of malformation syndromes and in defining the natural history of these conditions. Measurements allow objectivity in assessing individual features as part of the diagnostic process. Appearances can be deceiving, so specific criteria for features that can be reasonably measured have been established that permit consistency in determining whether a particular observation exceeds the limits of normal. The determination of short stature and microcephaly requires length (height) and head circumference measurements greater than 2 SD below the mean for a given age; ocular hypertelorism requires an interpupillary measurement greater than 2 SD above the mean; and macroorchidism requires a testicular volume (determined by comparison with volume beads or derived from length and width measurements) of greater than 2 SD above the mean. These criteria give more precision to the terms *short stature, small head, wide-spaced eyes,* and *large testes.*

Medical anthropometry is rarely used per se to make a diagnosis but is used rather to define a specific anatomic feature. Even the composite of multiple measurements in a patient with Down syndrome would be less diagnostic than a gestalt of Down syndrome gained through the eyes of an experienced examiner or the laboratory observation of the underlying chromosome aberration by a cytogeneticist. Initially, most patterns of malformation were delineated with little attention to measurement of specific features. After a sufficient number of individuals with a specific syndrome has been ascertained, measurements have sometimes confirmed the presence of the component features reported and sometimes documented that the feature is not a part of the syndrome or is found inconsistently.

Measurements of human anatomy assume greatest importance when considered in relationship to other measurements. Three types of comparisons are commonly used. One is a population reference, one a self-reference, and one a combination of the two. The population reference compares the measurement from one individual with measurements from a significant sample of others from the same population (those of the same race, sex, age, and so forth). The self-reference compares the measurements of one feature of an individual with other measurements from the same individual at the same time. This type of comparison detects disharmonic growth of various parts of the anatomy, an important characteristic of many syndromes and dysplasias. Features with disharmonic growth are often designated with the adjective *relative.* Thus an individual may have a normal-sized head but have "relative macrocephaly" in relation to height, a finding that can be helpful in distinguishing different conditions with short stature. The combination reference compares measurements from the same individual at different ages with growth curves prepared from measurements from individuals in the same population. This allows the individual's measurement to be assessed in relation to his or her own prior and future measurements and also in relationship to those of the population.

Standard growth references for a population can be longitudinal[1-4] (derived from multiple measurements from the same individuals at intervals over a period of years) or cross-sectional[5-11] (derived from single measurements from a large number of individuals covering the ages desired, usually collected at one time). Although longitudinal growth references may be most desirable, they require the tracking of a large cohort of subjects throughout the growth years. With few exceptions, the references available are cross-sectional.

Measurements made during the prenatal period have become increasingly important with the advent of ultrasonography. Prenatal ultrasound was initially used mainly to determine gestational age based on biparietal diameter. Present day ultrasound equipment can be used both to measure bony landmarks and to provide a view of soft tissues, nervous system, heart, kidneys, and other viscera. These advances in visualization of the fetus have allowed ultrasonographers to become "intrauterine dysmorphologists." Since most major malformations can be detected in utero with ultrasound, prenatal diagnosis has been expanded beyond those defects reflected in chromosome or biochemical abnormalities in the amniotic fluid and amniotic fluid cells. Ultrasound has also provided a large body of growth data regarding the normal embryo and fetus.[4]

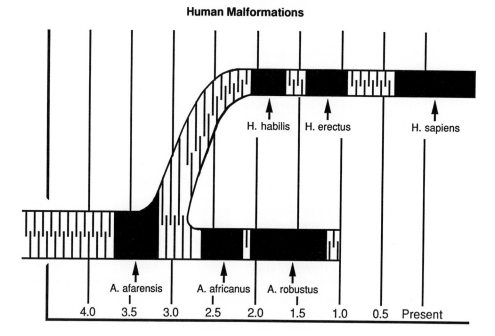

MILLIONS OF YEARS

Fig. 13–1. Time chart showing the evolution of humans during the past 4 million years.

Anthropometry

Anthropometry concerns primarily the measurements of the topography of human anatomy. It also includes various constructs that can be derived from these measurements (e.g., brain volume, surface area, and so forth can be calculated from topographic measurements) and a limited number of nontopographic measurements (e.g., weight, color, texture). Radiographic, sonographic, and magnetic resonance imaging techniques permit measurements of internal anatomy previously possible only during surgery or postmortem examination.

Images of our ancestors' appearance and how they functioned has been provided by anthropometric studies. These reconstructions derive primarily from the fragments of human skeleton and teeth that have been found in sedimentary deposits at various locations around the world. Contemporary anthropology examines the likenesses and differences found in humans now existing. Medicine uses anthropometry as a monitor of general well-being, as a diagnostic tool for human anomalies, and, to a limited extent, as a predictor of human behavior.

Early humans

Measurements of fossil remains have been used to delineate the appearance of early humans and their evolutionary descendants. The divergence of pongids (great apes) and hominids occurred over 4 million years ago.[12] The hominid line has since undergone significant morphologic changes in the spine, skull, pelvis, long bones, and feet, which accompanied the achievement of bipedal locomotion. Based on the configuration of the skeleton and teeth, anthropologists can determine the appearance of these primitive beings and can suggest the composition of their diet, their social behavior, and their intelligence.[12–17]

The work of anthropologists like Louis Leakey and Donald Johanson has provided a clearer picture of early human

ancestors.[12,16] *Australopithecus afarensis,* exemplified by Lucy, a 3.5-million-year-old skeleton discovered by Johanson, probably represents the oldest hominid ancestor found to date. Johanson and Edey[12] suggest that the *Homo* genus diverged from the hominids subsequent to *A. afarensis* (Fig. 13–1). Artistic reconstruction of the craniofacies of *A. afarensis* revealed a small, flattened cranium, forward-jutting lower face, flat nose, prominent supraorbital ridges and eyes, and a relatively sparse covering of facial hair (Fig. 13–2). The latter feature in the dark-skinned equatorial inhabitants is presumed to be secondary to a predominance of sweat glands in the face to assist in dissipating heat. The shape and size of the alveolar arch and teeth figure prominently in distinguishing early humans from apes (Table 13–1).

With the passing millennia, hominids acquired a more fully erect posture and grew substantially in size (Table 13–

Fig. 13–2. Representation of skulls from *A. afarensis* to *H. sapiens* showing the marked modification of the cranium and face that has occurred during evolution. The skull of *A. afarensis* is redrawn from Johanson and Edey.[12] Compare with the time chart in Fig. 13–1.

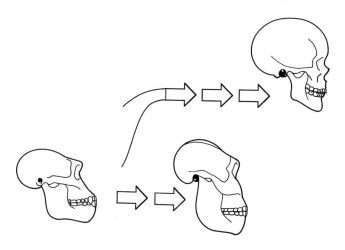

Table 13–1. Dental differences between apes and humans

	Apes (Pongidae)	Humans (Hominidae)
Maxillary arch	Canine and postcanine teeth form parallel rows; space between canine and incisors (diastema)	Dental arch curved contour No diastema
Canines	Large, conical, sharply pointed; pronounced sexual dimorphism; selective wear on sides and projection beyond postcanine teeth	Small, spatulate, blunt; no sexual dimorphism; wear flat from tip and no projection
Premolars	Unicuspid first premolars	Bicuspid first premolars
Molars	Wear uneven; second molars erupt after canines	Wear to flat surface; second molars erupt before canines

2). *Homo sapiens* emerged perhaps 3 million years ago and is distinguished as a unique species on the basis of fully erect posture, bipedal locomotion, longer growth period and slower rate of development, absence of premaxillary bone, well-marked chin, slight prognathism, prominent bony nose, outward rolled mucosal membrane forming the lip, lumbar spine curvature with a forward convexity, brain more than twice as large as the largest pongids, iliac fossae of the pelvis facing one another, short sacroiliac–acetabulum measurement, longer limbs and arms, nonopposable great toe set in line with other toes, transverse and longitudinal foot arches, scant body hair, and absence of tactile hairs.

Three major morphologic changes dominate the differences between apes and humans and between early hominids and late hominids. The *human foot* has evolved from a grasping structure to a support and balance structure. The hallux elongated in relation to the lateral toes and became parallel with them. The heel has extended posteriorly, and the flexible arch has developed to dampen the impact of walking. The trunk, neck, and head have achieved a vertical orientation, balanced on the lower limbs at the acetabulum. The *upright position* of the human body, which frees the upper limbs from pedal and clinging functions, has perhaps been the key to human ascent to dominance among the creatures. Standing upright permitted the hands to be used in combat, for portage, and for the shaping of tools and weapons. The *increased brain size* in relation to body mass and the decreased dependence on the mouth for protection and for object transport resulted in a considerable restructuring of the craniofacies, including the teeth. These morphologic changes accompanied, or perhaps permitted, functional advances, including effortless bipedal ambulation, speech, socialization, and the construction and use of tools and weapons.

The migration of humans throughout the world reflects an ability to adapt to geographic and climatic extremes. These adaptations require alterations in morphology such as changes in habitus, amount of hair, and skin color and thickness. Several "rules" relating to climatic adaptation have emerged. Body weight decreases, skin color darkens, and hair diminishes with the increasing environmental temperature. Body size usually increases and limb size decreases as the temperature of the habitat decreases. These changes may be accompanied by a lighter skin as well. More than mere curiosities, these adaptations explain some of the variabilities seen in the contemporary human races.

Modern humans

Modern humans date to about 50,000 years ago. If Johanson is correct, the *Homo* genus diverged from the australopithecenes about 3 million years ago. Thereafter the human line progressed through *Homo habilis* and *Homo erectus* before arriving at *H. sapiens* 200,000 years ago (Fig. 13–1). It is now thought that the Neanderthals were early *H. sapiens* who became extinct prior to the arrival of modern humans.

In comparison to their ancestors, modern humans have less robust skeletons and less muscle bulk. The brain is larger in absolute volume and in comparison to body size. The cranium forms a more conspicuous dome above the facies because of this. The facial profile has become flattened vertically, with less prominent jaws and teeth.

It should be considered that evolutionary changes are ongoing in humans but that, in the narrow window of time for which we have detailed information regarding humans, such changes will not likely be perceived. The dominant change in humans since the first written records were made (3000 BC to the present, about 250 generations) has been a change of scale. Humans have increased in stature, a phenomenon likely related to consistent and improved nutrition.

It is usual to categorize modern humans on a racial basis, i.e., on the basis of distinctive physical characteristics.[18] The predominant characteristics used are skin color, hair color and form, facial features, and habitus. Three major races, Caucasian, Negro, and Mongol, are acknowledged. A pure

Table 13–2. Body size[a] from *A. afarensis* to *H. sapiens*

	Time	Height (inches)	Weight (pounds)	Brain volume (cc)
A. afarensis	3.5 M BC	40–50	50–70	400–550[b]
H. habilis	2 M BC	48–60	60–100	500–800
H. erectus	1.5–2 M BC	60–66	80–140	700–1250
H. sapiens				
Neanderthal	200,000–50,000 BC	60–66	90–180	1000–1800
Modern	50,000 BC to present	60–74	100–220	1000–1800

[a]Measurements are estimated from the data of Brace and Montagu[13] and Johanson and Edey.[12]

[b]For comparison chimpanzee brains average 350 cc and gorilla brains average 550 cc.

Table 13–3. Racial differences in the incidence of congenital anomalies

Defect	Incidence in whites[a]	Incidence in blacks[a]
Anencephaly	9.5	2.5
Spina bifida	9.9	3.9
Tracheoesophageal fistula	1.1	0.0
Cleft lip ± cleft palate	8.7	3.1
Hypospadius	20.1	8.4
Clubfoot	29.2	16.2
Polydactyly	8.0	100.3

[a]Rates per 10,000 live births. From Erickson.[20]

racial phenotype is difficult, however, because of migration and admixing of the races.

It is evident that the incidences of many malformations differ according to race (Table 13–3).[19–21] Blacks, for example, have lower incidences of neural tube defects and cleft lip/cleft palate than do whites. Whether blacks have lower frequencies of gene mutations that contribute to these defects, whether they are exposed less frequently to causative environmental insults, or whether their phenotypes provide some specific or nonspecific resistance to these malformations is not known. Fraser[21] has suggested that the fullness of the perioral tissues offers protection against midfacial clefting.

Somatotyping

A number of attempts have been made to classify overall human physique because of evidence that different physiques can be associated with different temperaments and with predispositions to different diseases. The system that has gained the greatest attention is called somatotyping. This system, described by Sheldon and associates in the 1940s, recognizes three types of overall morphology.[22] Ectomorphy is characterized by general asthenia of the trunk and limbs with very little muscle and other soft tissue. The brain and skin surface area are relatively large compared with total mass. Mesomorphy is characterized by broad shoulders, heavily muscled chest and limbs, and little fat. Endomorphy is characterized by considerable fat involving the face, trunk, limbs,

and internal organs. Sheldon and colleagues[22] and others[23–25] have found that physique correlates strongly with personality, aggressiveness, success in various types of endeavor, and with predisposition to some medical ailments and social behaviors. Somatyping has also been employed to study Olympic athletes. Carter[24] used specific quantitative traits to arrive at a numerical ratio of the proportion of endomorphy, mesomorphy, and ectomorphy in a given athlete. As might be anticipated, those in certain sports tend to share physical attributes suited to that sport.

Throughout written history, there have been attempts to link the morphology of humans with their worth and position in society.[26–29] In Greek and Roman cultures, the human anatomy was celebrated in monumental works of art. In some cultures individuals with morphologic aberrations were given the status of gods.[26] In other cultures, infants born with similar aberrations were exposed or actively killed. In still other cultures, such individuals were exhibited as scientific and social curiosities.[27]

The first half of this century was marked by widespread attempts to correlate social qualities and behavior with human anatomy. In the United States, this racial/ethnic stereotyping was reflected in the limitation of certain races to immigrate (Immigration Act of 1924) and in the encouragement of peoples of Nordic ancestry to increase their reproduction relative to those of non-Nordic ancestry.[28] Similar views linking anatomic features and social worth were held in Europe and were expressed most dramatically in the Lebensborn program of the Third Reich.[29]

Dysmorphology

The study of abnormal morphology is in large part the study of disharmonic growth.[30–32] Individual morphologic features become distinctive because of their size in relation to other features around them. Downslanting palpebral fissures result from undergrowth of the malar region (zygoma) in relation to the frontal region (frontal bone). Micrognathia results from undergrowth of the mandible in relation to the maxilla. Macroglossia is overgrowth of the tongue in comparison to the oral cavity. This is not to say that absolute undergrowth or overgrowth does not occur in these circumstances, but only that the disharmony of growth is the phenomenon that provokes identification of features as dysmorphic. A large

Fig. 13–3. Normal distribution of features that vary among individuals. Sixty-eight percent of the population is between −1 and +1 SD; 95% is between −2 and +2 SD; 2.5% is below −2 SD; and 2.5% is above +2 SD.

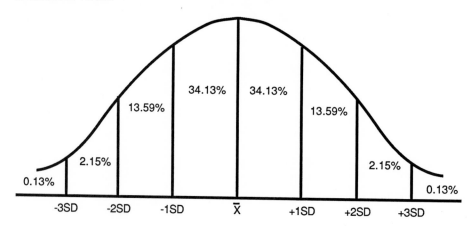

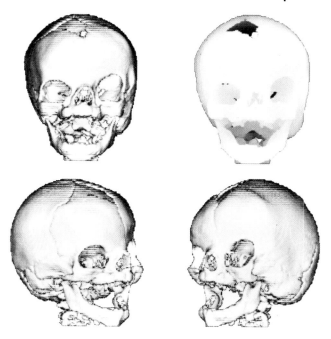

Fig. 13–4. Computed three-dimensional reconstruction of cranial tomography demonstrating skull with left coronal synostosis. Courtesy of Dr. Michael W. Vannier (Washington University Medical Center, St. Louis, MO).

tongue accommodated in a large mouth in a large craniofacies will not likely be singled out as a dysmorphic feature.

Dysmorphology employs both gestalt and measurements in assessing patients with anomalous development. Major anomalies pose little difficulty and in general do not require measurement. More subtle alterations of morphology may be discerned by the eye, but confirmation by measurement is reassuring to all concerned.

Standards and methods of measurement

The establishment of normal values for traits that vary continuously is based on the measurement of the trait in a large number of individuals. Unbiased estimates may be obtained by randomly sampling the population in question. In many cases, if sufficient data are accumulated, continuous variables are distributed in a manner that approximates a normal distribution curve. The distribution can be further described by two parameters, the mean and the standard deviation.[33] (The standard deviation is an estimate of the degree to which the trait varies from one individual to the next.)

Data that describe normal distributions have been well characterized mathematically and are available in tabulated form. This allows one to make initial generalizations about the distributions of the traits. For example, for a trait exhibiting a normal distribution, two-thirds or 68% of the observations will fall within ± 1 SD of the mean, and 95% will fall within ± 2 SD (Fig. 13–3).

Fig. 13–5. Three-dimensional reconstruction of computed tomography imaging of cranium of infant with osteogenesis imperfecta. Anteroposterior view (left) and vertex view (right) show marked deficiency of cranial ossification.

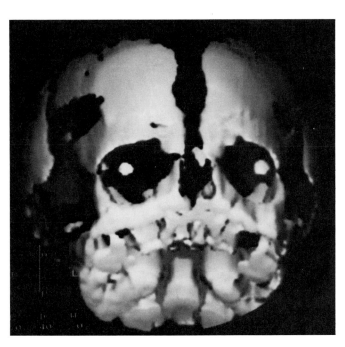

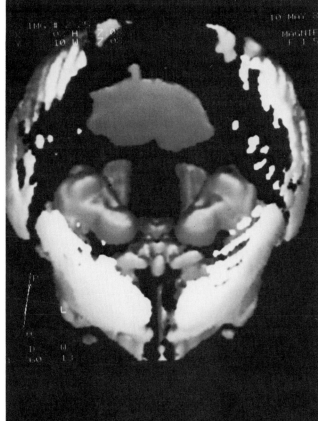

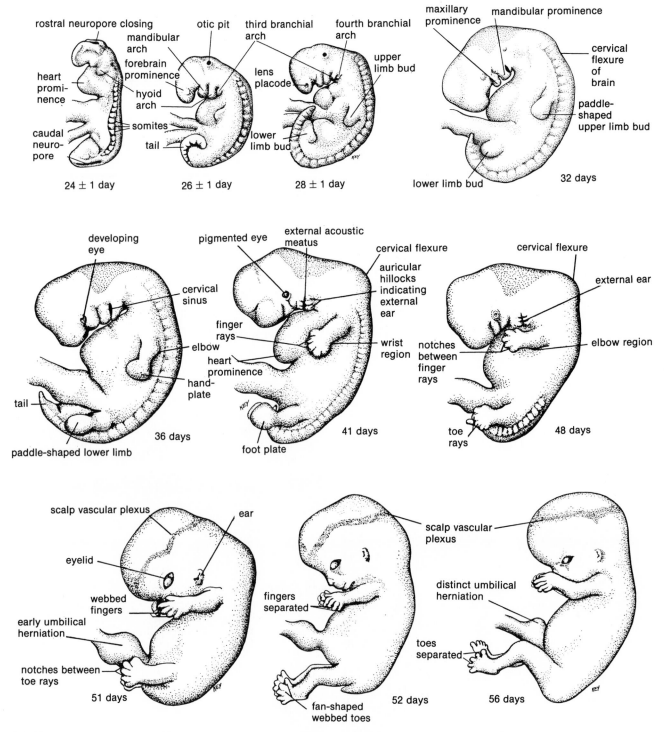

Fig. 13–6. Lateral appearance of embryos from days 24 to 56 (left) and frontal appearance of developing craniofacies from days 28 to 56 (right). Age expressed as day from ovulation, approximately day of conception. Data from Moore[48] and Patten.[49]

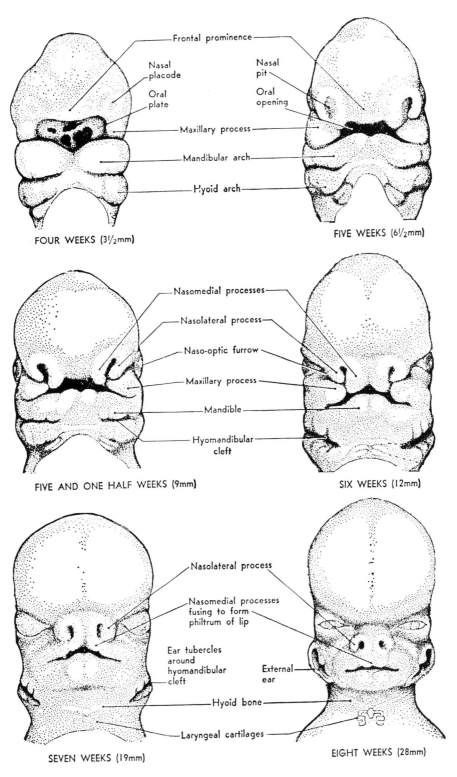

Frontal prominence

Nasal placode

Oral plate

Maxillary process

Mandibular arch

Hyoid arch

FOUR WEEKS (3½mm)

Nasal pit

Oral opening

FIVE WEEKS (6½mm)

Nasomedial processes

Nasolateral process

Naso-optic furrow

Maxillary process

Mandible

Hyomandibular cleft

FIVE AND ONE HALF WEEKS (9mm)

SIX WEEKS (12mm)

Nasolateral process

Nasomedial processes fusing to form philtrum of lip

Ear tubercles around hyomandibular cleft

Hyoid bone

Laryngeal cartilages

SEVEN WEEKS (19mm)

External ear

EIGHT WEEKS (28mm)

Fig. 13–6. Continued

225

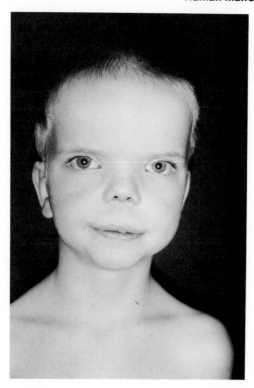 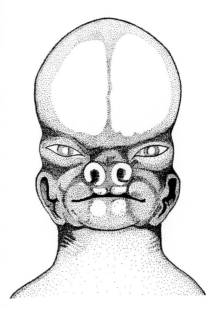

Fig. 13–7. Appearance of child with Robinow (fetal face) syndrome compared with a drawing of a fetal face at age 8 weeks. Photograph courtesy of Dr. Meinhard Robinow, Dayton, OH. Drawing after Patten.[49]

In many cases, abnormal physical measurements are arbitrarily considered to be those values that lie in the upper and lower 2.5% of the distribution or that are greater than 2 SD from the mean. Microcephaly is defined as a head circumference less than 2 SD below the mean, macrocephaly as greater than 2 SD above the mean. Functional deficits can be defined in these terms as well. Scores of less than 2 SD on standardized intelligence tests arbitrarily define mental retardation within our population.

A formidable body of human anatomic measurements (taken during the prenatal period and during infancy, childhood, and, to a lesser extent, adult life) has been accumulated.[4,10,11,34–36] It might be assumed that the growth standards were derived from data collected with rigidly controlled protocols, which entails placing the subject in a natural and relaxed position, having measurements taken by an experienced observer, and using the most precise instruments, (e.g. Calipers are used for taking measurements less than 30 cm, and rigid measuring devices [measuring table or stadiometer] are used for measuring length or height.) Certainly many of the standards were prepared in this optimal fashion. However, that is not always the case. It is advisable for the users of growth standards to become familiar with the population from which the data were collected, with the method of data collection, and with the number and experience of individuals collecting the data.

Growth references for certain uncommon populations may derive from pooled data. This applies particularly to growth references for skeletal dysplasias and syndromes.[9,10,37] The data may come from many sources, collected over a period of many years, and are usually collected by a number of

different observers in a number of different settings. Unfortunately, heterogeneity of the subject population may not be rigidly excluded. While such standards are not optimal, they may be the only reference available for certain populations.

Many genetic texts contain standards for growth during the childhood years but lack information on mature measurements. This deficiency is removed in part by the data in the Natick Anthropometric Survey.[36] In the latest (1988) survey, 132 different measurements were taken on 2208 females aged 18–50 yr and on 1774 males aged 17–51 yr. Seventy-eight percent of all subjects were aged 20–35 yr. The sample was composed of persons in the U.S. Army. Among the men, 66.1% were white, 25.8% black, and 3.8% Hispanic. Among the women, 51.6% were white, 41.8% black, and 2.6% Hispanic.

Obtaining accurate measurements is not easy. Features with clearly defined boundaries can be measured relatively precisely. Human topography is characterized by curvilinear structures and hence provides a greater challenge. Curvature of body surfaces, tone difference, and subject cooperation also influence the accuracy of measurements. Often the setting in which the person is evaluated does not permit the use of the most accurate instruments and may be compounded by insufficient lighting, lack of cooperation, and insufficient time to achieve the accuracy desired.

These difficulties aside, the clinician is called upon in a variety of settings to obtain measurements for use in diagnosis. Usually straight rulers and flexible tapes are the only measuring devices available. With knowledge of the proper anatomic landmarks and care in taking measurements, the clinician can make reliable observations under less than ideal

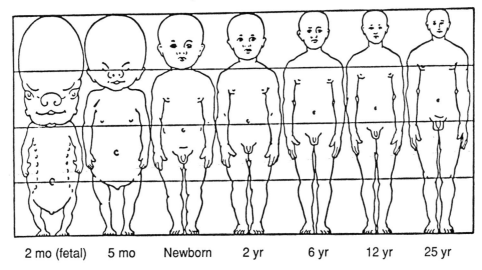

| 2 mo (fetal) | 5 mo | Newborn | 2 yr | 6 yr | 12 yr | 25 yr |

Fig. 13–8. Relative proportions of head, trunk, and extremities during different stages of growth. From Robbins et al.[51]

circumstances. That there is some limitation of comparison of these values with those carefully collected in the research setting must, however, be acknowledged.

Photogrammetry has been used as an alternative to direct measurement. Standardized photographs are taken to depict features of interest. A scale is included to permit various fea-

Fig. 13–9. Fetal weight, crown–rump (CR) length, and crown–heel (CH) length for days 56–168 postovulation. From Saul et al.[10]

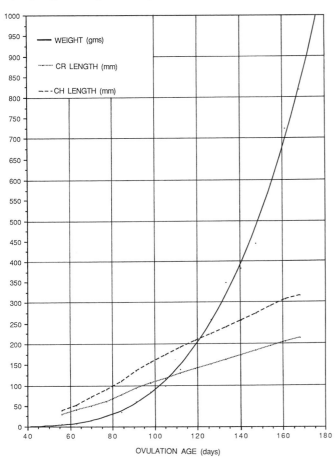

tures to be measured on the photograph. With the features converted into a two-dimensional image, measurements are easily made by hand or by computer. This method requires a standardized photographic assembly, is costly, and does not provide measurements immediately for the clinician.

Radiocephalometry provides another method for assessment of craniofacial anomalies.[38–40] Based on standardized positions and radiographic techniques, various landmarks of the craniofacial skeleton are identified and measurements taken. Radiocephalometry has utility in defining the anatomy in craniofacial syndromes and in planning reconstructive surgery. It requires standardized equipment, is tedious, and is not readily adaptable to most clinical settings.

Radiographs are also necessary for the measurement of most components of the skeleton. They permit individual bones to be measured for comparison to population data and permit one skeletal feature to be compared with others in the same individual. The latter use detects disharmonic growth. It has been most successfully employed in comparisons of the tubular bones of the hand, a procedure termed *metacarpophalangeal profile analysis*.[41] Most syndromes with abnormalities of the hands will have a more or less distinctive profile.

Computed tomography and magnetic resonance imaging can be used for two-dimensional viewing and for three-dimensional reconstruction of most anatomic parts (Fig. 13–4, 13–5).[42–46] The imaging systems give the clinician a view of many features that are normally hidden. Three-dimensional reconstructions are helpful in planning surgery and in projecting the results anticipated from surgery.

Embryonic and fetal growth

Measurements become important very early in pregnancy. The general well-being of the embryo and the fetus is often judged on size alone. Most insults to the rapidly growing prenatal organism will impair growth.

The embryonic period (especially weeks 2–8) has been divided into stages on the basis of size (greatest length or crown–rump length) and progress of morphologic develop-

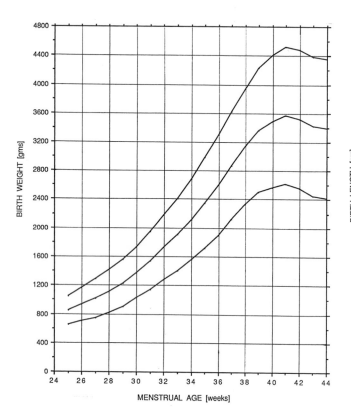

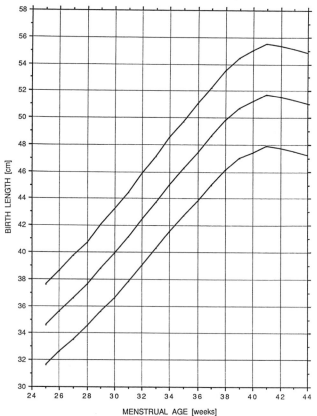

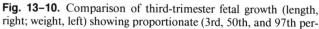

Fig. 13–10. Comparison of third-trimester fetal growth (length, right; weight, left) showing proportionate (3rd, 50th, and 97th per-centile) changes over time. From Saul et al[10] based on data from Usher and McLean.[54]

ment.[47] These stages, arbitrarily assigned, provide an orderly reference against which the growth and morphology of individual embryos can be compared.

The changes in proportion and scale of different body segments are among the most remarkable of prenatal events. Growth in the prenatal period is truly phenomenal, from a single celled organism weighing approximately 0.0000006 g at conception to a differentiated human being with billions of cells and weighing close to 3500 g at birth. Crown–rump length progresses from 0.4 mm at stage 7 (about 16 days postovulation) to 30 mm at stage 23 (end of embryonic period, about 56 days) to 51 cm at birth (about 280 days). Morphologic changes are equally impressive, particularly during the first 8 weeks. The lateral and frontal appearances of the morphologic changes in the face from days 24 to 56 are shown in Figure 13–6.

An understanding of the physical relationships between developing tissues and the proportions between these tissues can aid in the description of malformations and their etiology. For example, the Robinow syndrome is a condition with abnormal craniofacies, shortened extremities, and hypoplastic genitalia.[50] The facies resemble those present at the end of the embryonic or the beginning of the fetal period—hence the term fetal face syndrome, which has also been used (Fig. 13–7). The proportions present in this condition (macrocephaly, hypertelorism, and shortened extremities) suggest an arrest in morphologic development in the late embryonic stage with continued growth although disproportionate, from that stage onward. The cranium, face, and upper extremities maintain the relative proportion seen at 8 weeks

postconception instead of the normal relationships present at birth. To suggest an "arrest" of development is purely speculative but helps in the conceptualization of the abnormality. The illustration of Robbins et al.[51] beautifully depicts the relative proportions of head, trunk, and extremities at various ages (Fig. 13–8).

During the previable fetal period (8–24 weeks postovulation), a dramatic weight gain occurs in comparison to the length gain (weight increases approximately 164 times, and crown–rump length increases approximately 7 times; Fig. 13–9).[10,47] Once viability is possible (vaguely accepted as 24 weeks postovulation or 26 weeks gestation as calculated by the first day of the last menstrual period), linear growth and weight are roughly parallel (Fig. 13–10), with proportionate growth continuing until birth. Scammon and Calkins[35] have published measurements of numerous external features of more than 400 fetuses. These measurements can be used to assess anomalous growth in relation to gestational age or crown–heel length. Measurements of skeletal structures and of certain soft tissues and viscera have been made in utero during ultrasound examination.[4] Standard curves have been constructed from the measurements and provide a basis for prenatally identifying overall growth impairments or specific anomalies (Fig. 13–11).

Growth in infancy and childhood

Growth is a complex phenomenon, largely determined by the genetic constitution but also easily influenced by many

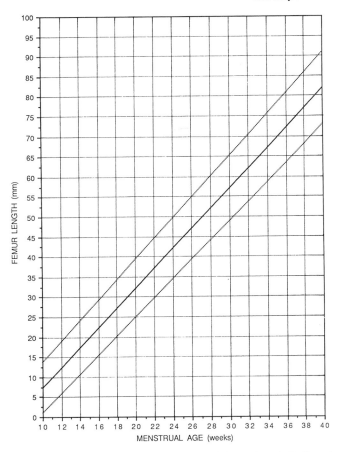

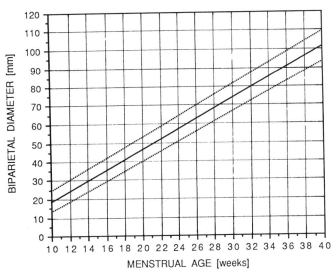

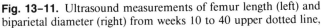

Fig. 13–11. Ultrasound measurements of femur length (left) and biparietal diameter (right) from weeks 10 to 40 upper dotted line, 97th percentile; solid line, 50th percentile; lower dotted line, 3rd percentile. From Saul et al[10] based on data of Elejalde and Elejalde.[4]

environmental insults.[52] Growth is mediated through hormonal stimulation of various tissues, particularly the chondrosseous skeleton. Nonspecific impairments of growth can be caused by a wide range of environmental influences, including nutrition, oxygen supply, infection, systemic disease, numerous drugs and chemicals, and emotional deprivation. Unlike prenatal environmental insults to growth, postnatal insults generally affect growth overall rather than that of isolated features. An exception to this generalization is the coarsening of lower facial features and gum hypertrophy caused by prolonged postnatal exposure to the hydantoins.[53]

Growth during infancy and childhood is expected to proceed at an orderly and predictable pace. Standards for growth of most anatomic features are available.[1–11,34,54,55] Feingold and Bossert[6] studied over 2400 individuals, newborn to age 14 yrs, and constructed growth curves for many different anatomic features. These and other growth references have been published in two recent books.[10,11] Most growth curves are prepared from measurements of a cross section of the population and with few exceptions are referenced against age.

Growth in individuals with skeletal dysplasias and malformation syndromes

Growth in many malformation syndromes, skeletal dysplasias, and metabolic disorders proceeds at a rate different from that of the general population. For most of these disorders,

insufficient cross-sectional or longitudinal data have been collected to permit the construction of growth curves.[9,10,37] For those conditions for which curves are available, growth can be monitored and the success of various treatments analyzed.

Growth curves for children with achondroplasia, the most common form of short-limb dwarfism, have been available since 1978 and are immensely useful in evaluating such patients. Horton et al.[9] collected growth data on over 400 patients with achondroplasia and constructed growth curves for stature, growth velocity, upper/lower segment ratios, and head circumference. The curves for stature and head circumference in Figure 13–12 demonstrate the marked discrepancy between the expected growth in achondroplasia and the normal growth in the general population. Following the growth of achondroplastic children using normal growth curves is of limited benefit, but comparisons with the growth curves of other children with achondroplasia can be very instructive. Individuals with achondroplasia usually have significant macrocephaly. Comparing their head growths to those of other individuals with achondroplasia can often reassure the family and thus avoid unnecessary diagnostic tests. Furthermore, if any growth-promoting intervention is used, the change in growth should be compared with that expected in achondroplasia without the intervention.

Meany and Farrer[37] have cataloged the information available on growth in a number of different genetic and congenital disorders. Their exhaustive tabulation reveals that all too often insufficient data are available to prepare clinically use-

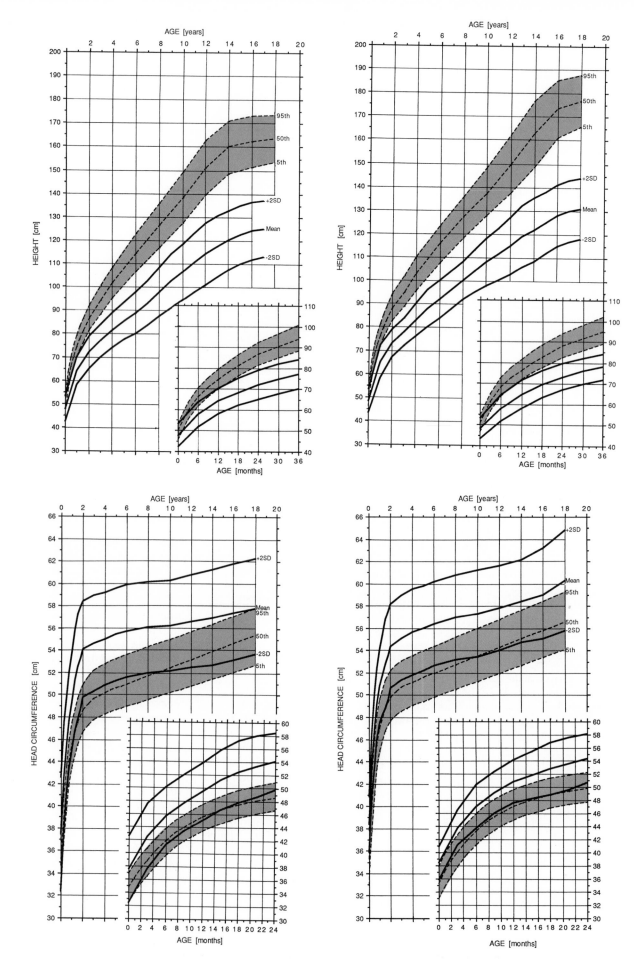

230

Table 13-4. Conditions for which growth curves are available[a]

Achondroplasia

Amyoplasia

Diastrophic dysplasia

Distal arthrogryposis

Down syndrome

Marfan syndrome

Multiple pterygium syndrome

Noonan syndrome

Pseudoachondroplasia

Sickle cell disease

Spondyloepiphyseal dysplasia

Williams syndrome

[a]From Saul et al.[10]

ful growth curves such as those available for achondroplasia. Table 13-4 lists those conditions for which growth information has been compiled and charts have been adapted for clinical use. The most useful curves are available in the collected works of Saul et al.[10] and Hall et al.[11] In many cases the available growth data must be considered preliminary because the studies did not include as many observations as broad collaborative studies have provided. Such broad studies are needed to understand the natural history of pathologic states and to provide the necessary information for counseling patients with abnormal growth and their families.

References

1. Tanner JM, Davies PSW: Clinical longitudinal standards for height and height velocity for North American children. J Pediatr 107:317, 1985.
2. Roche AF, Mukherjee D, Guo S, et al.: Head circumference reference data: birth to 18 years. Pediatrics 79:706, 1987.
3. Tanner JM, Whitehouse RH, Takaishi M: Standards from birth to maturity for height, weight, height velocity, and weight velocity: British children, 1965. Arch Dis Child 41:454, 613, 1966.
4. Elejalde BR, de Elejalde MM: The prenatal growth of the human body determined by the measurement of bones and organs by ultrasonography. Am J Med Genet 24:575, 1986.
5. Nellhaus G: Head circumference from birth to eighteen years: practical composite international and interracial graph. Pediatrics 41:106, 1968.
6. Feingold M, Bossert WH: Normal values for selected physical parameters: an aid to syndrome delineation. BDOAS X(13):135, 141, 153, 1974.
7. Hamill PVV, Drizd TA, Johnson CL, et al.: Physical growth: National Center for Health Statistics Percentiles. Am J Clin Nutr 32:607, 1979.
8. Merlob P, Sivan Y, Reisner SH: Anthropometric measurements of the newborn infant (27 to 41 gestational weeks). BDOAS XX(7):1, 1984.
9. Horton WA, Rotter JI, Rimoin DL, et al.: Standard growth curves for achondroplasia. J Pediatr 93:435, 1978.
10. Saul RA, Stevenson RE, Rogers RC, et al.: Growth References From Conception to Adulthood. Proc Greenwood Genet Center, Suppl 1, 1988.
11. Hall JG, Froster-Iskenius UG, Allanson JE: Handbook of Normal Physical Measurements. Oxford University Press, Oxford, 1989.
12. Johanson DC, Edey MA: Lucy: The Beginnings of Humankind. Simon and Schuster, New York, 1981.
13. Brace CL, Montagu MFA: Man's Evolution: An Introduction to Physical Anthropology. Macmillan, New York, 1965.
14. Birdsell JB: Human Evolution: An Introduction to the New Physical Anthropology, ed 2. Rand McNally, Chicago, 1975.
15. Hulse FS: The Human Species: An Introduction to Physical Anthropology, ed 2. Random House, New York, 1971.
16. Leakey LSB, Tobias PV, Napier JR: A new species of the genus *Homo* from Olduvai Gorge. Nature 202:7, 1964.
17. Coon CS: The Story of Man, Knopf, New York, 1962.
18. Coon CS, Garn SM, Birdsell JB: Races: A Study of the Problems of Race Formation in Man. Greenwood, Westport, CT, 1950.
19. Chung CS, Myrianthopoulos NC: Factors affecting risks of congenital malformations. BDOAS XI(10):1, 1975.
20. Erickson JD: Racial variations in the incidence of congenital malformations. Ann Hum Genet 39:315, 1976.
21. Fraser FC: The genetics of cleft lip and cleft palate. Am J Hum Genet 22:336, 1970.
22. Sheldon W, Stevens SS, Tucker WB: The Varieties of Human Physique. Hafner, Darien, CT, 1970.
23. de Garay AL, Levine L, Carter JEL: Genetic and Anthropological Studies of Olympic Athletes. Academic, New York, 1972.
24. Carter JEL: Physical Structure of Olympic Athletes. Part I. The Montreal Olympic Games Anthropological Project. S Karger, New York, 1982.
25. Glueck S, Glueck E: Physique and Delinquency. Harper Brothers, New York, 1956.
26. Ballantyne JW: Manual of Antenatal Pathology and Hygiene: The Embryo. Reprint. Jacob's Press, Clinton, SC, 1991.
27. Fiedler L: Freaks, Myths and Images of the Secret Self. Simon and Schuster, New York, 1978.
28. Haller MH: Eugenics: Hereditary Attitudes in American thought. Rutgers University Press, New Brunswick, NJ, 1963.
29. Thompson LV: Lebensborn and the eugenics policy of the Reichsführer-ss. Central Eur Hist 4:54, 1971.
30. Garn SM, Smith BH, LaVelle M: Applications of pattern profile analysis to malformations of the head and face. Radiology 150:683, 1984.
31. Stengel-Rutkowski S, Schimanek P, Wernheimer A: Anthropometric definitions of dysmorphic facial signs. Hum Genet 67:272, 1984.
32. Jones KL: Smith's Recognizable Patterns of Human Malformation, ed 4. WB Saunders, Philadelphia, 1988.
33. Snedecor GW, Cochran WG: Statistical Methods, ed 6. Iowa State University Press, Ames, 1967.
34. Brandt JM, Allen GA, Haynes JL, et al.: Normative standards and comparison of arthropometric data of white and black newborn infants. Dysmorph Clin Genet 4:121, 1990.
35. Scammon RE, Calkins LA: The Development and Growth of the External Dimensions of the Human Body in the Fetal Period. University of Minnesota Press, Minneapolis, 1929.
36. Gordon CC, Churchill T, Clauser CE: 1988 Anthropometric Survey of U.S. Army Personnel: Summary Statistics Interim Report. U.S. Army Natick Research, Development and Engineering Center, Natick, MA, 1989.
37. Meaney FJ, Farrer LA: Clinical anthropometry and medical genetics: a compilation of body measurements in genetic and congenital disorders. Am J Med Genet 25:343, 1986.
38. Broadbent BH: A new x-ray technique and its application to orthodontia. Angle Orthod 1:45, 1931.
39. Knott VB: Change in cranial base measures of human males and females from age 6 years to early adulthood. Growth 35:145, 1971.
40. Frias JL, King GJ, Williams CA: Cephalometric assessment of selected malformation syndromes. BDOAS XVIII(1):139, 1982.
41. Poznanski AK: The Hand in Radiological Diagnosis. WB Saunders, Philadelphia, 1984, p 31.

Fig. 13-12. Composite of growth curves for individuals with achondroplasia: stature (top) and head circumference (bottom). Females, left; males, right. Shaded areas represent normal growth; mean ± 2 SD are shown for achondroplasia. From Saul et al[10] based on data of Horton et al.[9]

42. Vannier MW, Marsh JL, Warren JO: Three-dimensional CT reconstruction images for craniofacial surgical planning and evaluation. Radiology 150:179, 1984.

43. Vannier MW, Gutierrez FR, Laschinger JC, et al.: Three-dimensional magnetic resonance imaging of congenital heart disease. RadioGraphics 8:857, 1988.

44. Geist D, Vannier MW: PC-based 3-D reconstruction of medical images. Comput Graphics 13:135, 1989.

45. Vannier MW, Knapp RH, Offutt CJ, et al.: Computers in radiology. Curr Imaging 1:128, 1989.

46. Vannier MW, Marsh JL: Three-dimensional reconstruction. In: Otolaryngology—Head and Neck Surgery: Update I. CW Cummings, et al., eds. CV Mosby, St. Louis, 1989, p 28.

47. O'Rahilly R, Müller F: Developmental Stages in Human Embryos. Carnegie Institution of Washington, Washington, DC, 1987, Publication 637.

48. Moore KL: Before We Are Born: Basic Embryology and Birth Defects, ed 3. WB Saunders, Philadelphia, 1988.

49. Patten BM: Human Embryology, ed 3. McGraw-Hill, New York, 1968.

50. Robinow M, Silverman FN, Smith HD: A newly recognized dwarfing syndrome. Am J Dis Child 117:645, 1969.

51. Robbins WJ, Brody S, et al.: Growth. Yale University Press, New Haven, 1928.

52. Lowrey GH: Growth and Development of Children, ed 6. Year Book Medical, Chicago, 1973, p 51.

53. Johnson JP: Acquired dysmorphic craniofacial features associated with chronic phenytoin therapy. Proc Greenwood Genet Center 3:114, 1984.

54. Usher R, McLean F: Intrauterine growth of live-born Caucasian infants at sea level: standards obtained from measurements in 7 dimensions of infants born between 25 and 44 weeks of gestation. J Pediatr 74:901, 1969.

55. Lubchenco LO, Hansman C, Boyd E: Intrauterine growth in length and head circumference as estimated from live births at gestational ages from 26 to 44 weeks. Pediatrics 37:403, 1966.

14

Molecular Approach to Understanding Human Malformations

GOLDER N. WILSON

> We cannot doubt that the most urgent need of modern embryology is a series of advances of a purely theoretical, even mathematico-logical nature. Only by something of this kind can we redress the balance which has fallen over to observation and experiment; only by some such effort can we obtain a theoretical embryology suited in magnitude and spaciousness to the wealth of facts which contemporary investigators are accumulating day by day.
>
> J. Needham, *A History of Embryology*[1]

Prospects for a molecular dysmorphology

A molecular biology of malformations would be greatly aided if the clinical science of dysmorphology could draw upon basic embryology for a clear set of rules. One could then group malformations much as the cardiologist categorizes heart failure: physiologic rules of pressure and flow differentiate high- versus low-output forms and provide a conceptual approach to therapy. Unfortunately, a theoretical embryology, particularly as it might explain human malformation, remains as distant today as it did in 1959. Dysmorphology has done much to enrich embryology but has received little in return; progress has occurred mostly by exploiting genetic or teratogenic anomalies rather than by deriving shape from embryologic principles. Indeed, genetics, through its concept of coded instructions, offers the best solution to Needham's lament. The much-ridiculed preformationalists were correct in saying that there was a microscopic human present in the egg—what they lacked was the concept of coded instructions. When the codes producing protein conformation from amino acid sequence, cell architecture from protein complex, and organ from cell interaction are as well understood as that from DNA to protein, then a comprehensive theory of embryology will be available. Environmental interaction (epigenesis) and evolutionary comparisons (phylogenesis) will provide the variables needed to test and define the theory, but its essence will be a branching molecular program.

What are the steps required to deduce an organism, given its genomic sequence? In contemplating this problem, with all its exciting potential for new design, several dilemmas of modern embryology come to mind. There is first a problem of information. Genomic complexity of higher organisms is exemplified by the enormity of space that will be required even to print the complete human sequence. A metric familiar to the readers of this chapter article is the McKusick catalog.[2] Over 200 volumes equivalent to the informational portion of the 1991 edition would be required merely to print the nucleotides, and another 30 volumes would be needed for a McKusick-style index. The ability to comprehend this sequence, even when compiled, is so far limited to amino acid codons, some structural RNAs, and a few regulatory signals (i.e., TATA boxes and splice junctions). Even the dramatic ability to study each level of genetic expression, illustrated in Figure 14–1, is dwarfed by the sheer number of molecules and loci that must be defined. An average gene size of 40 kilobase pairs (40 kb) predicts 100,000 genes in man and mouse, variably expressed in over 200 types of at least 10^{14} total cells.[3] Clearly those genes relevant to embryogenesis will be a subset of the total, but weaving diverse facts about receptors, cell adhesion molecules, or proto-oncogenes into a coherent tapestry of molecular embryogenesis is a formidable endeavor.

More cryptic than genome sequence may be the ciphers relating gene to cell to tissue structure. As Fulton[4] has pointed out, any cell is more like a crystal than a solution of freely diffusible molecules. Internal protein concentrations in red blood cells (35% by weight) or muscle cells (23% by weight) are more similar to the volume occupied by protein in a crystal (10%–80%) than to the dilute solutions often studied in laboratories. Indeed, many of the enzymes comprising classic biochemical pathways such as the Krebs cycle probably are associated in loose complexes that facilitate substrate transfer; more visible compartments include the Golgi, mitochondria, or peroxisomes. Knowledge of the mechanisms governing cell organization is confined to a few trafficking signals such as the carboxyterminus of peroxisomal proteins. Even the cytoskeleton, which consumes more than 35% of cell protein synthesis,[5] is understood more by its components (microtubules, intermediate filaments) than by its overall organization. There is much to learn about molecular and subcellular topology before the shape of an organism can be easily deduced.

At the intercellular level, aggregation has been related to specific adhesion molecules,[6] but regulation of lineage and differentiation is less well understood. Certain embryonic regions seem autonomous, as though the genetic program specifies fate regardless of their neighbors; others interact with their surroundings and exhibit enormous plasticity or compensation for injury. Adding to this unpredictability of cell–cell interaction is the physiologic level of embryogenesis;

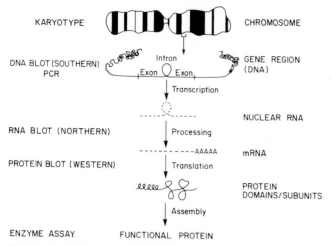

Fig. 14–1. Molecular analysis of genetic disease. The different levels available for genetic analysis and the techniques employed are illustrated. Note the increased precision (even the smallest chromosomal band defined by prometaphase analysis will contain 1 million base pairs of DNA) and diversity of modern methods (chromosome band, gene, transcription, processed RNA, structural protein, functional protein).

Table 14–1. Molecular approaches to characterizing genes responsible for human malformations

Candidate genes

Functional analysis (i.e., collagen)

Evolutionary homology (i.e., homeodomain)

Linkage disequilibrium (i.e., TGF-α)

Genetic mapping

Genomics (trait linked to known locus)

Anonymous loci (RFLPs, VNTRs)

Homozygosity (recessive traits; imprinted regions)

Physical mapping

Interstitial chromosome deletions

Chromosome translocations/inversions

Fragile sites

emerging forces due to circulation, excretion, or limb movement mold shape in ways that seem far removed from the genomic sequence. Rather than a gene specifying the position of each small blood vessel, bristle, or sweat pore, some randomness of outcome subject to boundaries and constraint must occur. Thus fingerprint patterns will relate roughly to genes determining fingerpad height, but the exact print varies between individuals. Even if the genomic instructions can be precisely delineated, there will be an inherent variability in the resulting embryo. This is the perspective of Waddington[7] as emphasized recently by Shapiro.[8]

The last barrier to a universal theory of embryogenesis is in fact the beginning. The zygotic genome does not begin life naked but is clothed by germ cell and egg. Even the simplest viral genomes rely on host cell organization to construct their elegant icosahedrons. In *Caenorhabditis elegans* and other nematodes, the very first cell division is asymmetric, yielding the AB (neurons) and P_1 (muscle, gonads) cells destined to initiate completely different lineages. In *Drosophila,* an asymmetric distribution of nurse cells imparts orientation to the egg that will be realized in anteroposterior and dorsoventral coordinates. The egg is a complex crystal with an endowment of specific gene modifications and maternally derived molecules—only from this starting point can a path from genome to organism be accurately charted. Yet, like the modifications introduced by phylogenesis or teratogenesis, the patterning of genome expression by parental history can be understood through comparison and experimental perturbation.

In summary, then, the best hope for a unifying theory of embryogenesis lies in defining the cascade of molecular interactions that connect genome to phenotype. Genetic anomalies offer the high road to genomic understanding provided both phenotype and inheritance are precisely delineated. This statement does not imply that the enormous plasticity and reparative potential of development can be entirely summarized by gene structure, but that genetic pathways provide a basic skeleton for the flesh of developmental inter-

action. In this chapter are discussed various approaches to characterizing genetic anomalies at the DNA level, as summarized in Table 14–1. Following a review of molecular technology, linkage and candidate gene approaches are described from a clinical perspective. Finally, a current map of human dysmorphogenetic loci is presented as an index of present and future progress in this area.

Primer of molecular biology as applied to human genetic disease

As illustrated in Figure 14–1, molecular biology has provided direct access to the human genome and unified previously discrete areas of genetics. Recombination distances, chromosomal bands, and amino acid sequences are now all related by the same medium of DNA base pairs—only the scales differ. This section is a brief review of DNA technology organized into nine basic components. More detailed treatments have been published by Watson et al.[9] and by Sambrook et al.[10] Since molecular biology has acquired a jargon that is often more formidable than the actual concepts, a glossary of key terms is provided as an introduction.

Allele: The usual definition (alternative forms of a gene occupying the same locus on homologous chromosomes) may be extended to include DNA differences detected by restriction endonucleases. For example, cleavage of the β-globin locus with the enzyme *Hpa* I may yield a larger (allele 1) or smaller (allele 2) fragment.

Anonymous DNA fragments or markers: A fragment of DNA isolated at random without reference to any particular gene or chromosomal location. Production and mapping of multiple anonymous DNA fragments allows markers to be distributed over the entire genome and facilitates mapping of disease loci. By convention, anonymous human DNA fragments are named according to chromosome location (i.e., 12 or X), copy number (single S, repetitive Z), and a number of identity (i.e., DXS42).

ASOs: Allele-specific oligonucleotides. Single-stranded DNA segments that are synthesized to hybridize to one DNA sequence (allele) but not to another, i.e., ASO for the M and Z sequences of the α_1-antitrypsin gene.

Bases or base pairs: The size unit (bp, base pairs; kb, kilobase pairs; mb, megabase pairs) commonly employed for RNA or DNA so that their lengths are interconvertible; i.e., a 30 kb DNA fragment will be completely transcribed as a 30 kb RNA.

cDNA: Complementary DNA. A single-stranded DNA molecule copied from messenger RNA (mRNA) utilizing reverse transcriptase and a poly-T primer that initiates synthesis at the poly-A region of the mRNA. The intervening sequences (introns) present in most genes will be absent from cDNA since they are removed from the mRNA by RNA processing (splicing).

Cloning: Deriving a population from a single isolate, whether as a composite replicative molecule (recombinant DNA cloning), single cell (cell cloning), or single individual (organismal cloning).

Complement: A DNA or RNA strand that matches a known strand but has opposite base pair sequence (A instead of U/T, C instead of G) and polarity such that the two strands can anneal to form a perfect hybrid. In experiments the known strand is often called the *template* or *sense strand* and its complement the *antisense strand* (in the case of duplex DNA), *primer* (in the case of synthetic oligonucleotides), or *transcript* (in the case of transcription into RNA)

Complexity: Number of independent DNA or RNA molecules represented in a sample. It is desirable, for example, that cDNA libraries be of high complexity so that mRNA molecules of low tissue abundance are represented.

Denaturation: Conversion of double-stranded DNA to its complementary single strands by heat or ionic strength.

DNA transfection/transformation: Uptake of purified viral (transfection) or cellular (transformation) DNA by cultured cells.

Dot-blot: Format for detection of DNA or RNA sequences by nucleic acid hybridization. Serial dilutions of various cell extracts (target sequences) are applied to a membrane (nitrocellulose or equivalent) using a modified 96 well microtiter dish as guide. The membrane is then hybridized to the desired DNA/RNA fragment (probe), and the target sequences are quantitated by autoradiology or colorimetric detection.

Exon: Segments of DNA coding for protein using a three-nucleotide amino acid code (codons).

Genome: The complete set of genes in a cell or organism.

Hybridization (renaturation): Reaction of a DNA or RNA molecule with a complementary molecule to form a duplex structure.

Intron: Segments of DNA (also known as *intervening sequences*) that interrupt protein-coding regions and are spliced out of nuclear RNA during maturation of messenger RNA.

Library: A population of recombinant DNA clones constructed so as to include a comprehensive collection of source DNA. A genomic library will optimally contain at least one copy of every DNA sequence in the genome.

Linkage disequilibrium: State of two genes, polymorphic sites, or mutations occurring together more frequently than expected by chance. A haplotype or framework consists of two or more restriction fragment alleles that exhibit disequilibrium and segregate as a group (i.e., *Tag* I allele 1, *Bam* HI allele 2, *Eco* RI allele 2).

Northern blot: A pun on the name of Southern to indicate gel electrophoresis, capillary transfer, and hybridization of RNA.

Oligo: Oligonucleotide. A single-stranded segment of DNA that is often produced by a DNA synthesizer.

PCR: Polymerase chain reaction. Can be used in a variety of formats to amplify a specific DNA or RNA sequence from a complex mixture.

Primer: An oligonucleotide that is complementary to a small segment of a single-stranded DNA or RNA and is used to initiate synthesis of a complete second strand.

Probe: A DNA, RNA, or synthetic oligonucleotide labeled with radioactivity or biotin to detect complementary sequences in a sample by hybridization.

Restriction endonuclease: Bacterial enzymes that cleave double-stranded DNA at specific sites (recognition sequences) of four to six nucleotides. The recognition sequences are often palindromes in the sense of GAATTC on one strand and CTTAAG on the complementary strand.

RFLP: Restriction fragment length polymorphism. Inherited variation at a DNA region that happens to occur within the recognition sequence for a restriction endonuclease. Digestion of the DNA region will then produce different restriction fragment lengths in different individuals. Once the variable region is sequenced, then the more cumbersome techniques of gel electrophoresis and Southern blotting can be replaced by PCR and dot-blot hybridization with ASOs.

Sequence: As a noun, the order and identity of nucleotides (bases) that comprise a DNA or RNA segment. As a verb, to determine that order through chemical or enzymatic methods. The term *sequences* often refers to a collection of DNA or RNA segments; e.g., ribosomal DNA sequences are highly GC rich.

Southern blot: A technique for gel electrophoresis, capillary transfer, and hybridization of DNA developed by E. M. Southern.

Stringency: The ionic strength or temperature of a hybridization reaction that determines the degree of identity required for two complementary molecules to hybridize. Low stringency will allow considerable mismatching (i.e., for evolutionary studies), while high stringency requires exact sequence identity before a stable hybrid will form (i.e., for ASO and PCR).

Vector: A plasmid or bacteriophage molecule that has been engineered to facilitate cloning of DNA segments. The sequences to be cloned, i.e., sequences from the β-globin region, are often termed *target sequences.*

VNTRs: Variable number of tandem repeats. Regions of DNA where a short sequence is variably repeated in head-to-tail fashion. Restriction enzymes with recognition sites bracketing the variable region will produce a single fragment that varies in size according to the number of repeats. Restriction enzymes cleaving within the variable region will produce an extremely complex array of fragments specific for each person (minisatellites, DNA fingerprinting).

Western blot: Pun on the name of Southern representing gel electrophoresis, capillary transfer, and antibody detection of proteins.

DNA hybridization

The elegance of the Watson-Crick structure was based not only on the symmetry of the double helix but also on its genetic information. Each strand is complementary to the other and can form a template for replacement copies. When the DNA duplex is subjected to suitable conditions of salt,

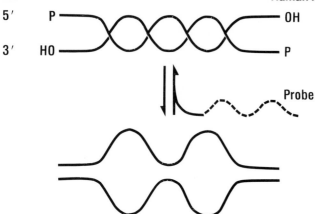

5′ P _____ OH
3′ HO _____ P

Probe

Fig. 14–2. DNA hybridization. Two complementary DNA strands are shown with reverse polarity from 5′ to 3′. Suitable conditions of heat or temperature cause renaturation into separate strands. Hybridization is the reverse reaction, with a radiolabeled probe substituting for one of the DNA strands.

pH, or temperature, the stacking forces and hydrogen bonds between strands are disrupted (Fig. 14–2). Conditions can then be reversed to allow reassociation or reannealing of the denatured strands. A hybridization reaction involves substituting labeled DNA or RNA for one strand (dotted line) so that reassociation can be quantitated based on how much radioactivity is incorporated into the duplex. The radioactive segment of RNA or DNA is called a *probe*. Many variations of hybridization reactions have been devised in which labeled duplex has been discriminated from unreacted probe using single-strand-specific nucleases or hydroxyapatite chromatography. The simplest and most sensitive have involved binding denatured DNA to a solid support such as nitrocellulose membranes. Unreacted probe can then be washed away using care to maintain the duplex. The amount of hybridization is then quantitated autoradiographically by exposing the membrane to x-ray film. A similar reaction can be performed on a tissue section or metaphase karyotype using the slide as solid support. The slide is then dipped into photographic emulsion to quantitate the amount of probe bound after hybridization and washing. The synthesis of probes from chemically modified nucleotides, i.e., those containing biotin, allows colorimetric detection of hybridization using the appropriate reagents (i.e., avidin coupled to horseradish peroxidase).

Two major variables affect hybridization: the complexity of the nucleic acid sample and the stringency of the hybridization conditions. Nucleic acid samples from higher organisms will contain complex mixtures of gene sequences in concentrations that are proportionate to gene copy number. For a given temperature and DNA concentration, the hybridization rate for a certain DNA probe will depend on the number and dosage of complementary genes in the DNA sample. Sequences present multiple times in the genome will have a higher effective concentration and reassociate more rapidly, than sequences present only once in the genome. These kinetic properties were the basis of the hybridization analyses that first identified repetitive sequences in animal genomes. Even with modern methods for synthesizing highly radioactive probes, detection of genes present only once per genome may require 2–3 days of autoradiography after hybridization. Since the kinetics of hybridization depend directly on the number of genes represented in the nucleic acid sample, complexity is a useful measure of completeness for recombinant libraries assembled from cellular RNA or genomic DNA.

Stringency describes the salt and temperature conditions used for hybridization. Low stringency allows hybrids to form even when there are mismatches between nucleotides on the two strands. Low stringency hybridization may be useful in noting regions of evolutionary homology or in identifying divergent gene families. High stringency conditions (salt and temperature near those that cause dissociation) can prevent hybridization if there is a single mismatch between strands of 20–25 nucleotides. This is very useful diagnostically if one wishes to distinguish a normal gene region from that containing a point mutation.

The synthesis of probes can be performed in several ways. Before the advent of recombinant DNA technology, only DNA or RNA molecules that occurred naturally in high abundance and purity could be used for labeling. Examples included viral DNA, ribosomal DNA, which was highly amplified in amphibian oocytes, and globin mRNA, which comprised a large fraction of the RNA in mammalian reticulocytes. Most probes are now synthesized directly based on DNA sequence information (oligonucleotide probes) or prepared by labeling cloned DNA segments. In the latter case, a deoxyribo- or ribonucleotide precursor is incorporated into a primed elongation reaction using the cloned gene as template. Enzymes include reverse transcriptase to synthesize probes from mRNA, DNA polymerase to fill in nicked recombinant DNA molecules (nicked translation), or RNA polymerase for transcribing recombinant molecules spliced next to specialized recombinant molecules designed from bacteriophages or plasmids (vectors). Terminal transferase and other enzymes can be used to place labeled "ends" on unlabeled DNA duplexes or single-stranded oligonucleotides.

DNA restriction

An armamentarium of over 200 commercially available bacterial enzymes has been assembled that recognizes specific nucleotide sequences in duplex DNA. Restriction endonucleases are named for their bacteria of origin, such as *Escherichia coli* (*Eco* RI) or *Bacillus amylofaciens* (*Bam* HI). Restriction endonucleases cleave at a palindromic four to six base pair sequence and produce DNA molecules with overlapping (staggered) or blunt ends. These ends will ligate with the ends of other DNA fragments produced by the same endonuclease, allowing splicing to produce new fragment combinations (recombinant DNAs). As illustrated in Figure 14–3, restriction of a DNA segment coupled with agarose gel electrophoresis to separate the products by size allows the localization of restriction sites on the DNA. Fragment sizes are calculated in base pairs, kilobase pairs, or megabase pairs according to their scale. A map is then drawn orienting the DNA in the 5′ → 3′ direction corresponding to RNA transcription. Frequently the duplex is represented by a single line with boxes to indicate important regions. For diploid organisms, any restriction map should really be given in duplicate to represent the two chromosomes, but in practice one cognate map is shown with arrows indicating variable sites among one or more individuals. Such variable sites are called *restriction polymorphisms*. A restriction map provides an ob-

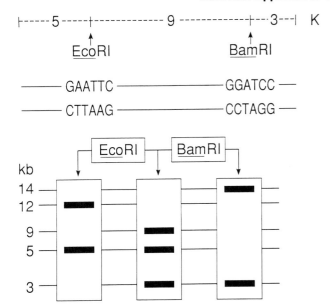

Fig. 14–3. DNA restriction. Restriction of a hypothetical 17,000 base pair (17 kb) DNA segment with the restriction endonucleases *Eco* RI and *Bam* HI is followed by size separation on agarose gels and construction of a restriction map. The middle lane represents the gel electrophoretic pattern expected from cleavage of the DNA segment with both *Eco* RI and *Bam* HI.

vious guide for recombinant DNA cloning of the chromosomal region or for examining mutations that alter restriction site patterns. Less obvious in the beginning was their utility as markers for mutant genes, chromosomal regions, or individual identity.

To pick out the restriction fragments of a specific gene from those of all other parts of the genome, a method for transferring DNA from gel to solid support was devised (Fig. 14–4). The procedure (Southern transfer) is accomplished by denaturation of the DNA within the gel and sandwiching it between a paper wick and a nitrocellulose membrane. Buffer is pulled from wick to membrane by capillary action, leaving an exact imprint of the gel on the membrane. Hybridization to a radioactive probe for the gene of interest then highlights fragments of that gene within the size-separated array of other genomic fragments. The resulting restriction map provides a preliminary estimate of gene size and becomes the blueprint for DNA cloning. An important application of Southern transfer techniques to facilitate the evolutionary comparisons mentioned below is the so-called zoo blot, which examines for gene homology among the DNA of multiple species.

DNA cloning

DNA fragments liberated by restriction endonucleases can be incorporated into specially constructed plasmid or bacteriophage molecules that have been cleaved with the same enzyme (Fig. 14–5). Recombinant DNA technology offers the

Fig. 14–4. Analysis of DNA by Southern blotting. The upper left displays tissue DNA that has been purified and contains a gene region (box) that has been cloned in a suitable vector. The DNA is cleaved with restriction endonuclease (dashed line), and the mixture of restriction fragments is applied to an agarose gel. Four lanes of the gel are shown, which could contain the same DNA sample cleaved with different restriction endonucleases or DNA samples from four individuals that are restricted with the same endonuclease. After electrophoresis to separate the restriction fragment mixtures according to size, the DNA within the gel is denatured with base and transferred to a nitrocellulose membrane by capillary filtration. Hybridization with a solution of radioactively labeled probe (filled box) followed by washing and autoradiography reveals the location of restriction fragments (bands) from the gene of interest. If the DNAs were from different individuals, then this particular gene probe and restriction endonuclease may have demonstrated a restriction fragment length polymorphism (different fragment sizes in different lanes).

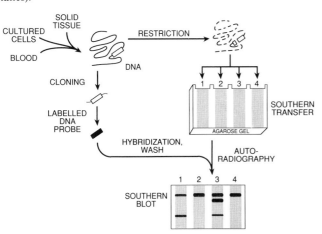

Fig. 14–5. DNA cloning. A target DNA such as that from the human genome is cleaved with a restriction endonuclease (vertical lines) to generate a wide array of fragment sizes. Vector DNA cleaved with the same endonuclease has staggered DNA ends identical to the target fragments. Recombination of target and vector DNA ends generates a random library of vector molecules, each of which contains a specific target fragment. Screening the library of recombinant DNA molecules with a DNA or RNA probe for the gene of interest allows the identification of a recombinant molecule with the desired target DNA fragment (recombinant selection). This recombinant vector is then amplified manyfold by growth in bacteria, and multiple copies or "clones" of the recombinant are available for preparation and study of the target DNA fragment.

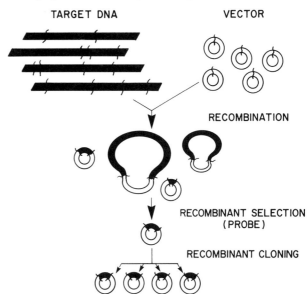

Table 14–2. Size limits of DNA separation and cloning methods

DNA fragment size	Separation method	Cloning vector
0–500 bp	Acrylamide gels	M13 bacteriophage
0.5–5 kb	1%–2% Agarose gels	Plasmids, lambda bacteriophage
5–15 kb	0.8% Agarose gels	Plasmids, lambda bacteriophage
10–30 kb	0.8% Agarose gels Pulsed-field gels	Cosmids
50 kb–3 mb	Pulsed-field gels	Yeast artificial chromosomes

advantage of transferring eukaryotic genes from a complex genomic environment (high complexity) to the simple genome of prokaryotic vectors. An Audubon of cloning vectors is now available for the variety of DNA sizes and restriction endonuclease configurations encountered in gene cloning (Table 14–2). Improvements in pulsed-field gel electrophoresis allow application of Southern transfer techniques to very large DNA fragments (50 kb to 3 mb). Newly developed yeast artificial chromosome (YAC) vectors can incorporate the large DNA restriction fragments visualized by pulsed-field electrophoresis and allow the rapid characterization of large chromosomal regions.

Various techniques for gene cloning have been perfected over the past 15 years. If a nucleic acid probe for a gene is available, then a library of all possible DNA restriction fragments from a genome is created in a suitable bacteriophage, plasmid, or yeast vector. Plating of the library on Petri dishes is followed by transfer of individual colonies to a membrane and identification of the desired DNA clones by hybridization and autoradiography. If a probe is not available, but the protein product is known, antibodies can be used to screen specialized "expression" libraries wherein each recombinant colony expresses a segment of protein corresponding to its spliced DNA fragment. Alternatively, if a portion of amino acid sequence is known for the protein, a combination of oligonucleotides can be synthesized that covers all the coding possibilities for that amino acid sequence. Screening of complementary DNA or genomic libraries can then be performed with the labeled mixture of oligonucleotide "guessmers." By employing either the direct cloning methods based on gene products or the indirect methods based on linkage and rearrangement (discussed below), it is possible to clone almost any gene.

Structural analysis of cloned DNA segments

Once a target region of the genome is cloned, it must be characterized to ensure correspondence with predicted properties. Direct restriction analysis can examine for the presence of sites predicted from genomic Southern blot analysis and provide the basis for subcloning the region into sequencing vectors such as M13 bacteriophage. Figure 14–6 shows the concept behind DNA sequencing and synthesis. The DNA segment is asymmetrically labeled or terminated at successive nucleotides in four separate reactions. Each reaction specifically examines one of the four nucleotides. Fractionating DNA fragments from the four reactions in parallel on a polyacrylamide gives bands corresponding to nucleotide positions. The nucleotide sequence can then be read directly by

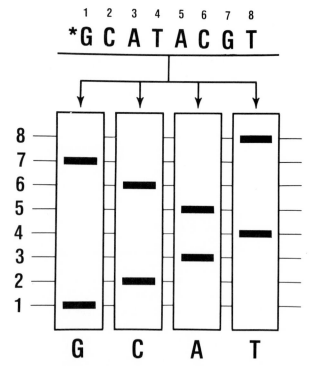

Fig. 14–6. DNA sequencing and synthesis. A hypothetical DNA single strand (oligonucleotide) containing 8 bp is labeled at one end (asterisk) and divided into four aliquots. The aliquots are separately cleaved by chemical reagents specific for one of the four dideoxynucleotides and the products run in parallel on an acrylamide sequencing gel that separates them according to size. After autoradiography to determine the position of all labeled fragments, the fragment sizes derived from each aliquot indicate the distance of the cleavage site (i.e., that specific dideoxynucleotide) from the labeled end. The DNA sequence can therefore be read by scanning from the bottom (smallest fragment) to the top of the autoradiogram. Once the sequence is known, portions of that sequence can be synthesized chemically (bottom) to provide primers for further sequencing or polymerase chain reactions.

scanning up the gel (Fig. 14–6). Once a DNA sequence is characterized, oligonucleotides identical or complementary to the sequence can be chemically synthesized for use as probes (Fig. 14–6, bottom). Individuals working in efficient laboratories can generate about 5000 nucleotides of DNA sequence per week. For genomic clones that were isolated through antibodies to their protein product, the determination of a DNA sequence compatible with the protein amino acid sequence establishes clone identity. For genomic regions isolated via proximity to a locus for which a DNA probe is available, a sequence interval that lacks termination codons (open reading frame [ORF]) is a provisional candidate for the gene of interest.

Functional assays of cloned DNA segments

Once DNA cloning, restriction analysis, and sequencing have provided a map for gene structure and organization, assays are required to relate DNA sequence to cellular and/or developmental function. The cloned gene or a portion thereof is transferred to a vector that promotes integration/expression of the gene in an in vivo system. These range from the uptake and expression of recombinant DNA into live cells to the microinjection of cloned segments into embryos

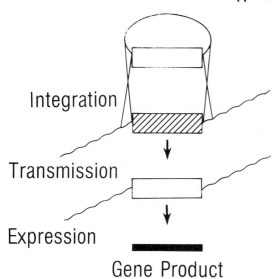

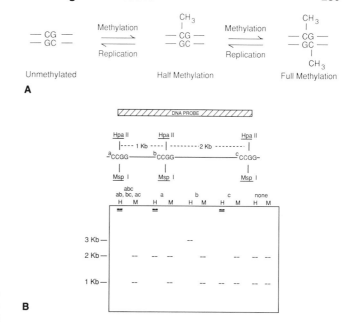

Fig. 14–7. Gene transfer. The three steps involved in obtaining synthesis of a cloned gene product are illustrated. Site-specific gene replacement is illustrated, meaning that the cloned gene (empty box) is inserted at exactly its normal genomic location with excision of the host copy (hatched box). In practice, specific insertion or replacement has been achieved for very few genes using specialized vectors ("constructs"). More commonly, multiple transgenes are inserted without targeting to their normal genomic location. A second step for expression in cells or transgenic animals is to ensure transmission of the gene to daughter cells or offspring; this has been a vexing problem with mutated mouse embryonic carcinoma cells and many other constructs. Finally, transcriptional, splicing, and/or protein processing signals compatible with the host must be included in the construct or insertion site to obtain normally regulated synthesis of functional product (solid bar).

Fig. 14–8. Restriction analysis of DNA methylation. A. Interconversions involved with de novo, half, and full methylation at deoxycytidine residues in double-stranded DNA. These conversions are catalyzed by methylase or demethylase enzymes and usually occur at the dinucleotide CpG. B. A hypothetical DNA region with CCGG recognition sequences a, b, and c for restriction endonucleases *Hpa* II/ *Msp* I. The enzyme *Hpa* II cuts only at unmethylated CCGG, whereas *Msp* I cuts regardless of methylation. Below this map is a Southern blot indicating the expected restriction fragments according to which combinations of CCGG sites are methylated in the DNA. Paired digestion with *Hpa* II (H) and *Msp* I (M) endonucleases can thus discriminate between multi-site, single site, and no methylation of the genomic DNA.

(Fig. 14–7). A useful technique for defining regulatory sequences involved in gene expression is to place upstream sequence regions from the gene of interest and fuse them with the bacterial chloramphenicol transacetylase (CAT) gene using specially engineered plasmids (constructs). The presence of viral sequences in these vectors promotes rapid integration into animal cells, and the regulatory effects of upstream sequences can be deduced from their efficiency in promoting cellular CAT activity. Systematic alteration of these regulatory gene sequences is performed by in vitro mutagenesis to confirm their necessity for CAT expression/repression. A map of nucleotide regions critical for transcriptional regulation of a gene can then be defined. Analysis by gene transfer has culminated in the production of transgenic mouse embryos in which developmental expression and effect can be determined. Constructs fusing the gene of interest to the bacterial β-galactosidase gene allows embryonic expression to be directly visualized by staining the embryo with chromogenic substrates, and this method has recently been applied as a general way to identify developmentally regulated genes in the mouse.[11] The manipulation of mouse embryogenesis as an avenue to understanding human dysmorphology is discussed in more detail below.

Study of DNA methylation by restriction analysis

The modification of gene activity through DNA methylation and chromatin structure may represent an additional level of developmental regulation. Methylation of DNA at the 5 position of cytosine was recognized in 1948 by Hotchkiss, and most methylated cytosines were shown by nearest neighbor analysis to occur at CpG doublets (Fig. 14–8A). Study of methylation patterns within specific DNA regions became possible when restriction endonucleases that recognized the same DNA sequence (isoschizomers; i.e., *Hpa* II and *Msp* I in Fig. 14–8B) but differed in their ability to cut methylated DNA were characterized. Cleavage at a restriction site by the methyl-insensitive nuclease but not by its companion enzyme becomes an assay for methylation (example in Fig. 14–8B). Using paired digestions and standard Southern blotting, reproducible and tissue-specific patterns of DNA methylation were soon defined. Furthermore, there was a good parallel between gene activity and lack of methylation, although the role of undermethylation as a cause or consequence of gene expression is still unclear. Since methyl groups might be introduced early in embryogenesis and maintained during subsequent replications, this seemed a likely candidate for the progressive gene inactivation that appears as a prominent theme in development.[12] Exogenous viral genomes introduced into mouse embryos were both repressed and methylated, while treatment of embryos with the methylation inhibitor 5-azacytidine reactivated enzymes that had been repressed earlier in development.[13] Yet the evolutionary distribution of DNA methylation raises questions about any universal role in development. Only 20% of lower vertebrate DNA is methylated compared with 80% in mammalian cells.

Drosophila has essentially no methylated DNA. Another caution is that experiments with 5-azacytidine may involve effects other than inhibition of methylation.

Evidence relating DNA methylation and gene expression has also been gathered from studies of mammalian X-chromosome inactivation. DNA isolated from inactive X chromosomes will not transform cells deficient in the X-encoded activity hypoxanthine phosphoribosyltransferase (HPRT). This inactivation is associated with increased methylation of the HPRT gene and can be reversed by the methylation inhibitor 5-azacytidine.[14] Restriction enzymes that simultaneously discriminate between DNA polymorphisms and DNA methylation provide consistent information in heterozygous females. Methylation at alternative X-linked polymorphisms is random, as predicted by the Lyon hypothesis for random X-chromosome inactivation. If structural rearrangement of one X chromosome is present, a condition known to cause preferential inactivation of the normal X, then at least a portion of methyl groups differs between the translocated and normal X chromosomes. There is not always a consistent correlation between the gene on the inactive X and hypermethylation, however; some genes on the inactive X are undermethylated. Complicating this issue is the fact that within a given gene only certain CpG sites are specifically methylated amidst a background methylation that does not exhibit regulatory change. An intriguing observation regarding DNA methylation is its differential pattern in maternal and paternal complements of the zygote genome.[15] DNA methylation may thus provide physical evidence for the genetic phenomenon of imprinting.

Locating genes by DNA linkage

It follows from Mendel's laws that diploid organisms have a pair of alleles at each locus that are transmitted to offspring with equal probability. Linkage exploits the deviations from Mendelian probabilities that occur because of the packaging of genes on chromosomes.[16] A diploid individual with alleles a_1a_2 at one locus and b_1b_2 at another may not produce the 1:1:1:1 ratios of each possible gamete (i.e., a_1b_1, a_1b_2, a_2b_1, a_2b_2) predicted by Mendel's laws. If only the combinations a_1b_1, a_2b_2 are produced, then it is likely that loci a and b lie on the same chromosome and exhibit genetic linkage. The establishment of linkage groups is thus an important tool for gene mapping. The exclusive production of gametes a_1b_1 and a_2b_2 also indicate that the alleles a_1–b_1 are located on one chromosome (in phase), while the alleles a_2–b_2 lie together on the other. Once phase is established, then the recombinant gametes a_1b_2 and a_2b_1 can be sought as an indication of chromosomal crossing-over between locus a and locus b. The proportion of recombinant gametes allows a quantitative estimate of linkage: the recombination fraction, or theta (Θ), is the ratio of recombinant over all possible gametes, i.e., $a_1b_2 + a_2b_1/\Sigma a_nb_n$ for the example above. A recombination fraction of 50% indicates no linkage, while 0% indicates complete linkage. The physical correlate of Θ is genetic distance, meaning that the higher the recombination fraction, the larger the interval of DNA separating the two loci. Each 1% of recombination is equivalent to 1 centiMorgan (cM) or about 10^6 bp over short distances, but the plateau of 50% recombination for infinite distance emphasizes that the correlation between Θ and distance is not strictly linear. It varies with sex, distance, and chromosomal region.[16]

The most straightforward linkage study is the two-point analysis in which a phenotype or locus of unknown location is examined for linkage to a reference locus. An early example from dysmorphology was linkage of the locus responsible for nail-patella syndrome to the ABO blood group locus on chromosome 9. If one considers this problem, it is intuitively obvious that both heterozygosity for ABO alleles and access to large families will maximize the opportunities to correlate inheritance of the syndrome with blood type. Children of a type O individual with nail-patella syndrome will not contribute linkage information, since both chromosomes would have identical O alleles. Both heterozygosity and phase must be established before recombinants can be identified. The number and frequency of different alleles at a locus are thus predictive of its value in linkage studies; a polymorphism information content (PIC) value can be calculated, which ranges from 0 for invariant loci to almost 1 for the HLA system.[17]

Family size influences the accuracy of linkage studies, since recombinants may be under- or overestimated in small samples. A maximal likelihood approach has been developed as a statistical measure of linkage which takes into account the number of individuals, pedigree structure, and informativeness in a linkage study.[16] For any given Θ, the likelihood $L(\Theta)$ of genotype segregation in the pedigree is related to the likelihood of no linkage (Θ = 50%). If one recombinant is noted among five offspring of an AB, nail-patella father, then the likelihood of no linkage = $L(0.5)$ = $\Theta(1 - \Theta)^4$ = $(0.5)^5$ = 0.031. The likelihood for a recombination rate of 10% becomes $L(0.1)$ = $(0.10)(0.90)^4$ = 0.066. One can proceed to calculate $L(\Theta)$ for various Θ until the value of Θ that is most consistent with the pedigree is identified (20% as shown in Table 14–3). This result is more meaningfully expressed as a ratio of $L(\Theta)$ to $L(0.5)$, known as the *odds for linkage,* and is usually converted to a logarithm so that values from different families can be added (multiplying the likelihoods). The logarithm of the odds (lod) ratio or lod score is thus $Z(\Theta)$ = $\log_{10}[L(\Theta)/L(0.5)]$.[16] As shown in Table 14–3, $Z(\Theta)$ values corresponding to a standard range of Θ values are calculated and the maximum $[Z(\Theta)]$ evaluated as evidence for or against the hypothesis of linkage. Computer programs such as LIPED or LINKAGE[16] are normally employed for these calculations. Maximal $Z(\Theta)$ values at Θ = 0.5 argue against linkage, while $Z(\Theta)$ values above 3 (odds ratio 10^3) are considered significant for linkage with the specified recombination fraction of Θ. In the nail-patella syndrome example of Table 14–3, $Z(\Theta)$ is a maximal 0.42 at Θ = 0.2, indicating that six to seven more families (35–40 offspring) with this structure would be needed to reach a lod score of 3. The actual recombination fraction measured between the ABO and nail-pa-

Table 14–3. Logarithm of the odds (lod) scores for various Θ values in the case of one recombinant and four nonrecombinants[a]

Θ	$1 - \Theta$	$(1 - \Theta)^4$	$\Theta(1 - \Theta)^4$	$\Theta(1 - \Theta)^4/0.031$	$Z(\Theta)$
0.01	0.99	0.96	0.0096	0.31	−0.5
0.1	0.9	0.66	0.066	2.13	0.33
0.2	0.8	0.41	0.082	2.64	0.42
0.3	0.7	0.24	0.072	2.32	0.37
0.4	0.6	0.13	0.052	1.70	0.23

[a]Note that the likelihood of no linkage $L(0.5)$ = $(0.5)(0.5)^4$ = 0.031 in this example and that the most plausible value of Θ is 0.2 since this optimizes $Z(\Theta)$ = $\log L(\Theta)/L(0.5)$ = 0.42. See text for further details.

tella syndrome loci is about 10%, which would produce a Z(Θ) above 3 with only 15 informative offspring.

Multi-point linkage is highly complex because of the numbers of potential recombinants and the assumptions required about gene order. As summarized by Ott,[16] n loci can be ordered in n!/2 ways, where each two symmetric orders are counted as one gene order. A more tractable approach is to assemble a tentative gene order by comparing recombination fractions between paired loci. The likelihood of this gene order can then be compared with that for other arrangements.[16] Once a gene order is established, the mapping of new loci using one of the known markers is much more straightforward. This explains the tremendous acceleration of genetic linkage and mapping studies that has occurred through the use of anonymous DNA markers.

Variation in DNA sequence as revealed by restriction endonucleases and Southern blotting has provided a systematic approach to genetic linkage. It is estimated that humans differ from one another at a minimum of 1 in every 4–500 bp; these variable sites represent single nucleotide changes or contain variable numbers of sequences that repeat in tandem (VNTRs). Point mutations, if they lie within a recognition sequence, may alter the length of DNA restriction fragments (restriction fragment length polymorphisms [RFLPs]), as shown in Figure 14–9. VNTRs produce a larger array of DNA restriction fragment sizes because of their iterated repeats and are more likely to be heterozygous. A prominent use of VNTRs is the DNA fingerprinting used in paternity and forensic testing.

Figure 14–9 illustrates a standard RFLP analysis in which the genotypes XX, ZX, and ZZ are predicted by the DNA restriction pattern of a neighboring locus. The boxed chromosomal region represents a polymorphic gene region for which a DNA probe is available. The pattern of restriction fragments visualized by Southern blotting, hybridization, and autoradiography may then be evaluated for linkage to the locus determining phenotypes X or Z. In the family depicted in Figure 14–9, the parental 11 kb RFLP allele segregates with allele X, while the 7 + 4 kb allele (extra restriction site) segregates with allele Z. Testing of all family members for X/Z and 11/7 + 4 kb status allows the calculation of a lod score as discussed above. The power of DNA analysis consists of the unlimited number of such probes that can be derived from known genes or even anonymous regions of DNA.

Randomly cloned DNA segments can be evaluated for polymorphism by restriction experiments employing multiple enzymes and several families. The use of restriction enzymes that contain the highly mutable CpG sequence in their recognition sites optimizes the chance of finding an RFLP. Cloned DNAs that detect frequent polymorphisms in the population (high PIC value)[17] are then assigned a chromosomal location by linkage analysis to reference markers or by hybridization to DNA from somatic cell hybrids containing single human chromosomes. Over the past decade, DNA probes derived from over 1000 known or anonymous loci have been characterized so as to saturate the entire human genome. Once a locus has been linked to a DNA marker, then the known DNA segment becomes a bridge to the unknown DNA region by successively cloning overlapping DNA segments and "walking" along the chromosome (Fig. 14–10). Linkage studies are facilitated if a chromosomal deletion or translocation has been seen in association with the

Fig. 14–9. Linkage analysis using RFLPs. An anonymous DNA probe (empty box) reveals the alternative restriction site configurations illustrated on the two chromosomes of a heterozygote. If this RFLP is located near a disease locus with the genotypes X (normal) and Z (abnormal), then for a given family the restriction patterns revealed by the anonymous probe are predictive of the genotypes XX, XZ, and ZZ. The accuracy of diagnosis depends on the degree of linkage (proximity of probe and disease locus), often expressed by a lod score. For certain genes such as that causing cystic fibrosis or sickle cell anemia there is linkage disequilibrium in the region, and the 11 kb fragment might always occur in phase with the normal allele X as shown, allowing diagnosis without determination of phase through a family study.

Fig. 14–10. Identifying disease loci by chromosome jumping. A known locus (black region) for which a probe is available can be utilized to characterize an unknown locus causing a particular phenotype (stippled region) through chromosome rearrangements that juxtapose the loci. Isolation of overlapping genomic DNA clones (chromosome walking) provides access to the unknown locus. This locus can then be definitively related to the phenotype by demonstrating linkage or linkage disequibrium with RFLPs (see Fig. 14–9) or by sequencing to demonstrate mutations using the polymerase chain reaction (see Fig. 14–11).

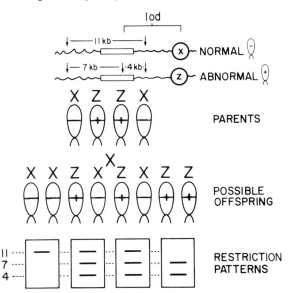

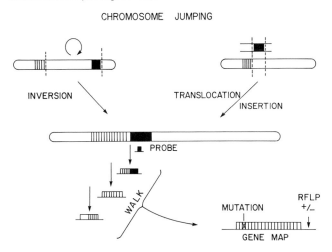

phenotype in question (see Identifying genetic loci through chromosomal rearrangements, below). DNA probes that detect RFLPS or VNTRs in the area of rearrangement can then be used for linkage studies in affected families. If no physical clue is available to guide linkage studies, then an assemblage of anonymous DNA probes that covers all 24 chromosomes must be tested until one probe exhibits linkage with the trait. This approach, using anonymous probes, is that outlined in the classic paper of Botstein et al.[17]

A recent example of linkage studies with DNA probes is the identification and characterization of the gene responsible for cystic fibrosis mutation. The approach first involved linkage of cystic fibrosis with anonymous DNA fragments on chromosome 7q, then the construction of a library of overlapping DNA segments from that chromosomal region, and finally the demonstration of expression, evolutionary conservation, and mutation of the putative cystic fibrosis gene[18]. Early experience with DNA diagnosis of cystic fibrosis using RFLP analysis demonstrated a phenomenon also evident at the β-globin and phenylalanine hydroxylase loci: a particular configuration of restriction sites occurred more frequently in individuals who had the abnormal mutation. If Figure 14–9 is examined once again, it can be seen that the 11 kb fragment happens to occur on the same chromosome as the X allele in this individual. Examination of unaffected and affected family members is necessary to determine this configuration (linkage phase), and the cosegregation of the 11 kb and X alleles may occur only within this family. If the two loci were equilibrated in the population, i.e., if there were no selective forces prohibiting their crossover or favoring their association, then families in which the 11 kb fragment is in phase with allele Z should be as frequent as families in which it is in phase with allele X. If this is not true, then the loci are in linkage disequilibrium (allele association), and a certain restriction fragment size becomes predictive for a genotype without the need for a linkage study to determine phase of marker and allele.

When several RFLPs are studied along a chromosomal region that exhibits disequilibrium, there is often a constellation of preferred restriction fragment sizes, referred to as a *haplotype* by analogy to the HLA locus. For example, if there are five RFLPs with the alternative fragment sizes a_1 and a_2, b_1 and b_2, and so forth, surrounding a locus of interest, then the abnormal genotype might be highly associated with the haplotype $a_1 b_2 c_1 d_2 e_1$. This highly specific combination among 2^5 possibilities would constitute very convincing evidence of allele association. The hemoglobinopathies illustrate the value of linkage disequilibrium, beginning with a specific *Hpa* I polymorphism that was predictive of the sickle cell mutation and continuing with highly specific haplotypes or "frameworks" of RFLPs that are predictive of various thalassemia mutations. In certain populations, the haplotype of RFLPs surrounding the α- or β-globin genes is so diagnostic that the gene mutation itself need not be verified.[19] The association of particular RFLP alleles with a certain trait suggests either genetic linkage or a pathogenetic relationship between the two loci. Known RFLPs from candidate genes may thus be initially evaluated for disequilibrium in individuals with a certain genetic or polygenic malformation without the need to evaluate family members. This approach has been applied to cleft palate as described below under Linkage, linkage disequilibrium, and homozygosity.

Identifying genetic loci using candidate genes

In several inborn errors of morphogenesis, a candidate gene may be implicated by the pathogenesis of the disorders. Examples include skeletal dysplasias such as osteogenesis imperfecta type I, which were long suspected to involve defects in collagen genes. Once a candidate gene is proposed, just as when an RFLP has been localized near a putative locus, a search for DNA alterations in affected patients must be conducted. One approach would be to examine affected patients for linkage disequilibrium of RFLP haplotypes surrounding the putative locus. This would confirm a relationship between locus and phenotype. A more direct approach involves screening for deletions of the locus in affected patients. Deletions will produce a strikingly rearranged restriction pattern by Southern blotting if the appropriate probes and restriction enzymes are used. It is too soon to know the overall frequency of gene deletions in human mutation—they range from about 50% in large genes like that causing Duchenne muscular dystrophy to a low percentage in the gene causing α_1-antitrypsin deficiency. If a deletion is not present, then demonstration of a mutation requires exhaustive DNA sequencing to look for single nucleotide or pauci-nucleotide changes. Fortunately, a new technology is available that greatly simplifies this approach and will find wide use in the detection and diagnosis of inherited malformations.

The polymerase chain reaction (PCR)[20] allows the amplification of a specific DNA region from a complex template such as human genomic DNA (Fig. 14–11). The method requires knowledge of the DNA sequence so that a pair of oligonucleotides can be synthesized that are complementary to each end of the target region. These oligonucleotides are oriented so that their 3′ ends will be facing each other and their 5′ ends will form the borders of the amplified DNA fragment (Fig. 14–11A). After the oligonucleotide primers anneal to the genomic DNA sample, one copy of the target region is synthesized using deoxynucleotides and a heat-stable DNA polymerase. The resulting duplexes are then heated to separate the strands and to allow a second cycle of primer annealing. During multiple cycles of heating and cooling, each amplified fragment in turn becomes a template and contributes to the chain reaction (Fig. 14–11A). The development of a heat-stable polymerase eliminated the need for new additions during each cycle and allowed the reaction to be mechanized. A new instrument, a thermal cycler, can produce up to 1 μg of a specific gene region from 0.5–1 μg of human genomic DNA in 3 hr. This represents over a 1 million-fold purification from surrounding sequences and can be performed on 20–30 different individuals simultaneously. Limitations of the PCR technique include the size of the fragment that can be amplified (less than 10 kb under most circumstances) and variable quantitation (the amount of amplified product is to always proportionate to the amount of initial template).

Most useful to date among the many applications of PCR is the ability to compare gene structure among individuals or species without the need for repetitive gene cloning. Once the gene sequence is defined using recombinant DNA clones from a single individual, oligonucleotide primers can be synthesized that allow study of that gene region in multiple individuals. Since the PCR product is abundant enough to be seen as a band after gel electrophoresis and ethidium bro-

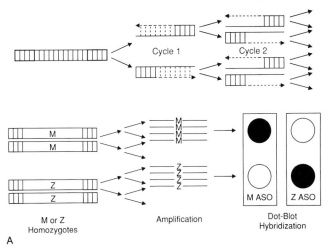

A

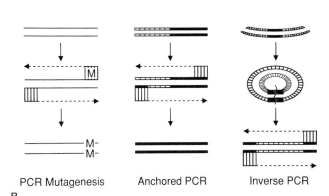

B

Fig. 14–11. The polymerase chain reaction. A. The basic PCR re-action is diagrammed showing a double-strand DNA segment with known sequence at both ends. Oligonucleotides (15–30 bp) comple-mentary to these end sequences can prime synthesis of an entire sec-ond strand using DNA polymerase or reverse transcriptase if the template is RNA. After the two strands are duplicated, a chain re-action can be initiated by incorporating successive cycles (20–30) of strand separation (heat denaturation), primer annealing, and poly-merization to amplify the initial two strands over 1 million-fold. B. PCR can be employed for the detection of alleles by employing bracketing primers to amplify the appropriate gene region, then ap-plying the amplified DNA to a membrane for "dot-blot" analysis.

Parallel incubation of duplicate blots with allele-specific oligonucle-otide probes (ASO) can distinguish genotypes by hybridization with M only (genotype *MM*), Z only (genotype *ZZ*), both (genotype *MZ*, data not shown), or neither (alternative alleles, data not shown). C. Variations of the PCR reaction, including primers engineered to produce a single base change in the amplified product (PCR muta-genesis), walking from a known region (filled lines) to an unknown end (stippled end) by attaching a synthetic primer (anchored PCR) and walking both directions from a known region by restriction, cir-cle formation, and polymerizing across the unknown region using primers for the known region (inverse PCR).

mide staining, deletions can be directly detected by noting an altered PCR product size. The PCR product can also be ap-plied to a nitrocellulose membrane in a dot-blot format and hybridized with allele-specific oligonucleotide probes as shown in Figure 14–11B. Rapid screening of many individ-uals for well-defined mutations such as the M, S, or Z alleles at the α_1-antitrypsin locus is then feasible. If there are no de-letions or altered restriction endonuclease sites detected within the PCR product, then DNA sequencing of the prod-uct may be performed to screen for single base pair changes. The PCR reaction itself may be used for sequencing by in-cluding an excess of one primer over the other to produce a single-stranded, asymmetrically labeled product.[20]

If the candidate gene has not yet been sequenced, then PCR can facilitate recombinant cloning using a partial amino acid sequence of the candidate gene product. Oligo-nucleotide mixtures based on possible coding sequences for the amino acids can be used to amplify a portion of the can-didate gene from a cDNA library.[20] Even though most of the degenerate oligonucleotides will not have the correct se-quence, a few correctly matched molecules are sufficient to prime amplification of a PCR product that will be specific for the gene in question. This product can then be labeled and used as a probe to isolate a complete cDNA molecule. After the cDNA has been characterized, specific regions of the gene can be examined for mutation in affected individuals using PCR. Although PCR is tremendously powerful in the detec-tion of well-characterized mutations, it is more cumbersome to scan large gene regions for novel mutations. The size limit of about 10 kb is particularly bothersome for large genes with numerous introns, although "multiplex" reactions employ-ing several sets of primers may allow simultaneous amplifi-cation and scrutiny of multiple exons.

PCR also is useful in identifying embryologically impor-tant genes in lower organisms so that they can be tested for structural and functional conservation in man. Since mis-matches of one base can be tolerated in either primer without altering the chain reaction, PCR can be used to introduce mutations into any cloned sequence for subsequent analysis in transgenic animals (Fig. 14–11C). As an example, the *Wnt*-1 protooncogene sequence was altered to increase or ab-late its expression in *Xenopus* oocytes and shown to have a role in embryonic axis determination.[21] In a similar manner, PCR allows detection of very small amounts of mRNA at early embryologic stages by employing reverse transcriptase and the appropriate oligonucleotide primers.[20] Once a gene has been shown to have an important role in the embryology of diverse organisms, its conservation in humans can be tested by Southern analysis under conditions of reduced hy-bridization stringency and then by PCR. Those regions of the gene that are shown to be conserved by Southern analysis can be used to prime the amplification and characterization of poorly conserved regions. Molecular analysis of the structure and variation of the corresponding human genes can then be conducted in the appropriate patients without the need for laborious cloning experiments.

Identifying genetic loci through chromosomal rearrangements

As diagrammed in Figure 14–10, the discovery of a chro-mosomal rearrangement in conjunction with an inherited condition provides both location of and access to the causa-tive gene. In lower organisms such as *Drosophila* or *C. ele-gans,* rearrangements of repetitive DNA elements called *transposons* may be induced at random and segregants screened for any morphogenetic phenotype. Since the phenotype will have been produced through disruption of the causative gene by a transposon, the latter becomes a "tag" for isolating the responsible gene. Transposon tagging has been utilized to isolate nematode mutations causing complex phenotypes such as *uncoordinated* for which pathogenesis and likely candidate genes were unknown.[22] In *Drosophila,* the homeobox was discovered by finding a fly with a homeotic phenotype produced by a pericentric inversion. The inversion transected the homeobox-containing gene and joined it with a known locus for which a probe was available. Using the approach diagrammed in Figure 14–10, the unknown locus (Antennopedia) was then characterized by isolating overlapping genomic clones extending from the known locus (chromosome walking).[22] Recently, a powerful transposon tagging system employing the *Drosophila* P element allowed the efficient isolation of any genetically determined phenotype in that organism.[22] These "chromosome jumping" techniques for juxtaposing known DNA with unknown morphogenetic mutations explain the rapid progress in the molecular embryology of lower organisms.

Genetic analysis of human dysmorphogenetic loci

After reviewing the technology for characterizing altered DNA structure, it can be seen that inherited malformations offer a powerful tool for unraveling the molecular developmental program. This does not diminish the considerable insights of teratogenesis, such as that provided by retinoid exposure in man, or the perspective of evolution in providing candidate genes for scrutiny in human developmental disorders. However, the large number of genetic malformations in man provides an immediate route to embryologically relevant genes. A recent survey[23] reveals the striking contribution of Mendelian genetics to human malformation. Review of the McKusick[2] catalog disclosed 1040 multiple defect syndromes and 721 isolated malformations that had been reported to follow a Mendelian pattern of inheritance. Of the nonchromosomal syndromes listed by Jones,[24] 176 had presumed Mendelian inheritance, 39 were of unknown etiology, and 11 were due to teratogens.[23] This list does not include the many single defects such as cleft palate that exhibit multifactorial etiology and thus probably involve one or more genetic loci of major effect. Also, the significant number of couples with infertility or multiple miscarriages not due to chromosomal or infectious causes undoubtedly will provide another source of developmentally significant mutations.

Linkage, linkage disequilibrium, and homozygosity

If a single malformation or syndrome has been shown to follow Mendelian inheritance, and families are available for study, then the array of approaches listed in Table 14–1 can be followed to identify the causative gene. These approaches will be laborious for the next few years, but will be greatly facilitated when a complete sequence and set of probes representing the entire human genome are available. The mapping approach involves linkage of a genetic malformation to a specific gene or chromosomal region. Once the genomic region is identified, more refined analysis can pinpoint the particular gene(s) involved. Early examples involved the use of polymorphic proteins, such as the linkage of nail-patella syndrome and ABO blood type loci discussed above. The utility of DNA markers is illustrated by progress in the genetic and physical mapping of neurofibromatosis.[25] Several chromosome regions were first excluded as the site of the NF-1 gene by an international collaborative study employing both conventional markers and RFLPs. As genetic mapping converged on the 17q region, two balanced translocations localized the NF-1 gene to 17q11 and provided a physical means of ordering nearby RFLPs. It is clear that a dominant disorder such as neurofibromatosis, with its relatively high frequency and multigenerational pedigrees, is a more tractable example than will be many rare or recessively inherited malformations.

The extensive genetic map compiled for the X chromosome has also been used to good advantage in localizing certain inborn errors of morphogenesis. X-linked hypohidrotic ectodermal dysplasia has been localized to the Xq11–Xq21.1 region by linkage with several anonymous RFLPs and a balanced X/9 translocation.[26] The Lowe oculocerebrorenal syndrome has been linked to the anonymous RFLP DXS42 near Xq24–26.[27] A balanced translocation has also helped to localize this disorder to the Xq25 region. Closely linked RFLPs for many other X-linked malformation syndromes are also available, including fragile X, nonspecific X-linked mental retardation, and severe combined immunodeficiency syndromes. A notable application of DNA linkage has focused on an X-linked form of ankyloglossia and secondary cleft palate.[28] Utilizing a large Icelandic pedigree, linkage to probes in the Xq21 region has been accomplished and substantiated by the presence of an interstitial deletion at this region in one affected individual. This approach to a gene involved in palatal fusion can be contrasted with that described next.

Ardinger et al.[29] have exploited the phenomenon of linkage disequilibrium to demonstrate an association of cleft palate with certain DNA polymorphisms surrounding the transforming growth factor-α (TGF-α) gene. Initial screening of 80 subjects with cleft palate and 102 unrelated controls using 12 RFLPs at five receptor or growth factor loci identified a disequilibrium at the TGF-α locus. Three RFLPS near the TGF-α gene were employed to assign haplotypes, and one (designated C2A2B2) was heterozygous in 16% and homozygous in 3% of cleft palate individuals compared with 5% and 1%, respectively, of control individuals.[29] It is not yet clear whether this is an association comparable to that between HLA B27 and ankylosing spondylitis or a linkage in the sense of proximity to or identity with a locus of major effect for cleft palate. Linkage studies in cleft palate families can now be performed to resolve this question. If linkage is confirmed, then a search for mutation can be conducted by the methods described below. This is a first example of a molecular approach that in theory is applicable to any malformation/syndrome exhibiting polygenic or Mendelian inheritance for which suitable candidate genes are available.

A final approach for localizing dysmorphogenetic genes using RFLPs is to search for homozygosity. In tumors such as retinoblastoma an important molecular change accompanying carcinogenesis is the loss of heterozygosity at suppessor loci. A patient heterozygous for a suppressor gene mutation may develop active retinoblastoma through loss of the normal allele through deletion, recombination, or monosomy of the 13q14 region. At the molecular level, homozygosity can be recognized by RFLP identity under certain circumstances, and such techniques have revealed identity of 13q14 RFLPs in a patient's retinoblastoma tumor cells despite heterozygosity in constitutional DNA.[30] Such acquired homozygosity has become a potent indicator for tumor suppressor genes in other tumors. A similar approach is possible in two categories of inherited birth defects. The first is exemplified by two patients with cystic fibrosis and unusually severe growth retardation who had uniparental disomy for chromosome 7.[31] Such occurrences may be reasonably common and produce a homozygous chromosome region that can be related to the presence of an inherited malformation. If these chromosomal regions are also subject to imprinting, there may be atypical malformations or growth delay in addition to the inherited defect. The second approach derives from the observation of Greenberg et al.[32] based on the theory of Lander and Botstein.[33] Individuals afflicted with recessively inherited malformations and consanguineous parents will have homozygosity surrounding the causative locus due to common descent. Several such parent–offspring groups will suffice to map the abnormal, homozygous region using a panel of RFLPs.

Chromosomal rearrangements

For humans, one is dependent on serendipity to obtain informative rearrangements, but recent advances illustrate Pasteur's comment that "fortune favors the prepared mind." Several inherited malformation syndromes for which the presumptive genes have been localized by balanced translocations are listed in Figure 14–16, below. These include Greig syndrome, Ivemark syndrome, and certain X-linked disorders as discussed above. Interstitial deletions of chromosomes have also been useful in relating malformation phenotypes to specific chromosomal regions. The association of Langer-Giedion syndrome with region 8q, of Prader-Willi and Angelman syndromes with 15q, of Miller-Dieker syndrome with 17p, and of DiGeorge anomaly with 22q all exemplify the rewards of careful cytogenetic analysis (Fig. 14–16). Because many of these cytologically visible deletions span a region of sufficient size to include multiple loci, they produce "contiguous gene deletion" syndromes[34] and may represent aggregate phenotypes. Interstitial deletions of the X chromosome in males are particularly illustrative of this concept—a patient with Duchenne muscular dystrophy also had adrenal hypoplasia and McLeod phenotype due to X chromosome deletion.[35] Deletions producing chondrodysplasia punctata[36] and/or combining X-linked adrenoleukodystrophy with color blindness have also been described.[37] The opportunity provided by these rearrangements is epitomized by cloning of the Duchenne muscular dystrophy gene. Worton et al.[38] exploited an X-autosome translocation that joined the Duchenne muscular dystrophy gene to ribosomal DNA, and Monaco and Kunkel[39] utilized the interstitial deletion described above[35] to enrich for the deleted genes in normal DNA. These advances certainly justify prometaphase karyotyping of selected patients with genetic malformation syndromes. Although such studies should certainly be classified as research, the eventual value to all patients invites their inclusion under a "molecular correlations" category in cytogenetic laboratory budgets as a necessary tool for maintaining technical competence and modern service. A caveat in the use of chromosomal rearrangements is to distinguish single gene effects from those due to cytogenetically unbalanced duplications and deletions.

Identification of human dysmorphogenetic loci using developmentally relevant genes in lower organisms

The finding that genes of significance in the embryology of lower organisms may exhibit sequence similarity to those of man offers a singular opportunity for understanding human malformations. The terms *homology* and *homolog* are used only to indicate sequence similarity; they do not here imply common descent. It should be recognized that exon shuffling and gene duplications can produce sequence similarities between genes that have no ancestral or functional relationship. Similarities produced by these processes can be termed *paralogies,* but this distinction is not relevant in a brief review. It is important to recognize, however, that sequence similarities among genes imply no conservation of the embryologic mechanisms that they regulate. The finding of human homeobox genes similar in sequence and arrangement to their homologs in *Drosophila* does not imply a similar developmental role. The wide phylogenetic distance and difference in embryology between these organisms almost guarantees altered function. Even highly conserved embryologic processes such as gastrulation must be stringently examined at the molecular level: does gastrulation reflect common inheritance of an extremely efficient device or convergent demand for apposing nonequivalent cell layers in embryos? Gerhart[40] suggests that mechanisms for gastrulation are really quite heterogeneous across phyla. Another example may be the two-dimensional "discs" for pattern generation in tissues ranging from the *Drosophila* imago to mammalian primitive streak or limb differentiation; this may reflect a common need for diffusable signals or a two-coordinate system for specifying positional information.[41] The molecules involved may be quite different. Elinson[42] has also challenged conventional wisdom regarding the conservation of early embryogenesis. The use of model systems such as *C. elegans* for all nematodes, *Mus musculus* for all mammals, and so forth, also may give the erroneous impression of conservation. Yet there are enormous differences in the early development of vertebrates, illustrated nicely by Elinson's comparison[42] of early development in three vertebrates—salamander, chick, and human.

Despite these caveats, DNA sequence homology offers the brightest hope for molecular insights into human malformations. That genes of similar structure are involved in the embryology of diverse phyla, that the mouse has become an embryologic *E. coli* to be manipulated at will, foreshadow a golden age of human dysmorphology.

Gene families in development

Several genes that regulate embryogenesis in lower organisms have homologs in the mammalian genome (Table 14–4).[43] Two themes unite these different sequences, that of DNA-binding proteins and that of protooncogenes or growth

Table 14–4. Gene families in development[a]

Domain(s)	Human	Mouse	Xenopus	Drosophila	C. elegans
Homeobox	S, E	S, E, F	S, E, F	S, E, F	
Paired box		S, E,	S	S, E, F	
Zinc finger	S	S, E,	S	S, E,	
EGF cassettes	S, E, F	S, E, F		S, E, F	S, E, F (lin-12)
Wnt-1	S, E	S, E	S, E, F (axis)	S, E, F (wingless)	
c-rel	S	S		S, E, F (dorsal)	

[a]S, structural homology; E, embryonic expression; F, embryologic function.

factors. Several families of homeobox genes are known in *Drosophila,* including those characteristic of the Antenno-pedia and Bithorax clusters, of the engrailed or paired genes, and of the caudal maternal effect gene. The hunchback and Kruppel genes of *Drosophila* contain a second family of DNA sequences called a *zinc finger* region, which was first recognized in the *Xenopus* transcription factor IIIA.[43] There is a close relationship among the various *Drosophila* ho-meobox genes and transcription factors, such as the Oct-2 protein, which regulates mammalian immunoglobulin syn-thesis; all are DNA-binding proteins, and many autoregulate their own expression. It is also clear that DNA-binding pro-teins have general regulatory functions that may not relate specifically to embryonic development. Again it must be stressed that the finding of sequence similarity does not imply functional homology.

If one views homeotic genes as mediating switches be-tween alternative developmental states (i.e., antennae to legs), then this category includes the *Notch* locus in *Drosoph-ila,* which mediates an early choice between nerve and epi-thelial cell states.[44] The *Notch* gene contains highly charac-teristic cysteine-rich repeating units that were first discovered in epidermal growth factor and later demonstrated in the het-erochronic *lin*-12 gene of *C. elegans.*[44] A view of homeotic genes as growth factors fits with the induction of products containing homeobox domains by retinoic acid in mouse te-ratocarcinoma cells or during amphibian limb regenera-tion.[45] Furthermore, several genes first discovered through their role in tumorigenesis have been shown to have key roles in development (Table 14–4). An attractive parallel between *Wnt*-1 protooncogene function and symmetry—segment polarity in *Drosophila,*[43] axis formation in *Xenopus,*[21] and situs in man—is discussed below. The early pattern gene *dor-sal* in *Drosophila* is homologous to the protooncogene *c-rel.*[43] These homologies raise the exciting prospect that several candidate genes are in hand that can be matched with human malformation syndromes. A caveat to this approach is to re-alize that most of the pattern genes defined in lower organ-isms have been lethal mutations, a fact that should focus at-tention on chromosomally normal human abortuses as much as liveborn malformed infants. Transgenic experi-ments in mice and frog oocytes should aid in the matching of pattern genes discovered in lower organisms with their phe-notypes in humans. To interpret and guide such endeavors properly, it is worthwhile to consider some properties of de-velopment in these lower organisms with an eye to their dif-ferences from humans. An excellent summary of these dif-ferences from the viewpoint of genetics can be found in the text by Wilkins.[22]

Model systems

Caenorhabditis elegans

Caenorhabditis elegans is a free-swimming nematode that was developed as a biological system by Sidney Brenner and his colleagues (for reviews, see refs. 22, 46). The organism measures about 1 mm in adult life and consists of several thousand cells. It is sexually dimorphic but normally repro-duces as a self-fertilizing hermaphrodite with five pairs of au-tosomes and two X chromosomes. Male offspring arise through nondisjunction of the X chromosomes, the key de-termining factor apparently being a 5/1 rather than a 5/2 au-tosome/sex chromosome ratio. The *C. elegans* haploid ge-nome contains 8×10^7 bp and has over 1000 identified genes that have been mapped to the six chromosomes. Embryogen-esis includes four larval stages lasting about 10 hr at room temperature, and the transparent embryo has allowed exten-sive visualization of cell lineage so that the pathway from zy-gote to each adult cell is precisely known. Additional advan-tages include rapid genetic crosses (3 days), an overlapping cosmid library from which any genomic region can be iso-lated, and the occurrence of transposons every four cosmid lengths that provide physical markers and a route to charac-terizing morphogenetic mutations.

The facility of genetic and cell lineage manipulation in *C. elegans* has allowed the characterization of mutations affect-ing almost every aspect of development. From 200 to 1100 mutatable loci in this estimated 4000 locus genome affect early embryogenesis and are of maternal effect; the genotype of the mother determines the phenotype of her offspring. The first maternal effect mutation to be analyzed was actually in a mollusk and specifies the direction of shell coiling.[22] Strict maternal effect mutations are required only during early em-bryogenesis and cannot be rescued by normal paternal al-leles. Partial maternal effect mutations can affect both early and later stages of embryogenesis and exhibit paternal rescue (i.e., 100% normal offspring with homozygous normal fa-ther, 50% normal with heterozygous father). An interesting phenomenon of maternal effect genes is that expression of both diploid copies may be required for normal function, re-flecting perhaps the requirement for abundant gene product in the oocyte. The *par* maternal effect mutations of *C elegans* cause the normal asymmetry of the first egg cleavage to be-come symmetric. In the most severe mutants, the lack of ini-tial asymmetry produces a disorganized ball of cells that ar-rests at the 1000 cell stage. Less severe mutants produce disordered migration of germ cells and a phenotype of female or male sterility. More than 60% of mutations affecting early embryogenesis in *C. elegans* present the latter phenotypes, a fact that should be remembered when considering causes of human infertility and early miscarriages.

Other mutations of interest in *C. elegans* include the *glp*-1 mutation, which alters the lineage derived from the AB cell, the larger of the asymmetric daughter cells generated by the first egg cleavage. Mutation of the *glp*-1 product causes AB pharyngeal precursors to become nerve cells instead, a switch characteristic of homeotic mutations. The *lin*-12 mutation mediates cell-type switching between vulvar cell precursors and, as described above, has been cloned to reveal homology to epidermal growth factor. The *mab*-5 mutation affects multiple cell lineages that comprise posterior structures. This mutation thus has the characteristic that might be expected for a gene regulating a code for positional information, and its molecular structure should be most interesting. Finally, the *ced* mutants are among an interesting series of mutations affecting neurogenesis in *C. elegans.* This primitive nervous system contains only 302 neurons but includes 118 cell types. Since the effect of each mutation can be mapped precisely in terms of nerve cell lineage, they may provide models for examining nerve interactions in human retardation syndromes. Because nearly 20% of developing nerve cells undergo cell death during *C. elegans* development, mutations that altered this cell death pattern produced easily visible phenotypes. Certain of these *ced* mutants also alter cell death in other tissues, suggesting that cell death involves a common pathway applicable to all cells in this organism. It will be fascinating to search for homologs of these genes in mammals since it has been hypothesized that cell death, like cell growth, may be regulated by highly conserved protooncogenes.

Drosophila

The control of segmentation in *Drosophila* represents the premier achievement of molecular developmental biology, and the rapid progress in this genetically manipulable organism will undoubtedly present many more candidate genes of possible relevance to man. Like *C. elegans, Drosophila* embryogenesis involves a series of larval forms but has vastly increased complexity. The first larval stage has over 10,000 cells compared with the 2500–3500 in *C. elegans,* and the *Drosophila* adult has over 1 million cells. The *Drosophila* genome has 1.65×10^8 bp, more than twice the size of *C. elegans,* and an estimated 10,000 complementation groups. There are three autosomes and one pair of sex chromosomes with sexual reproduction. The maternal RNA in the *Drosophila* egg has a complexity equal to 10% of the genome, and the early part of embryogenesis is totally dependent on the oocyte genome. Zygote expression begins during the formation of a peripheral syncytium of nuclei in the egg cytoplasm; more than 13 divisions occur without segregation of cytoplasm, resulting in a final number of 4600–6300 nuclei per embryo. Membranes proliferate and surround the nuclei to produce the cellular blastoderm (about 3.5 hr postfertilization) followed by gastrulation and differentiation to produce the first larval stage (instar). The first instar larva (imago) hatches from the egg case at about 24 hr after fertilization, and during each of three larval stages certain regions, called *imaginal discs,* proliferate but remain undifferentiated. The imaginal discs are diploid compared with the bulk of larval tissues, which are polyploid, and these are the source of many adult structures formed during the final stage of metamorphosis.

As in *C elegans,* at least 10% of the loci in *Drosophila* are thought to be expressed in the oocyte; i.e., they will present as strict or partial maternal effect mutations.[22] Several of these loci are essential for determining early egg pattern and for specifying the coordinates upon which later compartments and segments are based. While studies on other insects first presented evidence for two polar centers that specify anterior and posterior regions of the egg, it was the elegant genetic analysis of Nusslein-Volhard et al.[47] in *Drosophila* that clarified the mechanisms and structure of the genes involved. Removal of cytoplasm from the anterior or posterior egg poles has global effects on *Drosophila* embryogenesis, while removal of lateral cytoplasm has little effect. If anterior cytoplasm is replaced by that from the posterior pole, an embryo with two "tail" regions results; a complementary experiment produces the opposite phenotype. Corresponding to the surgical effects of the polar regions are a group of mutations, i.e., *bicaudal, caudal,* that abolish the ability of the anterior pole to direct formation of anterior structures. Other groups of mutations, i.e., *oskar* (lacking posterior structures) or *dorsal* (lacking dorsal structures), affect the posterior, dorsal, or ventral egg determinants. The molecular mechanisms of these egg pattern genes is yet to be defined. Most exhibit maternal effect, and two have interesting DNA sequence regions—a homeobox domain in the *caudal* gene and homology to the *c-rel* protooncogene in the *dorsal* gene, as mentioned above.

Once the egg coordinates are determined, a new group of genes act to subdivide the embryo into smaller compartments. Each segment of the mature fly is composed of an anterior and posterior compartment that reflects the combined expression of different sets of gap, pair-rule, and segmentation genes. Gap gene mutations (*Kruppel, hunchback, knirps*) delete contiguous groups of segments—their products are expressed over large regions. Pair-rule genes (*paired, engrailed, fushi tarazu*) interfere with the specification of anterior and posterior compartments—they often produce half the number of segments. Finally, the segment polarity genes (*wingless, gooseberry, hedgehog*) establish the orientation of anterior and posterior compartments. The *wingless* mutation produces a mirror-image duplication of the posterior compartment in each segment, thus ablating the anterior thoracic segment compartment that forms the wings. As mentioned above, certain of these genes have zinc finger regions, homeodomains, and homologies to mammalian protooncogenes that make them of potential relevance to higher organisms (Table 14–4).[43]

After the number of orientation of body segments have been determined, the classic homeotic loci act to specify the identity of each segment. These genes were first identified by their mutational phenotypes. The geneticist Bateson first named them *homoeotic* mutations to indicate that they replace one body structure with a normal structure drawn from another body region. The shortened term *homeotic* mutation is now applied rather broadly to mutations that substitute one cell fate for another.[44] Insects may be susceptible to morphologic substitutions, since a phenocopy (heteromorphosis) occurs during crayfish regeneration where an amputated antenna may be replaced by a leg.[1] When the two major clusters of homeotic genes were cloned by utilizing chromosome rearrangements, their structure revealed some striking correlations. First, the number of homeotic genes correlated exactly with the number of body segments. Second, the order of genes on the chromosome and their temporal expression during embryogenesis observed the same linear order as the segments that they controlled. This supported the combinatorial model that Lewis had deduced from genetic experiments—the most anterior segment requires expression of gene "a" to specify its identity; the next, "a + b"; the next, "a + b + c"; and so forth. The third correlation was an amino acid domain (about 60 amino acids or 180 bp of DNA) shared by most of the homeotic loci. This expressed region, the homeobox, was later shown to be present in some of the early egg pattern genes (*caudal*) as well as numerous other organisms from *Xenopus* to mouse to humans. Furthermore, the homeobox is representative of a diverging gene family, since other *Drosophila* segmentation genes such as *engrailed* or *paired* have a slightly different version of the homeodomain. These latter domains are also found in higher organisms, although their organization is less well characterized. The organizations of the Antennopedia homeobox genes (class I homeobox) in mouse and human show the same striking features as their *Drosophila* homologs: they are spaced at similar intervals along the chromosome, and their linear order predicts their temporal order of expression in the embryo.[48] Also similar is the fact that mammalian homeobox expression is primarily in the nervous system like those of *Drosophila;* the expression of one HOX3 locus (mouse loci are abbreviated Hox; human loci, HOX) is confined to a specific region of the human embryonic spinal cord.

Mus musculus

Higher mammals have two sex-specific stages of germ cell maturation, that producing primary oocytes or spermatocytes and that producing gametes at sexual maturity. Mouse primary germ cells are present in the allantois at 7.5 days postconception; they then migrate through the hindgut and up the dorsal mesentery to the germinal ridge. By 11 days postconception they have expanded from 10–100 cells to the 2500–3500 oogonia or spermatogonia, which will fuel subsequent reproductive cycles. During each mouse cycle, small groups of oocytes and follicular cells are stimulated to enlarge and synthesize a large component of maternal RNA. Proportionally more mouse oocyte RNA (10%) is stored as messenger RNA than in the oocyte RNA of sea urchins or frogs (about 1%). Early cleavage in mouse and other mammals is complete (holoblastic) and symmetric; it involves rotation of the cleavage axis at the two-cell stage when one blastomere divides longitudinally and the other equatorially. Another characteristic event of mammalian development is "compaction" of the eight cell morula to form a more spherical cluster. By 3.5 days, the morula has developed into a blastocyst with an outer trophectoderm (TE) of about 45 cells and an inner cell mass (ICE) of 15 cells. Also unique in mammals is a rapid degradation in oocyte RNA corresponding to relatively early activation of the zygotic genome; by 24 hr postfertilization there is a 40% decline in maternal RNA, which reaches 60% by the blastocyst stage. The zygotic genome is activated by the two cell stage, suggesting that strict maternal effect mutations will be rare in mammals—those that occur

may be partially rescued by normal paternal gene (zygotic) expression.

Subsequent events in mouse development include primitive streak formation by 6.5 days and completion of organogenesis by 14 days in a 21 day gestation period. Atypical in mouse embryogenesis relative to other mammals is the inversion of germ layers, which occurs at the "egg cylinder" stage (about 6 days).[21] While such differences and 70 million years of evolutionary distance complicate comparisons of mouse and humans, the ability to manipulate cells and genes in mouse embryos is a great attribute of this experimental system. Over 300 inbred lines are available that allow pure mutant "cultures," and almost 1000 loci have been mapped to the 20 mouse chromosomes. The haploid DNA content (3×10^9 bp) is equivalent to that of man and represents a 20-fold jump in complexity over that of *Drosophila*. An unusual feature of rodent genomes is a large α-satellite gene family, which comprises 10% of the DNA. Otherwise, many loci mapped in both mouse and human are syntenic—they occupy homologous positions relative to each other and with regard to the respective chromosome maps. The potential for cellular and genetic manipulation of the mouse is now reviewed (and is summarized in Fig. 14–12).

The frequent appearance of teratomas in certain inbred strains of mice has provided another method for constructing chimeras.[49] These teratomas gave rise to cell lines (embryonal carcinoma [EC] cells) that form derivatives of all three germ layers when cultured in vitro. The ability of EC cells to substitute for natural embryonic cells was demonstrated by numerous injection experiments. EC cells with several distinc-

Fig. 14–12. Manipulation of mouse embryogenesis to produce analogs of human diseases. First, embryo transfer allows development of foster pups in unrelated mothers to sort out genetic effects from maternal environment (left). Second, a cloned gene (black) can be introduced into unaffected animals (white) through oocyte injection, embryo transfer, and breeding of offspring to produce transgenic strains (left center). Third, blastocysts may be removed, dissociated to produce cultured embryonic stem cells, and subjected to mutagenesis through gene transfer or biochemical techniques (upper right). Mutated cells can then be reinjected into blastocysts to form chimeric offspring after embryo transfer (right center). The chimeras are then bred to yield stable transgenic lines with the desired phenotype (bottom center). Transgenes introduced into oocytes or embryonic stem cells may produce altered phenotypes through their own expression or through disruption of host genes at their site of integration.

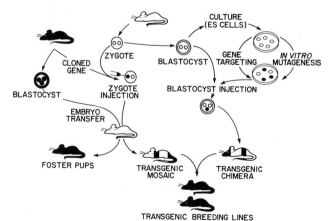

tive surface or enzymic markers provided the majority of tissues in one chimeric mouse embryo dubbed "Terry-Tom".[49] Unfortunately, the frequency of chimeric animals obtained using EC cells is a variable 5%–60%. The variability explains why attempts to construct mutants with this technique, such as an animal model for Lesch-Nyhan syndrome via injection of HPRT-deficient cells, have been frustrated because of correction by normal cells in the chimeras. An additional problem has been the establishment of breeding colonies with EC cell–derived chimeras. Because these cells generally have sex chromosome aneuploidy, their contribution to germ cells is very inefficient.

A more promising development for cell transplantation is the ability to culture embryo-derived totipotential cells (embryonal stem [ES] cells), which then form chimeras containing much higher proportions of donor cells in their tissues (Fig. 14–12, right). ES cells are derived from early blastomeres and have been shown to maintain their normal karyotypes in culture.[50] The attempt to construct a mouse with deficiency of HPRT was successfully performed by mutagenesis of ES cultures, injection of HPRT-deficient cells into blastocysts, and production of offspring with complete HPRT deficiency. Unfortunately, these mice have no neurologic symptoms analogous to human Lesch-Nyhan syndrome, perhaps indicating a difference in purine metabolism.[51] The chimeric animals did transmit the mutation, however, indicating that establishment of breeding mutant mouse lines was feasible with ES cells. Furthermore, HPRT-deficient ES cells can be corrected by transformation and homologous recombination with an intact HPRT gene. Theoretically, any mutation introduced into ES cells can be tested for viability and phenotype in whole animals through blastocyst injection and monitoring of embryos or offspring (Fig. 14–12). Breeding lines can then be established for mutations compatible with survival and fertility.

A third technique for manipulating mouse embryogenesis is through gene transfer. Recombinant retroviral infection of embryos, direct injection of DNA into a pronucleus of the zygote, or introduction of recombinant DNA into embryonic stem (ES) cells are the three current methods for constructing transgenic mice (Fig 14–11).[51] Recombinant molecules have also been successfully introduced into EC cells, but the lack of germ cell colonization in chimeras derived from EC cell lines has limited the usefulness of this approach. Microinjection of cloned DNA into the egg pronucleus usually produces up to 100 head-to-tail repeated copies of the transgene at a single site on the host genome. Although transfection is highly efficient and stable, expression is high in most derived tissues, and germ cell uptake is achieved, the inserted sequences often catalyze rearrangement of host sequences at the site of integration. These rearrangements and the multiple transgene copies may complicate cloning of the chromosomal integration site. Retroviral introduction of foreign genes, on the other hand, targets a single copy of the transgene to one chromosomal site with minimal rearrangement. Blastocysts may be exposed directly to virus or cocultivated with viral-infected cells before transfer to pseudopregnant animals. Cloning of the integration site is much easier, but germ line uptake is poor. DNA transfection or retroviral transduction may also be used to introduce transgenes into ES cells, and access to the germ line has been demonstrated. Further work with this promising system is required to ascertain its efficiency of integration and expression.

In addition to revealing signals for tissue-specific gene expression, transgenic constructs have provided markers for certain chromosomal regions and cell lineages in the embryo. Transgenes inserted into specific X chromosome regions can be assessed for inactivation and have provided proof for a pseudoautosomal region of the X that escapes inactivation. Genomic imprinting has been studied using transgenes that become differentially methylated and/or transcribed according to whether they are transmittted from the father or mother. Comparison of the transgene and its flanking host sequences for these characteristics should clarify the extent and nature of the imprinting process.[51] Lineage studies may be done simply by marking a blastomere with proviral gene copies and noting the distribution of this marker at later embryonic stages. One experiment in this vein produced an estimate of 8 ICM cells that give rise to the entire mouse embryo. More complex strategies place a toxic gene in precursor cells such that offspring have ablated tissues corresponding to their derived lineage. Inducible toxins would allow such studies to be extended to cell lineages that are essential for survival. A similar functional strategy has been used to augment embryonic growth through transgenic growth hormone genes or to produce tumors through transgenic oncogenes.

Homologous dysmorphogenetic loci in humans and mouse

Any review of murine genetic disease should begin by mentioning the "mouse clinic" held annually at the Jackson Laboratories.[52] The extensive linkage group conservation between the human and mouse genetic maps offers hope that many homologous mutations will exist even if their terminal phenotypes are quite different. A mouse with muscular dystrophy has already been discovered, and conservation of the X chromosome among all mammals indicates that many more homologous X-linked mutations will be found. Even though the mouse HPRT deficiency does not reproduce the human neurologic symptoms, it has been useful in designing strategies for gene replacement by homologous recombination. Mouse homologs of human genetic malformations that have not yet been mapped can potentially be used to identify and isolate the corresponding human genes.

The many genetic loci described in mice (about 1100) represent about one-fourth of the genetic diseases described in humans after many more years of detailed scrutiny.[52] Although the initial murine mutations presented obvious changes in external appearance, recent biochemical screening after large-scale mutagenesis has extended the spectrum of recognized genetic disease. For example, five mutations at the catalase locus were discovered after biochemical screening of 12,306 progeny from irradiated fathers. Some mouse diseases have been recognized before their human counterparts, such as a form of inherited microcytic anemia. Others have been constructed based on the human mutation. The mouse procollagen $\alpha 1$ gene was altered by in vitro mutagenesis to contain a single nucleotide substitution identical to that causing type II osteogenesis imperfecta in humans. Expression of the altered mRNA even at a 10% level in transgenic mouse caused a dominant perinatal lethal condition quite similar to the human disease.[51] Mouse diseases imitating human diabetes, exocrine pancreatic deficiency, androgen resistance (testicular feminization), pituitary dwarfism, hypothyroidism, T- and B-cell immune deficiences, anemias, thalassemias, hemoglobinopathies, muscular dystrophies, and neurologic degenerative diseases have all been recognized. The fact that phenotypes are different between organisms may even be an advantage if the mutation affects homologous gene regions. Defining the reasons for milder symptoms and later onset in the mdx mouse, despite its genetic identity to certain human Duchenne muscular dystrophy mutations, may give insight into therapy of the human disorder.

Extensive homology between malformation syndrome affecting mouse and humans is documented by Winter[53] (Table 14–5). Numerous mouse mutants cause defects of the neural tube or caudal skeleton. The prevailing defect is a shortened tail, but associated sacral defects may provide human correlations. Danforth's *short tail,* for example, may have renal agenesis, anal atresia, and missing sacral vertebrae reminiscent of human caudal regression. Mutations of the T locus on chromosome 17 also fall into this category. Mouse mutations affecting the axial skeleton resemble human disorders of segmentation such as the Jarcho-Levin syndrome, while those affecting limbs resemble many human defects including the autosomal recessive Roberts syndrome (Table 14–5). *Limb deformity* (*ld*) is similar to Cenani-Lenz syndrome in humans while *oligosyndactyly (Os)* with concurrent kidney hypoplasia is reminiscent of human acrorenal syndromes.

A variety of craniofacial syndromes have been defined in mice that include the *extra toes* (*Xt*) mutation with polydactyly and facial clefts reminiscent of human Greig syndrome (Table 14–5).[53] The *first arch* mutation (*far*) may be expressed asymmetrically on suitable backgrounds and resem-bles human hemifacial microsomia. Mouse skeletal dysplasias include models for osteopetrosis, cleidocranial dysplasia, achondrogenesis, and osteogenesis imperfecta; mutants producing ectodermal abnormalities are also of interest because of the variety of mechanisms responsible. *Dominant megacolon* (*Dom*) is similar to human Waardenburg syndrome and suggests neural crest alteration, *Tabby* (*Ta*) involves a pure X-linked ectodermal dysplasia, and *sparse fur* (*spf*) is the mouse version of human ornithine transcarbamylase (OTC) deficiency (Table 14–5). Two mouse syndromes are associated with situs defects, but unfortunately only the *iv* mutant has been well characterized. Winter[53] has made an important contribution in noting over 80 syndromes with mouse/human homology, and his computerized malformation data bases for both mouse and humans will aid in future comparisons.

Production of malformation syndromes in transgenic mice

Specific transgenic mouse models with implications for human morphogenesis are as yet few but illustrate the tremendous potential of this approach. Of interest in the latter regard are the production of mice with conditions resembling human hamartoses (syndromes with multiple benign and malignant growths). Multiple hemangiomas were produced by the introduction of polyomavirus into germ line cells, skin tumors were produced in bovine papillomavirus transgenic animals, and neurofibromas were produced by a human T-cell leukemia viral transgene.[51] The resemblance of the latter transgenic mouse to human neurofibromatosis emphasizes the relevance of transgenic technology to human genetic disease and dysmorphology. Also important are strategies for introducing expressed copies of genes that are known to be

Table 14–5. Parallels between human and murine malformation syndromes[a]

Malformation type	Mouse	Human
Neural tube/sacral defects	*Bent tail (Bt)*	Spina bifida
	Loop tail (Lp)	Caudal regression
	Danforth's *short tail (Sd)*	
	Splotch (Sp)	
	Curly tail (ct)	
Axial defects	*Rib-fusion (Rf)*	Jarcho-Levin (AR)
	Malformed vertebrae (Mv)	Spondylocostal dysplasias (AD, AR)
	Amputated (am)	
Limb defects	*Limb deformity (ld)*	Cenani-Lenz (AR)
	Luxoid (lu)	Limb defects
	Strong's luxoid (1st)	
	Oligosyndactyly (Os)	Acrorenal syndromes
Craniofacial defects	*Extra toes (Xt)*	Greig syndrome (AD)
	First arch (far)	Hemifacial microsomia
Pigmentary anomalies	*Dominant megacolon (Dom)*	Waardenberg syndrome (AD)
	Piebald (s)	Piebald trait (AD)
Polyasplenia/situs defects	*Situs inversus viscerum (iv)*	Kartagener syndrome (AR)
	Visceral inversion (vi)	Ivemark syndrome (AR)
Ectodermal defects	*Bare patches (bpa)*	Chondrodysplasia punctata (XL)
	Pupoid (pf)	Cocoon fetus (?AR)
	Tabby (Ta)	Christ-Siemens-Touraine (XL)
	Sparse fur (spf)	OTC deficiency (XL)

[a]For the mouse, lower case symbols imply recessive mutants, upper case dominant. *Bare patches, tabby* and *sparse fur* are X-linked. Human syndromes are listed as autosomal dominant (AD), recessive (AR), or X-linked (XL). Homology of the genes causing respective murine-human syndromes has only been proven for *sparse fur* and OTC deficiency.

important for the development of lower organisms. Balling et al.[45] have recently demonstrated that expression of a chimeric Hox 1.1 transcript (a fusion of the mouse homeobox 1.1 gene product with an actin promoter) produced offspring with craniofacial malformations resembling the *far* mutation. Of interest was the early demise of these offspring, which brings to mind the respiratory complications of first arch malformations in humans. Also reported but not commented on in their paper was the almost 100% affliction of F_1 offspring from transgenic mothers and the early embryonic expression of the Hox 1.1 transcript in these animals. Such characteristics are exactly those expected from an early pattern gene that is expressed in the oocyte and exhibits maternal effect. Similarity of these transgenic effects to the craniofacial malformations produced by retinoids in several species is also mentioned,[45] and this may correlate with the observation that Hox gene products are induced by retinoids in mouse teratocarcinoma cells.

In addition to rational strategies for examining candidate genes through functional transgene constructs, serendipitous mutations may be generated by transgene insertions. Production of an abnormal development phenotype by transgene insertion immediately provides a tag for characterization of the insertional mutation analogous to the "transposon tagging" discussed for lower organisms. An extremely interesting insertional mutant that illustrates the limits of clinical nomenclature is the Mov 13 strain produced by interruption of type I collagen sequences through insertion of a murine leukemia virus genome.[51] The proviral insertion alters DNA methylation and interferes with type I collagen transcription. In homozygous transgenic embryos, this mutation produces disruption of multiple blood vessels and is lethal by midgestation. Thus vascular disruption, a category of human dysmorphogenesis that usually implies sporadic etiology, may in fact be the end result of a Mendelian mutation. Another interesting transgenic insertion mutant was produced using a modified human myc oncogene.[54] Limb deformities were produced after the initial heterozygotes (one inserted copy) were bred to produce homozygotes (two inserted copies). The chromosomal insertion site was cloned and mapped to a region of mouse chromosome 2 where the recessive *limb deformity* locus (*ld;* Table 14–4) had been recognized by classic breeding studies. The spectrum of anomalies in the transgenic mice corresponded well with mutants at this classically defined locus, and a route to cloning the responsible allele(s) was provided.[54]

Clinical guidance of molecular applications

The importance of a clinical perspective is often neglected in the biological sciences, yet the contributions of clinical analysis to basic genetics and molecular biology are considerable. Garrod's concept of inborn errors, the molecular insights provided by sickle cell hemoglobin, and the recent renaissance of peroxisomes because of Zellweger syndrome are just a few examples. In the area of dysmorphology, one attempts to go beneath the surface complexity of malformations and recognize dysmorphogenetic mechanisms. The resulting concepts are best thought of as frameworks for organizing phenomena, undoubtedly imprecise and subject to modification as new data arise. For example, consideration of developmental hierarchy implies that early errors in embryo-

genesis may have multiple later consequences—hence the clinical concepts of sequence, malformation, disruption, and so forth, used to distinguish primary, intrinsic dysmorphogenetic processes from secondary, extrinsic ones. The user expects overlap of these processes in actual situations and imprecision once the cellular and molecular levels are reached, but the conceptual framework categorizes malformations and provides hypotheses for experimental exploration. Future directions in the molecular understanding of dysmorphology are now described according to four conceptual frameworks: pattern formation (or topogenesis), hierarchy, heterochrony, and homeostasis. These frameworks are proposed not as exclusive or exhaustive possibilities but as examples that may facilitate the analysis of human malformations.

Pattern formation in human embryogenesis

Three major aspects of morphogenesis are nicely summarized by Robert Steele[55] in a review of oncogenes and development. The form of an organism is determined by three chracteristics: the number of cell types, the amount of each cell type, and the arrangement of cell types in space. These characteristics depend on the corresponding processes of cell division, cell differentiation, and topogenesis or pattern formation. Each level of development, from the interactions of molecules to those of cell, organ, and organism, may be considered according to these frameworks of multiplication, transformation, and spatial arrangement. Remembering von Baer's laws, the most general characteristics of organisms are specified early in embryogenesis. The initial task of pattern formation, specifying the basic body plan, is thus an early part of the molecular program that will be shared by like organisms. As discussed previously, molecules responsible for early topogenesis in *Drosophila* are the egg and, when altered, present as maternal effect mutations.[47] Similar mutations affect related arthropods.[22] The genesis of each organ may also be considered an exercise in pattern formation that begins with a group of equivalent precursor cells. In larval organisms such as the *Drosophila* imago, undifferentiated regions (imaginal discs) are set aside that form new adult organs. In vertebrates, the limb buds represent a similar group of undifferentiated cells. These regions, like the initial zygote or morula, require some mechanism for spatial orientation. Pattern formation is a recurring theme in the embryo, and it is possible that a similar coding system is used to provide spatial orientation for diverse embryonic regions. This is the concept of positional information: "The rules, laws, or principles for the expression of genetic information in terms of pattern and form will be as general, universal, elegant, and simple as those that now apply to molecular genetics."[56]

Most embryologic systems will have preexisting constraints that specify pattern—the cytoplasmic organization and imprinted DNA of the oocyte are examples. Embryologic structures often begin as homogenous groups of cells within boundaries; it may be difficult to determine if ancestral differences among the cells or differences in the boundaries orient subsequent differentiation. Wolpert[56] has emphasized the importance of boundary regions and pointed out their special properties in various phyla. Their effects may include the high frequency of human midline defects[57] and phenomena such as interaction–interference in human twinning.[58] Can positional information arise de novo in a group of cells rather than being specified by prior (i.e., zygotic) organization? Theoretical models have shown that random variation in a few properties among a group of cells are sufficient to initate pattern. In 1952, Turing illustrated such effects based on chemical interaction–diffusion, and his model may explain the cyclic AMP–mediated aggregation of *Dictyostelium* cells during their initial aggregation en route to an organized fruiting body.[3] It is worth considering which human defects might involve disordered positional information rather than abnormal growth of differentiation. Particularly intriguing would be multiple anomaly syndromes with disordered pattern formation as a theme; the "disorganization" mutant in mice[53] might be one candidate.

As seen from the review of topogenesis in lower organisms, initial specification of the body plan in humans and other mammals is likely to occur early in development, perhaps even prior to fertilization. There is abundant messenger RNA in the mouse oocyte that may include the first instructions for anteroposterior, dorsoventral, and bilateral asymmetries that occur later in embryogenesis. Human conjoined twinning demonstrates that some positional information exists in the early embryonic disc, since the phenomenon of interaction–interference occurs if the two anteroposterior axes of conjoint twins are closely aligned.[58] It is important to recognize that alterations of the basic body plan are likely to present as early or undetected miscarriages (infertility) so that couples with these problems who have undergone negative screening for routine causes become candidate carriers of pattern gene mutations. If, as in lower organisms, some of these pattern genes are components of oocyte RNA, then they may exhibit strict or partial maternal effect and be present only in the female member of the couple under study. Certainly the presence of genes in the human genome that are homologous to those directing pattern in lower organisms provide intriguing candidate probes with which to analyze suspect couples and families.

Situs determination in humans is a good example of pattern formation. Situs abnormalities range from complete situs inversus to the polyasplenia spectrum, which includes anomalies of lungs, heart, intestine, and spleen.[59] At least two autosomal recessive conditions have been delineated with situs abnormalities—the Ivemark and Kartagener syndromes. The latter condition may be caused by abnormal cilia, but Ivemark syndrome patients as well as the phenotypically homologous *iv* mouse mutants do not have ciliary abnormalities. This suggests at least two types of genes involved in situs determination, and a recently observed family with a balanced translocation points to the location for one human gene. A mother and fetus had the same balanced 12/13 translocation, but only the fetus had malformations consistent with Ivemark syndrome.[60] The translocation breakpoints were at 13p13 and 12q13, marking the 12q13 breakpoint as the region of interest because 13p consists of repetitive DNA. If one assumes a causal rather than a chance association between translocation and phenotype, then the discordance in mother and fetus might be explained by unmasking of an autosomal recessive locus for Ivemark syndrome at 12q13. Another causal explanation for the phenotypic discordance would be that the rearranged gene at 12q13 exhibits maternal effect. Close to the 12q13 breakpoints are two genes homologous to those controlling segmentation in *Drosophila*—the HOX3 locus homologous to the Antennopedia homeobox and the human *Wnt*-1 locus homologous to

the segment polarity gene *wingless* (see Fig. 14–16, below). It is intriguing that increased *Wnt*-1 expression causes axis bifurcation in *Xenopus* embryos,[21] since translocation is a well-known route for activating oncogene expression in the development of certain cancers. Molecular characterization of the 12/13 translocation breakpoints should distinguish among these possiblities and perhaps identify a human gene of importance in early embryonic pattern and reproductive failure.

Hierarchy—the interpretation of morphologic complexity

Eldredge[61] has stressed the value of hierarchy in evolutionary thinking. He suggests two hierarchies of relevance, that of units (gene–organism–deme–species) and that of networks (protein–organism–population–community). Hierarchy in ontogeny is illustrated in Figure 14–13. An ontogenetic sequence (O), depicted as a progression from structure a to structure c, involves a cascade of intracellular and extracellular processes. Homeostatic networks of genes (G) and metabolites (M), like surface interactions or topologic constraints (T), are outside of cells. A mutation or teratogen affecting structure a will have necessary effects on b and c as well, including other structures that have a as precursor (represented by diverging arrows). One mutation can thus have multiple effects even if it is not pleiotropic in the genetic or biochemical sense: embryos are hierarchical systems that can amplify single insults, and phenotype is a compromise between these hierarchical effects and the constraints regulating them. In the peroxisomal disorders, the dysmorphologic consequences of hypotonia (bitemporal hollowing, tented upper lip) cannot be ascribed to a single gene per se, but reflect the hierarchical sequence of gene mutation–peroxisomal aberration–altered lipid metabolism–brain abnormality–hypotonia.[62] While obvious in some contexts, the hierarchical nature of embryogenesis must be explicitly stated to avoid oversimplification in others.

Because the clinician is forced to deal with dysmorphology from the "outside," attempting to work from phenotype to molecule or gene and not having the experimental luxury of following "inside" mutation to exterior phenotype, a descriptive nomenclature has been an inevitable and important tool in approaching malformations. Although clinical terms such as *the developmental field concept*[63] may attract hostility from molecular biologists because of their mechanistic imprecision, the recognition that certain malformations will occur together in different etiologic contexts is a hierarchical perspective important for classification.

As an example of the hierarchical mechanisms that separate malformations into categories for investigation, the term *dysplasia* has been particularly useful for molecular analysis. Dysplasias imply diffuse disorders of histiogenesis that are often conceptualized as derangements of structural molecules. Exploration of this category has rewarded biology with new molecular insights into development, highlighted by advances in the skeletal dysplasias. Mutations of the type I collagen genes in osteogenesis imperfecta have become prototypes for relating molecules to morphogenesis.[64] The pathway from the two genes proα_1 (COL1A1) and proα_2 (COL1A2), each with over 500 exons and complex RNA processing, to the procollagen chains cleaved by N-terminal protein processing, then to triple helix formation and assembly of collagen fibrils, and then to extracellular matrix synthesis

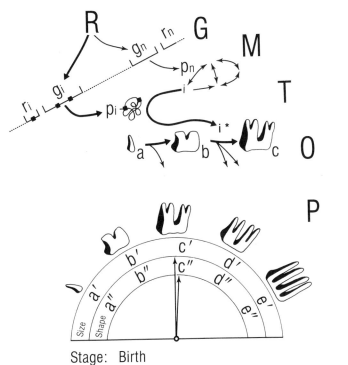

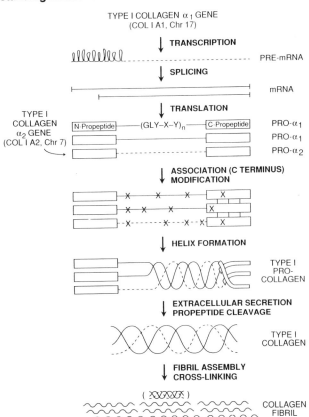

Fig. 14-13. Levels of developmental regulation. A hypothetical developmental sequence is shown (O) in which the precursor structure (a) progresses to more complex structure (b, c) through action of an invaginating factor (i*). Normal development in this species produces structure c at birth with size and shape coordinates c' and c". Changes in this developmental sequence can be represented by a modified clock model.[65] Earlier expression of factor i* will produce greater septation (i.e., coordinates d" or e") at a comparable developmental stage (birth is illustrated); delayed expression will produce a minimally septated structure (i.e., coordinates a", b"). Altered tissue response to i* or altered conversion of i to i* would produce equivalent changes, indicating that heterochrony is a mode of change that may encompass several mechanisms. The branching arrows in the developmental sequence indicate that derivative fields may also be influenced by factor i* because of the hierarchical nature of embryogenesis. Controls upon the final shape of structure c include regulation (R) of two genes (g_n, g_i) that mediate i activation, interactions at the gene level (G), metabolic networks of i-related molecules (M), and topologic constraints (T) that might influence the range of allowable septation, i.e., blood supply, tissue strength, external pressure. Heavy arrows highlight the major pathways by which factor i* expression can be altered (genes r_i and g_i controlling catalytic protein p_i) as opposed to modifying loci (r_n, g_n) conceived as having homeostatic functions. From Wilson.[66]

Fig. 14-14. Hierarchy of collagen gene expression. The type I collagen genes $pro\alpha_1$ (COL1A1) and $pro\alpha_2$ (COL1A2) encode the synthesis of pre-mRNAs with over 50 introns that are spliced to form mature mRNAs. Alternative splicing may result in mRNAs of different sizes. Procollagens with gly–X–Y amino acid repeats except for N- and C-terminal propeptides are translated. These associate in a triple helix consisting of 2 α_1 and 1 α_2 chains as directed by the conformation and structure of C-propeptides. Modifications consisting of sulfhydryl links, hydroxylations, and glycosylations then occur before movement to the Golgi apparatus for extracellular secretion. Once outside the cell, the propeptides are cleaved and the triple helices align into a larger repeating structure constituting the collagen fibril. Defects at each level of collagen expression are known and may be associated with "procollagen suicide" (destabilization of the triple helix through production of an abnormal procollagen precursor) or "hypermodification" if protein synthesis or secretion is slowed.

at the growth plates of cartilaginous bone provides numerous steps for mutations to produce the final common phenotype of bone fragility and thin sclerae (Fig. 14–14). In general, mutations that allow synthesis of a structurally abnormal $pro\alpha_1$ or $pro\alpha_2$ chain are more severe than mutations that decrease the amounts or ablate the synthesis of these chains. Synthesis of one abnormal collagen chain causes "protein suicide" by destroying the integrity of the triple helix and leading to degradation of both chains.[64] Thus, unlike the situation with many hemoglobinopathies and thalassemias, a point mutation affecting procollagen structure is often more severe than gene deletions or rearrangements that completely block transcription. Since the C-termini of procollagen molecules provide the nuclei for triple helix formation, mutations in these

regions cause the most severe forms of osteogenesis imperfecta. Mutations in the N-termini usually lead to the different phenotype of type VII Ehlers-Danlos syndrome. A further surprise from the molecular studies is that many severe cases of osteogenesis inperfecta, previously thought to be autosomal recessive, are actually instances of new mutations or germinal mosaicism with autosomal dominant inheritance. Thus the clinical delineation that provided the osteogenesis imperfectas for biochemical study gained an enormous return in diagnostic precision. The reciprocal value of clinical and scientific expertise is beautifully illustrated by the lessons of collagen metabolism.

As mentioned above, another group of dysplasias that emphasizes the need for a heirarchical view of morphogenesis is the peroxisomal disorders. First recognized as a disparate group of morphologic and/or biochemical alterations, these diseases were unified by the observation of peroxisomal deficiency in Zellweger syndrome.[62] The morphologic (brain, eye, ear, liver, kidney, bone defects) and metabolic (fatty acid, plasmalogen, bile acid, pipecolic acid, phytanic acid pathways) changes in Zellweger syndrome have become prototypic of a new category of recessive metabolic dysplasias that share deficiencies of multiple or pleiotropic peroxisomal proteins. Several of these disorders also have a common facial appearance and thus provide one of the first conditions in which dysmorphology may be explained at the biochemical and molecular levels. Molecular insights in this category again will provide a rich return on clinical investment. New concepts such as the intracellular topogenesis of peroxisomal proteins through a C-terminal tripeptide signal and the dual catalytic and structural roles of certain peroxisomal proteins provide new models for disease (for review, see ref. 62). It should be noted, however, that the metabolic dysplasias mainly affect fetal processes rather than embryonic ones. Understanding of early pattern formation is likely to come from other approaches.

Altered developmental timing—heterochrony

Heterochrony refers to a simple change in the timing of a developmental process. Minor changes in the timing of key events can produce striking asynchrony of the embryo. Delay or decreased action of a limb growth factor, for example, might produce an organism with drastically altered height and body proportions. Large changes in phenotype may be produced by subtle alterations in gene expression; from an evolutionary perspective, small inputs may lead to large outputs and produce discontinuous change.[65] A simple method for recognizing heterochrony is provided by the clock model of Gould.[65] The embryologic sequence (O) in Figure 14–13 reflects both growth and the action of an invaginating factor i to produce a septated structure. Progress in differentiation can be represented as a clockface with hands for size and shape—these follow the respective coordinates $a'c'$ and $a''c''$ as the gestation proceeds. Certain mutations in gene g_i might inactivate i and produce a developmental arrest with coordinates $c'a''$—a literal example might be lissencephaly, in which delay of septation relative to other developmental processes produces a brain typical of an earlier fetal stage. Numerous malformations resemble earlier embryonic structures and can be conceptualized as simple developmental arrests.[66] Alternatively, earlier activation or greater activity of factor i would produce a structure with accelerated septation (coordinates $c'e''$). Polymicrogyria would be the literal example of heterochrony by acceleration. The value of heterochrony as a concept is that it separates anomalies resulting from simple delay or acceleration of a developmental pathway from those of truly aberrant structure (not found in the normal embryo). A simple regulatory molecule such as a growth factor or hormone is implied for single malformations representing developmental arrests or for syndromes consisting mainly of growth asynchrony. In *C. elegans,* several heterochronic mutations have been characterized, including the *lin*-12 gene described above with sequences homologous to epidermal growth factor.[67] An example in humans may be the relation of Russell-Silver phenotype and the insulin-like growth factor-1 receptor (see below).

In addition to the large number of birth defects that present as developmental arrests, certain chromosomal and teratogenic disorders illustrate the operation of heterochrony by developmental retardation. Clinodactyly, certain dental anomalies, delayed maturation of liver function, delayed increase of somatomedin-like activity, and many other manifestations are typical of Down syndrome, and a delayed switch from fetal to adult hemoglobin, persisting hypersegmentation of neutrophils, and persistence of fetal muscles are typical of trisomy 13.[66] These multiple examples of asynchrony or dysmaturation in aneuploidy are consistent with the hypothesis of increased developmental variability from the perspective of time. While the imbalanced genome provides a route for molecular analysis in the chromosomal disorders, the phenomenon of heterochrony may provide an experimental approach in other syndromes for which no molecular defect is known. A relevant category would be the teratogenic disorders, since these must be understood through perturbation of the genetic program rather than by studying mutations.

Infants of diabetic mothers are known to experience a two- to three-fold increased risk for malformations, including developmental arrests such as holoprosencephaly.[66] Various other indices of delayed development include immature pulmonary surfactants, defective calcium homeostasis, persistent jaundice, and a delayed switch for fetal to adult hemoglobin. Fetal growth is delayed in both human and rodent diabetic pregnancy if poor control is manifested early; these are the fetuses at high risk for malformation. Developmentally regulated molecules such as renal β-glucuronidase in rodents provide markers for the teratogenic process through their altered developmental profiles.[68] In a sense, such developmentally regulated molecules are analogous to RFLPs in that their alternate states (delay vs. normal) may correlate with malformations, and they may be followed proximally to the primary events in embryogenesis that are responsible for asynchrony. Maternal serum α-fetoprotein is such a marker, since its increase is delayed (producing lower values at a given gestational age) in diabetic or chromosomally abnormal pregnancies. The perspective of heterochrony focuses molecular analysis on the primary causes producing developmental asynchrony (i.e., growth factors) rather than on a specific alteration of α-fetoprotein metabolism. Eventually, the primary causes of delayed fetal growth and development in early diabetic pregnancy may be discovered.

Homeostasis and the molecular analysis of aneuploidy

Developmental homeostasis has important consequences for both ontogeny and phylogeny. Morphologic change is not continuous and random, but constrained along certain channels allowed by the embryonic network comprising each organism. Waddington[7] referred to this as "canalization" and illustrated the concept as grooves on a surface that would constrain a rolling object from random direction. There is an attractive correlation between the polygenic inheritance (gene networks) implied for many human birth defects and the evolutionary theory of punctuated equilibrium.[65] In each case, a threshold model predicts tolerance of accumulated mutations in a constrained pathway until compensation fails and an altered morphology (birth defect or new species) results. Canalization has two immediate consequences for molecular embryology. First, mutations acting on the embryo will not be equivalent in their effect; the same mutation may be buffered to produce minimal effects in one individual but cause a defect on a different genetic background. Identical mutations at a locus of major effect for an anomaly exhibiting polygenic inheritance may thus be present in both affected and unaffected individuals. Second, the same gene may be involved in producing a family of defects or syndromes according to the combinations of modifying alleles.

A controversy has developed over the role of altered developmental homeostasis in aneuploid phenotypes.[8,69–71] One hypothesis, which might be called the *additive model*, extrapolates from the Mendelian tradition and focuses on genes a–e within the aneuploid segment (Fig. 14–15). Aneuploid phenotypes are merely aggregates of single gene effects, such that gene a causes defects A_1, A_2; gene b causes B_1; . . . gene e causes E_n. The implication is that the aneuploid phenotype can be reconstructed experimentally in a series of animals or patients containing triplicated copies of genes a–e in isolation. A contrasting view, which might be termed the *interactive hypothesis*,[8,69–71] regards most signs or symptoms of the aneuploid condition as network properties that reflect homeostasis and equilibrium of multiple genes within the outside of the aneuploid region (i.e., genes x–z in Fig. 14–15). An increased dosage of gene a, f, or i in isolation might produce no phenotypic alterations, but that of agh together could produce anomalies B–D. There is not a one-to-one correspondence of anomalies with triplicated genes—for example, the aneuploid segment agh may produce trait B only for individuals with allele x_1 rather than x_2. Implicit assumptions of the additive hypothesis derive from the simpler mechanisms of biochemical genetics. These include colinearity (one gene–one anomaly), continuity (aneuploid phenotypes are caused by "minimal chromosome regions" with precise borders), and dosage effects (150% levels of gene product may be as severe as the 0%–5% levels commonly implicated in autosomal recessive disorders). These three assumptions may simply not hold in the etiology of complex phenotypes such as chromosomal syndromes.[71]

Very different experimental implications derive from the additive and interactive hypotheses. The additive view has promoted mouse trisomy 16 as a model for Down syndrome.[72] While these mammalian trisomies have conspicu-ous similarities, there are also prominent phenotypic differences because of nonhomologous material and rearrangement of gene order of the larger mouse chromosome. Refinement of the model has been attempted by constructing transgenic mice with copies of human genes from the pertinent region of chromosome 21. The first such construct, a mouse transgenic for the human superoxide dismutase gene,[73] does provide the first test of 3/2 dosage of a specific gene against a representative background. The only phenotypic effect noted was an alteration of tongue neuromuscular junctions as reported in human Down syndrome.[73,74] There are unfortunately no data examining the incidence of this anomaly in other mouse or human aneuploidies that would bear upon the specificity of this alteration. Since the same tongue neuromuscular changes occur later in normal mouse development, the defect may be a nonspecific effect of the altered developmental timing which is so typical of mammalian aneuploidies.[66]

Very different molecular approaches might derive from the interactive hypothesis, since developmentally relevant genes outside of the aneuploid segment can be implicated in the phenotype. For example, a tantalizing correlation exists between a locus associated with familial Alzheimer disease on chromosome 21 and the ubiquitous incidence of Alzheimer neuropathology in Down syndrome. Unfortunately, recent studies have demonstrated that both the Alzheimer gene and that for amyloid precursor protein are located outside of the "minimal region" for Down syndrome on chromosome 21.[72] This discrepancy is difficult to incorporate within the assumptions of discrete boundaries and single gene effects implied by the additive hypothesis, but altered regulation of proximal genes by distal trisomy is not at all incompatible with the interactive hypothesis. The interactive perspective focuses attention not only on protooncogene sequences such as ets-1 on 21q for a role in the malformations characteristic of Down syndrome, but also on candidate pattern genes located outside of chromosome 21.

The interactive hypothesis would also suggest alternative studies of aneuploidy in animal models. The report of Vekemans and Trasler[75] illustrates this different perspective by showing an increased incidence of cleft palate when mouse trisomy 19 was produced in a strain with genetic predisposition to cleft palate. The production of an atypical anomaly within the aneuploid phenotype by manipulation of the genetic background supports the idea of gene interaction and a role of genes outside of the aneuploid segment. It follows that the specific anomalies in a chromosomally abnormal offspring may sometimes indicate a genetic predisposition for that anomaly in the family.[76] As Shapiro[70] has emphasized, aneuploid phenotypes arise from a hierarchy of connections extending through gene, cell, and embryo so that any one anomaly may have a complex genetic and embryonic history. Experimental approaches to aneuploidy should not only focus on simplistic animal models or gene dosage comparisons, but should also derive from the wealth of observations and specimens available through clinical genetics.

Genomics of human malformations

As discussed in the beginning, the most likely approach to the molecular understanding of human malformations is through the characterization of inborn errors of morphogenesis. Figure 14–16 (see also Table 14–6) illustrates human

Fig. 14–15. Contrast between the additive (A) and interactive (B) hypotheses. In each diagram, gene loci are represented by lower case letters and phenotypic manifestations by the upper case. Arrows indicate relationships between gene dosage and phenotypic effects. Colinearity (phenotypic manifestation A corresponds to altered dosage of gene a) and continuity (minimum region a–e with sharp borders determines phenotype A–E) are implicit assumptions of the additive hypothesis (in A). The interactive hypothesis emphasizes the roles of outside loci (x–z) as well as network properties of genes within the triplicated segment (a–i) in generating the aneuploid phenotype (in B). See text for discussion.

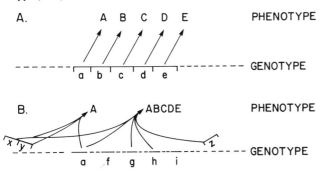

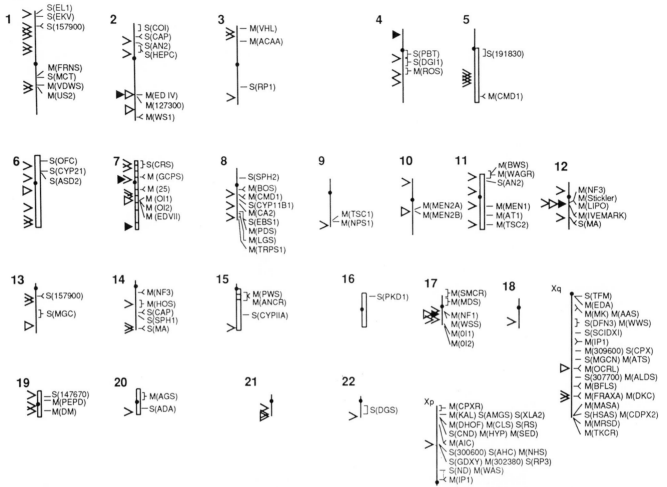

Fig. 14–16. Genomics of human malformations. Human chromosomes are represented by a line and centromere (circle) with provisionally mapped dysmorphogenetic loci indicated to the right. Each locus is denoted by its association with single (S) or multiple (M) malformations and by locus name or McKusick number (see Table 14–6). Loci mapped by balanced chromosomal translocations (—<), interstitial deletions (]—), or traditional linkage (—) are indicated. Locations are diagrammatic and not meant to specify locus order. To the left of each chromosome are interesting candidate genes such as protooncogenes/growth factors (>), collagen genes (▷), or homeobox clusters (▶). Many of the protooncogene locations correspond to common fragile sites. Thickened portions of the chromosomes are homologous to imprinted regions in the mouse (open box) or associated with imprinting in man (stippled)[50,82]. Questions marks indicate alternative map locations. The data and mapping format are mainly derived from McKusick[20] and from two recent reports.[60,83]

malformations for which genes have been mapped and a selection of potential candidate genes. The map illustrates some exciting advances but emphasizes by its sparsity the many genetic malformations that have yet to be localized. At least 88 genetic malformation syndromes and 64 isolated anomalies have been shown to be X-linked, allowing a rough comparison with the 952 syndromes and 657 single malformations listed as autosomal disorders by McKusick.[2,23] Assuming equal distribution, there would be about 73 dysmorphogenetic loci per autosome, suggesting either that these loci have a predilection for the X or that many autosomal malformations remain to be found. These types of questions—i.e., what proportion of the genome is concerned with morphogenesis, are these loci clustered in certain regions, and how do their number and organization correlate with evolution—are examples of genomic considerations for which the human record may provide important answers. Progress toward a genomics of dysmorphology is illustrated in Figure 14–16 where 74 of 1609 (4.6%) autosomal conditions and 43 of 152 X-linked conditions are mapped to specific chromosomal bands. Accelerated progress on the X chromosome reflects the many available DNA markers and provides an important justification for the Human Genome Project.

Although the prime use of an expanding human map will be for malformations exhibiting Mendelian inheritance, molecular applications to polygenic conditions[29] and chromosomal rearrangements[60] will also be facilitated. An example of how the genome map can aid molecular analysis is provided by the recent work of Francke and colleagues[77] on the ring 15 syndrome, which bears some resemblance to the Russell-Silver phenotype.[78] Affected children have prenatal and postnatal growth retardation as well as other minor dysmorphology and developmental delay. The gene for the insulin-like growth factor-1 receptor had been localized to the chromosome 15 terminus, precisely the region deleted during ring formation. Quantitative Southern analysis employing the IGF-1 receptor gene as probe demonstrated only one-half

Table 14–6. Disorders listed in Figure 14–16

Chromosome	Symbol	MIM no.	Disorder	Location	Type
1		157900	Möbius syndrome	?1p34	S
	EKV	133200	Erythrokeratoderma	1p34–36.3	S
	EL1	130500	Elliptocytosis	1p34–36.3	S
	FRNS	229850	Fryns syndrome	1q24	M
	US2	276901	Usher syndrome	1q32	M
	VDWS	119300	Van der Woude syndrome	1q32	M
2	COI	120200	Coloboma	2pter–p25.1	S
	CAP	115650	Anterior polar cataract	?2p25	S
	AN2	106200	Aniridia	?2p25	S
	HPEC	236100	Holoprosencephaly	2p21	S
	COL3A1	130050	Ehlers-Danlos type IV (ED IV)	2q31	M
		127300	Dyschondrosteosis	2q32	M
	WS1	193500	Waardenburg syndrome	2q37.3	M
3	VHL	193300	Von Hippel-Lindau syndrome	3p25–24	M
	ACAA	261519	Pseudo-Zellweger syndrome	3p23–22	M
	RP1	180380	Retinitis pigmentosa	3q21–24	S
4	PBT	172800	Piebald trait	4q12	M
	DGI1	125490	Dentinogenesis imperfecta	4q13–21	S
	ROS	180500	Rieger syndrome	4q23–27	M
5		191830	Renal agenesis	5q11–13	S
	GS	175100	Gardner syndrome	5q22–23	M
	CMD1	211970	Campomelic dwarfism	?5q33.1	M
6	OFC	119530	Orofacial cleft	6pter–p23	S
	ASD2	108800	Atrial septal defect	6p21.3	S
	CYP21	201910	21-Hydroxylase deficiency	6p21.3	S
7	CRS	123100	Craniosynostosis	7p21.2–.3	S
	GCPS	175700	Greig syndrome	7p13	M
	ZS	214100	Zellweger syndrome	7q11.23	M
	COL1A2	130060	Ehlers-Danlos type VII (ED VII)	7q21.3–22.1	M
	COL1A2	166200	Osteogenesis imperfecta I	7q21.3–22.1	M
	COL1A2	166210	Osteogenesis imperfecta II	7q21.3–22.1	M
8	SPH2	182900	Spherocytosis	8p11	S
	BOS	113650	Branchio-otic syndrome	8q13.3	M
	CMD1	211970	Campomelic dwarfism	?8q21.4	M
	CYP11B1	201710	11-Hydroxylase deficiency	8q21	S
	CA2	259730	Osteopetrosis-renal disease	8q22	M
	EBS1	131950	Epidermolysis bullosa, Ogna	8q24	S
	PDS	274600	Pendred syndrome	8q24	M
	LGS	150230	Langer-Giedion syndrome	8q24.11–.13	M
	TRPS1	190350	Trichorhinophalangeal syndrome	8q24.12	M
9	TSC1	191100	Tuberous sclerosis	9q33–4	M
	NPS1	161200	Nail-patella syndrome	9q34	M
10	MEN2A	171400	Multiple endocrine neoplasia 2A	10q21.1	M
	MEN2B	162300	Multiple endocrine neoplasia 2B	10q21.1	M
11	BWS	130650	Beckwith-Wiedemann syndrome	11pter–p15.4	M
	AN2	106200	Aniridia	?11p13	S
	WAGR	194070	WAGR	11p13	M
	MEN1	131100	Multiple endocrine neoplasia 1	11q13	M
	AT1	208900	Ataxia-telangiectasia	11q22–3	M
	TSC2	191090	Tuberous sclerosis	11q23	M
12		162200	Neurofibromatosis III (NF 3)	?12q13	M
	COL2A1	108300	Stickler syndrome	12q13.1–.3	M
		208530	Ivemark syndrome	12q13.1	M
	LIPO	151900	Multiple lipomatosis	12q13–4	M
		158330	Müllerian aplasia (MA)	12q14	S
13	MGC	249200	Hirschsprung disease	?13q22.1–32.1	S
14	NF3	163300	Neurofibromatosis III	?14q13	M
	SPH1	182870	Spherocytosis	14q22	S
	HOS	142900	Holt-Oram syndrome	14q23–24.2	M
	CAP	115650	Anterior polar cataract	?14q24	S
		158330	Müllerian aplasia	14q31	S

(continued)

Table 14–6. Disorders listed in Figure 14–16 (*Continued*)

Chromosome	Symbol	MIM no.	Disorder	Location	Type
15	PWS	176270	Prader-Willi syndrome	15q11	M
	ANCR	234400	Angelman syndrome	15q11–13	M
	CYP11A	201710	20,22-Desmolase deficiency	15q21	S
16	PKD1	173900	Adult polycystic kidney disease	16p13.12–.31	S
17	MDS	247200	Miller-Dieker syndrome	17p13.3	M
	SMCR	182290	Smith-Magenis syndrome	17p11.2	M
	NF1	162200	Neurofibromatosis I	17q11.2	M
	WSS	193500	Watson syndrome	17q11.2	M
	COL1A1	166200	Osteogenesis imperfecta I	17q21.31–22.05	M
	COL1A1	166210	Osteogenesis imperfecta II	17q21.31–22.05	M
18					
19		147670	Acanthosis nigricans	19p13	S
	PEPD	170100	Prolidase deficiency	19c—q13.11	M
	DM	160900	Myotonic dystrophy	19q13	M
20	AGS	118450	Alagille syndrome	20p11.2	M
	ADA	102700	Adenosine deaminase deficiency	20q12	S
21					
22	DGS	188400	DiGeorge anomaly	22q11	S
	NF2	101000	Neurofibromatosis II	22q11	S
Xp	KAL	308700	Kallmann syndrome	Xp22.32	M
	CPXR	302950	Chondrodysplasia punctata	Xp22.32	M
	DHOF	305600	Focal dermal hypoplasia	Xp22.31	M
	AMGS	301200	Amelogenesis imperfecta	Xp22.1–.3	S
	CLS	303600	Coffin-Lowry syndrome	Xp22.1–.2	M
	CND	304730	Corneal dermoids	Xp22.1–.2	S
	AIC	304050	Aicardi syndrome	Xp22	M
	HYP	307800	Vitamin D-resistant rickets	Xp22	M
	RS	312700	Retinoschisis	Xp22	S
	SEDL	313400	Spondyloepiphyseal dysplasia	Xp22	M
	XLA2	300310	X-linked agammaglobulinemia	Xp22	S
		300600	Åland eye disease	Xp21.2–.3	S
	AHC	300200	Adrenal hypoplasia	Xp21.2–.3	S
	NHS	302350	Nance-Horan syndrome	Xp21.1–22.3	M
	GDXY	306100	XY gonadal dysgenesis	Xp21–22	S
		302380	Catel-Mantzke syndrome	Xp21–22	M
	RP3	312610	Retinitis pigmentosa	Xp21	S
	ND	310600	Norrie disease	Xp11.4	S
	IP1	308300	Incontinentia pigmenti	?Xp11.2	M
	WAS	301000	Wiskott-Aldrich syndrome	Xp11–11.3	M
Xq	TFM	313700	Testicular feminization	Xcen–q13	S
	EDA	305100	Ectodermal dysplasia	Xq12.2–13.1	M
	MK	309400	Menkes disease	Xq12–3	M
	AAS	305400	Aarskog syndrome	Xq13	M
	DFN3	304400	Deafness with stapes fixation	Xq13–21.1	S
	WWS	314580	Wieacker-Wolff syndrome	Xq13–21	M
	SCIDXI	300400	Severe combined immune deficiency	Xq13.1–21.1	S
	IP1	308300	Incontinentia pigmenti	?Xq21	M
		309600	Allan-Herndon-Dudley syndrome	Xq21	M
	CPX	303400	Cleft palate-ankyloglossia	Xq21	S
		309300	Megalocornea	Xq21.3–22	S
	ATS	301050	Alport syndrome	Xq22–24	M
	OCRL	309000	Lowe syndrome	Xq25	M
	BFLS	301900	Börjeson-Forssman-Lehmann syndrome	Xq26–27	M
	ALDS	300700	Albinism-deafness syndrome	Xq26.3–27.1	M
	FRAXA	309550	Martin-Bell syndrome	Xq27.3	M
		307700	Agenesis of parathyroids	Xq26–27	S
	HSAS	307000	Hydrocephalus	Xq28	S
	CDPX2	302960	Chondrodysplasia punctata	Xq28	M
	DKC	305000	Dyskeratosis congenita	Xq28	M
	MRSD	309620	Christian syndrome	Xq28	M
	TKCR	314300	Goeminne syndrome	Xq28	M
		303350	MASA syndrome	Xq28	M

the number of copies of this gene in DNA from certain ring 15 patients;[77] this deficiency may explain the growth delay and possibly other dysmorphology of the ring 15 syndrome. Since only one homolog of the chromosomes 15 needs to be affected to produce the syndrome, the results imply that autosomal dominant cases of Russell-Silver phenotype might exist, and such have been reported.[79] Another explanation for the effects of ring 15 might be through imprinting. Figure 14–16 illustrates the regions of human chromosomes that, based on their homologs in the mouse might be expected to be imprinted. In the case of chromosome 15, evidence for imprinting has also been garnered in humans (see Chapter 15). The author speculates that imprinted regions will *not* necessarily be conserved between species, drawing upon his prediction that the similarities between the trisomy 3q and Brachmann-de Lange syndromes will be due to imprinting of the distal 3q region.[80]

This chapter is basically an argument for the synergistic potential of human clinical and molecular genetics. It behooves the clinician to preserve DNA from unusual patients, preferably in the form of transformed lymphoblast cultures. While some question the scientific value of descriptive specialties such as dysmorphology, clinical delineation is the complement of genomic sequencing that may one day provide the link between morphology and molecules. Once the complete human genomic sequence is known, then a repository of clinically defined malformations becomes a tremendous resource for interpretation that will rival that of any organism. Each malformed patient represents an important opportunity for analysis, even if the clinical syllogisms seem vague when contrasted with the precision of molecular technology. As stated by the controversial geneticist Richard Goldschmidt[81] some years ago:

Progress in biology is derived from cooperation of observation, experiment, and constructive thinking and none of these can claim primacy. A good observation may lead to results which a meaningless experiment cannot achieve, and a good idea or analysis may accomplish with one strike what a thousand experiments cannot do. This truism, obvious as it is in the history of all sciences, is frequently forgotten in this era of overestimation of new techniques, which are tools of progress only when in the hands of constructive thinkers. We must therefore take whatever material is available in any field and try to use it to its full extent, subject to critical evaluation.

References

1. Needham J: A History of Embryology. Arno, New York, 1975 (reprint of 1959 edition).
2. McKusick, VA: Mendelian Inheritance in Man, ed 9. Johns Hopkins University Press, Baltimore, 1991.
3. Bonner JT: On Development. The Biology of Form. Harvard University Press, Cambridge, 1974.
4. Fulton AB: How crowded is the cytoplasm? Cell 30:345, 1982.
5. Jockusch B, Fuchtbauer A, Wiegand C, et al.: Probing the cytoskeleton by microinjection. In: Molecular Biology of the Cytoskeleton. JW Shay, ed. Plenum, New York, 1986, p 1.
6. Edelman GM: Topobiology: An Introduction to Molecular Embryology. Basic Books, New York, 1988.
7. Waddington, CH: Canalization of development and the inheritance of acquired characters. Nature 150:563, 1942.
8. Shapiro BL: Down syndrome—a disorder of homeostasis. Am J Med Genet 33:146, 1983.
9. Watson JD, Tooze J, Kurtz DT: Recombinant DNA: A Short Course. Scientific American Books, New York, 1983.
10. Sambrook J, Fritsch EF, Maniatis T: Molecular Cloning: a Laboratory Manual. Cold Spring Harbor Laboratory, Cold Spring Harbor, NY, 1989.
11. Gossler A, Joyner AL, Rossant J, et al.: Mouse embryonic stem cells and reporter constructs to detect developmentally regulated genes. Science 244:463, 1989.
12. Caplan AI, Ordahl CP: Irreversible gene expression model for control of development. Science 201:120, 1978.
13. Ravin A, Riggs AD: DNA methylation and gene function. Science 210:604, 1980.
14. Liskay RM, Evans RJ: Methylation and non-random X inactivation. Proc Natl Acad Sci USA 77:4895, 1982.
15. Surani AZ, Reik W, Allen ND: Transgenes as molecular probes for genomic imprinting. Trends Genet 4:59, 1988.
16. Ott J: Analysis of Human Genetic Linkage. Johns Hopkins University Press, Baltimore, 1985.
17. Botstein D, White RL, Skolnick M, et al.: Construction of a genetic linkage map in man using restriction fragment length polymorphisms. Am J Hum Genet 32:314, 1980.
18. Kerem B-S, Rommens JM, Buchanan JA, et al.: Identification of the cystic fibrosis gene: genetic analysis. Science 245:1073, 1988.
19. Weatherall DJ: The New Genetics and Clinical Practice. Oxford University Press, Oxford, 1985.
20. White TJ, Arnheim N, Erlich HA: The polymerase chain reaction. Trends Genet 5:179, 1989.
21. McMahon AP, Moon RT: Ectopic expression of the proto-oncogene int-1 in *Xenopus* embryos leads to duplication of the embryonic axis. Cell 58:1075, 1989.
22. Wilkins AS: Genetic Analysis of Animal Development. John Wiley & Sons, New York, 1986.
22. Cooley L, Delley R, Spradling A: Insertional mutagenesis of the *Drosophila* genome with single P elements. Science 244:1221, 1988.
23. Wilson GN: Genomics of human dysmorphogenesis. Am J Med Genet 42:187, 1992.
24. Jones KL: Smith's Recognizable Patterns of Human Malformation. WB Saunders, Philadelphia, 1988.
25. Collins FS, Ponder BAJ, Seizinger BR, et al.: Invited editorial: the von Recklinghausen neurofibromatosis region on chromosome 17—genetic and physical maps come into focus. Am J Hum Genet 44:1, 1989.
26. Zonana J, Clarke A, Sarfarazi M, et al.: X-linked hypohidrotic ectodermal dysplasia: localization within the region Xq11-21.1 by linkage analysis and implications for carrier detection and prenatal diagnosis. Am J Hum Genet 43:75, 1989.
27. Reilly DS, Lewis RA, Ledbetter DH, et al.: Tightly linked flanking markers for the Lowe oculocerebrorenal syndrome, with application to carrier assessment. Am J Hum Genet 42:748, 1988.
28. Williamson R: The molecular genetics of complex inherited diseases. Br J Cancer 58(Suppl IX):14, 1988.
29. Ardinger HH, Buetow KH, Bell GI, et al.: Association of genetic variation of the transforming growth factor-alpha gene with cleft lip and palate. Am J Hum Genet 45:348, 1989.
30. Weinberg RA: Finding the anti-oncogene. Sci Am Sept:44, 1988.
31. Spence JE, Perciaccante RG, Greig GM, et al.: Uniparental disomy as a mechanism for human genetic disease. Am J Hum Gen 42:217, 1988.
32. Greenberg F, Hejtmancik JF, Caskey CT; Homozygosity mapping of autosomal recessive dysmorphologic syndromes: a proposal for collaboration and DNA banking. Proc Greenwood Genet Center 8:163, 1989.
33. Lander E, Botstein D: Homozygosity mapping of autosomal recessive disease using RFLPs. Science 236:1567, 1987.
34. Schmickel RD: Contiguous gene deletion syndromes: a component of recognizable syndromes. J Pediatr 109:231, 1986.
35. Francke U, Ochs HD, de Martinville B, et al.: Minor Xp21 chromosome deletion in a male associated with expression of Duchenne muscular dystrophy, chronic granulomatous disease, retinitis pigmentosa, and McLeod syndrome. Am J Hum Genet 37:250, 1985.
36. Curry CJR, Magenis RE, Brown M, et al.: Inherited chondrodysplasia punctata due to a deletion of the terminal short arm of an X chromosome. N Engl J Med 311:1010, 1984.
37. Sack GH Jr, Raven MB, Moser HW: Color vision defects in adrenomyeloneuropathy. Am J Hum Genet 44:794, 1989.
38. Worton RG, Duff C, Sylvester JE, et al.: Duchenne muscular dystrophy involving translocation of the dmd gene next to ribosomal RNA genes. Science 224:1447, 1984.
39. Monaco AP, Kunkel LM: A giant locus for the Duchenne and Becker muscular dystrophy gene. Trends Genet 3:33, 1987.

40. Gerhart JC: The cellular basis of morphogenetic change—group report. In: Evolution and Development. JT Bonner, ed. Springer-Verlag, Berlin, 1982, p 259.

41. Horn HS; Adaptive aspects of development—group report. In: Evolution and Development. JT Bonner, ed. Springer-Verlag, Berlin, 1982, p 215.

42. Elinson RP: Change in developmental patterns: embryos of amphibians with large eggs. *In:* Development as an Evolutionary Process. RA Raff, EC Raff, eds. Alan R Liss, New York 1987, p 1.

43. Dressler GR, Gruss P: Do multigene families regulate vertebrate development? Trends Genet 4:214, 1988.

44. Bender WJ: Homeotic gene products as growth factors. Cell 43:559, 1985.

45. Balling R, Mutter G, Gruss P, et al.: Craniofacial abnormalities induced by ectopic expression of the homeobox gene *Hox 1.1* in transgenic mice. Cell 58:337, 1989.

46. Kenyon C: The nematode *Caenorhabditis elegans.* Science 240:1448, 1988.

47. Nusslein-Volhard C, Frohnhofer HG, Lehmann R: Determination of anteroposterior polarity in *Drosophila.* Science 238:1675, 1987.

48. Ferguson-Smith AC, Fienberg A, Ruddle FH: Isolation, chromosomal localization, and nucleotide sequence of the human *HOX 1.4* homeobox. Genomics 5:250, 1989.

49. Martin GR: Teratocarcinomas and mammalian embryogenesis. Science 209:768, 1980.

50. Solter D: Nuclear transfer in mammalian embryos: role of paternal, maternal, and embryonic genome in development. In: Developmental Genetics of Higher Organisms: a Primer in Developmental Biology. GM Malacinski, ed. Macmillan, New York, 1988, p 441.

51. Jaenisch R: Transgenic animals. Science 240:1468, 1988.

52. Leiter EH, Beamer WG, Shultz LD, et al.: Mouse models of genetic diseases. BDOAS XXIII(3):221, 1987.

53. Winter RM: Malformation syndromes: a review of mouse/human homology. J Med Genet 25:480, 1988.

54. Woychik RP, Stewart TA, Davis LG, et al.: An inherited limb deformity created by insertional mutagenesis in a transgenic mouse. Nature 318:36, 1985.

55. Steele R: Oncogenes, proto-oncogenes, and development. In: Developmental Genetics of Higher Organisms: a Primer in Developmental Biology, GM Malacinski, ed. Macmillan, New York, 1988, p 53.

56. Wolpert L: Positional information and pattern formation. Curr Top Dev Biol 6:183, 1971.

57. Opitz JM, Gilbert EF: CNS anomalies and the midline as a developmental field. Am J Med Genet 12:443, 1982.

58. Machin GA, Sperber GH: Lessons from conjoint twins. Am J Med Genet 28:89, 1987.

59. Opitz JM: Editorial comment. Am J Med Genet 21:175, 1985.

60. Wilson GN, Stout JP, Schneider NR, et al.: Balanced chromosome 12/13 translocation and situs abnormalities: homology of early pattern formation in man and lower organisms? Am J Med Genet 38:601, 1991.

61. Eldredge N: Unfinished Synthesis: Biological Hierarchies and Modern Evolutionary Thought. Oxford University Press, New York, 1987.

62. Wilson GN: Clinical manifestations of peroxisomal disorders. Proc Greenwood Genet Center 8:112, 1989.

63. Opitz JM: The developmental field concept. Am J Med Genet 21:1, 1985.

64. Byers PH, Bonadio JF: The molecular basis of clinical heterogeneity in osteogenesis imperfecta. In: Metabolic and Genetic Disease in Pediatrics. J Lloyd, CR Scriver, eds. Butterworths, London, 1985, p 56.

65. Gould SJ: Ontogeny and Phylogeny. Belknap Press, Cambridge, 1977.

66. Wilson GN: Heterochrony and human malformation. Am J Med Genet 29:311, 1988.

67. Ambros V, Horwitz HR: Heterochronic mutants of the nematode *Caenorhabditis elegans.* Science 226:409, 1984.

68. Wilson GN, Howe M, Stover J: Delayed developmental sequences in rodent diabetic embryopathy. Pediatr Res 19:1340, 1985.

69. Epstein CJ: Specificity versus nonspecificity in the pathogenesis of aneuploid phenotypes. Am J Med Genet 29:161, 1988.

70. Shapiro BL: The pathogenesis of aneuploid phenotypes: the fallacy of explanatory reductionism [letter to the editor]. Am J Med Genet 33:146, 1989.

71. Wilson GN: The karyotype/phenotype controversy: genetic and molecular implications of alternative hypotheses. Am J Med Genet 36:500, 1990.

72. Avraham KB, Schickler M, Sapoznikov D, et al.: Down's syndrome: abnormal neuromuscular junction in tongue of transgenic mice with elevated levels of human Cu/Zn-superoxide dismutase. Cell 54:823, 1988.

73. Epstein CJ: Down syndrome (trisomy 21). In: The Metabolic Basis of Inherited Disease, ed 6. CR Scriver, AL Beaudet, WS Sly, D Valle, eds. McGraw-Hill, New York, 1989, p 291.

74. Korenberg JR, Pulst S-M, Neve RL, et al.: The Alzheimer amyloid precursor protein maps to human chromosome 21 bands q21.105–q21.05. Genomics 5:124, 1989.

75. Vekemans M, Trasler T: Liability to cleft palate in trisomy 19 mouse embryos. J Craniofac Genet Dev Biol (Suppl 2):235, 1986.

76. Wilson GN, Mian A, de Chadarevian J-P, Vekemans M: Effect of aneuploidy and neoplasia on human ribosomal DNA inheritance. Am J Med Genet Suppl 3:121, 1987.

77. Francke U, Darras BT, Ozcelik T, et al.: Loss of IGF-1 receptor gene in patients with ring 15 chromosome is related to severe postnatal growth failure. Proc Greenwood Genet Center 8:159, 1989.

78. Wilson GN, Sauder SE, Bush M, et al.: Phenotypic delineation of ring chromosome 15 and Russell-Silver syndromes. J Med Genet 22:233, 1985.

79. Duncan PA, Hall JG, Shapiro LR, et al.: Three-generation dominant transmission of the Silver-Russell syndrome. Am J Med Genet 35:245, 1990.

80. Wilson GN, Hieber VC, Schmickel RD: The association of chromosome 3 duplication and the Cornelia de Lange syndrome. J Pediatr 93:783, 1978.

81. Goldschmidt R: The Material Basis of Evolution. Yale University Press, New Haven, 1982 (reprint of 1940), p 184.

82. Nadeau JH: Maps of linkage and synteny homologies between mouse and man. Trends Genet 5:82, 1989.

83. Schwartz CE, Ulmer J, Brown A, et al.: Allan-Herndon syndrome II. Linkage to DNA markers in Xq21. Am J Hum Genet 47:454, 1990.

15

Future Directions and Expectations

JUDITH G. HALL

This chapter briefly explores some of the advances in developmental biology[1] that appear to be relevant to a better understanding of early human development. Each species has unique variations, but the themes are recurrent and comparisons are very helpful. Classically, the fruit fly, frog, and chick have been used for developmental experiments, but more recently the nematode, mouse, and zebra fish have been used as models for specific aspects of development. The advent of in vitro fertilization in humans has allowed the study of very early fertilization and cleavage in human embryos as well. Improved prenatal diagnostic techniques are providing a window to early human embryonic and fetal growth. Traditionally, early development has been studied by the use of teratogens or genetic mutants. When a poison or teratogen was used, its effects were observed and interpreted as blocking normal development. When a mutant strain was utilized, an abnormality in development was observed and recognized to disturb normal development. It is worth pointing out that most of the mutants that have been used for studies in animals would be lethal early in human development. Only relatively subtle congenital anomalies are compatible with live birth and survival in humans. Nevertheless, a review of the state of the art of developmental genetics gives a framework in which to consider the congenital anomalies and syndromes that are observed in humans.

As in the rest of clinical genetics, the unusual case, the experiment of nature, may give the most insight into normal processes. We can expect, in the future, that epidemiology, improved prenatal diagnosis, teratogenic experimentation, and further animal work will make a major impact on our understanding of human congenital anomalies. However, those areas are covered elsewhere in this volume, and thus the aim of this chapter is primarily to look at mechanisms that are being defined by the advances in developmental and molecular genetics.

Cell lineage

Once the egg has been fertilized and the new zygote created, the question of what the fate of the daughter cells in each cell division will be becomes an area of great interest. In lower animals, such as frogs and fruit flies, much of the fate of specific cells is determined by the cytoplasm laid down in the egg by the mother. Within the egg there is polarization of various substances at the two ends of the egg prior to fertilization. These concentrations determine the fate of the cells that develop in specific areas. Perhaps the best example of preprogrammed cell lineage is the nematode, for which a diagram of cell division can be made that precisely outlines the fate of every daughter cell. If one cell is obliterated, the loss of func-

tion or structure can be predicted with great accuracy. In higher animals, there is apparently less determination by individual cells and greater influence from the surrounding environment.[2] There is more interaction between cells and more flexibility in the ultimate fate of specific cells. It is important to distinguish between the developmental fate (the pattern of differentiation that a cell expresses in one particular circumstance) and the developmental potential (the range of fates that a cell is capable of expressing). It appears in lower animals that there is very little range of fates, whereas in higher animals there is the ability to catch up and make up for lost cells at certain times in development.[3]

The backbone of cell lineage experiments is to follow a "marked" cell during development. This is usually done either (1) by producing chimeras, in which two types of identifiable cells are mixed at a very early stage in development, such as the chick–quail chimeras in which the cell origin can be distinguished by cellular markers;[4] or (2) by actually marking a specific cell in early development with vital dyes or radioactivity. More recently, a variety of tissue types have become available that allow construction of chimeras in which the cell origin can be identified.[5] These kinds of experiments have led to an understanding of (1) cell lineage and cell commitment in early mammalian development and (2) the contribution that various tissues make to organ development. In addition, by targeting cells for removal or death, the effect of the loss of a particular cell, or cell type, and the tolerance at various stages in embryologic development for that kind of loss can be observed. These studies allow the identification of particularly important cell lines such as germ cells or neural crest cells and the observation of the migration and differentiation of a particular cell line.[5,6] It appears that cells have surface markers that identify their origins and current status. These surface markers interact with various environmental signals and change as the status of the cells changes.[7] The cell adhesion markers are a good example.[8]

Pattern formation, segmentation, and cell orientation

In early embryonic development, cells grow rapidly, creating a multicellular organism. The cells of many species go through a process of reorganization called *gastrulation,* with the subsequent development of three basic tissue types: ectoderm, mesoderm, and endoderm. In order for this to happen, the organism must have a plan or orientation. In *Drosophila,* the orientation of cells to produce patterns of anterior/posterior, ventral/dorsal, and segmentation are programmed in a very specific way.[9] Enormous progress has been made in understanding, on a molecular basis, the embryonic processes leading to segmentation. These involve a very complex interaction of temporal and spacial relationships.[10] In early *Drosophila* embryogenesis, specific genes are expressed in cells that specify positions. There are several different phases to this specification and require communication between cells. Each cell in a segment of the developing *Drosophila* will have expressed the same unique set of gene products. The ventral and dorsal parts of the segment will have also expressed another different set of genes "marking" the cells in various ventral/dorsal areas as well. The adult insect body is composed of serially repeated units or body segments, with superimposed patterns according to the position of a particular segment.

In *Drosophila,* many of the gene products that determine specific segments are already present in the egg and relate to the anterior versus the posterior pole of the egg. This type of cytoplasmic organization has not yet been documented in mammalian eggs, but most of the genes involved in the process of embryonic pattern formation in *Drosophila* are conserved in evolution, making it likely that they also play a role in producing segmentation in higher animals as seems to be the case in mice.[10,11] The process in *Drosophila* that involves anterior/posterior as well as dorsal/ventral patterns involves identifiable protein markers, including a variety of homeotic genes in the cells that define a particular area. By a series of interactions the boundaries of various segments are delineated, and the cells from that segment "know" their identity. The boundaries of gene expressions are determined by an early-acting series of genes that interact with each other and with the gradient laid down in the egg.

Chemical gradients seem to be used as well in limb development to orient the cells as to their position and ability to respond. Body segments that will be involved in limb development thus become further specialized with additional gradients superimposed (e.g., vitamin A receptor concentration on cell membranes).[1] Thus the early pattern formation of the embryo allows differentiation of specific segments and areas that then leads to the ability of the cells in those areas to undergo more specific differentiation of tissue types and organ development. Early pattern formation is essential to developing complex organisms, and the genes that produce the patterns appear to have been preserved through evolution.

Differentiation to specific cell types and organ types

The processes by which cells differentiate and the time frame in which that differentiation remains partial or becomes complete is as yet poorly understood, but it appears that cell surface markers and receptors play a very important role in the progressive determination of cell types.[12] A great deal is being learned about the particular proteins (both cell surface and intracellular) that are unique to a particular cell type. It has become clear from the work in bone marrow stem cells that there are various degrees of differentiation and potentiality. It is thought that cell adhesion molecules play a major role in the process of self-identity.[8] The fact that cell adhesion molecules are closely related to immunologic molecules also suggests that they play a role in cellular recognition. Both the environment (particularly the surrounding cells) and the po-

sition of a particular cell among other cells also play a role in producing that cell's identity. In addition, growth factors (both circulating and local) and the presence of receptors on the cell surface of particular tissues seem to prime the cells to become a particular type of differentiated cell. A great deal is being learned about the factors present in the eye that play a role in induction of tissues, factors in the central nervous system that lead to migration and differentiation of specific areas, and factors in the limb with regard to the role of gradients.[1]

In each body area, there are numerous subtypes of cells that are necessary for the formation of a particular organ. Some subtypes of cells are multipotential; others are very specific in their role. At what point in development or what leads to loss of potential is not clear for most cell types. To have regeneration of a tissue, undifferentiated cells must be present.

In addition to the development of specific cell types for different tissues, the development of organs is a unique process.[13] In the early embryo multiple organs are being developed at the same time, and this development appears to be time specific. This time specificity is described as a threshold after which the same influences have little or different effects. The processes that lead to a group of cells working together in a very specialized way to produce a particular organ and maintain it is far from understood. Ideally, if an organ is diseased or lost, it could be regenerated. At this point in time, bone marrow, skin, and liver show good potential for regeneration; however, the mechanisms even here are poorly understood. The study of differentiation and organ formation has great importance for the therapy of the infant with malformations.

Growth factors

There are many kinds of growth factors that play extremely important roles in development.[14-16] Cytokines lead to tissue differentiation and growth. Once a particular tissue type is differentiated it appears to be responsive to still other growth factors. Our understanding of growth factors during embryologic development has been heightened during the last few years by the study of oncogenes, that is, tumor-producing genes. It turns out that most of the oncogenes code for gene products that are found in the course of normal embryologic development. Many of these growth factors were first isolated because they were present in increased amounts in cancer tissues, but it has become clear that they play a role in normal embryologic development first and foremost. Growth factors usually only have an effect on a tissue if the tissue has receptors for that factor. Thus the regulation of effect is primarily through the presence or absence of receptors.

For the most part, a particular growth factor will occur at several different times in several different tissues during the course of development. In other words, that factor and its receptor get used over and over again to produce different effects in different systems at different times.

Endocrinologists subdivide growth factor effects into hormonal (exert widespread effects by distribution through the circulation), paracine (exert localized effects in the general vicinity of production), and autocrine (exert direct effects only on the cell producing the growth factor). It appears that all of these modes of affecting cell growth and turnover are used during embryologic development in different tissues.

The powerful role that growth factors play during development is just being appreciated. With the advent of molecular and immunologic techniques that enable these factors and their receptors to be traced during the course of development, a map of their effects in various tissues at various times can be developed. There is great interest in the use of growth factors after birth for increased wound healing, for decreasing the mass of abnormal growths such as hemangiomas, and for encouraging normal growth as in short stature, healing of fractures, and hypoplasia of structures.

Many of the growth factors have names that reflect the tissue in which they were initially discovered, but the names may not actually reflect their primary function in normal development. In addition, many growth factors are being found to have structural similarities and/or to be parts of families. Seven specific families have been identified: insulin, epidermal growth factor, platelet-derived growth factor, heparin, absorbable interferon, interleukins, and transforming growth factors. These families have similar structures and functions.

The interesting aspect of these growth factors is that they appear not only to lead to increase growth of a tissue but also may change its fate and/or differentiation. It is quite clear that knowledge about growth factors will contribute to a greater understanding of cell–cell interactions and differentiation during development.

Cell biology

The study of developmental biology includes an understanding of gene expression and regulation.[1] Clearly these processes as well as the control involved in the processes are very important in the course of development. Very little is known at this time concerning control mechanisms that regulate gene expression or control DNA processing. Furthermore, little is known about how proteins assemble in the cell once they are produced and whether this assembly may be different from cell type to cell type. It is quite clear already that a particular gene may have alternative splicing, giving different products, and that the gene products themselves are processed in many ways before they are ready to assemble. Further developments in this area will surely help to define the specific gene products involved in both normal and abnormal development as well as how their production is controlled.

Programmed cell death

It has been suspected for a long time and now is quite clear that cell death during embryogenesis is a normal part of differentiation.[17] For instance, in the limb the loss of tissue between digits, and in the brain the loss of cells that do not have multiple intracellular connections, are now recognized to be normal events in development. It is not yet clear how frequently programmed cell death occurs in other tissues or what determines the events that lead to cell death.[18] Clearly, overzealous cell death can lead to loss of important tissue, while lack of cell death at certain times in development can

lead to tissue that is susceptible to malignancy (i.e., DES vaginal dysplasia). However, the role of programmed cell death in normal and abnormal development is not fully understood at this time.[19]

Heterochrony and atavism

Normal embryologic and fetal development occur within a very specific framework of time.[20] The timetable of particular events varies from tissue to tissue and from organism to organism. In some situations, a particular developmental process may occur gradually so that at one time very few cells have completed the process, while at another time most cells have. Alternatively, there appear to be threshold phenomena in embryologic development in which all cells have to have accomplished a change at a particular time for development to proceed normally.

It has been suggested that as part of evolution particular stages of embryologic development may be delayed in some organisms to allow for expansion of that phase. Certainly, what we consider to be the most highly developed animals have a long gestation and are relatively immature at the time of birth. The human infant, for instance, is very immature and dependent compared with other primates, and the human brain continues to grow and develop for 2 years after birth. Obviously if the embryonic time clock is out of synchrony congenital anomalies can occur in the form of both retention of structures that were meant to have been lost (atavisms)[21] and loss of structures that were meant to be preserved. It seems likely that a certain number of abnormalities that occur late in development in humans could fall into this category.

The role of function or use of a structure during normal development

At a relatively early stage in embryologic development, structures begin to function, i.e., the heart begins to beat, and limbs begin to move. The importance of function during normal embryonic development is not clear. However, at least in fetal life, it seems to be essential for normal development. For instance, in the development of the heart the contracting of the tubular heart tissue leads to its final shape.[22] The lungs will be underdeveloped at birth if in utero breathing has not occurred. The palate may not close completely if the tongue and jaw do not move into the correct position. Limbs will have contractures of the joints if there is lack of normal fetal movement of the limbs. Even the metabolic aspects of the gut, liver, and lung will not be ready for extrauterine function if they have not been functional in utero. It may well be that a large number of human congenital anomalies occurs secondary to failure of fetal tissues to function during in utero development.

Plasticity

The mammalian embryo appears to have an amazing ability to "make up" for a deficiency. For instance, monozygous twins are not half the normal size even though they started as one egg. In experimental work on mammalian tissue it would appear that there is a sensing system that gives feedback to how rapidly tissues ought to grow and to what extent they ought to grow.[23] For instance, the liver does not continue to grow indefinitely; thus there is flexibility, allowing catch-up growth but also some feedback mechanism of recognizing correct size. When a tissue regenerates, it grows back to a specific size.

It has been suggested that one of the distinctions between mammals and lower animals is how responsive the cells are to surrounding tissues and cells. This mechanism of interplay is poorly understood, but if missing would surely lead to undergrowth or overgrowth of particular tissues.

Maternal effects

In lower animals the term *maternal effects* is used to imply cytoplasmic effects (things that have been put into the egg before fertilization[1]), while in mammals and humans the term is used to imply an illness or an abnormal metabolic state in the mother. It is important to understand this distinction, since in embryologic development both types of influences can have a major effect.

Taking the maternal effect concept from low animals, the question is how much influence do cytoplasmic factors inherited from the mother have in modifying embryonic development in the human. At present, mitochondrial disease is the only type of cytoplasmic effect that has been studied in humans. But it would appear that other structures in the cytoplasm, such as the internal architecture of cells, spindle formation, peroxisomal budding, and so forth, may in fact be determined by what is present in the egg. Since these cell structures would be anticipated to have a major effect on cell growth and possibly on the function in specific tissues, it might be anticipated that these structures could play a major role in the production of congenital anomalies.

Maternal effects of the type described in humans, e.g., maternal illness or abnormal metabolic state, can also clearly influence embryonic and fetal development. This kind of effect is seen in disorders such as maternal phenylketonuria and maternal diabetes. However, the exact mechanisms leading to disturbances in the embryo/fetus are still poorly understood. The question is how many other maternal illnesses, heterozygous states, and metabolic imbalances can also produce deleterious effects in a developing embryo and/or fetus.

Nontraditional inheritance

The last few years have led to the realization that nontraditional forms of inheritance may play a very important role in embryonic development.

1. Mosaicism in both somatic cells and the germline have been recently documented. It now appears that mosaicism is very common, if not universal. However, its effects depend on the time at which a second cell develops and the tissue in which it occurs. Mosaicism can clearly lead to abnormal growth and function. Confined placental mosaicism is present in 2%–3% of all live births.[24]

2. Parent of origin or imprinting differences are being recognized in mammals in several ways: pronuclear transplantation, triploid phenotypes, chromosomal deletion syndromes, unipa-

rental disomy, loss of heterozygosity in childhood cancers, transgenic inheritance, and human specific diseases. The role of parent or origin differences during embryologic development is not fully appreciated. It appears that most housekeeping genes do not have parent of origin effects; however, other genes specific to tissues may have very major modifications depending on the parent of origin of the genetic information.[25]

3. Uniparental disomy, that is, the inheritance of both genes or chromosomes from a single parent, was thought not to occur but is now recognized to occur relatively frequently. It appears that it is tolerated in some parts of the genome relatively well and in others relatively poorly. It is a noninherited form of genetic disease.

4. Cytoplasmic, including mitochondrial, inheritance appears to be an important part of normal development, but its role in congenital anomalies is poorly understood.

Mapping and sequencing in the human genome

At present, there is a major effort being made to sequence the entire human genome.[26] Clearly that would identify numerous genes whose role and normal function are not yet known or even suspected. However, that will only be the beginning of real understanding, since once those genes have been identified their roles in development and in disease processes will need to be understood. The process of sequencing will give little insight into control, regulation, or interrelations of gene products.

Human/mouse homologies

Many homologies have been identified between the gene maps of humans and mouse.[27] Already the human/mouse homologous maps have allowed identification of areas of chromosomes that appear to be homologous in the two species. A grid has been developed that predicts where specific genes are mapped in the other species. Therefore, experiments that would never be considered in human development can be carried out in mice. Specific diseases can be produced in mouse strains, and genetically engineered therapies can be tested.

New techniques

The techniques of studying early embryonic development in lower animals and now in mammals are very complex. However, a number of recent developments suggest that many new types of observations will now be possible because of a combination of these new techniques.

1. DNA markers make it possible to identify the source of genetic information (i.e., from which parent or organism it has come). In situ techniques allow localization of particular genes or gene products within a cell and on a chromosome. Using monoclonal antibodies, it is possible to identify specifically various proteins or parts of proteins and to determine their localization within the cell. Cloning techniques allow development of large amounts of a particular compound so that it can be analyzed by traditional methods. Polymerase chain reactions allow the amplification of a very small amount (even a single strand) of a particular piece of DNA.

2. The formation of viable chimeras provides a model in which cell lineage can be traced and the roles of particular genes or

cell types can be determined. Chimeras may be constructed from quite unusual cell types such as parthenogenetic or transgenic lines. Embryonic stem cells that have had specific mutations inserted become very useful for understanding gene function.[28]

3. Transgenic mice have become a very powerful method with which to observe the regulation of individual genes. A specific gene is inserted into the male pronucleus of a fertilized egg and becomes incorporated into the DNA of the zygote.[1] By accident, as trangenic mice are made, disruption of normal genes[29] to produce mutations can occur. These mutations are often quite interesting to study.

4. Ablation experiments using molecular techniques allow the ablation of a particular gene product in a particular tissue. The effects of the presence or absence of that product at various stages in development can be studied.[1]

Clearly, there is a great deal known, both in general and in specific detail, about the many aspects of human anomalies. Research in the fields of perinatology, developmental biology, and developmental genetics holds great promise for increasing our understanding of these anomalies. With the many different molecular techniques and animal models, rapid progress is being made toward defining the elements in early development. It is becoming clear that the processes involved are extremely complex. Nevertheless, the observations being made are dramatic and, as more is learned, will surely help both to explain and to prevent human congenital anomalies.

References

1. Gilbert SF: Developmental Biology, ed 2. Sinauer Associates, Sunderland, MA, 1988.
2. Rossant J: Development of extraembryonic cell lineages in the mouse embryo. In: Experimental Approaches to Mammalian Embryonic Development. J Rossant, RA Pedersen, eds. Cambridge University Press, Cambridge, 1988, p 97.
3. Adamson ED: Cell-lineage-specific gene expression in development. In: Experimental Approaches to Mammalian Embryonic Development. J Rossant, RA Pedersen, eds. Cambridge University Press, Cambridge, 1988, p 321.
4. Balaban E, Teillet M-A, LeDouarin N: Approaches to the quail-chick chimera system to the study of brain development and behaviour. Science 241:1339, 1988.
5. Kimmel CB, Warga RM: Tissue-specific cell lineages originate in the gastrula of the zebrafish. Science 231:365, 1986.
6. Rossant J: Retroviral mosaics: a new approach to cell lineage analysis in the mouse embryo. Trends Genet 2:302, 1986.
7. Gardner RL: Cell allocation and lineage in the early mouse embryo. In: Cellular Basis of Morphogenesis. D Evered, J Marsh, ed. John Wiley & Sons, New York, 1989, p 172.
8. Edelman GM: CAMs and lgs: cell adhesion and the evolutionary origins of immunity. Immunol Rev 100:11, 1987.
9. Ingham PW: The molecular genetics of embryonic pattern formation in *Drosophila.* Nature 335:25, 1988.
10. Awgulewitsch A, Utset MF, Hart CP, et al.: Spatial restriction in expression of a mouse homoeo box locus within the central nervous system. Nature 320:328, 1986.
11. Kessel M, Balling R, Gruss P: Variations of cervical vertebrate after expression of a *Hox-1.1* transgene in mice. Cell 61:301, 1990.
12. Johnson MH, Maro B: Time and space in the mouse early embryo: a cell biological approach to cell diversification. In: Experimental Approaches to Mammalian Embryonic Development. J Rossant, RA Pedersen, eds. Cambridge University Press, Cambridge, 1986, p 35.
13. Walbot V, Holder N: Developmental Biology. Random House, New York; 1987, p 459.
14. Growth Factors. Br Med Bull 45:317, 1989.
15. Crumpton MJ, Dexter TM: Growth factors in differentiation and development; a discussion. Philos Tran R Soc Lond 327(1239):65, 1990.
16. Nilsen-Hamilton M: Growth Factors and Development. Academic, San Diego, 1990.
17. Cunningham TJ: Naturally occurring neuron death and its regulation by developing neural pathways. Int Rev Cytol 74:163, 1982.
18. Snow MHL: Cell death in embryonic development. In: Perspectives on Mammalian Cell Death. CS Potten, ed. Oxford University Press, Oxford, 1987, p 202.
19. Chalfie M, Wolinsky E: The identification and suppression of inherited neurodegeneration in *Caenorhabditis elegans.* Nature 345:410, 1990.
20. Wilson GN: Heterochrony and human malformation. Am J Med Genet 29:311, 1988.
21. Cantu JM, Ruiz C: On atavisms and atavistic genes. Ann Genet 28:141, 1985.
22. Clark EB: Cardiac embryology. Am J Dis Child 140:41, 1986.
23. Hay ED: Extracellular matrix, cell skeletons, and embryonic development. Am J Med Genet 34:14, 1989.
24. Hall JG: Review and hypotheses: somatic mosiacism: observations related to clinical genetics. Am J Hum Genet 43:355, 1988.
25. Hall JG: Genomic imprinting—review and relevance to human diseases. Am J Hum Genet 46:857, 1990.
26. Watson JD: The human genome project: past, present and future. Science 248:44, 1990.
27. Searle AG, Peters J, Lyon MF, et al.: Chromosome maps of man and mouse IV. Ann Hum Genet 53:89, 1989.
28. Robert EJ, Bradley A: Production of permanent cell lines from early embryos and their use in studying developmental problems. In: Experimental Approaches to Mammalian Embryonic Development. J Rossant, RA Pedersen, eds. Cambridge University Press, Cambridge, 1986, p 475.
29. Enver T, Raich N, Ebens AJ, et al: Developmental regulation of human fetal-to-adult globin gene switching in transgenic mice. Nature 344:309, 1990.

Subject Index